Biomaterials, Bioengineering and Sustainability

Volume 5

There is an urgent need to address the current paradigm shifts in bioengineering for Human Health aiming the creation of breakthrough tissue engineered products, manufacturing technologies and effective regenerative treatments for tackling different diseases/disorders in a personalized manner. Yet, the excessive costs and wastes related to the development and production of biomaterials and advanced therapy medicinal products, and the increasing use of plastics in cell culture methods and animal derived reagents has recognized the importance of decreasing the direct carbon footprint and thus, implement sustainable principles and solutions in the innovation ecosystem. The main goal of the volumes in Biomaterials, Bioengineering and Sustainability series is to catapult and consolidate new concepts and solutions towards the development of the next-generation of sustainable and eco-friendly biomaterials and tissue engineering and regenerative medicine approaches. Each volume will focus on the latest developments dealing with the identification of new sources of sustainable or recycled biomaterials, providing ideas for green technologies and methods that can be applied for biomaterials advanced processing and scaffolding strategies, and applications in biofabrication, tissue engineering, regenerative medicine, and drug delivery systems. It also aims to include the exploitation of renewable and sustainable source of human cells applied for cell therapies or in combination with sustainable biomaterials. The develop complex in vitro 3D/4D models and dynamic cell culture systems will be other subjects to be further explored from a sustainable perspective. This series aims to attract the contributions of leading experts in bioengineering, cell biology, materials engineering, and environmental sciences.

Maurice N. Collins • Mario Culebras
Editors

Sustainable Biopolymers and Composites for Biomedical Applications

Springer

Editors
Maurice N. Collins
School of Engineering, Health Research
Institute and Bernal Institute
University of Limerick
Limerick, Ireland

Mario Culebras
Institute of Materials Science
University of Valencia
Valencia, Spain

ISSN 2731-751X ISSN 2731-7528 (electronic)
Biomaterials, Bioengineering and Sustainability
ISBN 978-3-031-91971-8 ISBN 978-3-031-91972-5 (eBook)
https://doi.org/10.1007/978-3-031-91972-5

This Springer imprint is published by the registered company Springer Nature Switzerland AG
The registered company address is: Gewerbestrasse 11, 6330 Cham, Switzerland

Contents

Letter from the Editors: Sustainable Biopolymers and Composites for Biomedical Applications

1

Maurice N. Collins and Mario Culebras

This book, *Sustainable Biopolymers and Composites for Biomedical Applications*, provides a comprehensive vison that delves into the growing convergence between sustainability and biomedical research. With increasing awareness of the crucial need for more environmentally and low carbon footprint materials, this book addresses the enormous potential of biopolymers and composites in the biomedical field.

The biomedical industry has long been reliant on synthetic polymers for various applications, such as: polyethylene (PE), polyethylene glycol (PEG), polyvinyl alcohol (PVA), polyacrylic acid (PAA), polyacrylamide (PAM), polyvinylamine (PVAm) and polyvinylpyrrolidone (PVP) ranging from medical devices to drug delivery systems. However, the environmental impact of these materials all of them derived from petroleum-based resources has motivated novel research lines that involves the use of more sustainable alternatives. In this context, biopolymers, derived from natural resources such as: food waste and lignocellulosic biomass, offer a promising solution. In addition, the possibility to use these biopolymers as matrices for developing advanced composite materials, novel functional materials, with additional benefit of some biopolymers containing cell signaling ability for

M. N. Collins (✉)
School of Engineering, Health Research Institute and Bernal Institute, University of Limerick, Limerick, Ireland

Research Ireland Centre for Advanced Materials and BioEngineering Research (AMBER), Dublin, Ireland

Research Ireland Bioeconomy Research Centre BiOrbic, Dublin, Ireland
e-mail: maurice.collins@ul.ie

M. Culebras (✉)
Institute of Material Science, (ICMUV) University of Valencia, Valencia, Spain
e-mail: Mario.culebras@uv.es

M. N. Collins, M. Culebras (eds.), *Sustainable Biopolymers and Composites for Biomedical Applications*, Biomaterials, Bioengineering and Sustainability 5,
https://doi.org/10.1007/978-3-031-91972-5_1

next generation tissue engineering, drug delivery and wound healing applications, are now paving the way for future innovations that align health advancements and environmental challenges.

This book brings together contributions from leading experts in the fields of polymer science, materials engineering, biomedical research, and sustainability. Through the chapters, we explore the properties, design, and functionalization of sustainable biopolymers, and the ways in which they can be engineered to meet the specific demands of biomedical applications. We cover a wide range of topics, including lignocellulosic derived polymers, microbial-synthesized materials, nanocomposites, and the how these materials can be incorporated in biomedical systems/devices.

Our goal with this publication is not only to highlight the current state of research but also to inspire further advancements in this rapidly evolving field. We believe that the synergy between sustainable materials and biomedical science/engineering holds the potential to impact directly in the manufacturing of the next generation of medical devices, prosthetics, drug delivery systems, while reducing significantly the environmental footprint whilst contributing to the circular economy of the biomedical sector.

We are grateful to our contributors for sharing their expertise and insights, and we hope that readers will find this book to be a valuable resource in both academic and professional settings. Whether you are a researcher, an engineer, a healthcare professional, or simply someone passionate about sustainable innovation, we believe this volume will broaden your understanding of the intersection between biomedicine and sustainability.

Current Trends in Sustainable Biopolymers for Biomedical Engineering and Pharmaceutical Applications

2

Seda Ceylan, İsmail Kutlugün Akbay, and Didem Demir

Abstract

Polymeric materials, which are used in many areas in our daily lives, have the potential to have negative impacts on the environment throughout their life cycle, including resource depletion, non-renewability, and solid waste generation. Therefore, it is important to identify sustainable ways and methods. Biopolymers, which are in the class of polymers and are of biological origin, as can be understood from the bio suffix in the name, have an important place among the materials evaluated with a sustainability approach. Researchers and professionals across a wide range of disciplines are very interested in biopolymers because they represent a leading class of functional materials appropriate for high-value applications. Interdisciplinary research is important to understand the fundamental and applied aspects of biopolymers to address various complex issues related to health and well-being. In order to reduce environmental impact and dependence on fossil fuels, much effort has been made to replace synthetic polymers with biodegradable materials, especially those derived from natural resources. In this context, many types of biopolymers have been developed to meet the needs of ever-expanding applications. These biopolymers are used in the biomedical and pharmaceutical industries and are expanding their use day by day due to their unique properties. This chapter focuses on the various uses of biopolymers in the

S. Ceylan (✉)
Department of Bioengineering, Adana Alparslan Türkeş Science and Technology University, Adana, Türkiye
e-mail: sceylan@atu.edu.tr

İ. K. Akbay
Department of Engineering, Mersin University, Chemical Engineering, Mersin, Türkiye

D. Demir
Department of Chemistry and Chemical Process Technologies, Tarsus University, Mersin, Türkiye

M. N. Collins, M. Culebras (eds.), *Sustainable Biopolymers and Composites for Biomedical Applications*, Biomaterials, Bioengineering and Sustainability 5,
https://doi.org/10.1007/978-3-031-91972-5_2

biomedical and pharmaceutical industries and provides a future outlook for the biopolymer industry.

Keywords

Biopolymers · Biomedicine · Nanocarriers · Biocompatibility · Sustainability

2.1 Introduction

Polymers and polymeric materials, which used frankly in the last century throughout the world, have been used extensively for its beneficial parameters for most of the cases from household applications to biggest industrial sites all over the world (Namazi 2017). Unfortunately, even though with its wonderful properties such as, lightweight, durability, impact resistance, price, etc., its degradation and breaking down to little pieces with the daily usage of these type of materials could be massive impact to both environment and health of the living beings (Webb et al. 2012). Microplastics (Kukkola et al. 2024), monomer migration (Pilevar et al. 2019) and Great Pacific garbage patch (Connan et al. 2021) are one of the few examples of the recent problems of the daily use of polymer and polymeric materials. Most of the problem mainly caused by the single-use plastics (Herweyers et al. 2023).

Even with the current technology and science, polymer and polymeric materials, especially synthetic ones are still used heavily and daily throughout the world (Zhong et al. 2020). To solve the abovementioned problems and not changing anything about the daily user preferences and comfort, having similar-properties alternatives to single-use, synthetic polymers and polymeric materials is a crucial task for the current and next generation.

One of the top categories for the single-use polymers and polymeric materials are medical and pharma applications. With its urgent and important reasons of the single use, changing the usage scenarios of the medical product and components does not seem possible in the near future (Romero et al. 2020; Zaharescu and Varca 2022). Finding better alternatives for medical and pharma applications is not an easy task with its important usage areas and risks.

Using a similar material for medical and pharma applications to forfeit the predecessor is a first way to match its criteria. Biopolymers could be a similar alternative to polymers and polymeric materials that can be game changing to especially the single-use medical and pharma applications (Getahun et al. 2024). With this approach, sustainable and biocompatible alternatives could be found with overachieved properties. Biopolymers, which can be derived from natural and synthetic sources, can be used with this purpose with its marvelous properties (Smith et al. 2016). Coming from nature, biopolymers could be more compatible to its uses medical and pharma applications rather than its alternative polymer and polymeric materials. And with its sustainable production cycle, it could be possible to produce and obtain without any problem in the future (Vinod et al. 2020).

Biopolymers or nature derived polymers and polymeric materials are materials that can be derived from or by from natural products such as plants, flowers, trees or animals, insects, aquatic creatures, and their by-products (Christian 2016). Biopolymer can be either synthesized from or can be derived directly from its source. Because it is possible derivation directly from its source, biopolymers are used without knowledge over centuries (Rendón-Villalobos et al. 2016). Therefore, with its cultural heritage of the past, most of the biopolymers can be divided into possible groups, with their possible usage scenarios for medical and pharma applications. Thus, biopolymers could also be a starting point for the medical and pharma research.

In this chapter, sustainable biopolymers for biomedical engineering and pharma applications are discussed thoroughly with the current trends in medical and pharma applications and research. Sustainability and availability of the biopolymers for biomedical engineering and pharma applications is also explained with the application areas of the last decade. With the increasing of the single-use plastic waste every day, finding sustainable and biologically compatible alternatives is a very important task and we believe that this could be the starting point of the researchers working on this manner.

2.2 Biopolymers and Sustainability

Polymers are macromolecules with high molecular weight formed by the combination of monomers, the smallest building blocks. They can be synthetic or natural depending on their source. Biopolymers can be considered in the class of natural polymers, but what distinguishes the two is that not all biopolymers are biodegradable (Caillol 2021). Biopolymers are organic substances obtained from living organisms or their by-products and are structurally known as large macromolecules consisting of a multitude of repeating units (Nazrun et al. 2024; Jaya et al. 2022). These repeating units encompass amino acids, saccharides, and fatty acids, which may also contain diverse chemical side chains. Structurally, biopolymers can be obtained naturally or synthetically and can be classified according to both the type of raw material used and the method chosen. In this direction, the method of obtaining biopolymers on the basis of raw materials is schematised in Fig. 2.1.

Biopolymers can be classified into two principal categories: those derived from natural sources and those produced through synthetic routes. The former encompasses polymers derived from plants, animals, and microorganisms sourced from natural environments, whereas the latter involves the polymerisation of bio-based monomers. Natural biopolymers obtained from plant and animal sources can be in polysaccharide, protein or lipid structure according to the presence of repeating units within themselves. Examples of polysaccharides are chitin/chitosan, starch, alginate, pectin, gum, cellulose and their derivates. Protein-based biopolymers are classified into two principal categories: animal and plant proteins. Animal proteins include casein, collagen, gelatin, keratin and silk, whereas plant proteins include wheat gluten, zein and soy proteins. Biopolymers with a lipid structure include

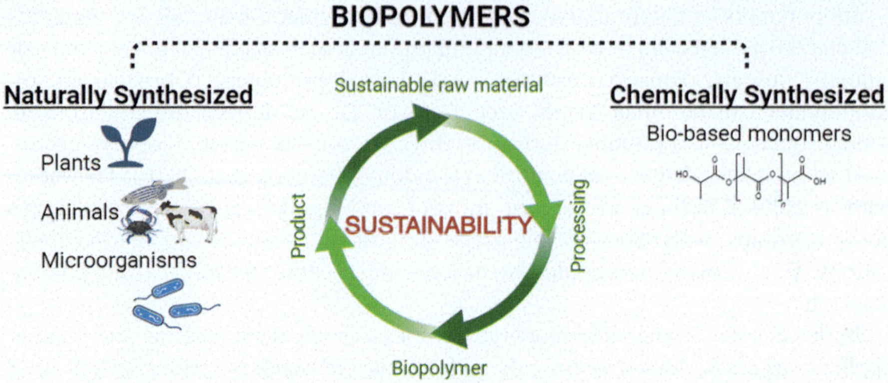

Fig. 2.1 Classification based on the method of obtaining biopolymers on the basis of raw materials

beeswax, oils and free fatty acids. In addition, the category of natural biopolymers includes polyhydroxyalkanoates, bacterial cellulose, xanthan, and pullulan, which are synthesised directly by microorganisms (Perera et al. 2023; Zubair et al. 2021).

On the other hand, synthetic polymers produced after a series of chemical reactions using bio-based monomers are also considered as biopolymers. In the light of the developments in the biotechnology industry, especially driven by biomass fermentation technologies, bio-based aliphatic and aromatic polyesters have been successfully synthesised using a wide variety of monomers such as diols, diacids, hydroxyacids, lactones, erephthalic acid, 2,5-furandicarboxylic acid, and vanillin monomers (Zhang et al. 2021). The main source of these bio-based aliphatic monomers are starch, cellulose and vegetable oil biomasses.

The suffix -bio, which is the root of the word biopolymer, indicates that these materials have a biological origin as are natural structures. They are highly advantageous in overcoming the limitations of synthetic polymers, which are currently available and used effectively in many applications. The production of conventional petroleum-based polymers, defined as synthetic polymers, requires large amounts of energy and resources. Indeed, given that certain chemical-based synthetic polymers are toxic to humans, animals, plants and microbial cells, and biopolymers have been introduced as an alternative in order to make polymers suitable for biomedical applications (Jeevanandam et al. 2022). In recent years, the synthesis of polymers from renewable resources with a sustainability approach has become an important area of industrial and academic interest as a viable solution to the depletion of fossil fuels, the increasing threat to the environment (Zhang et al. 2021).

The keyword "sustainability" encountered here covers the design, manufacture and utilisation of polymers and polymer production processes that are efficient, effective, safe and more environmentally sound when considered from the perspective of the polymer industry. Therefore, in the context of ensuring sustainability as a fundamental problem to which solutions are being sought worldwide, studies on the production of polymers used in almost all sectors today as biodegradable, recyclable and compostable materials using widely available renewable and recyclable resources continue with great interest. In this context, although biopolymers obtained from natural resources with a sustainability approach are used in a variety of sectors, including agriculture, automotive, electricity and building, they are regarded as a principal functional material class for high-value applications such as the food and medical industry. In particular, their similarities to living systems, biocompatibility, biodegradability and non-toxicity due to their obtaining from natural sources show biopolymers as unique candidates that can be evaluated for medical applications such as drug delivery, tissue regeneration, wound healing and the field of pharmacy. Thus, the following sections of this review are designed to introduce biopolymers with potential for use in the biomedical and pharmaceutical industries, and to review the current studies on the evaluation of these biopolymers for both application areas.

2.2.1 Natural Sources

Polymers produced by natural resources spontaneously during the life cycle or as a result of the processing of natural resources through a number of chemical reactions are called biopolymers. Among biopolymers, self-existing polymer sources in nature are animals, plants and microorganisms.

2.2.1.1 Animal-Derived

The most widely used animal-derived biopolymers are chitin, chitosan, hyaluronic acid (hyaluronan), collagen, gelatin, keratin, agarose and silk fibroin-based polymers. These polymers are biodegradable, relatively less toxic and renewable, and are therefore of great importance in the biomedical and pharmaceutical applications. When evaluated in terms of sustainability, the production of biopolymers from animal sources constitutes a very important area in terms of both the direct use of animal resources naturally found in nature within ethical frameworks and the prevention of threats that may arise to the environment when animal waste is not disposed of appropriately (Tarafdar et al. 2021).

Chitin, found in the shells of crustaceans and skeletons of insects, is one of the most widely used animal-derived biopolymers. The chitin molecule is a polysaccharide comprising 2-acetylamino-2-deoxy-D-glucose units connected by β-glycosidic bonds at position 1,4. Chitin exhibits three polymorphic varieties, designated α, β, and γ (Flórez et al. 2023; Piekarska et al. 2023). The differences in crystal structure resulting directly influence the processing capabilities of chitin. The inherent ordered structure and strong intramolecular and intermolecular interactions limit the solubility of chitin in most organic solvents and water, thus limiting its utilisation. The deacetylation process developed here enables the conversion of chitin to chitosan, which is soluble in acidic solutions. Chitosan, a derivative of chitin, consists of glucosamine and N-acetylglucosamine and is a reactive copolymer due to its functional amino groups (Nirmal et al. 2024; Demir et al. 2016). The most renewable animal sources for chitin and chitosan biopolymers are crustacean waste collected from the marine industry (Amiri et al. 2022). The annual industrial production of chitin from marine industry waste, which has a chitin content in the range of approximately 15–40%, has been estimated to be approximately 1×10^{11} tonnes (Je and Kim 2006; Triunfo et al. 2022). Given the challenges currently facing the marine industry, including issues with supply chains, fluctuations in availability, and environmental concerns, there is a growing need to identify alternative sources of chitin. In this regard, insects are also regarded as a promising alternative source of chitin (ur Rehman et al. 2023; Hahn et al. 2020). The most studied insect species here is the black soldier fly (*Hermetia illucens*) (Triunfo et al. 2022; Khayrova et al. 2024; Adamaki-Sotiraki et al. 2024) and recent studies have shown that chitosan extracted from insect species can be successfully used in biomaterial production (Lee et al. 2024).

Collagen, the most abundant protein in animal connective tissues, is another important biopolymer (Felix et al. 2019). The primary amino acids that constitute collagen are proline, glycine, and hydroxyproline. Collagen is composed of protein fibrils that are wrapped in a triple helix structure, which is formed by the combination of these amino acids (Goldberga et al. 2018; Shoulders and Raines 2009). It has considerable industrial potential for use in pharmaceuticals and biomedical materials due to its favourable properties, including strong biocompatibility, high degradability, low antigenicity, treating orthopedic diseases, skin injuries and ophthalmic diseases, promoting nerve regeneration and anti-aging capability (Rezvani Ghomi et al. 2021; Zhou et al. 2023). The principal sources of commercial collagen are cattle, pig and other mammalian animal by-products derived from land animals. Additionally, marine organisms such as sponges, jellyfish, molluscs (including mussels, squid, cuttlefish and octopus), and fish also contain collagen. Fish collagen is more readily absorbed by the body and has a higher bioavailability than collagen derived from pigs or cows. It is also more acceptable to the general public due to certain religious beliefs such as Islam, Judaism and Hinduism (Fatiroi et al. 2023; Coppola et al. 2021).

Gelatin, derived from collagen through hydrolysis, is one of the highly versatile biopolymer with a wide range of applications in the food, pharmaceutical, and biomedical industries. Global demand for gelatin reached 620.6 kilotonnes in 2019, up from 412.7 kilotonnes in 2015. This growth is projected to continue, with an anticipated increase of approximately 6% volume between 2020 and 2027 (Aksun Tümerkan 2021). The global gelatin market is driven by an increase in demand food, pharmaceuticals and cosmetic sectors. It is employed as gelling agent in food products, as coating for capsules and as stabiliser for emulsions in pharmaceuticals, as binder and gelling agent in cosmetics. Additionally, it is a frequently preferred polymer in the production of biomaterial development such as wound dressings (Seifi et al. 2024), drug delivery systems (Yaman et al. 2024) and scaffolds for tissue regeneration (Kemençe and Bölgen 2017).

Keratin is an animal protein that has recently attracted significant interest within the field of biopolymers. As a fibrous protein which contains diverse amino acid sequences within its structure, exhibits a broad range of functional properties. Its primary characteristics can be described as renewable, sustainable, biocompatible and biodegradable. Keratin can be sourced from a variety of animal based materials, including feathers, hair, wool, animal claws and nails (Saha et al. 2019). As an example of the extraction of keratin from wool fiber materials with a sustainability approach, the work done by Goyal et al. can be examined. In the study, keratin was obtained by treating the wool with urea and L-cysteine and then subjecting it to dialysis, and the resulting keratin was used to create casting films and electrospun fibrous membranes with the help of gelatin, alginate and polyacrylonitrile polymers (Goyal et al. 2022).

2.2.1.2 Plant Derived

The development of plant-based biopolymers represents a shift in the use of materials from predominantly synthetic polymers and plastics. In this regard, although it is predominantly employed as a bioplastic in the packaging industry (Ghasemlou et al. 2024), it is also extensively utilized in the production of biomaterials (Iravani and Varma 2019) and in the pharmaceutical field (Opriş et al. 2024). Plants are capable of naturally producing a range of biopolymers, including starch, cellulose, carrageenan, alginate, pectin, tragacanth, lignin, silk, elastin and rubber.

Cellulose, the primary component of plant cell walls, is the most prevalent biopolymer on Earth. It is a linear polysaccharide constituted of glucose units bonded together by acetal linkages between the carbon atoms C1 and C4 of glycopyranose rings (McNamara et al. 2015). The primary sources of cellulose are agricultural by-products, including fruits, vegetables, forest residues, and plant matter. Cellulose represents approximately 1.5×10^{12} tonnes of annual biomass production and is regarded as an almost inexhaustible source of renewable raw materials, in line with the growing demand for environmentally friendly and biocompatible products (Klemm et al. 2005). Due to their distinctive properties, biodegradability, and outstanding physical and mechanical properties, cellulose, nanocellulose, and their derivatives occupy an important position in biological applications. In particular, the shortcomings of cellulose, including its vulnerability to microbial attack, sensitivity to moisture and insolubility in water, have prompted the development of cellulose derivatives. Derivatives of cellulose, including cellulose acetate, cellulose sulphate, nitrocellulose, carboxymethyl cellulose, ethyl cellulose and methyl cellulose, have been synthesised by replacing the hydroxyl groups of cellulose with other functional groups, including acids, oxides and chlorides (Pourmadadi et al. 2023; Seddiqi et al. 2021).

Pectin is another of the most common plant-based biopolymers. Although pectin is typically employed as emulsifying, stabilizing, gelling and thickening agent in the food industry (Vanitha et al. 2019), it has also garnered attention for its potential applications in biomedical and pharmaceutical field. From a chemical perspective, it is a heteropolysaccharide comprising D-galacturonic acid units connected by α-(1–4) glycosidic bonds (Pierce et al. 2020). The raw materials for pectin as a biopolymer are citrus peels or apple pomace, which are by-products of fruit juice production. Furthermore, sugar beet waste from sugar production, sunflower seeds used to extract oil, cocoa husks and potato pulp can also be employed in the production process (Akin-Ajani et al. 2021).

Starch, as another biopolymer, is one of the promising feedstocks for the continued use of biopolymers due to its relatively low cost, renewability and abundant availability. Its chemical structure contains two types of polymers, linear amylose and branched amylopectin. Starch can be easily converted to thermoplastic in the presence of platicisers such as glycerol, citric acid, sorbitol and maleic anhydride and at high temperatures (90–180 °C) (Agarwal et al. 2023; Dang and Yoksan 2015). This use attracts a lot of attention from an environmental and economic point of view, especially as it is an alternative to plastics in terms of sustainability. Conversely, properties such as swelling power, solubility, gelatinisation, rheological properties, mechanical behaviour and enzymatic digestibility indicate the potential for starch utilisation in biological applications. It is employed in a variety of capacities within the pharmaceutical industry, serving as a diluent, disintegrant, lubricant, binder, and lubricant (Phukan and Nongkhlaw 2022). In biomedical applications, it is utilized as a raw material in the fabrication of drug-release systems, wound dressing materials, and scaffolds (Kaur et al. 2007a).

2.2.1.3 Microorganism Derived

Microorganism-derived biopolymers are a class of polymers formed by the combination of monomers obtained by consuming carbon sources during the growth of any living organism, including algae, bacteria and fungi. Extracellular polymeric substances (EPS) and polyhydroxyalkanoates (PHAs) are regarded as microbial biopolymers. The microbial production process of biopolymers utilises sludge, wastewater, agricultural waste and soft carbon sources such as glucose, sucrose and fructose. EPS is employed for the biosorption of nutrients, heavy metals and a multitude of chemical reactions due to its distinctive amphiphilic, gelling and biocompatible nature. PHA is utilised in the medical sector and in the production of green plastics due to its biodegradable properties (Gupta et al. 2020).

2.2.2 Synthetic Sources

Synthetic biopolymers, which can be game changing with their alterable properties, can be obtained from natural sources or can be synthetically obtained from different sources via chemical reactions or chemical processes (Asuwin Prab et al. 2023). Also, biodegradation of this biopolymers is crucial for its usability in the selected areas. Last decade is very remarkable for synthetic biopolymers over natural polymers for its distinguish properties such as stability and durability and also over with other types of polymers. Synthetic biopolymers mostly used for its abovementioned properties for biomedical engineering and pharma applications, because at the end of the day, hygiene and stability of the single-use products matters the most (Attama et al. 2009).

Even with their functionality and tuneable properties, synthetic biopolymers need to be chemically enhanced to improve their cell and other living tissue interactions for biomedical engineering and pharma applications (Reddy et al. 2021). Thus, synthetic and natural biopolymers can be also used to improve their weaknesses and get better with the composite approaches. Moreover, not only a weakness improvement but also multi-functional properties with the bio-composites can be achieved (Mtibe et al. 2021).

To name a synthetic polymer to be synthetic biopolymer, one must be biodegradable and non-biobased. With their predictable and reproducible properties such as molecular weight, polydispersity index and tensile strength, most of the synthetic biopolymers are used to improve the biomedical engineering and pharma applications (Kluge and Mauck 2011). Poly ethylene glycol (PEG), Poly vinyl alcohol (PVA), Poly lactic acid (PLA), Poly ethylene oxide (PEO) and Poly caprolactone (PCL) are the few examples of the synthetic biopolymers for the biomedical engineering and pharma applications.

One of the most used polymers in the synthetic biopolymers is PEG. Biocompatible, immunogenic nature of the PEG is the main reasons for the usage for biomedical engineering and pharma applications. Most of the studies consists of cross-linkage with polymeric chains with PEG. These types of processes mainly affected the synthetic biopolymer PEG with the properties of diffusion, mechanical properties, biological degradation and so on (Das et al. 2023a). PEG based biopolymers can be enhanced with other types of materials to improve its biological and mechanical properties such as polymers or ceramics and nanoparticles and can be used in biomedical engineering and pharma applications as well as medical devices (Khan et al. 2023).

PVA is also one of the most studied biopolymers of the last decade. Water soluble, nontoxic, biocompatible nature of this polymer is main reason for the extensively studied. Adhesive, emulsify and film forming and self-gel forming properties are favoured for wound patches, skin repair, dialysis and drug delivery systems (Mallakpour and Rashidimoghadam 2018). One of the most important aspects of the PVA is the hydrophobic and hydrophilic parts of the polymers, this leads to very wide spectrums of applications for the biomedical engineering and pharma applications (Verma et al. 2023). Also, water solubility of the PVA can be altered with the hydrolysation and polymerization degree. Highly hydrolysed PVA (>95%) needs to be dissolved around 90 °C with aquatic conditions, partly hydrolysed PVA (<87%) could be easily dissolved with water (Tsou et al. 2016). Solubility is an important part of the biomedical engineering and pharma applications, and this leads to many different usage scenarios.

PLA is one of the most used biodegradable, aliphatic polyester that can be used in as a biopolymer for the biomedical engineering and pharma applications. It can be derived as lactic acid from various natural based renewable sources such as, sugarcane, tapioca and starch (Mukherjee et al. 2023). Due to unharmful nature of the degradation products of PLA, it can be used for numerous biomedical engineering and pharma applications without any issue (Ghalia and Dahman 2017). Different forms of PLA could be made for processing with different chiral forms of lactic acid. Poly-l-lactic acid, poly-d-lactic acid and poly-d,l-lactic acid is the just a few examples of different forms of lactic acid (Lasprilla et al. 2012). This could be used to improve the biomedical engineering and pharma applications with different needs.

PEO is the longer molecular form of PEG, is one of the highly used biodegradable and hydrophilic biopolymer with antigen, immunogen and cell adhesion properties. Containing both hydrophilic and hydrophobic groups, and non-ionic nature, is an important part of this polymer. Solubility in cold water and organic solvents is also important part of this synthetic biopolymer (Gelardi et al. 2016).

PCL is very different with the abovementioned biopolymers with a very low glass temperature and melting point. On the other hand, because it is a hydrophobic biopolymer, usage scenarios are also different as PCL can be degraded up to one year in vivo (Savioli Lopes et al. 2012). Therefore, it is widely used as a synthetic biopolymer for biomedical engineering and pharma applications, especially the bone tissue engineering thanks to its biocompatible and durable nature (Zaroog et al. 2019).

PU is one of the most used, single-use medical device for biomedical engineering and pharma applications such as veins, arteries, connections and valves. It is also used as tissues for biomedical engineering and pharma applications for its excellent properties for blood vessels, skin, cartilages and so on (Chavarría-Gaytán et al. 2010). Therefore, bacterial adhesion resistance of the PU is a very important part of the production of biomedical engineering and pharma applications with PU, to overcome this type of bacterial and protein activity of the PU, inserting bioactive compounds via composite materials are developed with polymers, metals and ceramic materials in the last years (Wendels and Avérous 2021).

Other than this options, many synthetic biopolymers can be list here, but none of them going to be the most desired structure, composition, mechanical strength and biocompatibility. Also, selecting a synthetic biopolymer for selected biomedical engineering and pharma applications not going to be suitable for most. Cell suitability, cell activation, bacterial and protein adhesion, tissue repairing, tissue suitability, reusability and price are the most important parameters of the selected synthetic biopolymers for biomedical engineering and pharma applications. Other than its unique and highly rated properties, synthetic biopolymers could also have a bad properties like low cell adhesion, to overcome this type of disadvantages, composite materials, copolymerization and blending with other biopolymers could reduce the risk of the using synthetic biopolymers. New methods for production of biomedical engineering and pharma applications such as 3D printing could also boost the usage of synthetic biopolymers.

2.3 Application Areas

Rapid population development worldwide has resulted in an exponential rise in the usage of short-lived, throwaway items that wind up in landfills. Globally, the usage of non-biodegradable materials seriously harms the environment. Since they are completely biodegradable, polymers made from wood, other fibre crops, or agricultural waste have the potential to be a component of a sustainable circular economy (George et al. 2020; Bari et al. 2021). In addition, natural biological sources such as plants, animals, microorganisms, and agricultural wastes are the source of biopolymers. They can be chemically synthesised from plant sources such corn, rice, wheat, potatoes, sorghum, yams, cassava, bananas, corn, tapioca, cotton and barley, or from monomeric components like sugars, oils and amino acids. Cattle are the primary animal supply; marine sources include fish, corals, sponges, lobsters, and shrimps; microbial sources include yeasts, fungus, and algae (Udayakumar et al. 2021). They have been investigated for a range of applications in the industrial, biomedical, pharmaceutical, drug-delivery, tissue engineering, medications, tablets, adhesives, paper, food, cotton, and rayon sectors, including sorption, due to their abundance, high tolerance, high thermal stability, non-toxicity, antibacterial activity, antifungal activity, biocompatibility, and biodegradability, among other unique qualities like strong adsorption capacities and ease of functionalization (Das et al. 2023b).

Recent developments in natural polymers have piqued attention across a range of industries because of their improved qualities and simplicity in commercialization. For an enhanced impact of these biopolymers as composites, readily available natural polymers such as collagen, keratin, chitosan, silk, and elastin can also be combined with synthetic polymers. Thus, the current trend is characterised by an increasing focus on polymers, biopolymers, and the combination of synthetic and biopolymers. The use of biopolymers and biopolymer composites in biomedical engineering and pharmaceutical applications are covered in this section (Chaabouni et al. 2014; Ling et al. 2018).

2.3.1 Biomedical Engineering

Biopolymers have recently shown exceptional advantages over traditional plastic polymers so long as they are applied in ways that improve functionality and provide value to human existence. As a result, biopolymers have drawn a lot of interest due to their unique tunable properties that make them appealing in a variety of applications and play a significant role in day-to-day living (Biswal 2019). When creating materials for use in biomedical applications, adjustable features like biodegradability, biocompatibility, renewability, affordability, and availability are crucial. Biopolymers may provide materials with these kinds of properties. Aside from these characteristics, target-oriented applications might be produced by modifying the polymer components to develop smart biopolymers (Arif et al. 2022). In this section of the review, we will examine the most commonly used biopolymers for biomedical engineering in detail.

Because of its many functionalization options, gelatin can be easily and successfully crosslinked. It can also be combined with other materials (such as metal nanoparticles, carbonaceous materials, minerals, and polymeric materials with desired functional properties) to create hybrid materials with enhanced thermo-mechanical, physio-chemical, and biological properties. Due to their distinct functional characteristics, gelatin-based hydrogels and nanocomposite hydrogels can be used in a variety of technological, biological, and environmental applications (Kumari et al. 2010; Balaji et al. 2018). For medical textile application, researchers studied on to create intelligent drug-eluting nanofibrous matrices that may be used as a starting point in the production of medical textiles (Ali et al. 2023). In other words, gelatin has exceptional performance and tremendous promise in a wide range of biomedical applications involving wound healing, drug administration, biosensing, and tissue regeneration because of its special qualities and ease of manufacture.

Regarding this, collagen is a natural fibrous protein that is crucial for tissue repair because it creates the biological environment needed for cell development and facilitates the adhesion, migration, and proliferation of cells (Morissette Martin et al. 2019). Due to their inherent gel-forming capacity, physicochemical characteristics, superior biocompatibility, and biodegradability, collagen is extremely popular options for the creation of cryogels. Collagen-based cryogels has demonstrated potential for application in biomedicine and have been effectively used as three-dimensional cell culture platforms.

Brown algae naturally produce alginate, a polysaccharide with a number of advantageous qualities, such as increased availability, affordability, strong biocompatibility, low cytotoxicity, and ease of gelation in the presence of divalent cations (Kumar et al. 2017). Because of its widespread availability, high compatibility, low cytotoxicity, low cost, and simplicity of gelation, alginate, a polysaccharide produced from brown seaweed, has been thoroughly studied as a biomaterial for several biomedical sciences as well as tissue engineering (Contessi Negrini et al. 2019; Hu and Lo 2021).

In contrast, elastin-derived peptides are synthetic biopolymers that have a similar conformation and structure to elastin but are soluble in aqueous media. Because of their biological activities and physicochemical properties, elastin and related peptides may be used as biomaterials to develop a variety of biomedical devices, such as scaffolds, hydrogels, and drug delivery systems for tissue engineering. Elastin is one of the main components of the extracellular matrix; in addition to contributing to cellular signalling, it offers resistance and elasticity to a wide range of human tissues and organs (Varanko et al. 2020). In addition to these, the essential and adaptable properties of the elastin-like polypeptides enable them to produce a variety of nanostructures, including nanoparticles (Lima et al. 2022).

Chitosan is one of the most attractive biopolymers in this field because of its promising properties for biomedical engineering applications, such as biodegradability, biocompatibility, and non-toxicity. As a result, chitosan and its derivatives are gaining significant interest in a wide range of biomedical applications (Hamedi et al. 2022). The current research presents several chitosan-based bioadhesives, both passive and active, and their various external stimuli response structures, including pH, light, and thermoresponsive systems (Fan et al. 2016). A variety of bioadhesive methods using chitosan as the primary polymer component or adhesive agent were also given in Table 2.1, along with some examples. Additionally included are chitosan-based bioadhesives and their possible uses in medicine for hemostatic, wound dressing, suture-free surgery, and medication delivery systems. The outcomes validated the chitosan bioadhesives' capacity for wound healing, hemostasis,

Table 2.1 The most commonly used biopolymers and their applications

Biopolymer	Application	Ref
Gelatin	Medical textile, tissue engineering, wound dressing, organ-on-a-chip, and biosensing	Jiang et al. (2021), Loiola et al. (2017), Wang et al. (2022), Gungor et al. (2021)
Collagen	Wound healing, Cell culture, tissue engineering, cell signalling	Razavi et al. (2020), Andonegi et al. (2020), op't Veld et al. (2018), Goodarzi et al. (2019)
Alginate	Encapsulated Cell Therapy, Tissue engineering, Wound dressing, islet cells	Orive et al. (2003), Nah et al. (2019), Lee et al. (2012)
Elastin	Tissue Engineering, Wound Dressing, Ocular disorders, Nanotechnology	Sharma et al. (2021), Pereira et al. (2021), Fernández-Colino et al. (2019)
Chitosan	Bioadhesives, tissue engineering, Ocular disorders, Hemostatic applications	Balakrishnan et al. (2017), Liu et al. (2021), Shou et al. (2020), Dudhani and Kosaraju (2010), Demir and Bölgen (2017), Ruprai et al. (2019)
Silk	Tissue engineering, wound dressing, nanotechnology, Stem cell engineering, Devices, biosensors	Xie et al. (2015), Lin et al. (2022), Liang et al. (2020), Ma et al. (2022)
Starch	Cosmetics, Wound dressing, Tissue engineering	Ounkaew et al. (2020), Kartik et al. (2021), Qamruzzaman et al. (2022)
Cellulose	Tissue engineering, devices, Ocular disorders, Cellular labelling and bioimaging, biosensors	Hasanin (2022), Mali and Sherje (2022)
Poly hydroxy alkanoates (PHA)	Tissue engineering,medical implants,diagnostic devices	Ansari et al. (2021), Kalia et al. (2023)

and bioadhesion, as well as their enormous potential for use in biomedical applications (Xu et al. 2019).

Owing to its exceptional biological activities and tunable chemical-physical characteristics, silk sericin a naturally occurring protein derived from silkworm cocoons—has been thoroughly investigated and employed in the biomedical profession (Liu et al. 2022). Furthermore, sericin's many functional groups derived from its diverse amino acid makeup enable it to be cross-linked and chemically altered to create adaptable constructions that operate as substitute matrices in biological applications. Sericin has recently been included into a range of bulk constructions (films, hydrogels, scaffolds, conduits, and devices) as well as micro-nano formulations for tissue engineering and regenerative medicine (Qi et al. 2018). We explain the many types of silk sericin, comprehensively summarise its features, and show how they might be used in both newly established and future biological applications presenting research articles.

Starch can be used for a wide range of biomedical and pharmaceutical applications because to their distinct physicochemical and functional properties, which have been extracted from various botanical sources such as corn, potatoes, rice and wheat. When choosing a starch source for unique applications, factors including swelling power, solubility, gelatinization, rheological qualities, mechanical behaviour, and enzymatic digestibility are crucial (Kaur et al. 2007b). Table 2.1 shows the different applications of biopolymers.

Cellulose is a linear biopolymer which is composed of nanofibrils, thus having a large surface area. In addition to plants, other sources of cellulose include bacteria, algae, fungus, and mammals; the sole animal source of cellulose being tunicates. Because of its distinct physicochemical characteristics and excellent biocompatibility, cellulose-based biomedical materials are gaining interest (Seddiqi et al. 2021). Therefore, cellulose-based biomaterials represent a novel material with great potential for usage in large-scale biomedical applications, either on their own or in combination with additional additives. They are also employed in a number of biological processes, including tissue engineering, wound dressing, and medication administration.

The polymers known as polyhydroxyalkanoates (PHAs) are produced sustainably by bacterial fermentation in the presence of limited nutrients. It is possible to adjust PHAs' mechanical characteristics as well as their degradation profile (Gregory et al. 2022). It might take the place of polymers made from petroleum as an environmentally beneficial substitute. In addition, (PHAs) used as biomaterials in medical equipment, including patches, sutures, and other items and help in reducing the plastic pollution that surged abruptly due to the COVID-19 waste (Pramanik 2023).

2.3.2 Pharmaceutical Applications

Scientists, the medical community, and business have all shown a significant deal of interest in the use of biopolymers in research, particularly in recent years. Due to the advantages of using biopolymers as edible coatings and films in the food sector, natural drug encapsulating materials have found practical uses. This study focuses on the invention, uses, and advantages of biopolymers in the pharmaceutical industry and as encapsulating materials for probiotics and other controlled drug delivery systems (Gheorghita et al. 2021).

A family of naturally occurring biopolymers known as polysaccharides have attracted a lot of interest because of their special qualities, which make them appealing for use in a variety of applications. In the pharmaceutical industry, cellulose which is belong to polysaccharide family is commonly used excipient as an anticaking agent, stabilizer, texture modifier, and drug delivery system, nanoparticulate drug delivery systems coating materials for tablets or capsules that shield them from light, moisture, and other environmental elements (Jabeen and Atif 2024; Sganzerla et al. 2021). In addition these, drug delivery systems composed of biopolymers that may react to various environmental stimuli, such as temperature, pH, and enzymes, to release the medication at the appropriate time and place are known as stimulus-responsive biopolymeric drug delivery matrices.

Alginate is another often utilised biopolymer that may be modified to react to pH, temperature, and ion stimuli. Drugs have been delivered to the skin, lungs, and gastrointestinal system using matrices based on alginate (Prasad et al. 2018).

Nanocarrier systems also have been widespread in recent years. In another research, alginate modified with doxorubicin and alginate modified with glycyrrhetinic acid were combined to create self-assembled polysaccharide nanocarriers, which were then utilised to treat liver cancer (Guo et al. 2013). Collagen-based nanocarriers have been used in brain-specific and genetic material delivery because of their notable biocompatibility and low antigenicity. In an attempt to treat neurological illnesses, one research used the gelling process of type I collagen hydrogel in situ to transport glial-derived growth factors to the central nervous system (Posadas et al. 2016). In addition, theophylline (THF)-encapsulated type I collagen-based nanocarriers have been utilised to transport medications through the oral and pulmonary routes (Nagarajan et al. 2014).

PLA, sometimes referred to as polylactide, is a naturally occurring polyester derived from renewable resources such fermented sugarcane, corn starch, and cassava plants. Chemical recycling and polymerisation transform PLA into biodegradable bioplastics. Adenocarcinomic human alveolar basal epithelial cells (A549 cells) were shown to have effectively internalised PLA nanocarriers in the literature, and it was clear that these cells showed outstanding drug transport efficiency (da Luz et al. 2017) .

Polyhydroxyalkanoates, PHAs, are aliphatic polyesters made by a variety of bacteria via the process of biosynthesis. But they only appear when the microorganisms have an abundance of carbon sources and there is a noticeable lack of other macromolecules. Polyhydroxybutyrate, PHB, is produced by a wide variety of microorganisms, and enzymes may readily break them down for a more beneficial nutritional supplement. In another research study, curcumin was encapsulated in PHB nanoparticles and delivered over an extended period of time. Additionally assessed were the antibacterial and anticancer properties. Different test were used to further validate the anticancer activity of the curcumin-loaded PHB nanoparticles (Senthilkumar et al. 2018).

Plants provide pectin, a polysaccharide that is used in many different products. Pectin and pectin-based nanocomposites have drawn the attention of many researchers due to their natural availability, biocompatibility, biodegradability, nontoxicity, flexibility, and enhanced structural and functional features. A few in vivo investigations verified that pectin's physicochemical properties affected cholesterol metabolism. More significantly, when howthorn pectin is taken as opposed to pectin hydrolyzates, the chemical structure of pectin has a big role in lowering the levels of cholesterol in the liver and plasma (Zhu et al. 2015).

Polycaprolactone, PCL is another class of aliphatic polyesters that are obtained by the catalytic polymerization of a cyclic ester known as caprolactone. A research objective was to use $scCO_2$-assisted drying of reverse emulsions to produce PCL nanoparticles loaded with progesterone for use in drug delivery systems in with the aim of resolving issues with conventional solvent evaporation of emulsions used in the production of polymeric nanoparticles (Guilherme et al. 2014).

2.4 Future Perspective and Conclusion

Future advances in applying various biopolymeric systems in therapeutics applications, with the inclusion of the capability to scale up with controlled and targeted properties, could be a crucial step for the future as the proper nanocarrier is essential to carry the genetic or DNA material to the targeted site. Since they will be utilised more in biological systems, effective processing techniques for extracting such biopolymeric systems must be given top priority. It is also strongly proposed that computational models be incorporated to understand the impacts on the material profile, including the degradation profile and the trafficking of polymeric nanoparticles within and outside of cells for further commercialisation. In order to bring about a revolutionary breakthrough in biomedical materials, extensive research on the surface and functionalisation of biopolymers, such as nanocellulose, may be necessary. This is because surface or chemical modification may drastically change the properties of the cell-material interaction. The encouraging findings from recent research included in this review will pave the way for the creation of more sophisticated smart biopolymers with regulated functional characteristics, therefore establishing a foundation for the development of more effective biopolymers for use in biomedical and pharmaceutical applications.

References

Adamaki-Sotiraki C, Abenaim L, Mannucci A, Rumbos CI, Bedini S, Castagna A, Conte G, Tognocchi M, Dolianitis V, Athanassiou CG, Conti B (2024) Performance of Hermetia illucens (Diptera: Stratiomyidae) larvae reared on organic waste diets and pupal chitin and chitosan yield. Environ Sci Pollut Res 31:37366–37375. https://doi.org/10.1007/S11356-024-33545-X/TABLES/4

Agarwal S, Singhal S, Godiya CB, Kumar S (2023) Prospects and applications of starch based biopolymers. Int J Environ Anal Chem 103:6907–6926. https://doi.org/10.1080/03067319.2021.1963717

Akin-Ajani OD, Okunlola A, Akin-Ajani OD, Okunlola A (2021) Pharmaceutical applications of pectin. In: Pectins – the new-old Polysaccharides. https://doi.org/10.5772/INTECHOPEN.100152

Aksun Tümerkan ET (2021) Sustainable utilization of gelatin from animal-based agri–food waste for the food industry and pharmacology. In: Valorization agri-food wastes by-products recent trends, innovations sustainability challenges. Academic Press, pp 425–442. https://doi.org/10.1016/B978-0-12-824044-1.00041-6

Ali IH, Elkashlan AM, Hammad MA, Hamdi M (2023) Antimicrobial and anti-SARS-CoV-2 activities of smart daclatasvir-chitosan/gelatin nanoparticles-in-PLLA nanofibrous medical textiles; in vitro, and in vivo study. Int J Biol Macromol 253:127350

Amiri H, Aghbashlo M, Sharma M, Gaffey J, Manning L, Moosavi Basri SM, Kennedy JF, Gupta VK, Tabatabaei M (2022) Chitin and chitosan derived from crustacean waste valorization streams can support food systems and the UN Sustainable Development Goals. Nature Food 3(10):822–828. https://doi.org/10.1038/s43016-022-00591-y

Andonegi M, Las Heras K, Santos-Vizcaíno E, Igartua M, Hernandez RM, de la Caba K, Guerrero P (2020) Structure-properties relationship of chitosan/collagen films with potential for biomedical applications. Carbohydr Polym 237:116159. https://doi.org/10.1016/j.carbpol.2020.116159

Ansari S, Sami N, Yasin D, Ahmad N, Fatma T (2021) Biomedical applications of environmental friendly poly-hydroxyalkanoates. Int J Biol Macromol 183:549–563. https://doi.org/10.1016/j.ijbiomac.2021.04.171
Arif ZU, Khalid MY, Sheikh MF, Zolfagharian A, Bodaghi M (2022) Biopolymeric sustainable materials and their emerging applications. J Environ Chem Eng 10:108159. https://doi.org/10.1016/j.jece.2022.108159
Asuwin Prab RG, Bajaj G, John AE, Chandran S, Kumar VV, Ramakrishna S (2023) A review on the recent applications of synthetic biopolymers in 3D printing for biomedical applications. J Mater Sci Mater Med 34. https://doi.org/10.1007/S10856-023-06765-9
Attama AA, Uzochukwu IC, Onunkwo GC (2009) An overview of synthetic biopolymers in drug delivery. In: Biopolymers in drug delivery: recent advances and challenges, pp 122–130. https://doi.org/10.2174/978160805078910901010122
Balaji AB, Pakalapati H, Khalid M, Walvekar R, Siddiqui H (2018) Natural and synthetic biocompatible and biodegradable polymers. https://doi.org/10.1016/B978-0-08-100970-3.00001-8
Balakrishnan B, Soman D, Payanam U, Laurent A, Labarre D, Jayakrishnan A (2017) A novel injectable tissue adhesive based on oxidized dextran and chitosan. Acta Biomater 53:343–354
Bari E, Sistani A, Morrell JJ, Pizzi A, Akbari MR, Ribera J (2021) Current strategies for the production of sustainable biopolymer composites. Polymers (Basel) 13:1–15. https://doi.org/10.3390/polym13172878
Biswal T (2019) Biopolymers for tissue engineering applications: a review. Mater Today Proc 41:397–402. https://doi.org/10.1016/j.matpr.2020.09.628
Caillol S (2021) Special Issue "Natural Polymers and Biopolymers II". Molecules 26. https://doi.org/10.3390/MOLECULES26010112
Chaabouni E, Gassara F, Brar SK (2014) In: Brar SK, Dhillon GS, Soccol CR (eds) Biopolymers synthesis and application BT – biotransformation of waste biomass into high value biochemicals. Springer New York, New York, pp 415–443. https://doi.org/10.1007/978-1-4614-8005-1_17
Chavarría-Gaytán MC, Olivas-Armendáriz I, García-Casillas PE, Martínez-Villafañe A, Martínez-Pérez CA (2010) Synthesis and characterization of polyurethane scaffolds for biomedical applications. Mater Res Soc Symp Proc 1243:127–132. https://doi.org/10.1557/PROC-1243-19/METRICS
Christian SJ (2016) Natural fibre-reinforced noncementitious composites (biocomposites). Woodhead Publishing. https://doi.org/10.1016/B978-0-08-100038-0.00005-6
Connan M, Perold V, Dilley BJ, Barbraud C, Cherel Y, Ryan PG (2021) The Indian Ocean "garbage patch": empirical evidence from floating macro-litter. Mar Pollut Bull 169. https://doi.org/10.1016/J.MARPOLBUL.2021.112559
Contessi Negrini N, Bonnetier M, Giatsidis G, Orgill DP, Farè S, Marelli B (2019) Tissue-mimicking gelatin scaffolds by alginate sacrificial templates for adipose tissue engineering. Acta Biomater 87:61–75. https://doi.org/10.1016/j.actbio.2019.01.018
Coppola D, Lauritano C, Esposito FP, Riccio G, Rizzo C, de Pascale D (2021) Fish waste: from problem to valuable resource. Mar Drugs 19:116. https://doi.org/10.3390/MD19020116
da Luz CM, Boyles MSP, Falagan-Lotsch P, Pereira MR, Tutumi HR, de Oliveira Santos E, Martins NB, Himly M, Sommer A, Foissner I (2017) Poly-lactic acid nanoparticles (PLA-NP) promote physiological modifications in lung epithelial cells and are internalized by clathrin-coated pits and lipid rafts. J Nanobiotechnol 15:1–18
Dang KM, Yoksan R (2015) Development of thermoplastic starch blown film by incorporating plasticized chitosan. Carbohydr Polym 115:575–581. https://doi.org/10.1016/J.CARBPOL.2014.09.005
Das A, Debnath A, Banerjee K, Bhattacharjee S, Deb A, Chatterjee S, Mondal A (2023a) Nanoparticles in bone tissue engineering. In: Nanostructured materials for tissue engineering. Elsevier, pp 427–456. https://doi.org/10.1016/B978-0-323-95134-0.00012-2
Das A, Ringu T, Ghosh S, Pramanik N (2023b) A comprehensive review on recent advances in preparation, physicochemical characterization, and bioengineering applications of biopolymers. Springer Berlin Heidelberg. https://doi.org/10.1007/s00289-022-04443-4

Demir D, Bölgen N (2017) Synthesis and characterization of injectable chitosan cryogel microsphere scaffolds. Int J Polym Mater Polym Biomater 66:686–696. https://doi.org/10.1080/00914037.2016.1255614

Demir D, Öfkeli F, Ceylan S, Bölgen N (2016) Extraction and characterization of chitin and chitosan from blue crab and synthesis of chitosan cryogel scaffolds. J Turkish Chem Soc Sect A Chem 3:131–144. https://doi.org/10.18596/jotcsa.00634

Dudhani AR, Kosaraju SL (2010) Bioadhesive chitosan nanoparticles: preparation and characterization. Carbohydr Polym 81:243–251

Fan B, Xing Y, Zheng Y, Sun C, Liang G (2016) pH-responsive thiolated chitosan nanoparticles for oral low-molecular weight heparin delivery: in vitro and in vivo evaluation. Drug Deliv 23:238–247

Fatiroi NS, Jaziri AA, Shapawi R, Mokhtar RAM, Noordin WNM, Huda N (2023) Biochemical and microstructural characteristics of collagen biopolymer from unicornfish (Naso reticulatus Randall, 2001) bone prepared with various acid types. Polymers 15:1054. https://doi.org/10.3390/POLYM15041054

Felix M, Romero A, Guerrero A (2019) Collagen as a potential biopolymer for the production of porous matrices (scaffolds) with application in tissue engineering. In: Materials for biomedical engineering: absorbable polymers, pp 217–244. https://doi.org/10.1016/B978-0-12-818415-8.00008-5

Fernández-Colino A, Wolf F, Rütten S, Schmitz-Rode T, Rodríguez-Cabello JC, Jockenhoevel S, Mela P (2019) Small caliber compliant vascular grafts based on elastin-like recombinamers for in situ tissue engineering. Front Bioeng Biotechnol 7:340

Flórez M, Cazón P, Vázquez M (2023) Selected biopolymers' processing and their applications: a review. Polymers (Basel) 15. https://doi.org/10.3390/POLYM15030641

Gelardi G, Mantellato S, Marchon D, Palacios M, Eberhardt AB, Flatt RJ (2016) Chemistry of chemical admixtures. In: Science and technology of concrete admixtures, pp 149–218. https://doi.org/10.1016/B978-0-08-100693-1.00009-6

George A, Sanjay MR, Srisuk R, Parameswaranpillai J, Siengchin S (2020) A comprehensive review on chemical properties and applications of biopolymers and their composites. Int J Biol Macromol 154:329–338. https://doi.org/10.1016/j.ijbiomac.2020.03.120

Getahun MJ, Kassie BB, Alemu TS (2024) Recent advances in biopolymer synthesis, properties, & commercial applications: a review. Process Biochem 145:261–287. https://doi.org/10.1016/J.PROCBIO.2024.06.034

Ghalia MA, Dahman Y (2017) Biodegradable poly(lactic acid)-based scaffolds: synthesis and biomedical applications. J Polym Res 24. https://doi.org/10.1007/S10965-017-1227-2

Ghasemlou M, Barrow CJ, Adhikari B (2024) The future of bioplastics in food packaging: an industrial perspective. Food Packag Shelf Life 43:101279. https://doi.org/10.1016/J.FPSL.2024.101279

Gheorghita R, Anchidin-Norocel L, Filip R, Dimian M, Covasa M (2021) Applications of biopolymers for drugs and probiotics delivery. Polymers (Basel) 13. https://doi.org/10.3390/polym13162729

Goldberga I, Li R, Duer MJ (2018) Collagen structure-function relationships from solid-state NMR spectroscopy. Acc Chem Res 51:1621–1629. https://doi.org/10.1021/ACS.ACCOUNTS.8B00092/ASSET/IMAGES/LARGE/AR-2018-00092K_0005.JPEG

Goodarzi H, Jadidi K, Pourmotabed S, Sharifi E, Aghamollaei H (2019) Preparation and in vitro characterization of cross-linked collagen–gelatin hydrogel using EDC/NHS for corneal tissue engineering applications. Int J Biol Macromol 126:620–632. https://doi.org/10.1016/j.ijbiomac.2018.12.125

Goyal S, Dotter M, Diestelhorst E, Storck JL, Ehrmann A, Mahltig B (2022) Extraction of keratin from wool and its use as biopolymer in film formation and in electrospinning for composite material processing. J Eng Fiber Fabr 17. https://doi.org/10.1177/15589250221090499/ASSET/IMAGES/LARGE/10.1177_15589250221090499-FIG14.JPEG

Gregory DA, Taylor CS, Fricker ATR, Asare E, Tetali SSV, Haycock JW, Roy I (2022) Polyhydroxyalkanoates and their advances for biomedical applications. Trends Mol Med 28:331–342

Guilherme MR, Mauricio MR, Tenorio-Neto ET, Kunita MH, Cardozo-Filho L, Cellet TSP, Pereira GM, Muniz EC, da Rocha SRP, Rubira AF (2014) Polycaprolactone nanoparticles containing encapsulated progesterone prepared using a scCO2 emulsion drying technique. Mater Lett 124:197–200

Gungor M, Sagirli MN, Calisir MD, Selcuk S, Kilic A (2021) Developing centrifugal spun thermally cross-linked gelatin based fibrous biomats for antibacterial wound dressing applications. Polym Eng Sci 61:2311–2322

Guo H, Lai Q, Wang W, Wu Y, Zhang C, Liu Y, Yuan Z (2013) Functional alginate nanoparticles for efficient intracellular release of doxorubicin and hepatoma carcinoma cell targeting therapy. Int J Pharm 451:1–11

Gupta J, Rathour R, Medhi K, Tyagi B, Thakur IS (2020) Microbial-derived natural bioproducts for a sustainable environment: a bioprospective for waste to wealth. In: Refining biomass residues for sustainable energy and bioproducts, Technol Adv Life Cycle Assessment, Econ, pp 51–85. https://doi.org/10.1016/B978-0-12-818996-2.00003-X

Hahn T, Tafi E, Paul A, Salvia R, Falabella P, Zibek S (2020) Current state of chitin purification and chitosan production from insects. J Chem Technol Biotechnol 95:2775–2795. https://doi.org/10.1002/JCTB.6533

Hamedi H, Moradi S, Hudson SM, Tonelli AE, King MW (2022) Chitosan based bioadhesives for biomedical applications: a review. Carbohydr Polym 282:119100. https://doi.org/10.1016/j.carbpol.2022.119100

Hasanin MS (2022) Cellulose-based biomaterials: chemistry and biomedical applications. Starch-Stärke 74:2200060

Herweyers L, Moons I, Barbarossa C, De Pelsmacker P, Du Bois E (2023) Understanding who avoids single-use plastics and why: a cross-country mixed-method study. J Clean Prod 414:137685. https://doi.org/10.1016/J.JCLEPRO.2023.137685

Hu T, Lo ACY (2021) Collagen–alginate composite hydrogel: application in tissue engineering and biomedical sciences. Polymers (Basel) 13. https://doi.org/10.3390/polym13111852

Iravani S, Varma RS (2019) Plants and plant-based polymers as scaffolds for tissue engineering. Green Chem 21:4839–4867. https://doi.org/10.1039/C9GC02391G

Jabeen N, Atif M (2024) Polysaccharides based biopolymers for biomedical applications: a review. Polym Adv Technol 35:1–23. https://doi.org/10.1002/pat.6203

Jaya B, Brajesh B, Antonella F, Giovanna LD, Amit K (2022) Biopolymer: a sustainable material for food and medical applications. Polymers (Basel) 14:1–22

Je JY, Kim SK (2006) Antimicrobial action of novel chitin derivative. Biochim Biophys Acta Gen Subj 1760:104–109. https://doi.org/10.1016/J.BBAGEN.2005.09.012

Jeevanandam J, Pan S, Rodrigues J, Elkodous MA, Danquah MK (2022) Medical applications of biopolymer nanofibers. Biomater Sci 10:4107–4118. https://doi.org/10.1039/D2BM00701K

Jiang C, Wang K, Liu Y, Zhang C, Wang B (2021) Using wet electrospun PCL/gelatin/CNT yarns to fabricate textile-based scaffolds for vascular tissue engineering. ACS Biomater Sci Eng 7:2627–2637

Kalia VC, Patel SKS, Lee J-K (2023) Exploiting polyhydroxyalkanoates for biomedical applications. Polymers (Basel) 15. https://doi.org/10.3390/polym15081937

Kartik A, Akhil D, Lakshmi D, Panchamoorthy Gopinath K, Arun J, Sivaramakrishnan R, Pugazhendhi A (2021) A critical review on production of biopolymers from algae biomass and their applications. Bioresour Technol 329:124868. https://doi.org/10.1016/j.biortech.2021.124868

Kaur L, Singh J, Liu Q (2007a) Starch – A potential biomaterial for biomedical applications. In: Nanomaterials and nanosystems for biomedical applications, pp 83–98. https://doi.org/10.1007/978-1-4020-6289-6_5

Kaur L, Singh J, Liu Q (2007b) Starch – a potential biomaterial for biomedical applications. In: Mozafari MR (ed) Nanomaterials and nanosystems for biomedical applications. Springer Netherlands, Dordrecht, pp 83–98. https://doi.org/10.1007/978-1-4020-6289-6_5

Kemençe N, Bölgen N (2017) Gelatin- and hydroxyapatite-based cryogels for bone tissue engineering: synthesis, characterization, in vitro and in vivo biocompatibility. J Tissue Eng Regen Med 11:20–33. https://doi.org/10.1002/term.1813

Khan MUA, Aslam MA, Bin Abdullah MF, Hasan A, Shah SA, Stojanović GM (2023) Recent perspective of polymeric biomaterial in tissue engineering– a review. Mater Today Chem 34:101818. https://doi.org/10.1016/J.MTCHEM.2023.101818

Khayrova AS, Sazhnev NA, Korobovskaya DV, Lopatin SA, Kildeeva NR, Varlamov VP (2024) Isolation of chitosan-melanin complex from black soldier fly adults and obtaining nanofibrous materials based on it. Appl Biochem Microbiol 60:201–206. https://doi.org/10.1134/S0003683824020078/FIGURES/4

Klemm D, Heublein B, Fink HP, Bohn A (2005) Cellulose: fascinating biopolymer and sustainable raw material. Angew Chemie Int Ed 44:3358–3393. https://doi.org/10.1002/ANIE.200460587

Kluge JA, Mauck RL (2011) Synthetic/biopolymer nanofibrous composites as dynamic tissue engineering scaffolds. In: Advances in polymer science. Springer, Berlin, Heidelberg, pp 101–130. https://doi.org/10.1007/12_2011_142

Kukkola A, Chetwynd AJ, Krause S, Lynch I (2024) Beyond microbeads: examining the role of cosmetics in microplastic pollution and spotlighting unanswered questions. J Hazard Mater 476:135053. https://doi.org/10.1016/J.JHAZMAT.2024.135053

Kumar A, Lee Y, Kim D, Rao KM, Kim J, Park S, Haider A, Lee DH, Han SS (2017) Effect of crosslinking functionality on microstructure, mechanical properties, and in vitro cytocompatibility of cellulose nanocrystals reinforced poly (vinyl alcohol)/sodium alginate hybrid scaffolds. Int J Biol Macromol 95:962–973. https://doi.org/10.1016/j.ijbiomac.2016.10.085

Kumari A, Yadav SK, Yadav SC (2010) Biodegradable polymeric nanoparticles based drug delivery systems. Colloids Surf B: Biointerfaces 75:1–18. https://doi.org/10.1016/j.colsurfb.2009.09.001

Lasprilla AJR, Martinez GAR, Lunelli BH, Jardini AL, Filho RM (2012) Poly-lactic acid synthesis for application in biomedical devices – a review. Biotechnol Adv 30:321–328. https://doi.org/10.1016/J.BIOTECHADV.2011.06.019

Lee BR, Hwang JW, Choi YY, Wong SF, Hwang YH, Lee DY, Lee S-H (2012) In situ formation and collagen-alginate composite encapsulation of pancreatic islet spheroids. Biomaterials 33:837–845

Lee H, Kim J, Myung S, Jung TG, Han DW, Kim B, Lee JC (2024) Extraction of γ-chitosan from insects and fabrication of PVA/γ-chitosan/kaolin nanofiber wound dressings with hemostatic properties. Discov Nano 19:1–14. https://doi.org/10.1186/S11671-024-04016-6/FIGURES/7

Liang X, Li H, Dou J, Wang Q, He W, Wang C, Li D, Lin J, Zhang Y (2020) Stable and biocompatible carbon nanotube ink mediated by silk protein for printed electronics. Adv Mater 32:2000165

Lima LF, Sousa MGDC, Rodrigues GR, de Oliveira KBS, Pereira AM, da Costa A, Machado R, Franco OL, Dias SC (2022) Elastin-like polypeptides in development of nanomaterials for application in the medical field. Front Nanotechnol 4:874790

Lin M, Zheng Z, Yang L, Luo M, Fu L, Lin B, Xu C (2022) A high-performance, sensitive, wearable multifunctional sensor based on rubber/CNT for human motion and skin temperature detection. Adv Mater 34:2107309

Ling S, Chen W, Fan Y, Zheng K, Jin K, Yu H, Buehler MJ, Kaplan DL (2018) Biopolymer nanofibrils: structure, modeling, preparation, and applications. Prog Polym Sci 85:1–56. https://doi.org/10.1016/j.progpolymsci.2018.06.004

Liu C, Lei F, Li P, Wang K, Jiang J (2021) A review on preparations, properties, and applications of cis-ortho-hydroxyl polysaccharides hydrogels crosslinked with borax. Int J Biol Macromol 182:1179–1191. https://doi.org/10.1016/j.ijbiomac.2021.04.090

Liu J, Shi L, Deng Y, Zou M, Cai B, Song Y, Wang Z, Wang L (2022) Silk sericin-based materials for biomedical applications. Biomaterials 287:121638. https://doi.org/10.1016/j.biomaterials.2022.121638

Loiola LMD, Cortez Tornello PR, Abraham GA, Felisberti MI (2017) Amphiphilic electrospun scaffolds of PLLA–PEO–PPO block copolymers: preparation, characterization and drug-release behaviour. RSC Adv 7:161–172. https://doi.org/10.1039/C6RA25023H

Ma H, Li J, Zhou J, Luo Q, Wu W, Mao Z, Ma W (2022) Screen-printed carbon black/recycled Sericin@ fabrics for wearable sensors to monitor sweat loss. ACS Appl Mater Interfaces 14:11813–11819

Mali P, Sherje AP (2022) Cellulose nanocrystals: fundamentals and biomedical applications. Carbohydr Polym 275:118668. https://doi.org/10.1016/j.carbpol.2021.118668

Mallakpour S, Rashidimoghadam S (2018) Poly(vinyl alcohol)/carbon nanotube nanocomposites: challenges and opportunities. In: Biodegradable and biocompatible polymer composites: processing, properties and applications, pp 297–315. https://doi.org/10.1016/B978-0-08-100970-3.00010-9

McNamara JT, Morgan JLW, Zimmer J (2015) A molecular description of cellulose biosynthesis. Annu Rev Biochem 84:895. https://doi.org/10.1146/ANNUREV-BIOCHEM-060614-033930

Morissette Martin P, Grant A, Hamilton DW, Flynn LE (2019) Matrix composition in 3-D collagenous bioscaffolds modulates the survival and angiogenic phenotype of human chronic wound dermal fibroblasts. Acta Biomater 83:199–210. https://doi.org/10.1016/j.actbio.2018.10.042

Mtibe A, Motloung MP, Bandyopadhyay J, Ray SS (2021) Synthetic biopolymers and their composites: advantages and limitations—an overview. Macromol Rapid Commun 42:2100130. https://doi.org/10.1002/MARC.202100130

Mukherjee C, Varghese D, Krishna JS, Boominathan T, Rakeshkumar R, Dineshkumar S, Brahmananda Rao CVS, Sivaramakrishna A (2023) Recent advances in biodegradable polymers – properties, applications and future prospects. Eur Polym J 192:112068. https://doi.org/10.1016/J.EURPOLYMJ.2023.112068

Nagarajan U, Kawakami K, Zhang S, Chandrasekaran B, Nair BU (2014) Fabrication of solid collagen nanoparticles using electrospray deposition. Chem Pharm Bull 62:422–428

Nah H, Lee D, Heo M, Lee JS, Lee SJ, Heo DN, Seong J, Lim H-N, Lee Y-H, Moon H-J, Hwang Y-S, Kwon IK (2019) Vitamin D-conjugated gold nanoparticles as functional carriers to enhancing osteogenic differentiation. Sci Technol Adv Mater 20:826–836. https://doi.org/10.1080/14686996.2019.1644193

Namazi H (2017) Polymers in our daily life. Bioimpacts 7:73–74. https://doi.org/10.15171/BI.2017.09

Nazrun T, Hassan MK, Hossain MD, Ahmed B, Hasnat MR, Saha S (2024) Application of biopolymers as sustainable cladding materials: a review. Sustainability 16:27. https://doi.org/10.3390/SU16010027

Nirmal N, Demir D, Ceylan S, Ahmad S, Goksen G, Koirala P, Bono G (2024) Polysaccharides from shell waste of shellfish and their applications in the cosmeceutical industry: a review. Int J Biol Macromol 265:131119. https://doi.org/10.1016/J.IJBIOMAC.2024.131119

op't Veld RC, van den Boomen OI, Lundvig DMS, Bronkhorst EM, Kouwer PHJ, Jansen JA, Middelkoop E, Von den Hoff JW, Rowan AE, Wagener FADTG (2018) Thermosensitive biomimetic polyisocyanopeptide hydrogels may facilitate wound repair. Biomaterials 181:392–401. https://doi.org/10.1016/j.biomaterials.2018.07.038

Opriş O, Mormile C, Lung I, Stegarescu A, Soran ML, Soran A (2024) An overview of biopolymers for drug delivery applications. Appl Sci 14:1383. https://doi.org/10.3390/APP14041383

Orive G, Hernández RM, Gascón AR, Calafiore R, Chang TMS, De Vos P, Hortelano G, Hunkeler D, Lacík I, Shapiro AMJ (2003) Cell encapsulation: promise and progress. Nat Med 9:104–107

Ounkaew A, Kasemsiri P, Jetsrisuparb K, Uyama H, Hsu Y-I, Boonmars T, Artchayasawat A, Knijnenburg JTN, Chindaprasirt P (2020) Synthesis of nanocomposite hydrogel based carboxymethyl starch/polyvinyl alcohol/nanosilver for biomedical materials. Carbohydr Polym 248:116767

Pereira AM, da Costa A, Dias SC, Casal M, Machado R (2021) Production and purification of two bioactive antimicrobial peptides using a two-step approach involving an elastin-like fusion tag. Pharmaceuticals 14:956

Perera KY, Jaiswal AK, Jaiswal S (2023) Biopolymer-based sustainable food packaging materials: challenges, solutions, and applications. Foods 12:2422. https://doi.org/10.3390/FOODS12122422

Phukan M, Nongkhlaw FT (2022) Starch: an overview of its conventional and unconventional sources, pharmaceutical and industrial applications. Curr Trends Pharm Res 9:140–161

Piekarska K, Sikora M, Owczarek M, Jóźwik-Pruska J, Wiśniewska-Wrona M (2023) Chitin and chitosan as polymers of the future—obtaining, modification, life cycle assessment and main directions of application. Polymers 15:793. https://doi.org/10.3390/POLYM15040793

Pierce A, Zheng Y, Wagner WL, Scheller HV, Mohnen D, Tsuda A, Ackermann M, Mentzer SJ (2020) Pectin biopolymer mechanics and microstructure associated with polysaccharide phase transitions. J Biomed Mater Res Part A 108:246–253. https://doi.org/10.1002/JBM.A.36811

Pilevar Z, Bahrami A, Beikzadeh S, Hosseini H, Jafari SM (2019) Migration of styrene monomer from polystyrene packaging materials into foods: characterization and safety evaluation. Trends Food Sci Technol 91:248–261. https://doi.org/10.1016/J.TIFS.2019.07.020

Posadas I, Monteagudo S, Cena V (2016) Nanoparticles for brain-specific drug and genetic material delivery, imaging and diagnosis. Nanomedicine 11:833–849

Pourmadadi M, Rahmani E, Shamsabadipour A, Samadi A, Esmaeili J, Arshad R, Rahdar A, Tavangarian F, Pandey S (2023) Novel carboxymethyl cellulose based nanocomposite: a promising biomaterial for biomedical applications. Process Biochem 130:211–226. https://doi.org/10.1016/J.PROCBIO.2023.03.033

Pramanik N (2023) A tool for biomedical application: synthesis and modification of polyhydroxyalkanoates. Sustain Chem Pharm 32:101041. https://doi.org/10.1016/j.scp.2023.101041

Prasad K, Mondal D, Sharma M, Freire MG, Mukesh C, Bhatt J (2018) Stimuli responsive ion gels based on polysaccharides and other polymers prepared using ionic liquids and deep eutectic solvents. Carbohydr Polym 180:328–336

Qamruzzaman M, Ahmed F, Mondal MIH (2022) An overview on starch-based sustainable hydrogels: potential applications and aspects. J Polym Environ 30:19–50

Qi C, Liu J, Jin Y, Xu L, Wang G, Wang Z, Wang L (2018) Photo-crosslinkable, injectable sericin hydrogel as 3D biomimetic extracellular matrix for minimally invasive repairing cartilage. Biomaterials 163:89–104

Razavi M, Primavera R, Kevadiya BD, Wang J, Buchwald P, Thakor AS (2020) A collagen based cryogel bioscaffold that generates oxygen for islet transplantation. Adv Funct Mater 30:1902463

Reddy MSB, Ponnamma D, Choudhary R, Sadasivuni KK (2021) A comparative review of natural and synthetic biopolymer composite scaffolds. Polymers 13:1105. https://doi.org/10.3390/POLYM13071105

Rendón-Villalobos R, Ortíz-Sánchez A, Tovar-Sánchez E, Flores-Huicochea E, Rendón-Villalobos R, Ortíz-Sánchez A, Tovar-Sánchez E, Flores-Huicochea E (2016) The role of biopolymers in obtaining environmentally friendly materials. In: Composites from renewable and sustainable materials. IntechOpen. https://doi.org/10.5772/65265

Rezvani Ghomi E, Nourbakhsh N, Akbari Kenari M, Zare M, Ramakrishna S (2021) Collagen-based biomaterials for biomedical applications. J Biomed Mater Res Part B Appl Biomater 109:1986–1999. https://doi.org/10.1002/JBM.B.34881

Romero M, Macchione MA, Mattea F, Strumia M (2020) The role of polymers in analytical medical applications. A review. Microchem J 159:105366. https://doi.org/10.1016/J.MICROC.2020.105366

Ruprai H, Romanazzo S, Ireland J, Kilian K, Mawad D, George L, Wuhrer R, Houang J, Ta D, Myers S (2019) Porous chitosan films support stem cells and facilitate sutureless tissue repair. ACS Appl Mater Interfaces 11:32613–32622

Saha S, Arshad M, Zubair M, Ullah A (2019) Keratin as a biopolymer. In: Springer series on polymer and composite materials. Springer, Cham, pp 163–185. https://doi.org/10.1007/978-3-030-02901-2_6

Savioli Lopes M, Jardini AL, Maciel Filho R (2012) Poly (lactic acid) production for tissue engineering applications. Procedia Eng 42:1402–1413. https://doi.org/10.1016/J.PROENG.2012.07.534

Seddiqi H, Oliaei E, Honarkar H, Jin J, Geonzon LC, Bacabac RG, Klein-Nulend J (2021) Cellulose and its derivatives: towards biomedical applications. Cellulose 28:1893–1931. https://doi.org/10.1007/s10570-020-03674-w

Seifi S, Shahverdi M, Shaygani H, Shamloo A, Mohammadi K (2024) Fabrication of gelatin-based antibacterial bilayer wound dressing using direct writing and electrospinning methods. Int J Pharm 659:124274. https://doi.org/10.1016/j.ijpharm.2024.124274

Senthilkumar P, Dawn SS, Saipriya C, Samrot AV (2018) Surfactant (span20) influenced synthesis of polyhydroxybutyrate nanoparticles for hydrophobic drug delivery. Rasayan J Chem 11:1686–1695

Sganzerla WG, Ribeiro CPP, Uliana NR, Rodrigues MBC, da Rosa CG, Ferrareze JP, de Lima Veeck AP, Nunes MR (2021) Bioactive and pH-sensitive films based on carboxymethyl cellulose and blackberry (Morus nigra L.) anthocyanin-rich extract: a perspective coating material to improve the shelf life of cherry tomato (Solanum lycopersicum L. var. cerasiforme). Biocatal Agric Biotechnol 33:101989

Sharma A, Sharma P, Roy S (2021) Elastin-inspired supramolecular hydrogels: a multifaceted extracellular matrix protein in biomedical engineering. Soft Matter 17:3266–3290

Shou Y, Zhang J, Yan S, Xia P, Xu P, Li G, Zhang K, Yin J (2020) Thermoresponsive chitosan/DOPA-based hydrogel as an injectable therapy approach for tissue-adhesion and hemostasis. ACS Biomater Sci Eng 6:3619–3629

Shoulders MD, Raines RT (2009) Collagen structure and stability. Annu Rev Biochem 78:929. https://doi.org/10.1146/ANNUREV.BIOCHEM.77.032207.120833

Smith AM, Moxon S, Morris GA (2016) Biopolymers as wound healing materials. Wound Heal Biomater 2:261–287. https://doi.org/10.1016/B978-1-78242-456-7.00013-1

Tarafdar A, Gaur VK, Rawat N, Wankhade PR, Gaur GK, Awasthi MK, Sagar NA, Sirohi R (2021) Advances in biomaterial production from animal derived waste. Bioengineered 12:8247. https://doi.org/10.1080/21655979.2021.1982321

Triunfo M, Tafi E, Guarnieri A, Salvia R, Scieuzo C, Hahn T, Zibek S, Gagliardini A, Panariello L, Coltelli MB, De Bonis A, Falabella P (2022) Characterization of chitin and chitosan derived from Hermetia illucens, a further step in a circular economy process. Scientific Reports 12(1):1–17. https://doi.org/10.1038/s41598-022-10423-5

Tsou YH, Khoneisser J, Huang PC, Xu X (2016) Hydrogel as a bioactive material to regulate stem cell fate. Bioact Mater 1:39–55. https://doi.org/10.1016/J.BIOACTMAT.2016.05.001

Udayakumar GP, Muthusamy S, Selvaganesh B, Sivarajasekar N, Rambabu K, Sivamani S, Sivakumar N, Maran JP, Hosseini-Bandegharaei A (2021) Ecofriendly biopolymers and composites: preparation and their applications in water-treatment. Biotechnol Adv 52:107815. https://doi.org/10.1016/j.biotechadv.2021.107815

ur Rehman K, Hollah C, Wiesotzki K, Heinz V, Aganovic K, ur Rehman R, Petrusan JI, Zheng L, Zhang J, Sohail S, Mansoor MK, Rumbos CI, Athanassiou C, Cai M (2023) Insect-derived chitin and chitosan: a still unexploited resource for the edible insect sector. Sustainability 15:4864. https://doi.org/10.3390/SU15064864

Vanitha T, Khan M, Vanitha T, Khan M (2019) Role of pectin in food processing and food packaging. In: Pectins – extraction, purification, characterization and applications. https://doi.org/10.5772/INTECHOPEN.83677

Varanko AK, Su JC, Chilkoti A (2020) Elastin-like polypeptides for biomedical applications. Annu Rev Biomed Eng 22:343–369

Verma C, Quraishi MA, Alfantazi A, Rhee KY (2023) Biodegradable synthetic polymers in sustainable corrosion protection: present and future scenarios. Adv Ind Eng Polym Res 6:407–435. https://doi.org/10.1016/J.AIEPR.2023.04.005

Vinod A, Sanjay MR, Suchart S, Jyotishkumar P (2020) Renewable and sustainable biobased materials: an assessment on biofibers, biofilms, biopolymers and biocomposites. J Clean Prod 258:120978. https://doi.org/10.1016/j.jclepro.2020.120978

Wang W, Zhou Z, Liu N, Zhang X, Zhou H, Wang Y, Fang K, Wu T (2022) Improving biocompatibility of polyester fabrics through polyurethane/gelatin complex coating for potential vascular application. Polymers (Basel) 14:989

Webb HK, Arnott J, Crawford RJ, Ivanova EP (2012) Plastic degradation and its environmental implications with special reference to poly(ethylene terephthalate). Polymers 5:1–18. https://doi.org/10.3390/POLYM5010001

Wendels S, Avérous L (2021) Biobased polyurethanes for biomedical applications. Bioact Mater 6:1083–1106. https://doi.org/10.1016/J.BIOACTMAT.2020.10.002

Xie H, Yang W, Chen J, Zhang J, Lu X, Zhao X, Huang K, Li H, Chang P, Wang Z (2015) A silk sericin/silicone nerve guidance conduit promotes regeneration of a transected sciatic nerve. Adv Healthc Mater 4:2195–2205

Xu R, Ma S, Wu Y, Lee H, Zhou F, Liu W (2019) Adaptive control in lubrication, adhesion, and hemostasis by Chitosan–Catechol–pNIPAM. Biomater Sci 7:3599–3608

Yaman SM, Demir D, Bölgen N (2024) Design of gelatin cryogel scaffolds with the ability to release simvastatin for potential bone tissue engineering applications. Biomed Mater 19(5):055019

Zaharescu T, Varca GHC (2022) Radiation modified polymers for medical applications. Radiat Phys Chem 194:110043. https://doi.org/10.1016/J.RADPHYSCHEM.2022.110043

Zaroog OS, Borhana AA, Perumal SSA (2019) Biomaterials for bone replacements: past and present. Ref Modul Mater Sci Mater Eng. https://doi.org/10.1016/B978-0-12-803581-8.11442-0

Zhang Q, Song M, Xu Y, Wang W, Wang Z, Zhang L (2021) Bio-based polyesters: recent progress and future prospects. Prog Polym Sci 120:101430. https://doi.org/10.1016/J.PROGPOLYMSCI.2021.101430

Zhong Y, Godwin P, Jin Y, Xiao H (2020) Biodegradable polymers and green-based antimicrobial packaging materials: a mini-review. Adv Ind Eng Polym Res 3:27–35. https://doi.org/10.1016/J.AIEPR.2019.11.002

Zhou N, Liu Y-D, Zhang Y, Gu T-W, Peng L-H, Zhou N, Liu Y-D, Zhang Y, Gu T-W, Peng L-H (2023) Pharmacological functions, synthesis, and delivery progress for collagen as biodrug and biomaterial. Pharmaceutics 15:1443. https://doi.org/10.3390/PHARMACEUTICS15051443

Zhu R-G, Sun Y-D, Li T-P, Chen G, Peng X, Duan W-B, Zheng Z-Z, Shi S-L, Xu J-G, Liu Y-H (2015) Comparative effects of hawthorn (Crataegus pinnatifida Bunge) pectin and pectin hydrolyzates on the cholesterol homeostasis of hamsters fed high-cholesterol diets. Chem Biol Interact 238:42–47

Zubair M, Pradhan RA, Arshad M, Ullah A (2021) Recent advances in lipid derived bio-based materials for food packaging applications. Macromol Mater Eng 306:2000799. https://doi.org/10.1002/MAME.202000799

Green Synthesis of Sustainable Materials from Biomass for Bioengineering

3

Aditya Singh, Shubhrat Maheshwari, Sudarshan Singh, and Bhupendra G. Prajapati

Abstract

Biomass and sustainable raw materials play a pivotal role in driving industries towards the principles of green technology and sustainability. Nature offers a diverse range of renewable raw materials with distinct properties and chemical compositions. The intersection of green nanotechnology and biomedical sciences creates opportunities for extensive biological research and medical applications at the molecular and cellular levels, aiming to develop eco-friendly nano-systems that yield significant economic and social benefits with low environmental impact. This innovative concept also opens avenues for utilizing non-toxic reagents and metabolites from living organisms in the green synthesis of nano-systems, encompassing metallic nanoparticles, polymeric nanoparticles, and vesicular drug delivery. The simplicity, scalability, and cost-effectiveness of production, coupled with enhanced properties, position green synthesis of sustainable materials as promising candidates for bioengineering applications. In particular, biomedical and bioengineering processes stand to gain directly from

A. Singh
Department of Pharmacy, Faculty of Pharmacy, Integral University, Lucknow, India

S. Maheshwari
Faculty of Pharmaceutical Sciences, Rama University, Kanpur, Uttar Pradesh, India

S. Singh (✉)
Office of Research Administration, Chiang Mai University, Chiang Mai, Thailand

Faculty of Pharmacy, Chiang Mai University, Chiang Mai, Thailand

B. G. Prajapati
Shree. S. K. Patel College of Pharmaceutical Education and Research, Ganpat University, Kherva, Gujarat, India

Centre for Research Impact & Outcome, Chitkara College of Pharmacy, Chitkara University, Rajpura Punjab, India

M. N. Collins, M. Culebras (eds.), *Sustainable Biopolymers and Composites for Biomedical Applications*, Biomaterials, Bioengineering and Sustainability 5,
https://doi.org/10.1007/978-3-031-91972-5_3

applications harmonize with green principles remains compelling. The exploration of renewable resources and sustainable raw materials, coupled with advancements in green nanotechnology and biomedical sciences, paints a holistic picture of innovation that transcends traditional boundaries. This convergence holds the promise of not only addressing current environmental and health challenges but also contributing to a future where technology and sustainability coexist seamlessly for the benefit of humanity (Ojukwu and Nwaiwu 2023; Sharma et al. 2023).

3.2 Green Nanotechnology

Nanotechnology, as a multidisciplinary field as shown in Fig. 3.1, converges the expertise of chemists, biologists, physicists, and materials science engineers, serving as a pivotal enabling technology (Albert 2023; Katti 2013). The escalating utilization of nanostructured materials, however, has prompted valid concerns regarding potential environmental and public health ramifications (Upadhyay and Singh 2020). In response, a specialized subfield has emerged, focusing on the development of safe and ecologically sustainable solutions (Su et al. 2023).

At the forefront of mitigating the ecological footprint of nanotechnology lies the amalgamation of green chemistry principles into the framework of nanoscience, known as green nanotechnology. This paradigm seeks to redefine the creation, manufacturing, and utilization of nanomaterials through a lens of sustainability and environmental responsibility.

The tenets of green chemistry, rooted in the reduction of hazardous substances, the design of safer chemicals and materials, and the minimization of waste, serve as

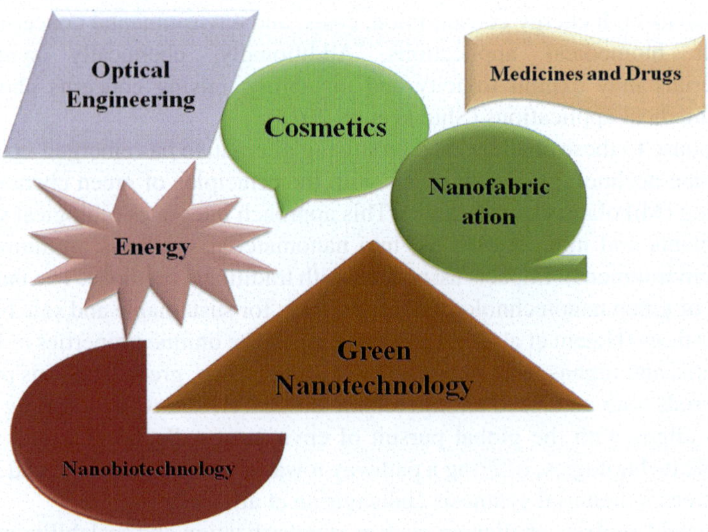

Fig. 3.1 Branches of green nanotechnology

the bedrock of green nanotechnology. The central ambition is to proactively address environmental and health concerns associated with nanomaterials throughout their lifecycle (Husain et al. 2023).

In the realm of green nanotechnology, innovative strategies are deployed to curtail the hazards posed by nanomaterials. Fundamental to this approach is the strategic substitution of environmentally benign alternatives for conventional, potentially harmful components. This involves the meticulous selection of nanomaterial precursors that exhibit minimal ecological and human health impacts, thereby contributing to the development of sustainable and safe nanomaterials (Shah et al. 2023). Simultaneously, a critical focus within green nanotechnology involves the optimization and modification of existing synthetic and processing methodologies. By scrutinizing the entire lifecycle of nanomaterials, from synthesis and production to utilization and disposal, the principles of green chemistry are applied to minimize resource consumption, waste generation, and environmental impact. The reevaluation and redesign of nanomaterial processes serve to enhance their overall sustainability, aligning with ecological and human health considerations (Zhang et al. 2023).

Green synthesis in biomedical engineering stands out as a transformative approach, weaving together the realms of nanotechnology and environmental consciousness. In this context, the advantages of green synthesis over conventional chemical methods are pivotal for the advancement of medical technologies (Zhang et al. 2023). The foremost attribute that distinguishes green synthesis is its inherent focus on biocompatibility. By employing natural compounds and biomolecules as precursors, green synthesis ensures that the resulting nanomaterials seamlessly integrate with biological systems. This is particularly crucial in biomedical applications where compatibility with living tissues and minimal adverse effects are paramount (Corsi et al. 2023). Moreover, the reduced toxicity associated with green-synthesized nanomaterials enhances their appeal in the biomedical field. Traditional chemical synthesis often entails the use of harsh solvents and reagents, leaving behind residues that can compromise the safety of medical interventions. In contrast, green synthesis methods leverage mild reaction conditions, mitigating the risk of toxicity and adverse reactions. This shift aligns with the overarching goal of biomedical engineering, which seeks to harness cutting-edge technologies without compromising patient safety (Fuku et al. 2023).

Sustainability is another compelling facet of green synthesis that resonates with the ethos of contemporary biomedical practices. The use of renewable resources and environmentally sustainable processes underscores a commitment to minimizing the ecological footprint associated with medical advancements. As the healthcare industry increasingly pivots towards sustainable solutions, green synthesis emerges as a proactive step towards aligning biomedical engineering with broader environmental goals (Dubey et al. 2022).

Cost-effectiveness further accentuates the appeal of green synthesis in biomedical applications. The simplicity of the synthesis process, coupled with the utilization of natural precursors, often translates to reduced production costs. This not only makes green-synthesized nanomaterials economically viable but also democratizes access to advanced medical technologies, a critical consideration in the global healthcare landscape.

Perhaps most intriguingly, green synthesis methods offer a pathway to nanomaterials with enhanced functionality (Kumar 2023). By drawing inspiration from the intricate properties of natural compounds, researchers can tailor nanomaterials for specific biomedical applications. This customization spans improved targeting mechanisms, finely tuned drug release kinetics, and augmented imaging capabilities. In essence, green synthesis not only meets the stringent requirements of biocompatibility and safety but also opens new avenues for innovation in biomedical engineering (Ojha et al. 2023).

The process of green synthesis is a meticulously orchestrated sequence of steps, each contributing to the eco-friendly and sustainable nature of the method. It commences with the judicious selection of green precursors, which may encompass a diverse array of natural sources ranging from plant extracts to microbial agents. The choice of precursors sets the tone for the entire synthesis process, emphasizing the departure from conventional, often more environmentally taxing, materials.

Continuing down the green synthesis pathway, the next crucial aspect involves the utilization of eco-friendly solvents. Conventional methods frequently rely on volatile organic solvents with adverse environmental impacts. Green synthesis opts for benign alternatives, such as water or non-toxic organic solvents, minimizing the ecological footprint of the process. This deliberate choice resonates with the overarching principles of green chemistry, where the entire life cycle of a product is considered in the pursuit of sustainability.

Temperature and energy conditions represent additional key parameters in green synthesis. Traditional methods often demand high energy inputs, contributing to the carbon footprint of the overall process. Green synthesis, on the other hand, prioritizes energy efficiency by employing milder reaction conditions. This not only aligns with sustainable practices but also underscores the economic viability of green-synthesized nanomaterials. Furthermore, the synthesis process in green nanotechnology often benefits from the catalytic properties of natural compounds, reducing the need for additional catalysts that might introduce toxicity or environmental hazards. The reliance on inherent catalytic capabilities aligns with the overarching goal of streamlining processes to be both efficient and environmentally friendly (Vargas et al. 2023).

3.3 Herbal Approach

The biological synthesis of metal and metal oxide nanoparticles using plant extracts represents a burgeoning field with significant environmental implications (Table 3.1). Copper nanoparticles, synthesized from magnolia leaf and clove extracts, exhibit stability and antibacterial properties (Tiwari et al. 2023). Palladium and platinum nanoparticles, derived from cinnamon bark, custard apple peel, and various plant extracts, showcase controlled morphologies and sizes. Titanium dioxide nanoparticles, synthesized from diverse plant sources, demonstrate larvicidal and

Table 3.1 Herbal drug loaded nanoparticles

Formulation	Activity	Active ingredients	Method of preparation	Reference
CPT encapsulated nanoparticles	Anticancer	Camptothecin	Dialysis method	Lu et al. (2023)
Artemisinin nano-capsules	Anticancer	Artemisinin	Self-assembly procedure	Manasa and Shivananjappa (2023)
Curcuminoids solid lipid nanoparticles	Anticancer	Curcuminoids	Micro-emulsion technique	Wani et al. (2023)
Berberine-loaded nanoparticles	Anticancer	Berberine	Ionic gelation method	Prabhakar et al. (2023)
Glycyrrhizic acid loaded nanoparticles	Antihypertensive and anti-inflammatory	Glycyrrhizin acid	Rotary-evaporated film ultrasonication method	Khoobchandani et al. (2020)

antibacterial activities. The eco-friendly nature of this green synthesis approach underscores its sustainable appeal, though challenges related to scalability and mechanistic understanding remain. Future research should prioritize optimizing synthesis conditions, exploring new plant sources, and evaluating the broader biological and environmental impacts of these nanoparticles. Overall, the field holds promise for advancing sustainable nanotechnology applications with diverse functionalities (Das and Sharangi 2020).

3.4 Green Synthesis of Metallic Nanoparticles for Pharmaceutical and Biomedical Engineering Application

The green synthesis of metallic nanoparticles (MNPs) represents a significant stride toward sustainable and environmentally benign practices in the realms of pharmaceutical and biomedical engineering. Traditional methods of MNP synthesis often involve the use of toxic chemicals, raising concerns about safety and environmental impact. In contrast, green synthesis methods leverage natural sources such as plants, microbes, and biomolecules, offering a cleaner and more eco-friendly approach. Plant-mediated synthesis involves using plant extracts as both reducing and stabilizing agents, exploiting phytochemicals in the nanoparticle formation process. Microbial synthesis utilizes microorganisms like bacteria and fungi, showcasing their ability to reduce metal ions and participate in nanoparticle synthesis (Vasanth et al. 2023). Other green approaches involve biomolecules such as proteins, peptides, and enzymes, contributing to the reduction and stabilization of MNPs. The characterization of green-synthesized MNPs involves techniques like XRD, TEM, and FTIR, providing insights into their structural properties. In pharmaceutical applications, these MNPs exhibit promise in drug delivery systems, offering controlled and targeted release, as well as demonstrating antimicrobial and anticancer properties. Biomedical engineering applications include the use of MNPs as contrast agents in imaging modalities like MRI and CT, and in biosensors for early disease detection. As the field advances, challenges related to scaling up green synthesis methods for large-scale production need addressing, and continuous exploration of innovative applications is crucial for unlocking the full potential of green-synthesized MNPs in advancing healthcare technologies.

Nanoparticles have been extensively investigated through various techniques to elucidate their size, crystal structure, elemental composition, and a multitude of other physical characteristics. Often, the examination of physical attributes necessitates the use of multiple techniques due to the distinct strengths and limitations inherent in each method (AlGabbani 2023). Combinatorial characterization becomes imperative to overcome the challenges posed by selecting the most appropriate method. Key criteria in nanoparticle characterization include size, shape, surface chemistry. These factors, along with organic ligands on their surfaces, can significantly influence other features and applications of nanoparticles. Additionally, magnetic procedures like SQUID, VSM, FMR, and XMCD offer specific insights tailored to different families of materials (Khafaga and Ewies 2023; Singh et al. 2023; Garcella et al. 2021; Chandra et al. 2022).

In the realm of antibacterial mechanisms, metal nanoparticles (MNPs) have shown promise in combating bacterial infections through electrostatic interactions, strong bonds with bacterial membranes leading to cell wall breakdown, enhanced permeability, and transfer of metal ions into the cell. MNPs and metal ions can induce reactive oxygen species (ROS) production, causing oxidative stress and disrupting the bacterial antioxidant defense system (Kandav and Sharma 2023). However, despite the myriad advantages of nanoparticles, certain drawbacks must be acknowledged. These include high production costs, the potential for inhalation leading to lung disease, and disruptions in homeostasis. Nanotoxicity, a burgeoning discipline of toxicology, explores the adverse effects of nanoparticles, often attributed to their highly reactive nature due to their small size. While plant extract nanoparticles present a promising avenue for green synthesis, challenges arise in identifying the functional molecules responsible for therapeutic purposes. The overall toxicity of green-produced nanomaterials *in vivo* remains a critical area for future research (Sandulovici et al. 2022).

In the synthesis of nanoparticles, various approaches are employed, with the chemical approach being a prominent method. This method involves metallic precursors, reducing agents (RAs), and stabilizing agents (SAs). The synthesis process plays a crucial role in determining the characteristics of nanoparticles, and understanding the chemical approach is essential for tailoring the properties of the resulting nanomaterials (Zhang et al. 2020). Nanoshells and nanocages have garnered significant attention in the field of nanotechnology, particularly for their potential applications in various biomedical contexts. In a study conducted by Neeves and Birnboim, a composite spherical particle composed of a metallic shell and a dielectric core was theorized to exhibit Localized Surface Plasmon Resonance (LSPR) modes, allowing for tunable wavelengths across a broad electromagnetic spectrum.

Subsequent work by Halas and Nordlander at Rice University demonstrated that silica-gold nano-shells could be positioned in the near-infrared region, where biomatter absorption is minimal. These nano-shells, created by depositing gold into amine-terminated silica spheres, showcased successful irreversible photothermal ablation of tumor tissue in both *in vitro* and *in vivo* settings (Vernet-Crua et al. 2023).

The intricate control required for the metallic shell's thickness and smoothness in conventional synthesis methods posed challenges. Nevertheless, the potential applications of nano-shells extended beyond tumor ablation. Halas and West explored their use in whole-blood immunoassays, demonstrating that nano-shells, when conjugated with antibodies, served as recognition sites for specific analytes, modifying the LSPR upon analyte interaction. This paved the way for multifunctional magnetic gold nano-shells (Mag-GNS) developed by Jaeyun et al., incorporating Fe3O4 nanoparticles for magnetic resonance imaging (MRI) and gold nanoshells for photothermal therapy. By linking antibodies to Mag-GNS, targeted cancer cell detection and elimination were achieved, highlighting the versatility of these nanostructures (Chaudhary et al. 2023a).

Similarly, gold nanocages, a novel class of nanostructures, were introduced by Xia and Coworkers. These hollow porous gold nanoparticles, formed by reacting silver nanoparticles with chloroauric acid, exhibited LSPR peaks in the near-infrared range. The tunability of these peaks, achieved through control of wall thickness and porosity, made gold nanocages promising for applications in drug delivery and controlled drug release. Their hollow interiors provided additional functionality, allowing for the incorporation of small objects such as magnetic nanoparticles, leading to the development of multifunctional hybrid nanostructures for diagnostic imaging and therapy (Cassani et al. 2023).

Transitioning to silver nanoparticles, these particles, ranging in size from 1 to 100 nm, have gained prominence in various biomedical applications. Efforts to incorporate silver nanoparticles into medical devices, such as bone cement and surgical instruments, underscore their versatility. Ionic silver, effective in wound treatment, has witnessed a shift toward replacing silver sulfadiazine in wound care. Samsung's introduction of Silver Nano, embedding silver nanoparticles on household appliance surfaces, further exemplifies their diverse applications.

In the realm of biomedical imaging, silver nanoparticles exhibit attractive physiochemical properties, drawing attention for Surface-Enhanced Raman Spectroscopy (SERS). Synthesis methods involve the reduction of silver salt with reducing agents, employing colloidal stabilizers like polyvinyl alcohol and poly(vinylpyrrolidone). Novel approaches, such as using β-d-glucose and starch, showcase the evolving methods in silver nanoparticle synthesis. Importantly, the size and shape of silver nanoparticles impact their efficacy; studies have demonstrated size-dependent interactions with viruses like HIV-1 (Sulaiman 2023).

While not as widely preferred as gold nanoparticles and nanoshells, silver nanoparticles have made a significant impact on modern medical science. The noble metals' unique properties ensure their continuous utilization as newer applications and protocols unfold, promising a dynamic future in the ever-evolving landscape of nanotechnology in healthcare.

Table 3.2 Metallic nanoparticles advanced application

Types of nanoparticles	Application	Technique	Reference
Multimodal imaging nanoparticles	Detection of even subtle differences between body tissues	CT	Cruse et al. (2022)
Iron oxide nanoparticles	Higher resolution	MRI	Yano et al. (2022)
Fe2O3, Gd2O3	Easy to perform	Ultrasound	Peng et al. (2009)
Gold and silver nanoparticles	Wide field of view	CT	Kamaraj et al. (2022)

One key area of focus is drug delivery. Metallic nanoparticles, such as gold and silver nanoparticles, can serve as efficient drug carriers. Their size allows for easy penetration into cells, and their surfaces can be functionalized to enhance biocompatibility and target specific tissues. By encapsulating drugs within these nanoparticles, controlled release systems can be designed, improving the therapeutic efficacy while minimizing side effects (Magdy et al. 2023).

In diagnostics, metallic nanoparticles play a crucial role, particularly in imaging techniques. Gold nanoparticles, for instance, exhibit strong surface plasmon resonance, making them excellent contrast agents for imaging modalities like computed tomography (CT) scans. Additionally, magnetic nanoparticles, often composed of iron oxide, are employed in magnetic resonance imaging (MRI), enabling precise and non-invasive visualization of tissues.

The field of theranostics, an integration of therapy and diagnostics, benefits significantly from metallic nanoparticles. Multifunctional nanoparticles can be designed to combine therapeutic agents with imaging capabilities, allowing for personalized medicine approaches. This convergence enhances treatment monitoring and facilitates a more targeted and efficient therapeutic intervention (Chaudhary et al. 2023b). Moreover, metallic nanoparticles find application (Table 3.2) in tissue engineering. They can be incorporated into scaffolds or coatings to improve the mechanical and biological properties of biomaterials. Silver nanoparticles, known for their antimicrobial properties, are often integrated into wound dressings and implant coatings to prevent infections and promote tissue regeneration.

In cancer therapy, the unique properties of metallic nanoparticles are harnessed for innovative approaches. Photothermal therapy utilizes the ability of nanoparticles, particularly gold nanorods or nano-shells, to absorb near-infrared light and convert it into heat. This localized hyperthermia selectively destroys cancer cells while minimizing damage to healthy tissues.

Despite their tremendous potential, challenges exist, such as concerns about the long-term biocompatibility and potential toxicity of metallic nanoparticles. Rigorous testing and comprehensive studies are essential to address these issues and ensure the safety of their biomedical applications (Sadanandan et al. 2023; Ameen et al. 2023; Setyawati et al. 2023).

3.5 Green Synthesis of Polymeric Nanoparticles Incorporated Bioactive Compounds

The green synthesis of polymeric nanoparticles incorporated with bioactive compounds is a burgeoning field with significant implications for pharmaceutical and biomedical engineering applications (Ruang-Areerate et al. 2022). This innovative approach, rooted in sustainable and environmentally conscious practices, addresses the growing need for efficient drug delivery systems and biocompatible materials. By utilizing plant extracts and biopolymers as precursors for nanoparticle synthesis, the process minimizes the use of harmful chemicals, aligning with the principles of green chemistry. The resulting polymeric nanoparticles serve as versatile carriers for bioactive compounds, offering controlled release and targeted delivery to specific cells or tissues. This strategy enhances the therapeutic effects of pharmaceutical agents, potentially reducing side effects and improving patient outcomes. In addition to its pharmaceutical applications, green-synthesized polymeric nanoparticles contribute to the advancement of biomedical engineering by allowing for the tailored engineering of nanoparticle properties (Tajik et al. 2022). This includes size, surface charge, and drug release kinetics, tailored to specific biomedical requirements. The integration of green synthesis with advanced technologies opens avenues for the development of multifunctional nanoparticles, capable of serving diagnostic, therapeutic, and imaging purposes simultaneously. In essence, green synthesis of polymeric nanoparticles incorporated with bioactive compounds represents a paradigm shift in drug delivery and biomedical materials, emphasizing sustainability and innovation in the pursuit of enhanced healthcare solutions.

The production process yields eco-friendly nanoparticles (Table 3.3) with improved stability, adaptability for clinical applications, and compatibility with biological systems. Organisms have evolved mechanisms to thrive in environments with high metal concentrations, modifying their chemical composition to mitigate toxicity (Kumawat et al. 2022).

Biological processes chemically reduce metal ions through dissimilatory metal reduction, where the enzyme undergoes oxidation, and the metal ion undergoes reduction. The resulting metallic nanoparticles are then safely extracted for further evaluation (Castro et al. 2022). Metal ions in an aqueous or soil sample adhere to the organism itself. Bacteria, fungi, and plants obtain peptides or cell walls bonded with metal ions, stabilizing the nanoparticles. The choice of biological approaches for nanoparticle synthesis is influenced by various factors, with the desired form of the metal nanoparticle being a crucial determinant. The limited selection of organisms is attributed to their inherent resistance against metals.

Recent strides in nanotechnology are poised to have a profound impact on pioneering therapeutic strategies. The ability to produce nanoparticles in the protein size domain opens up diverse biomedical applications, triggering responses and enhancing therapeutic effects with minimal undesirable consequences. While therapies for various diseases typically involve synthetic medicines with associated adverse effects, there is a growing inclination toward the use of phytochemicals known for their minimal side effects. Despite numerous advantages, green

Table 3.3 The fabrication of nanoparticles stems from the inherent resistance of organisms to specific metals

Bioactive	Type of polymers	Type of polymeric nanoparticles	Applications purpose	Reference
Rapamycin	PLGA	PLGA NPs	Anti-glioma activity	Suriyakala et al. (2022)
Fenofibrate (Feno)	PLGA	Nanospheres	Diabetic retinopathy	Abdel-Lateef (2022)
Fenofibrate (FF)	Anionic copolymers based on methacrylic acic and methyl methacrylate (Eudragit L 100)	Nano-capsule	Undefined oral delivery	Shanmugam et al. (2022)
Thymus vulgaris L. (Thyme oil)	Eudragit® L100-55	Nano-capsules	Antioxidant	Khan et al. (2022a)
Geraniol	PCL	Nano-capsule	Antioxidant	Park et al. (2012)
Rosmarinus officinalis L. (Rosemary oil)	Eudragit® L100-55	Nano-capsule	Antioxidant	Francia et al. (2022)
Paclitaxel (PTX)	PCL-PEG-PCL	Nano-capsules	Modulated chemotherapy	Wang et al. (2022a)
Amphotericin B (Amp B)	Biopolymer of PCL	Nanoprecipitation	Anti-leishmanial	Charelli et al. (2022)

nanotechnology encounters challenges, particularly in scaling up production. Currently limited to laboratory-scale experiments, translating findings into large-scale manufacturing processes poses difficulties (Dahlman et al. 2014; Bertrand et al. 2017; Bhattacharya et al. 2022; Dewangan et al. 2022).

Polymeric nanoparticles (NPs) have gained significant attention in recent years due to their unique properties stemming from their small size. These nanoparticles offer various advantages as drug carriers, including the potential for controlled release, protection of drugs and bioactive molecules against environmental factors, and enhancement of bioavailability and therapeutic indices (Fig. 3.2).

The process involves preparing an organic phase with a polar solvent (e.g., ethyl acetate) in which the polymer and drug are dissolved. This organic solution is emulsified in an aqueous phase containing a surfactant (e.g., polyvinyl acetate), resulting in nanodroplets. The solvent is then evaporated, and solidified nanoparticles are obtained, which can be washed, collected, and freeze-dried for long-term storage (Zafar et al. 2022; Cheng et al. 2022). This method is frequently used for nanosphere production, with nanoparticles ranging from 80 to 900 nm (Hussain et al. 2022; Li et al. 2022).

Polymeric nanoparticles (NPs) play a crucial role in drug delivery and various biomedical applications due to their unique properties (Sakhi et al. 2022). The characterization of these nanoparticles is essential for understanding their behavior, optimizing formulations, and ensuring their safety (Abruzzo et al. 2022).

The size of polymeric NPs, typically ranging from 100 to 300 nm, is a critical parameter. Dynamic and static light scattering, electron microscopy, and AFM are

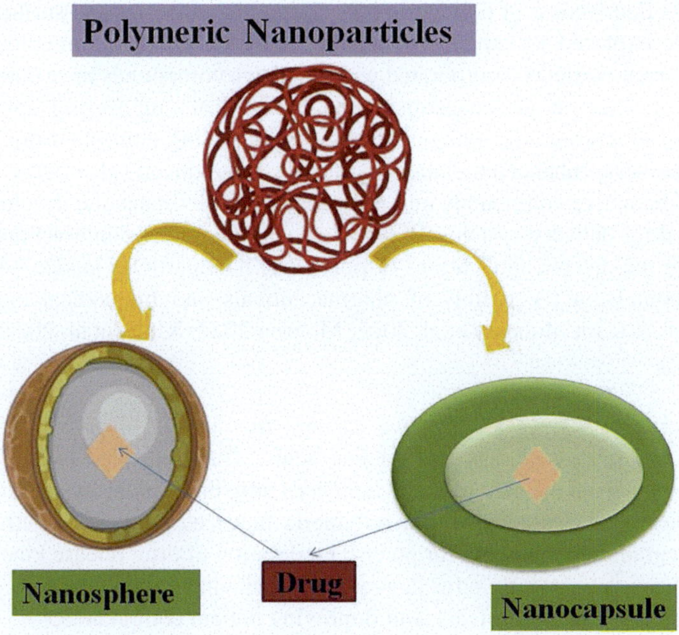

Fig. 3.2 Polymeric nanoparticles represent a promising avenue in drug delivery systems, offering tailored solutions for controlled release and enhanced therapeutic outcomes

commonly used techniques for size measurement (Seo et al. 2022). Polydispersity and unimodal size distribution are desired characteristics (Zhang et al. 2022). Atomic absorption spectroscopy and time-of-flight mass spectrometry aid in determining the chemical composition of polymeric NPs. The surface area of NPs influences reactivity and interactions. Gas adsorption methods, such as nitrogen adsorption, assess surface area. Surface chemistry is investigated through techniques like X-ray photoelectron spectroscopy and secondary ion mass spectroscopy. Zeta potential reflects the surface charge of particles, impacting their stability. Techniques like Doppler velocimetry determine particle velocity, from which zeta potential is calculated. Zeta potential values around ±30 mV contribute to colloidal suspension stability. Monitoring pH provides insights into the stability of nanoparticulate suspensions. Changes in pH may indicate polymer degradation or influence zeta potential, impacting electrostatic stability.

Physicochemical stability is crucial for industrial applications. Factors such as particle aggregation, polymer stability, and drug content affect stability. Drug association modes, whether adsorbed or dissolved, are estimated through various comparative studies. The toxicological effects of nanoparticles on various organisms and the environment are critical considerations. Challenges in nanoecotoxicology research include nanoparticle selection, understanding capture pathways, and identification of suitable organisms for experiments (Wen et al. 2022; Xiao et al. 2022). *In vitro* studies using cell lines assess cytotoxicity, while *in vivo* studies validate the safety and effectiveness of polymeric NPs. Targeting strategies and surface modifications are explored to enhance therapeutic efficacy while minimizing toxicity. Polymeric nanoparticles incorporated with bioactive compounds have emerged as a promising avenue in pharmaceutical and biomedical engineering applications. These nanostructures offer unique advantages, including controlled drug release, targeted delivery, enhanced therapeutic efficacy, and reduced side effects. The integration of bioactive compounds into polymeric NPs facilitates the development of advanced drug delivery systems, diagnostics, and therapeutic interventions. Here, we explore the diverse applications of polymeric nanoparticles loaded with bioactive compounds in the realms of pharmaceuticals and biomedical engineering (Wang et al. 2022b; Mohanty et al. 2022; Mohsen 2022; Xiong et al. 2022; Teixeira et al. 2022).

- Polymeric NPs serve as effective carriers for various bioactive compounds, including drugs, peptides, and nucleic acids. The controlled release of these compounds from the nanoparticles enhances drug bioavailability and therapeutic outcomes. Encapsulation within polymeric matrices protects bioactive agents from degradation, allowing for precise modulation of drug release kinetics. This capability is particularly advantageous for achieving sustained drug concentrations, minimizing side effects, and improving patient compliance.
- This targeted approach increases drug accumulation at the desired site, minimizing systemic exposure and improving treatment outcomes. Polymeric NPs offer a versatile platform for tailoring surface properties to achieve selective drug delivery in cancer therapy, inflammatory diseases, and other medical conditions.
- Polymeric NPs loaded with contrast agents or imaging probes play a crucial role in diagnostics.
- Polymeric NPs have shown promise in addressing challenges associated with drug delivery to the central nervous system. These nanoparticles can traverse the blood-brain barrier, delivering bioactive compounds to specific brain regions. This capability is particularly valuable for treating neurodegenerative disorders, brain tumors, and other neurological conditions.
- Incorporation of antimicrobial agents into polymeric NPs provides a targeted approach for combating infections. These nanostructures can enhance the stability and solubility of antimicrobial compounds, allowing for controlled release at infection sites. Polymeric NPs loaded with antibiotics, peptides, or antimicrobial agents demonstrate potential in the development of innovative strategies against bacterial, viral, and fungal infections.
- Polymeric NPs contribute to the field of tissue engineering by providing controlled release of growth factors, cytokines, and other bioactive molecules. These nanoparticles support cell proliferation, differentiation, and tissue regeneration. By mimicking the natural extracellular matrix, polymeric NPs facilitate the creation of biomimetic scaffolds for regenerative medicine applications.
- The use of polymeric NPs in vaccine delivery has gained attention for enhancing immune responses. Antigens and adjuvants can be encapsulated within these nanoparticles to improve antigen stability, controlled release, and immune

system activation. This approach holds promise for developing effective vaccines against infectious diseases and cancers.

- Polymeric nanoparticles have applications in cardiovascular medicine, particularly for targeted drug delivery to treat conditions such as atherosclerosis and thrombosis. The nanoparticles can be designed to release anticoagulant or anti-inflammatory agents at the site of vascular lesions, minimizing systemic side effects and improving the efficacy of treatment.
- Polymeric nanoparticles find applications in dentistry for targeted drug delivery and oral health management. They can be utilized to encapsulate antimicrobial agents, growth factors, or remineralizing agents for the treatment of dental caries, periodontal diseases, and other oral conditions. The controlled release of bioactive compounds contributes to improved dental therapies.
- Beyond healthcare, polymeric nanoparticles incorporated with bioactive compounds have potential applications in environmental remediation. These nanoparticles can be designed to remove pollutants, toxins, or heavy metals from water or soil. Functionalization of the nanoparticles allows for specific interactions with target contaminants, offering an innovative approach to address environmental challenges.
- Polymeric nanoparticles loaded with antioxidants or anti-inflammatory agents have applications in managing oxidative stress and inflammation-related diseases. These nanoparticles can scavenge free radicals, reduce inflammation, and promote tissue healing. The controlled release of bioactive compounds contributes to sustained therapeutic effects.

3.6 Regulatory Aspects of Green Synthesis Using Sustainable Materials

Green synthesis, characterized by environmentally friendly processes and the use of sustainable materials, has gained prominence in various scientific fields, including chemistry, materials science, and pharmaceuticals. While the potential benefits of green synthesis are substantial, there are important regulatory aspects that need to be considered to ensure the safety, efficacy, and compliance of products derived from such processes. This article delves into the regulatory landscape surrounding green synthesis, focusing on the use of sustainable materials. Green synthesis involves the development of products using eco-friendly methodologies, minimizing the use of hazardous substances and reducing environmental impact. In the context of sustainable materials, this often includes renewable resources, biodegradable compounds, and processes with low energy consumption (Madani et al. 2022).

Several regulatory agencies worldwide oversee the approval and regulation of products derived from green synthesis. In the United States, the EPA plays a crucial role in evaluating and regulating chemicals, ensuring they meet safety and environmental standards.

Green synthesis processes must align with EPA guidelines to receive approval for commercial use. European Chemicals Agency (ECHA) oversees chemical regulations in the European Union, including the Registration, Evaluation, Authorization, and Restriction of Chemicals (REACH) regulation. Green synthesis routes must adhere to REACH requirements, emphasizing the substitution of hazardous chemicals with safer alternatives.

Food and Drug Administration (FDA) for applications in pharmaceuticals and food, the FDA in the United States provides regulatory oversight. Green synthesis of pharmaceutical ingredients or food additives must comply with FDA regulations for safety and efficacy.

International Cooperation on Cosmetics Regulation (ICCR) facilitates cooperation among regulatory bodies overseeing cosmetics to ensure global harmonization (Becker et al. 2022).

Green synthesis of cosmetic ingredients must meet ICCR guidelines for safety and labeling.

Regulatory bodies require comprehensive toxicological studies to assess the safety of products derived from green synthesis. Sustainable materials must be thoroughly evaluated for potential health risks, and toxicity data should be submitted for regulatory review. Green synthesis emphasizes the use of materials with minimal environmental impact.

Regulatory submissions should include data on the biodegradability of substances to assess their ecological footprint. Products derived from green synthesis may qualify for eco-labels or certifications. Regulatory bodies often consider the environmental footprint and sustainability of the entire production process. Clear and accurate information about the green synthesis process, sustainable materials used, and environmental benefits must be provided on product labels. Misleading claims could lead to regulatory scrutiny and penalties.

Regulatory compliance extends to intellectual property laws (Saxe et al. 2022; Ma et al. 2022; Madani et al. 2022; Tran et al. 2022). Companies must ensure that their green synthesis processes are patentable and comply with relevant intellectual property regulations. Lack of standardized protocols for green synthesis poses a challenge for regulatory assessments. Efforts are underway to establish clear guidelines and criteria for evaluating the greenness of synthesis processes. Achieving global harmonization of regulations related to green synthesis is an ongoing challenge. Collaborative efforts among regulatory bodies aim to streamline processes and facilitate international acceptance (Khalil et al. 2022).

3.7 Challenges and Future Perspectives

One of the critical challenges in the widespread adoption of green-synthesized nanomaterials in biomedical applications is the establishment of comprehensive regulatory frameworks and safety standards. Current regulations often focus on traditionally synthesized materials and adapting them to the unique characteristics of green-synthesized nanomaterials is crucial. Establishing clear safety guidelines and ensuring adherence to ethical practices are essential steps to gain regulatory approval for medical applications. While green synthesis methods are designed to be environmentally friendly, the long-term impact of green-synthesized nanomaterials on ecosystems and biodegradability remains a concern. Continuous research is needed to assess the fate of these materials in the environment, ensuring that they do not pose risks to ecosystems over time (Choudhary et al. 2022; Pandit et al. 2022). Developing nanomaterials with enhanced biodegradability and minimal environmental persistence will contribute to sustainable practices. Green-synthesized nanomaterials offer a platform for multifunctional applications, where a single material can serve both diagnostic and therapeutic purposes. However, achieving precise targeting in vivo remains a challenge. Future research should focus on enhancing the specificity of these nanomaterials, ensuring they reach specific cells or tissues with minimal off-target effects. This will pave the way for personalized medicine and more effective therapeutic interventions. Overcoming the challenges in green nanotechnology requires interdisciplinary collaboration between scientists, engineers, clinicians, and regulatory experts. The integration of expertise from various fields is essential to address complex issues, ranging from synthesis methods to clinical applications. Establishing collaborative networks and research consortia will facilitate knowledge exchange and accelerate progress in the field. As with any emerging technology, addressing ethical considerations and gaining public trust are pivotal for the successful integration of green nanotechnology in biomedical applications. Transparent communication regarding the benefits and potential risks, as well as addressing societal concerns, will play a crucial role in shaping public perception. Ethical frameworks for the responsible development and use of green-synthesized nanomaterials need to be established. The evolving landscape of green nanotechnology necessitates a skilled workforce equipped with knowledge in nanoscience, green chemistry, and biomedical applications (Zhou et al. 2023; Aram et al. 2022; Karam et al. 2022). Educational programs and training initiatives should be developed to prepare scientists, engineers, and professionals to navigate the interdisciplinary challenges of this field. Investing in workforce development will contribute to the sustainable growth of green nanotechnology in biomedical sciences. Green-synthesized nanomaterials offer a unique opportunity for advancing precision medicine. By tailoring nanotherapeutics to individual patient profiles, these materials can enhance treatment efficacy while minimizing side effects. The future holds the promise of personalized nanomedicine, where green-synthesized nanoparticles are precisely designed to target specific genetic or molecular characteristics of diseases (Bhat et al. 2022).

The convergence of diagnostics and therapeutics, known as nanotheranostics, represents a promising avenue for green-synthesized nanomaterials. Future developments may focus on creating nanomaterials that not only deliver therapeutic agents but also act as imaging contrast agents, allowing for simultaneous diagnosis and treatment. This holistic approach could revolutionize disease management strategies. Green-synthesized nanomaterials can play a crucial role in addressing global health challenges, especially in resource-limited settings. The development of cost-effective and sustainable nanotherapeutics for diseases prevalent in these regions holds significant potential. Future efforts should aim at creating solutions that are accessible, affordable, and environmentally sustainable. The future of green nanotechnology hinges on continuous innovation in synthesis techniques. Advancements in understanding plant-matter interactions, microbial synthesis pathways, and bio-inspired approaches will expand the repertoire of green synthesis methods. Harnessing the full potential of natural resources and biomimicry will lead to the development of novel nanomaterials with enhanced properties (Saravanan et al. 2022; La Barbera et al. 2022; Sreenikethanam et al. 2022; Basit et al. 2023). Recognizing the societal and cultural dimensions of green nanotechnology is crucial for its acceptance and integration into diverse communities. Future research should explore the cultural implications of using green-synthesized nanomaterials, considering factors such as local beliefs, customs, and ethical considerations. Engaging with communities in the development process will contribute to socially responsible applications (Khan et al. 2022b). The long-term environmental impact of green-synthesized nanomaterials requires continuous monitoring and risk assessment. Future studies should focus on developing robust methodologies for assessing the environmental fate of these materials and their potential ecological implications (Sun et al. 2022).

3.8 Conclusions

The intricate interplay between sustainable raw materials, green nanotechnology, and biomedical sciences forms a compelling narrative of innovation, environmental responsibility, and potential advancements in various sectors. The integration of renewable resources into nanotechnology applications, guided by the principles of green chemistry, not only addresses environmental concerns but also propels the development of advanced technologies in biomedical engineering. The paradigm shift towards green synthesis methodologies represents a transformative approach, emphasizing biocompatibility, reduced toxicity, sustainability, and cost-effectiveness. Green-synthesized nanomaterials offer promising solutions in drug delivery systems, biosensors, and various biomedical applications. The amalgamation of green principles into nanotechnology aligns with contemporary biomedical practices, where compatibility with living tissues and safety are paramount considerations.

The exploration of renewable resources, sustainable raw materials, and green nanotechnology within the realm of biomedical sciences paints a holistic picture of innovation that transcends traditional boundaries. This convergence holds the promise of not only addressing current environmental and health challenges but also contributing to a future where technology and sustainability coexist seamlessly for the benefit of humanity. The journey towards this future is marked by challenges, yet the transformative potential of green nanotechnology in biomedical applications is indeed a beacon guiding us towards a more sustainable and ethically responsible era in scientific and technological advancement.

The challenges encountered in the development of green-synthesized nanomaterials for biomedical applications serve as catalysts for innovation. From standardization issues to scalability concerns, each challenge presents an opportunity for researchers to devise creative solutions. Collaborative efforts across disciplines are essential to address these challenges systematically and propel the field towards viable and sustainable solutions.

Green synthesis methods stand out as a cornerstone in the evolution of biomedical engineering. The inherent biocompatibility, reduced toxicity, and cost-effectiveness of green-synthesized nanomaterials contribute to their appeal in various applications. The synthesis of nanomaterials from natural sources offers a bridge between advanced technologies and environmentally conscious practices, fostering a synergy that holds great promise for the future. Green nanotechnology has the potential to address global health challenges by providing sustainable and accessible solutions. The development of cost-effective nanotherapeutics, especially in resource-limited settings, can revolutionize disease management. As the field advances, a focus on creating solutions that are not only scientifically innovative but also culturally sensitive and socially responsible is imperative.

The integration of green nanotechnology in biomedical applications necessitates a commitment to continuous monitoring and ethical considerations. Environmental impact assessments, risk evaluations, and adherence to safety standards are paramount in ensuring the responsible development and deployment of green-synthesized nanomaterials. Open communication and transparency with the public are essential elements in gaining trust and acceptance. The future of green nanotechnology in biomedical sciences is poised for exciting developments. Precision medicine, personalized nanotherapeutics, and the integration with advanced imaging technologies offer avenues for groundbreaking research. Sustainable nanotechnology is not just a scientific pursuit; it is a collective vision that requires ongoing interdisciplinary collaboration, education, and societal engagement. The convergence of technology and ethics is a defining characteristic of the green nanotechnology revolution. The field goes beyond scientific innovation; it embodies a commitment to ethical practices, environmental stewardship, and social responsibility. As green-synthesized nanomaterials make their mark in biomedical applications, this convergence will shape the ethical landscape of future technological advancements.

References

Abdel-Lateef MA (2022) Utilization of the peroxidase-like activity of silver nanoparticles nanozyme on O-phenylenediamine/H2O2 system for fluorescence detection of mercury (II) ions. Sci Rep 12(1):6953

Abruzzo A, Croatti V, Zuccheri G, Nicoletta FP, Sallustio V, Corazza E, Vitali B, Cerchiara T, Luppi B, Bigucci F (2022) Drug-in-cyclodextrin-in-polymeric nanoparticles: a promising strategy for rifampicin administration. Eur J Pharm Biopharm 180:190–200

Albert HM (2023) Nanotechnology: physicochemical and green synthesis, characterizations and applications. Perfect Writer Publishing

AlGabbani Q (2023) Nanotechnology: a promising strategy for the control of parasitic infections. Exp Parasitol 250:108548

Ameen F, Al-Maary KS, Almansob A, AlNadhari S (2023) Antioxidant, antibacterial and anticancer efficacy of Alternaria chlamydospora-mediated gold nanoparticles. Appl Nanosci 13(3):2233–2240

Aram E, Moeni M, Abedizadeh R, Sabour D, Sadeghi-Abandansari H, Gardy J, Hassanpour A (2022) Smart and multi-functional magnetic nanoparticles for cancer treatment applications: clinical challenges and future prospects. Nanomaterials 12(20):3567

Backx BP (2022) Green nanotechnology: only the final product that matters? Nat Prod Res 36(13):3507–3509

Basit F, He X, Zhu X, Sheteiwy MS, Minkina T, Sushkova S, Josko I, Hu J, Hu W, Guan Y (2023) Uptake, accumulation, toxicity, and interaction of metallic-based nanoparticles with plants: current challenges and future perspectives. Environ Geochem Health 27:1–5

Becker J, Manske C, Randl S (2022) Green chemistry and sustainability metrics in the pharmaceutical manufacturing sector. Curr Opin Green Sustain Chem 33:100562

Bertrand N, Grenier P, Mahmoudi M, Lima EM, Appel EA, Dormont F, Lim JM, Karnik R, Langer R, Farokhzad OC (2017) Mechanistic understanding of in vivo protein corona formation on polymeric nanoparticles and impact on pharmacokinetics. Nat Commun 8(1):777

Bhat SA, Sher F, Hameed M, Bashir O, Kumar R, Vo DV, Ahmad P, Lima EC (2022) Sustainable nanotechnology based wastewater treatment strategies: achievements, challenges and future perspectives. Chemosphere 288:132606

Bhattacharya S, Anjum MM, Patel KK (2022) Gemcitabine cationic polymeric nanoparticles against ovarian cancer: formulation, characterization, and targeted drug delivery. Drug Deliv 29(1):1060–1074

Cao J, Pan Y, Jiang Y, Qi R, Yuan B, Jia Z, Jiang J, Wang Q (2020) Computer-aided nanotoxicology: risk assessment of metal oxide nanoparticles via nano-QSAR. Green Chem 22(11):3512–3521

Cassani L, Marcovich NE, Gomez-Zavaglia A (2023) Seaweed bioactive compounds: promising and safe inputs for the green synthesis of metal nanoparticles in the food industry. Crit Rev Food Sci Nutr 63(11):1527–1550

Castillo-Henríquez L, Alfaro-Aguilar K, Ugalde-Álvarez J, Vega-Fernández L, Montes de Oca-Vásquez G, Vega-Baudrit JR (2020) Green synthesis of gold and silver nanoparticles from plant extracts and their possible applications as antimicrobial agents in the agricultural area. Nanomaterials 10(9):1763

Castro KC, Costa JM, Campos MG (2022) Drug-loaded polymeric nanoparticles: a review. Int J Polym Mater Polym Biomater 71(1):1–3

Chandra H, Kumari P, Yadav A, Yadav S (2022) Green biosynthesized metallic nanoparticles and future biomedical applications. In: Green nanomaterials for industrial applications. Elsevier, pp 93–105

Charelli LE, de Mattos GC, de Jesus S-BA, Pinto JC, Balbino TA (2022) Polymeric nanoparticles as therapeutic agents against coronavirus disease. J Nanopart Res 24:1–5

Chaudhary J, Tailor G, Yadav M, Mehta C (2023a) Green route synthesis of metallic nanoparticles using various herbal extracts: a review. Biocatal Agric Biotechnol 50:102692

Chaudhary J, Tailor G, Mehta C, Yadav M (2023b) An overview of biosynthesized metal nanoparticles via medicinal plant extracts of the Moraceae family. Biocatal Agric Biotechnol 52:102812

Cheng H, Jiang Z, Sun C, Wang Z, Han G, Chen X, Li T, Fan Z, Zhang F, Yang X, Lv L (2022) Protein stabilized polymeric nanoparticles inspired relay drug delivery for tackling post-chemotherapeutic metastasis. Chem Eng J 427:131672

Choudhary M, Jones JB, Paret ML (2022) Natural or green synthesis nanomaterials and impact on plant pathogens. In: Nanotechnology-based sustainable alternatives for the management of plant diseases. Elsevier, pp 5–29

Corsi I, Venditti I, Trotta F, Punta C (2023) Environmental safety of nanotechnologies: the eco-design of manufactured nanomaterials for environmental remediation. Sci Total Environ 864:161181

Cruse K, Trewartha A, Lee S, Wang Z, Huo H, He T, Kononova O, Jain A, Ceder G (2022) Text-mined dataset of gold nanoparticle synthesis procedures, morphologies, and size entities. Sci Data 9(1):234

Dahlman JE, Barnes C, Khan OF, Thiriot A, Jhunjunwala S, Shaw TE, Xing Y, Sager HB, Sahay G, Speciner L, Bader A (2014) In vivo endothelial siRNA delivery using polymeric nanoparticles with low molecular weight. Nat Nanotechnol 9(8):648–655

Das S, Sharangi AB (2020) Nanotechnology: a potential tool in exploring herbal benefits. In: Functional bionanomaterials: from biomolecules to nanoparticles. Springer, Cham, pp 27–46

Dewangan HK, Singh N, Kumar Megh S, Singh S, Lakshmi. (2022) Optimisation and evaluation of Gymnema sylvestre extract loaded polymeric nanoparticles for enhancement of in vivo efficacy and reduction of toxicity. J Microencapsul 39(2):125–135

Dubey SK, Parab S, Achalla VP, Narwaria A, Sharma S, Jaswanth Gowda BH, Kesharwani P (2022) Microparticulate and nanotechnology mediated drug delivery system for the delivery of herbal extracts. J Biomater Sci Polym Ed 33(12):1531–1554

Dutta D, Das BM (2021) Scope of green nanotechnology towards amalgamation of green chemistry for cleaner environment: a review on synthesis and applications of green nanoparticles. Environ Nanotechnol Monit Manag 15:100418

Fahmy SA, Preis E, Bakowsky U, Azzazy HM (2020) Palladium nanoparticles fabricated by green chemistry: promising chemotherapeutic, antioxidant and antimicrobial agents. Materials 13(17):3661

Falsini S, Bardi U, Abou-Hassan A, Ristori S (2018) Sustainable strategies for large-scale nanotechnology manufacturing in the biomedical field. Green Chem 20(17):3897–3907

Francia S, Shmal D, Di Marco S, Chiaravalli G, Maya-Vetencourt JF, Mantero G, Michetti C, Cupini S, Manfredi G, DiFrancesco ML, Rocchi A (2022) Light-induced charge generation in polymeric nanoparticles restores vision in advanced-stage retinitis pigmentosa rats. Nat Commun 13(1):3677

Fuku X, Dyosiba X, Iftikhar FJ (2023) Green prepared nanomaterials from various biodegradable wastes and their application in energy. Nano-Struct Nano-Objects 35:100997

Garcella P, Wijaya TH, Kurniawan DW (2021) Narrative review: herbal nanocosmetics for anti aging. J Pharm Sci Clin Res 8(1)

García-Quintero A, Palencia M (2021) A critical analysis of environmental sustainability metrics applied to green synthesis of nanomaterials and the assessment of environmental risks associated with the nanotechnology. Sci Total Environ 793:148524

Ghosh K, Satapathy SS, Ghosh S, Jauhari S, Kundu CN, Si S (2020) Green chemistry approach for gold nanoparticles synthesis using plant extracts: a potential material towards catalysis and biology. Adv Nat Sci Nanosci Nanotechnol 11(3):035012

Gilbertson LM, Zimmerman JB, Plata DL, Hutchison JE, Anastas PT (2015) Designing nanomaterials to maximize performance and minimize undesirable implications guided by the Principles of Green Chemistry. Chem Soc Rev 44(16):5758–5777

Hatem KH, Ahmed BM, Al-Noor TH (2023) Consciousness of green nanotechnology among chemistry scholars at the College of Education for Pure Sciences-Ibn Al-Haitham in Iraq. J Namib Stud Hist Politics Cult 33:1069–1081

Husain S, Nandi A, Simnani FZ, Saha U, Ghosh A, Sinha A, Sahay A, Samal SK, Panda PK, Verma SK (2023) Emerging trends in advanced translational applications of silver nanoparticles: a progressing dawn of nanotechnology. J Funct Biomater 14(1):47

Hussain Z, Pandey M, Thu HE, Kaur T, Jia GW, Ying PC, Xian TM, Abourehab MA (2022) Hyaluronic acid functionalization improves dermal targeting of polymeric nanoparticles for management of burn wounds: in vitro, ex vivo and in vivo evaluations. Biomed Pharmacother 150:112992

Iravani S, Varma RS (2020) Greener synthesis of lignin nanoparticles and their applications. Green Chem 22(3):612–636

Izvle NT, Trave KL (2020) Improvement of titanium dioxide nanoparticle synthesis with green chemistry methods using lemongrass (Cymbopogon citratus) extract. Mater Tehnol 54(6):755–759

Jahangirian H, Lemraski EG, Webster TJ, Rafiee-Moghaddam R, Abdollahi Y (2017) A review of drug delivery systems based on nanotechnology and green chemistry: green nanomedicine. Int J Nanomedicine:2957–2978. 12, 2957–2978. doi: 10.2147/IJN.S127683.

Kamaraj C, Karthi S, Reegan AD, Balasubramani G, Ramkumar G, Kalaivani K, Zahir AA, Deepak P, Senthil-Nathan S, Rahman MM, Islam AR (2022) Green synthesis of gold nanoparticles

Sandulovici RC, Carmen-Marinela M, Grigoroiu A, Moldovan CA, Savin M, Ordeanu V, Voicu SN, Cord D, Costache GM, Galatanu ML, Popescu M (2022) The physicochemical and antimicrobial properties of silver/gold nanoparticles obtained by "green synthesis" from willow bark and their formulations as potential innovative pharmaceutical substances. Pharmaceuticals 16(1):48

Saravanan A, Deivayanai VC, Kumar PS, Rangasamy G, Hemavathy RV, Harshana T, Gayathri N, Alagumalai K (2022) A detailed review on advanced oxidation process in treatment of wastewater: mechanism, challenges and future outlook. Chemosphere 308:136524

Saxe JK, Hoffman L, Labib R (2022) Method to incorporate green chemistry principles in early-stage product design for sustainability: case studies with personal care products. Green Chem 24(12):4969–4980

Seo BB, Kwon Y, Kim J, Hong KH, Kim SE, Song HR, Kim YM, Song SC (2022) Injectable polymeric nanoparticle hydrogel system for long-term anti-inflammatory effect to treat osteoarthritis. Bioact Mater 7:14–25

Setyawati MI, Wang Q, Ni N, Tee JK, Ariga K, Ke PC, Ho HK, Wang Y, Leong DT (2023) Engineering tumoral vascular leakiness with gold nanoparticles. Nat Commun 14(1):4269

Shah DJ, Sharma AS, Sharma VS, Vishwakarma VK, Sudhakar AA, Shrivastav PS, Varma RS (2023) Microcrystalline cellulose decorated with Fe3O4 nanoparticle catalysts for the microwave-assisted synthesis of Thioglyoxamides. ACS Appl Nano Mater 6(5):4005–4016

Shanmugam J, Dhayalan M, Savaas Umar MR, Gopal M, Ali Khan M, Simal-Gandara J, Cid-Samamed A (2022) Green synthesis of silver nanoparticles using Allium cepa var. aggregatum natural extract: antibacterial and cytotoxic properties. Nanomaterials 12(10):1725

Sharma A, Pal K, Saini N, Kumar S, Bansal D, Mona S (2023) Remediation of contaminants from wastewater using algal nanoparticles via green chemistry approach: an organized review. Nanotechnology 34:352001

Shukla S, Khan R, Saxena A, Patel A, Selvam S, Hussain CM (2023) Future of modern society: sustainability in green nanotechnology. In: Nanoremediation. Elsevier, pp 393–410

Singh A, Ansari VA, Ahsan F, Akhtar J, Khushwaha P, Maheshwari S (2021) Viridescent concoction of genstein tendentious silver nanoparticles for breast cancer. Res J Pharm Technol 14(5):2867–2872

Singh S, Sharma N, Shukla S, Behl T, Gupta S, Anwer MK, Vargas-De-La-Cruz C, Bungau SG, Brisc C (2023) Understanding the potential role of nanotechnology in liver fibrosis: a paradigm in therapeutics. Molecules 28(6):2811

Soltys L, Olkhovyy O, Tatarchuk T, Naushad M (2021) Green synthesis of metal and metal oxide nanoparticles: principles of green chemistry and raw materials. Magnetochemistry 7(11):145

Soni RA, Rizwan MA, Singh S (2022) Opportunities and potential of green chemistry in nanotechnology. Nanotechnol Environ Eng 7(3):661–673

Sreenikethanam A, Raj S, Gugulothu P, Bajhaiya AK (2022) Genetic engineering of microalgae for secondary metabolite production: recent developments, challenges, and future prospects. Front Bioeng Biotechnol 10:836056

Su L, Li J, Ran F (2023) Fabricating carbon-based electrode materials via uptake of amino nano-polystyrene into Pistia stratiotes roots for enhancing supercapacitance. Green Chem 25:9351–9362

Sulaiman M (2023) Factors influencing the green synthesis of metallic nanoparticles using plant extracts: a comprehensive review. Pharm Fronts 5:e117–e131

Sun S, He L, Yang M, Cui J, Liang S (2022) Facet junction engineering for photocatalysis: a comprehensive review on elementary knowledge, facet-synergistic mechanisms, functional modifications, and future perspectives. Adv Funct Mater 32(1):2106982

Suriyakala G, Sathiyaraj S, Babujanarthanam R, Alarjani KM, Hussein DS, Rasheed RA, Kanimozhi K (2022) Green synthesis of gold nanoparticles using Jatropha integerrima Jacq. flower extract and their antibacterial activity. J King Saud Univ-Sci 34(3):101830

Tajik S, Beitollahi H, Torkzadeh-Mahani M (2022) Electrochemical immunosensor for the detection of anti-thyroid peroxidase antibody by gold nanoparticles and ionic liquid-modified carbon paste electrode. J Nanostructure Chem 12(4):581–588

Teixeira A, Sárria MP, Pinto I, Espiña B, Gomes AC, Dias AC (2022) Protection against paraquat-induced oxidative stress by Curcuma longa extract-loaded polymeric nanoparticles in zebrafish embryos. Polymers 14(18):3773

Tiwari A, Joshi M, Kenwat R, Paliwal SR, Sulakhiya K, Paliwal R (2023) Nanophytomedicine: nanotechnology for herbal product development and value addition. In: Phytopharmaceuticals and herbal drugs. Academic Press, pp 197–212

Tran TV, Nguyen DT, Kumar PS, Din AT, Jalil AA, Vo DV (2022) Green synthesis of ZrO 2 nanoparticles and nanocomposites for biomedical and environmental applications: a review. Environ Chem Lett:1–23. 20(2),1309-1331; https://doi.org/10.1007/s10311-021-01367-9

Upadhyay AK, Singh DP (eds) (2020) Algae and sustainable technologies: bioenergy, nanotechnology and green chemistry. CRC Press

Vargas J, García L, Baena Y (2023) Nanotechnology and herbal products: advances and perspectives in the treatment of diabetes and some of its complications. Rev J Appl Pharm Sci 13(12):001–014

Vasanth S, Shree AA, Bhat J, Vemireddy BG, Bondu VK (2023) Role of herbal nanotechnology in triple negative breast cancer. J Pharm Negat Results:2913–2920. Vol-14; DOI: https://doi.org/10.47750/pnr.2023.14.S02.343

Vernet-Crua A, Cruz DM, Mostafavi E, Truong LB, Barabadi H, Cholula-Díaz JL, Guisbiers G, Webster TJ (2023) Green-synthesized metallic nanoparticles for antimicrobial applications. In: Nanomedicine. Woodhead Publishing, pp 297–338

Wang X, Fan Y, Yan J, Yang M (2022a) Engineering polyphenol-based polymeric nanoparticles for drug delivery and bioimaging. Chem Eng J 439:135661

Wang X, Gu Y, Li Q, Xu Y, Shi Y, Wang Z, Xia M, Li J, Wang D (2022b) Synergistic chemo-photothermal cancer therapy of pH-responsive polymeric nanoparticles loaded IR825 and DTX with charge-reversal property. Colloids Surf B: Biointerfaces 209:112164

Wani S, Rajput A, Pingale P (2023) Herbal nano-formulations: a magical remedy for management of fungal diseases. J Herb Med 42:100810

Wen M, Yu N, Wu S, Huang M, Qiu P, Ren Q, Zhu M, Chen Z (2022) On-demand assembly of polymeric nanoparticles for longer-blood-circulation and disassembly in tumor for boosting sonodynamic therapy. Bioact Mater 18:242–253

Xiao X, Teng F, Shi C, Chen J, Wu S, Wang B, Meng X, Essiet Imeh A, Li W (2022) Polymeric nanoparticles—promising carriers for cancer therapy. Front Bioeng Biotechnol 10:1024143

Xiong W, Guo Z, Zeng B, Wang T, Zeng X, Cao W, Lian D (2022) Dacarbazine-loaded targeted polymeric nanoparticles for enhancing malignant melanoma therapy. Front Bioeng Biotechnol 10:847901

Yano TA, Kajisa T, Ono M, Miyasaka Y, Hasegawa Y, Saito A, Otsuka K, Sakane A, Sasaki T, Yasutomo K, Hamajima R (2022) Ultrasensitive detection of SARS-CoV-2 nucleocapsid protein using large gold nanoparticle-enhanced surface plasmon resonance. Sci Rep 12(1):1060

Zafar A, Alruwaili NK, Imam SS, Alsaidan OA, Ahmed MM, Yasir M, Warsi MH, Alquraini A, Ghoneim MM, Alshehri S (2022) Development and optimization of hybrid polymeric nanoparticles of apigenin: physicochemical characterization, antioxidant activity and cytotoxicity evaluation. Sensors 22(4):1364

Zhang D, Ma XL, Gu Y, Huang H, Zhang GW (2020) Green synthesis of metallic nanoparticles and their potential applications to treat cancer. Front Chem 8:799

Zhang P, Xue M, Lin Z, Yang H, Zhang C, Cui J, Chen J (2022) Aptamer functionalization and high-contrast reversible dual-color photoswitching fluorescence of polymeric nanoparticles for latent fingerprints imaging. Sensors Actuators B Chem 367:132049

Zhang L, Zhang M, Mujumdar AS, Yu D, Wang H (2023) Potential nano bacteriostatic agents to be used in meat-based foods processing and storage: a critical review. Trends Food Sci Technol 131:77–90

Zhou W, Xin C, Chen Y, Mouhouadi RD, Chen S (2023) Nanoparticles for enhancing heavy oil recovery: recent progress, challenges, and future perspectives. Energy Fuel 37(12):8057–8078

Sustainable Materials for Tissue Engineering

4

Hajer Radhouani, Cristiana Gonçalves, Rui L. Reis, and Joaquim M. Oliveira

Abstract

Tissue engineering has emerged as a promising field with the potential to completely reinvent medical treatments and therapies for various diseases and conditions. Nevertheless, with the industry's progress, it is becoming increasingly evident that prioritizing sustainable materials is essential to speed up translation into the market/clinics. Sustainability and biomaterials complement each other, supporting the development of new sustainable materials through advanced technological processes. These biomaterials, either extracted from biological resources or produced using green technology, are drawing the attention of tissue engineering. Herein, we provide a thorough overview of the sustainable natural and synthetic biomaterials utilized in tissue engineering, focusing on the procedures used to extract and produce these materials and their characteristics and structures.

Additionally, it explores how these materials are employed in the biomedical field, especially for tissue engineering applications. Essential insights for current research and development in tissue engineering by combining advances in sustainable material science with biological information are also provided. The ultimate goal is to contribute to creating innovative, effective, and durable sustainable biomaterials for tissue engineering applications.

Hajer Radhouani and Cristiana Gonçalves contributed equally with all other contributors.

H. Radhouani (✉) · C. Gonçalves (✉) · R. L. Reis · J. M. Oliveira
3 B's Research Group, I3Bs – Research Institute on Biomaterials, Biodegradables and Biomimetics, University of Minho, Headquarters of the European Institute of Excellence on Tissue Engineering and Regenerative Medicine, AvePark, Parque de Ciência e Tecnologia, Zona Industrial da Gandra, Guimarães, Portugal

ICVS/3B's–PT Government Associate Laboratory, Braga/Guimarães, Portugal

M. N. Collins, M. Culebras (eds.), *Sustainable Biopolymers and Composites for Biomedical Applications*, Biomaterials, Bioengineering and Sustainability 5,
https://doi.org/10.1007/978-3-031-91972-5_4

Keywords

Sustainable materials · Tissue engineering · Natural biomaterials · Synthetic biomaterials · Biocompatibility · Biomedical applications

4.1 Introduction

Tissue engineering has emerged as a promising field with the potential to disruptively reinvent medical treatments and therapies for various diseases and conditions. Nevertheless, with the industry's progress, it is becoming increasingly evident that prioritizing sustainable solutions is required. Conventional tissue engineering techniques are concerning because they rely on finite resources and generate waste. Consequently, researchers are turning their attention to sustainable materials in tissue engineering. Sustainable biomaterials, such as natural and synthetic ones, are used in tissue engineering to create cellular growth and differentiation scaffolds. These biodegradable materials can offer temporary support without harm, reducing environmental effects and improving compatibility with biological systems. They also minimize patient rejection and adverse reactions, thus improving patient outcomes. Additionally, the effectiveness anticipated from sustainable biomaterials can help reduce healthcare costs by avoiding additional surgeries or treatments (Biswal et al. 2020).

Ultimately, biopolymers can offer a sustainable solution to reducing carbon footprints and energy consumption in today's industrial landscape (Shogren et al. 2019). These eco-friendly polymers can be easily recycled at the end of their lifespan, aligning with the principles of a circular economy. Their use in various industries, such as biomedical engineering and scientific research, has increased due to the raising concern on plastic pollution and the need for more environmentally friendly solutions. The rising demand for eco-friendly alternatives in today's industrial sector has increased interest in biopolymers as a sustainable solution (Al Mahmud et al. 2024). These ecologically friendly polymers help reduce carbon footprints and energy consumption and can be easily recycled at their end life, promoting a circular economy. As concerns over plastic pollution continue to escalate, industries such as biomedical engineering and scientific research are increasingly turning to biopolymers for their environmentally friendly properties (Aranda et al. 2023).

Promoting sustainability in tissue engineering reduces environmental impact. It can also improve the safety and efficacy of therapies for patients. The development of sustainable biopolymer-based biomaterials is crucial for tissue engineering, as they offer biodegradable scaffolds for tissue regeneration and drug delivery systems (Mahmud et al. 2023). These materials mimic the natural extracellular matrix (ECM), providing an optimal cell growth and tissue regeneration environment. As demand for sustainable solutions raises, integrating biopolymers into tissue engineering will play a critical role in shaping the future of healthcare and environmental conservation (Noro et al. 2024). Sustainable materials such as biodegradable polymers, decellularized tissues, and cell-derived ECM are extensively explored, offering transformative potential across various applications like bone regeneration, cartilage repair, skin substitutes, and vascular grafts (Joyce et al. 2021). Integrating sustainable practices in tissue engineering supports the transition towards a circular economy, promoting long-term sustainability and resilience. Employing natural materials such as decellularized plant tissues and renewable sources, particularly algae or fungi, researchers can create biocompatible scaffolds that promote regenerative therapies and contribute to the general objective of achieving a circular economy (Harris et al. 2021).

Essential factors to consider are the choice of biocompatible and biodegradable biomaterials derived from renewable or abundant natural sources. In addition, sustainable solutions prioritize energy-efficient industrial processes and waste reduction throughout production and disposal (Li et al. 2023). Efficiently using resources, such as limiting the consumption of growth factors and lowering the physical space required for tissue culture infrastructure, is of utmost importance. To achieve sustainability in tissue engineering, it is crucial to include circular economy ideas, such as recycling and reusing biomaterials and by-products, while responsible progress in science also imposes ethical considerations like animal care and adherence to regulatory frameworks.

Acquiring a comprehensive knowledge of the anatomy and structure of target tissues is crucial when trying to develop biomaterials that can effectively repair and regenerate tissues (Cao and Ding 2022). Development in biomaterial science, combined with cellular and molecular biology technologies, presents exciting opportunities for developing biomaterials with distinctive characteristics. Biomimetic materials are designed to mimic natural tissues' structure, composition, and functions. These materials incorporate biological compounds such as Collagen, elastin, and hyaluronic acid. These materials can improve different cells' functions, including attachment, growth, and specialization, by imitating living systems' structured arrangement and shifting patterns (Ma 2008).

Applying natural polymers in tissue engineering is increasing due to their biodegradability and compatibility with cells and enzymes. Advances in fabrication techniques, such as additive manufacturing and bottom-up methods, are crucial for sustainable materials development, enabling precise control over material properties and architecture. In fact, additive manufacturing makes three-dimensional printing of polymeric materials containing cells possible by producing living materials (Priks et al. 2020). The interdisciplinary approach of combining natural polymers with synthetic materials and advanced fabrication methods can create biomaterials that closely resemble human tissues, offering new opportunities for functional and biocompatible medical implants.

A comprehensive overview of sustainable materials used in tissue engineering approaches is provided herein (Fig. 4.1). It gives detailed information on the most typical natural and synthetic materials, emphasizing their chemical, structural, physicochemical, and biological characteristics. The crucial importance of sustainability in the development of tissue engineering by thoroughly analyzing existing research and prospects is also highlighted. It promotes a more responsible and forward-looking approach to medical innovation.

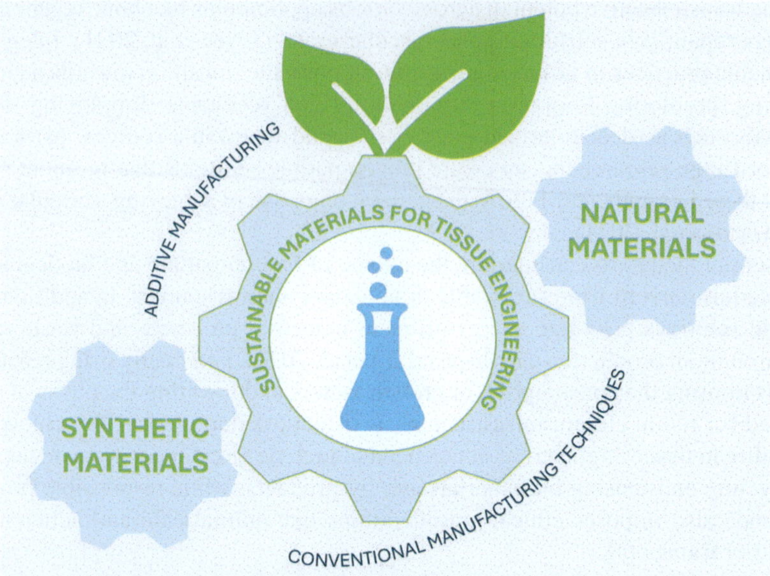

Fig. 4.1 Sustainable biomaterials for tissue engineering

4.2 Natural Biomaterials

4.2.1 Collagen

Collagen, a protein found in 1% to 2% of muscle tissue and 6% of robust and tendinous muscle weight, is synthesized by fibroblasts from pluripotential adventitial or reticulum cells (Rajabimashhadi et al. 2023; Owczarzy et al. 2020; Gorgieva and Kokol 2011). Collagen has unique structural characteristics, making it biodegradable, biocompatible, non-cytotoxic, and can be processed into various forms. Over 90% of Collagen is type I, found in bones, skins, tendons, vascular, ligatures, and organs (Aberoumand 2012). Collagen type I is crucial in maintaining tissue integrity through interactions with cell surfaces, other ECM molecules, and growth and differentiation factors. However, the abundance and proportion of types I and III Collagen can change due to age or injury (Jongjareonrak 2006).

Collagen is primarily found in several animal sources, including bovine skin, pig skin, and chicken waste. Its use is restricted due to religious and ethnic constraints, regulatory and quality control issues, and potential biological contaminants. Marine organisms have been identified as promising alternatives due to their availability, lack of disease risk, and high collagen profits (Li et al. 2004; Ogawa et al. 2003). Marine Collagen, sourced from fish scales and skin, is popular due to its similarity to human Collagen and minimal disease transmission risk, making it a suitable biomedical alternative (Rajabimashhadi et al. 2023).

Collagen is a fibrous protein that has a unique structural motif consisting of three parallel polypeptide strands coiling together in a right-handed triple helix (Fig. 4.2) and is essential for tissue strength and elasticity. It can be split into two independent groups: (i) Fibrillar collagens (I, II, III, V, XI, XIV, and XXVII) and (ii) non-fibrillar collagens (Owczarzy et al. 2020).

The collagen protein family exhibits mechanical strength due to its spatial structure, wide structure diversity, and unique super-helical structure, making it a valuable animal protein (Owczarzy et al. 2020).

The tropocollagen, or "collagen molecule," is a subunit of larger collagen aggregates. Each subunit is approximately 300 nm long and has a diameter of 1.5 nm. The collagen's structure, which is high in proline and hydroxyproline and has a strong sequence homology across genus and family line, is distinctive. The typical sequence follows the pattern Gly-Pro-Y or Gly-X-Hyp, (X and Y may be any of numerous other amino acid residues) (Gorgieva and Kokol 2011), having a very variable structure (Fig. 4.2).

Collagen production is a straightforward process in water, forming various matrix systems, including meshes, hydrogels, scaffolds, injectable solutions, and dispersions (Gorgieva and Kokol 2011). The three primary techniques for collagen extraction are neutral salt-solubilized Collagen, acid-solubilized Collagen, and pepsin-solubilized Collagen (PSC) (Aberoumand 2012). The PSC extraction method has been used to extract Collagen from various sources, including the skin of brown-stripe red snapper, albacore tuna, black drum, and sheepshead seabream skin, bone and scale, and fish waste material (Jongjareonrak 2006; Noitup et al. 2005; Li et al. 2004; Ogawa et al. 2003; Nagai and Suzuki 2000). The extraction procedure can be enhanced by adjusting parameters, with high temperatures being more advantageous for pilot scales (Noitup et al. 2005; Ogawa et al. 2003).

It is noteworthy that Collagen is considered a sustainable material because it is derived from natural, renewable sources and is biodegradable, making it environmentally friendly. Numerous efforts are being made to create biomimetically collagen-based macromolecules with diverse physicochemical properties and macromolecular arrangements for tissue engineering applications (Potaros et al. 2009; Silva et al. 2012). Collagen, first used in medical surgery in the late nineteenth century, has since become a significant biomaterial in clinical medicine, including injectable Collagen for tissue defects augmentation, haemostasis, burn dressings, hernia repair, bioprosthetic heart valves, vascular grafts, drug delivery systems, and nerve regeneration (Gorgieva and Kokol 2011). As technology advances, collagen-based biomaterials will continue to play a crucial role in modern healthcare.

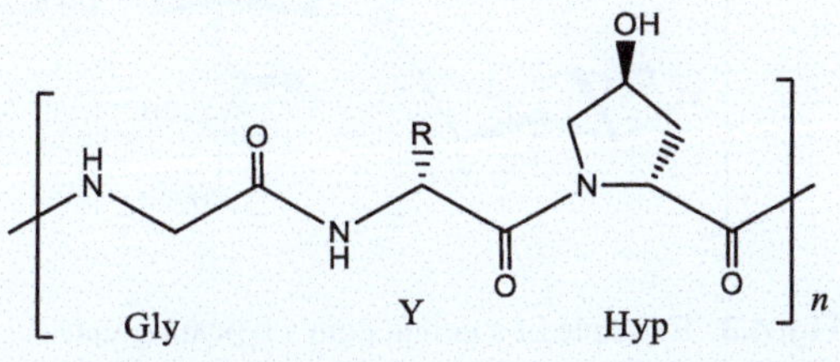

Fig. 4.2 Example of a collagen's repeating unit

Collagen type I is widely used in medical devices because it promotes biocompatible tissue regeneration. It's used in wound dressings and heart valve replacements, and its role in biomedical applications is expected to expand with further research (Burke et al. 1983). Collagen, when combined with chondrocytes and stem cells, promotes cartilage tissue growth and wound healing. Collagen-based scaffolds stimulate tissue regeneration and differentiation, making them versatile tools in tissue engineering. Collagen enhances the formation of functional tissues, making it a valuable biomaterial in regenerative medicine approaches (Parenteau-Bareil et al. 2010; Yudoh and Karasawa 2012; Kock et al. 2012; Zhang et al. 2009).

4.2.2 Gellan Gum (GG)

Gellan gum (GG), a sustainable macromolecule, is a polysaccharide produced by *Sphingomonas elodea*, a non-pathogenic bacteria. It has excellent biocompatibility and is often used with collagen-based scaffolds for tissue engineering applications. GG supports cell growth and regeneration, making it a key player in regenerative medicine (Osmalek et al. 2014; da Silva et al. 2008; Novac et al. 2014; Kang et al. 2015; Oliveira et al. 2010). Its versatility and biodegradability make it an attractive option for tissue engineering and regenerative medicine.

GG is a linear, anionic exopolysaccharide with a tetrasaccharide repeating unit of α-L-rhamnose, β-D-glucuronic acid, and two acyl groups bound to glucose residue (Osmalek et al. 2014; Novac et al. 2014; Prajapati et al. 2013) (Fig. 4.3). The composition is approximately 60% glucose, 20% rhamnose, and 20% glucuronic acid (Prajapati et al. 2013).

GG is produced through pure culture fermentation of *Pseudomonas elodea* carbohydrates, purified with isopropyl alcohol, dried, and milled, with efficiency influenced by media composition, pH, temperature, agitation rate, and oxygen availability (Prajapati et al. 2013). GG can be processed into hydrogels resistant to heat and acid, requiring a temperature of at least 70 °C and cooling to induce coil-to-helix transition. Deacetylated gellan gum can be produced by alkaline treatment,

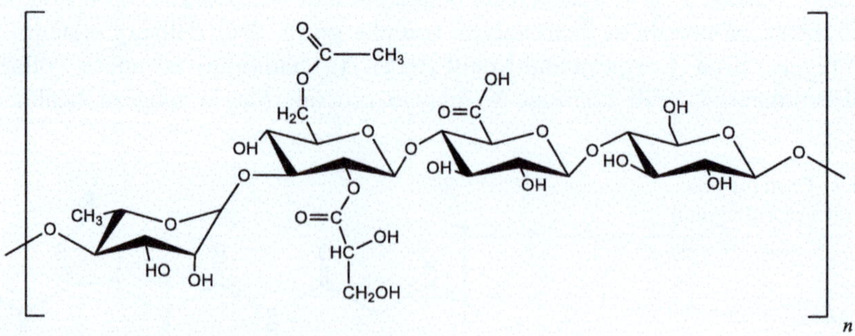

Fig. 4.3 Example of a gellan gum's repeating unit

resulting in rigid and brittle gels. Hot deacetylated gellan gum can also be clarified as an agar substitute (Osmalek et al. 2014; da Silva et al. 2008, 2014; Prajapati et al. 2013).

GG hydrogel is produced through *Pseudomonas elodea* pure culture fermentation of carbohydrates, then purified with isopropyl alcohol and dried and milled. Production efficiency varies with typical fermentation factors. The process involves a minimum temperature of 70 °C and subsequent cooling to trigger the transition from coil to helix (Osmalek et al. 2014; da Silva et al. 2008, 2014; Prajapati et al. 2013). Alkaline treatment is commonly used to eliminate the acetyl groups in native gellan gum, producing deacetylated gellan gum. The native gellan produces malleable gels that are easily molded, whereas the deacetylated gellan forms firm and fragile gels. GG can be further purified through hot filtration after deacetylation, making it a substitute for agar (Osmalek et al. 2014; Prajapati et al. 2013). GG is also a versatile agent used in food and cosmetics for gelling, stabilizing, and suspending. It has received FDA and EU approval for its use in tissue engineering. GG hydrogels have shown potential in noninvasive injectable applications but have some challenges, such as a high gelation temperature. However, GG hydrogels can be methacrylated for tunable properties without affecting biocompatibility, making them suitable for various tissue engineering applications. Despite these challenges, GG hydrogels have shown promise in different applications (Osmalek et al. 2014; Kang et al. 2015; da Silva et al. 2014; Coutinho et al. 2010). The combination of gellan gum and carboxymethyl chitosan forms a highly intricate gel that exhibits significant promise as a material for cartilage tissue engineering (Tang et al. 2012).

4.2.3 Chitosan

Chitosan is a naturally occurring biodegradable polysaccharide derived from chitin, the second most abundant natural polymer, making it a sustainable and renewable material. It consists of varying amounts of N-acetyl-2 amino-2-deoxy-D-glucose residues, which can be protonated for solubility in diluted acidic aqueous solutions. Its unique properties and applications in various fields make it a valuable material (Aranaz et al. 2021; Ibrahim and El-Zairy 2015). This linear polysaccharide is a copolymer of β(1–4) linked D-glucosamine and N-acetyl D-glucosamine residues. Chitin is a polysaccharide, a homopolymer comprised of 2-acetamido-2-deoxy-b--D-glucopyranose units (Dunne et al. 2014; Bhardwaj et al. 2011; Fang et al. 2014; Baran et al. 2012; Sionkowska et al. 2014) (Fig. 4.4).

Chitosan is soluble in dilute acids and has a strong positive charge due to protonation. It can be used as a physical crosslinking component in scaffold construction. It has favorable degradation kinetics and mimics glycosaminoglycan components. However, it is often blended with other polymers due to its poor mechanical properties and high swelling ability (Dunne et al. 2014; Bhardwaj et al. 2011; Sionkowska et al. 2014; Zhang et al. 2013; Bhardwaj and Kundu 2011).

Numerous studies report using CS and silk fibroin (SF) as natural materials for tissue-engineered scaffolds due to their biocompatibility, degradability, and

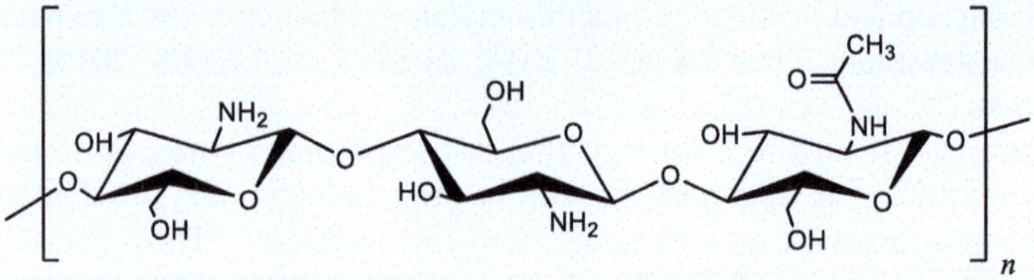

Fig. 4.4 Chitin main repeating unit

mechanical properties (Dunne et al. 2014; Bhardwaj and Kundu 2011; Lai et al. 2014; Silva et al. 2008; Mirahmadi et al. 2013). The SFCS scaffolds exhibit strong interactions between their synthetic and biological components, primarily promoted by hydrogen bonds. These scaffolds replicate the *in vivo* extracellular matrix with flexible biological, structural, and mechanical properties. Consequently, they reveal significant potential for repairing abdominal wall defects, healing skin wounds, and regenerating bone and tracheal cartilage, yielding promising results in laboratory settings and living organisms (Dunne et al. 2014; Sionkowska and Płanecka 2013). A study was conducted to test the efficacy of injecting alginate-chitosan beads dispersed in a hydrogel directly into the joint. The results were promising and indicated that this new dual-phase biomaterial could be a viable treatment option for osteoarthritis in humans (Oprenyeszk et al. 2013). The use of a polyelectrolyte poly(Lactide-co-Glycolide) (PLGA) with CS complex scaffold for *in vivo* cartilage repair using tissue engineering was studied. The scaffold maintained cellular proliferation, migration, and chondrogenic differentiation, regenerating hyaline cartilage for 12 weeks (Zhang et al. 2013). Moreover, hybrid chitosan/blood implants have been found to effectively heal cartilage defects by suppressing fibrocartilage scar tissue formation, promoting bone remodelling, and facilitating blood vessel migration and woven bone repair (Lafantaisie-Favreau et al. 2013; Bell et al. 2012; Mathieu et al. 2013).

4.2.4 Silk Fibroin (SF)

Silk fibroin (SF), a fibrous protein from the silkworm Bombyx mori, is the main structural component of silk, making up 70–90% of the fiber. It is a biopolymer composed of two proteins: hydrophobic fibroin and hydrophilic sericin. It is an amphiphilic block copolymer with a heavy chain of 12 repetitive units. SF is secreted by the silkworm into the posterior silk gland and stored in the middle gland before being spun out through the anterior silk gland. Sustainable silk fibroin has high mechanical properties, making it a desirable biomaterial for neural tissue engineering and neuroprotection in disorders such as stroke and Alzheimer's (Filippi et al. 2020).

Moreover, raw silk is composed of SF (75–85% w/w), glue-like coating sericin (17–25% w/w), wax and fats (1.5%), colorants, and mineral components (1%).

These rates depend on the species, origin, and culture conditions (Sionkowska et al. 2014). SF heavy chains (350–390 kDa) include a highly repetitive sequence of Gly-Ala-Gly-Ala-Gly-Ser, with less repetitive sequences of hydrophobic/aromatic residues and amorphous regions containing charged, polar, and bulky residues (Suzuki 2016) (Fig. 4.5). SF also has three crystal structures: silk I, silk II, and silk III (Lai et al. 2014; Hashimoto et al. 2015).

SF, the structural fiber protein, can be extracted cheaply from cocoons of wild and domesticated silkworms, spiders, wasps, honeybees, and ants. It is typically extracted from silk filaments produced by Bombyx mori silkworms. The silk fibers are degummed, rinsed with distilled water, air-dried, and dissolved in a ternary solvent. The regenerated SF solution is obtained through dialysis against distilled water and filtration at room temperature (Sionkowska et al. 2014; Jin et al. 2014a; Gong et al. 2014). This natural polymeric biomaterial has excellent permeability, mechanical properties, biocompatibility, and biodegradability and is being increasingly explored as a potential source for producing on-demand therapeutic materials and tissue engineering scaffolds despite its long-standing use as a textile fiber (Jin et al. 2014b; Tabatabai et al. 2015). In fact, besides the traditional use of SF in the textile industry, due to its excellent softness, hygroscopicity, and mechanical strength (Hashimoto et al. 2015), it has also been used as a surgical suture without any severe side effects. Moreover, SF is considered one of the best biomaterials for skeletal tissue regeneration due to its excellent biocompatibility, biodegradability, mechanical strength, high oxygen/water permeability, and minimal inflammatory reactions *in vivo* (Lai et al. 2014; Jin et al. 2014a; Saha et al. 2013). It can be processed into films, nonwoven nets, sponges, and hydrogels, which maintain the same properties (Foss et al. 2013; Zhang et al. 2007; Yan et al. 2012).

SF obtained from *Bombyx mori* silkworm is a promising scaffolding material for tissue engineering, specifically for cartilage and meniscus regeneration (Yan et al. 2012). Saha et al. (2013) discovered that Antheraea mylitta silk fibroin scaffolds are more chondroinductive, while *Bombyx mori* scaffolds are more osteoinductive, suggesting the potential for a multi-layered combination for osteochondral defect regeneration. SF materials, such as SF/hyaluronic acid 3D matrices, genipin cross-linked chitosan/SF sponges, and silk fibroin-chondroitin sulphate-sodium alginate porous hybrid scaffolds, have shown promising results in engineering strategies for bone regeneration (Silva et al. 2008; Jin et al. 2014a; Foss et al. 2013; Naeimi et al. 2014).

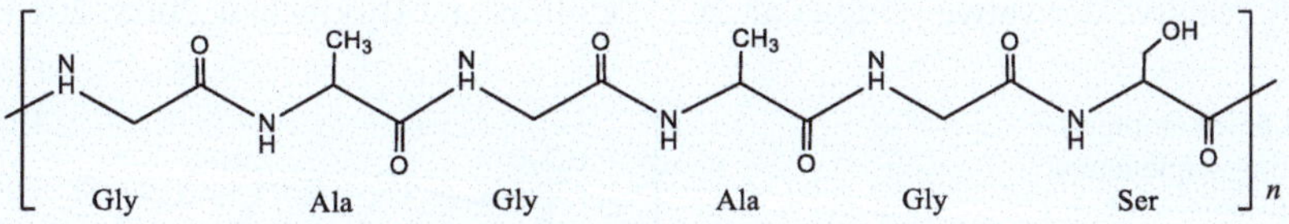

Fig. 4.5 Example of a repeating sequence of a crystalline region of SF protein heavy chains

4.2.5 Hyaluronic Acid (HA)

Hyaluronic acid, Hyaluronan or Hyaluronate (HA), is a linear, hydrophilic, polyanionic polysaccharide, naturally found as a high molecular weight glycosaminoglycan in the extracellular matrix, connective tissues, epithelial tissues, neural tissues, synovial fluid, vitreous humour, and umbilical cord (Ong et al. 2015; Zhao et al. 2014). HA is a polysaccharide with a molecular weight of up to six million Daltons, composed of repeating disaccharide units of β-1, 4-glucuronic acid, and β-1, 3-N-acetyl-D-glucosamine (Fig. 4.6). It is not synthesized in the Golgi apparatus, and catabolism occurs through hyaluronidase-mediated enzymatic degradation or chemical mechanisms (Shen et al. 2010).

Meyer and Palmer first isolated hyaluronic acid (HA) from the vitreous body in 1934 (Meyer and Palmer 1934a) .Today, it is produced through bacterial fermentation or extracted from various sources for commercial purposes. Extraction procedures are optimized to remove protein and minimize degradation. However, low yields and high polydispersity of HA products limit their use. The potential risk of contamination with proteins and viruses is reduced by using healthy tissues and extensive purification procedures (Meyer and Palmer 1934b; Murado et al. 2012; Boeriu et al. 2013).

Microbial HA manufacture at industrial scale was first achieved in the 1980s by Shiseido (Meyer and Palmer 1934a). Optimization of cultivation conditions, culture media, and strain improvement were performed to raise HA yield and quality. However, that technique is also limited due to mass transfer constraint triggered by the high viscosity of the fermentation broth. It is essential to highlight that bacterial fermentation produces HA with high molecular weight and purity, but the risk of contamination with bacterial endotoxins, proteins, nucleic acids, and heavy metals occurs (Boeriu et al. 2013; Liu et al. 2011).

Techniques used to derivatization the HA include sulphation, carbodiimide-mediated modification, esterification, hydrazide modification, crosslinking with polyfunctional epoxides, divinyl sulphone, and glutaraldehyde. HA products derived from esterification are more rigid, stable, hydrophobic, and less enzyme-resistant (Collins and Birkinshaw 2013). HA can be derivatized through carbodiimide-mediated modification, which allows covalent binding between carboxyl and amine groups. Carbodiimide reactions can be sensitive and result in acylurea, an unreactive intermediate. The yield of derivatized HA is also affected by these reactions. Sulphation can also result in HA. The crosslinking approach to engineer HA properties involves exposing it to a cross-linker or synthesizing a highly reactive derivative (Ong et al. 2015; Collins and Birkinshaw 2008, 2013).

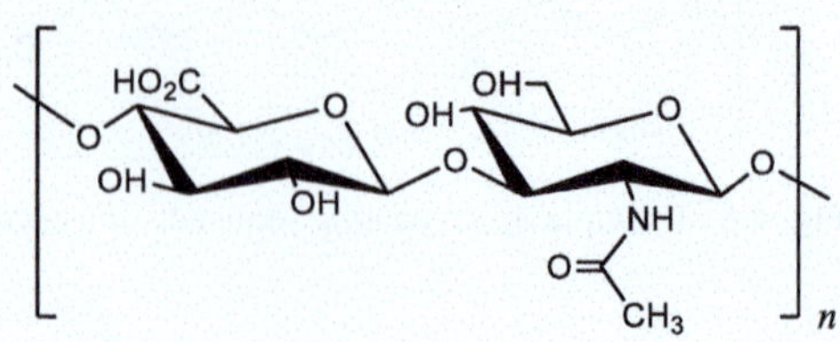

Fig. 4.6 Example of a repeating sequence of hyaluronic acid chains

HA's 3D structure with significant porosity and surface area benefits cell adhesion, extracellular matrix deposition, gas and nutrient transport, and metabolic product release. It is crucial for joint lubrication, nutrition, and preservation of cartilage (Collins and Birkinshaw 2013; Kang et al. 2009; Kim et al. 2011).

4.2.6 Alginate

Alginate, a natural polysaccharide, is widely used in textiles, agri-food, paper, cosmetics, biomedical, and pharmaceuticals. Its biological function is to form a structure-forming component in algae (Silva et al. 2012; Draget et al. 2005; Vauchel et al. 2009). Alginates are linear binary copolymers of (1 → 4) linked β-D Mannuronic acid (M) and α-L-glucuronic acid (G) residues of different compositions and sequences (Fertah et al. 2015). They are present in both salt and acid forms. The salt form is a significant cell wall component in all brown seaweeds, constituting up to 40–47% of the dry weight of algal biomass. For the acid form, it is a linear polyuronic acid and is mentioned as alginic acid (Nalamothu et al. 2014) (Fig. 4.7).

Haug and colleagues discovered the sequential structure of alginates through partial acidic hydrolysis and fractionation, separating alginate into three distinct fractions with varying compositions. The first two fractions contain homopolymeric G and M molecules, while the third fraction has equal proportions of both monomers and many MG dimer residues (Draget et al. 2005; Haug 1964; Haug and Larsen 1966; Haug et al. 1966; Andersen et al. 2012). The M/G ratio and block structure significantly influence alginates' physicochemical and rheological properties, which are biopolymers with industrial significance, often exhibiting high G content. Monomer sequence (M and G) can vary among algal species and different tissues of the same species. The M/G ratio and the block structure significantly affect alginates' physicochemical and rheological properties. These biopolymers with more industrial significance usually show high G content (Draget et al. 2005; Fertah et al. 2015).

Alginate is produced using cultures of *Pseudomonas* species or *Azotobacter* bacteria (*Azotobacter chroococcum* and *A. vinelandii*) (Vu et al. 2009). Alginate is also naturally found in the cell walls of brown seaweeds (Kloareg and Quatrano 1988). Alginate extraction from algal material involves an acidification step to remove contaminant glycans. The second step is neutralizing alginic acid with alkali to form water-soluble sodium alginate. After separation, the soluble sodium alginate is

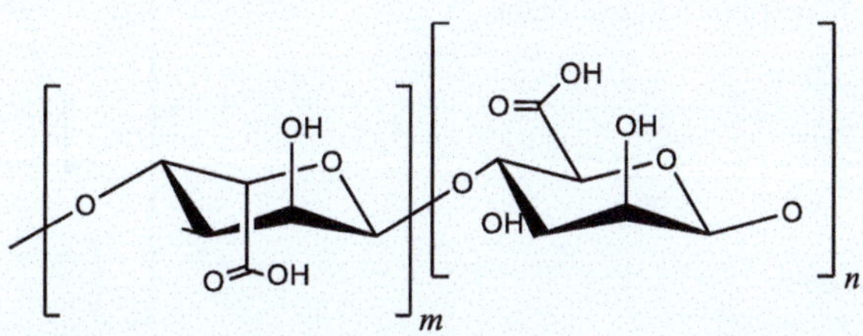

Fig. 4.7 Example of a repeating sequence of alginate chains

precipitated by alcohol, mineral acid, or calcium chloride, converted to sodium form if needed, and dried and milled. The algal raw material and the algae's age determine the colour of the extracted alginate, which can be controlled through bleaching. That method is optimized for sustainable and therapeutic applications (Silva et al. 2012; Draget et al. 2005). The main industrial applications of alginates are linked to their ability to crosslink with ions, retain water, gelling, viscosifying, and stabilizing properties (Nalamothu et al. 2014).

4.2.7 Chondroitin Sulphate (CS)

Chondroitin sulphate (CS) is an acid mucopolysaccharide found in various mammals, invertebrates, and some bacteria. It is a important part of the extracellular matrix and is the most frequent glucose amino glycan in cartilage, responsible for water retention and pressure resistance (Shi et al. 2014; Jerosch 2011). CS can be extracted from various natural sources, including terrestrial and marine species, using proteolytic digestion and purification methods (Michelacci and Dietrich 1976; Seno and Meyer 1963; Chen et al. 2000; Srinivasan et al. 1969; Karamanos et al. 1988; Vazquez et al. 2013; Sugahara et al. 1996; Borsig et al. 2007; Mano 2013; Kim 2015; Cole and Hall 2004). The most successful commercial products of CS, in terms of market volume and profits, are those related to cartilage regeneration, anti-inflammatory activity, and osteoarthritis (OA) (Vazquez et al. 2013).

CS is a polymeric carbohydrate comprising repeating disaccharide units of glucuronic acid and N-acetyl-galactosamine linked by β-(1 → 3) glycosidic bonds and sulphated in some carbon positions (CS not sulphated is CS-O) (Fig. 4.8). Also, it has a molecular mass of 20–60 kDa and has free carboxylic acid groups (suitable for carbodiimide-mediated functionalization). Tracheal and shark CS have varying chain sizes, with tracheal CS 20–25 kDa and shark CS 50–80 kDa; their concentration and composition depend on the organism and tissue (Shi et al. 2014; Lai et al. 2012).

The processes of CS isolation from cartilage have been established and generally include four phases: (1) cartilage hydrolysis, (2) proteoglycan core breakdown, (3) protein elimination and CS recovery, and (4) purification (Shi et al. 2014). The first two steps are typically conducted employing alkaline hydrolysis, subsequently combined with selective precipitation of GAG using cationic quaternary ammonium

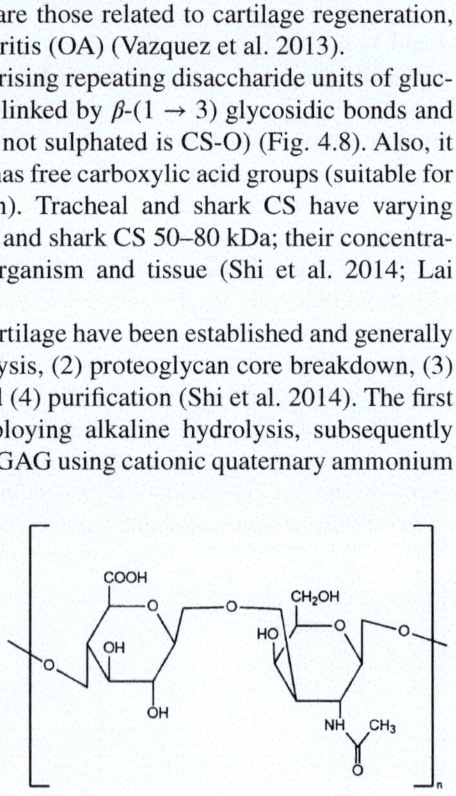

Fig. 4.8 Example of a repeating sequence of chondroitin sulphate chains

chemicals, non-ionic detergents, potassium thiocyanate or alcoholic solutions, deproteinization with trichloroacetic acid, and lastly the purification with gel filtration and ion-exchange and size-exclusion chromatography. Recently, Murado's research (Murado et al. 2012) showed the optimization of a fast and economical extraction method obtaining a purified CS product (99%) from skate cartilage wastes with a high concentration of 35–45 $g.L^{-1}$ (Shi et al. 2014).

The application of CS-based products depends on the purity and quality of GAG in commercial products. Low-cost and high-yield extraction procedures are crucial to maintain CS quality. Clinical applications require highly concentrated and pure CS, which controls OA symptoms like inflammation and pain, impedes disease progression and prevents enzymes like hyaluronidase in synovial fluid (Shi et al. 2014; Jerosch 2011). CS also improves synovial cells' hyaluronic acid production, thus increasing viscosity and synovial fluid levels.

4.2.8 Cellulose

Cellulose, a fundamental and sustainable component of green plants' cell walls, is produced by all plant matter and secreted by certain bacteria, prokaryotes, freshwater and marine algae (Ong et al. 2015). It is the most abundant renewable and biodegradable polymer. Cellulose is one of the many beta-glucan compounds with the formula $(C_6H_{10}O_5)n$. It is a polycarbohydrate of a combination of cellubiose units, formed by two anhydroglucose subunits (Fig. 4.9). This polysaccharide possesses the distinctive property of being incapable of being produced from or broken down into monosaccharides through hydrolysis. That unique property results from the cellulose structure and its elaborate hydrogen bond network that prevents this polysaccharide from melting or dissolving in common solvents. Such a complex is responsible for the high mechanical properties of cellulose, which are crucial for its natural function and are suitable for composite reinforcement applications (Orellana 2013).

Cellulose represents a promising candidate to be converted to derivatives. The purification and isolation of cellulose comprise several steps, including a pulping process, partial hydrolysis, dissolution, re-precipitation, and extraction with organic solvents. Purification and isolation processes often lead to cellulose degradation and oxidation through reactions with acids and bases (Ong et al. 2015).

A cellulose polymer allows chondrocyte proliferation and exhibits biocompatibility, and an injectable product based on hydroxypropyl methylcellulose hydrogel

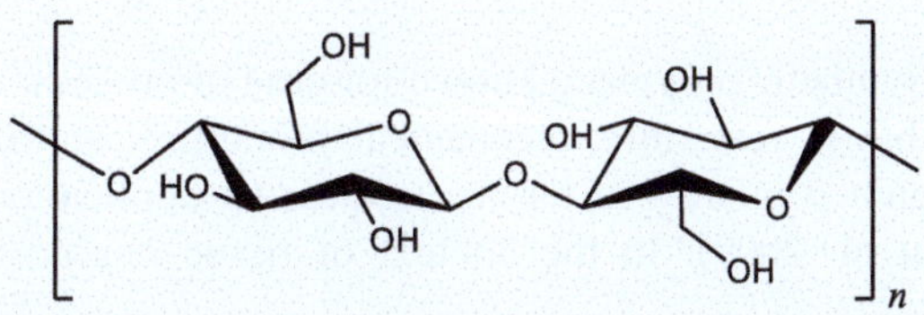

Fig. 4.9 Example of a repeating sequence of cellulose chains

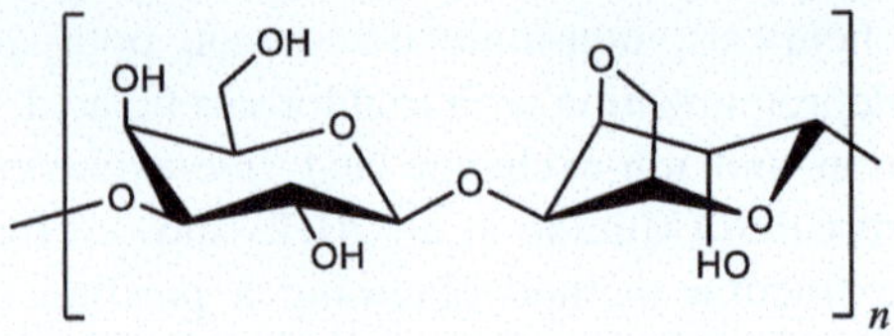

Fig. 4.10 Example of a repeating sequence of agarose chains

can be used for 3D chondrocyte culture for articular cartilage repair (Muller et al. 2006; Vinatier et al. 2009).

4.2.9 Agarose

Agarose, a natural polysaccharide from red seaweed, is used for tissue regeneration due to its biocompatibility, adjustable mechanical properties, and hydrogel-like properties. Its sustainability is also attributed to its biodegradable nature and potential for renewable marine resource sources. It can be efficiently extracted from red algae, particularly those belonging to the genera Gelidium and Gracilaria (Lebbar et al. 2018). Agarose is a linearly composed polymer of repeating units of agarose, a disaccharide comprising residues from L-galactose and D-galactose (Fig. 4.10).

Agarose is widely utilized in various scientific disciplines due to its unique gel-forming properties and ability to form a porous matrix when dissolved in hot water and cooled (Vinatier et al. 2009).

Agarose gels, obtained through temperature changes, form a crosslinked alginate matrix through ionic bonding. It's used for chondrocyte culture and cartilage tissue engineering. High-concentration agarose can be used for in vitro compression to understand chondrocyte response (Zhang et al. 2009; Yodmuang et al. 2015; Khanarian et al. 2012; Zignego et al. 2014). Moreover, agarose implantation containing chondrocytes or mesenchymal stem cells (chondrocyte- or MSC-laden hydrogels) in osteochondral defects, which ensures physiologically relevant mechanical properties, allowing to repair tissue containing collagens and proteoglycans. Despite its promising performance, agarose has been poorly studied *in vivo* due to its inhibitory effect and inability to degrade *in vivo*, which prevents graft integration with the host tissue (Vinatier et al. 2009; Yodmuang et al. 2015; Khanarian et al. 2012). Furthermore, cartilage tissue formation within an agarose hydrogel is complicated by an inability to customize agarose scaffold structure and composition (Yodmuang et al. 2015).

4.3 Synthetic Biomaterials

Synthetic polymers, known for ease of process, chemical modification, biocompatibility, versatility, mechanical properties, and controllable biodegradability, have gained interest in tissue engineering applications in the last few decades (Zhang et al. 2009). In the context of tissue engineering, the currently used synthetic polymers are polylactic acid (PLLA), which exists in both L and D forms, polyglycolic acid (PGA), and their copolymer poly-lactic-co-glycolic acid (PLGA). The 3D matrices can be manufactured with these biodegradable polymers, which the FDA has approved. The subsequent topics will cover various instances of synthetic biomaterials (Zhang et al. 2009) with bioactive molecules for enhanced functionality (Djukić-Vuković et al. 2019; Capuana et al. 2022).

4.3.1 Poly(Lactic-Co-Glycolic Acid) (PLGA)

PLGA is a polypeptide with no antigenicity or immunogenicity (Fig. 4.11). It possesses good biological and physico-chemical properties (non-toxic, hydrophilic, and biodegradable) (Zhang et al. 2013). It is frequently used in drug delivery systems, tissue engineering, and medical implants. PLGA undergoes breakdown into non-toxic by-products, making it a safe choice for various biomedical uses.

PLGA can be synthesized through copolymerizing lactic and glycolic acids with a catalyst under controlled conditions. Due to its favourable properties, PLGA can be further processed into various forms, such as nanoparticles, microparticles, or scaffolds for biomedical applications. PLGA is known as a copolymer composed of lactic acid and glycolic acid. It is known for its antigenicity, immunogenicity, and non-toxic, hydrophilic, and biodegradable properties. This sustainable material offers a promising solution for developing eco-friendly medical devices and treatments. In contrast to traditional polymers, poly(lactic-co-glycolic acid) stands out for its biodegradability and compatibility with living tissues.

Interestingly, PLGA is among the most typical biomaterials being exploited in bone/cartilage tissue engineering strategies. However, conventional PLGA does not mimic important properties of biological tissue, including cartilage tissue (Zhu et al. 2014), which is why it is commonly studied as a complex component with other compounds.

A PLGA–P188–PLGA matrix microdevice was developed with an efficient, easy-to-handle and represents an injectable tool for cartilage repair (Morille et al. 2013). PLGA/chitosan polyelectrolyte complex also possesses excellent potential as a scaffold for cartilage tissue engineering (Zhang et al. 2013). It was found that it is feasible to repair articular cartilage using a single-layer porous PLGA structure with no exogenous cells and that cartilage regeneration can be improved further by applying short-term continuous passive motion (Chang et al. 2012). Moreover, Eswaramoorthy et al. showed that sustained PTH(1–34) release from PLGA microspheres suppresses osteoarthritis progression in rats (Eswaramoorthy et al. 2012).

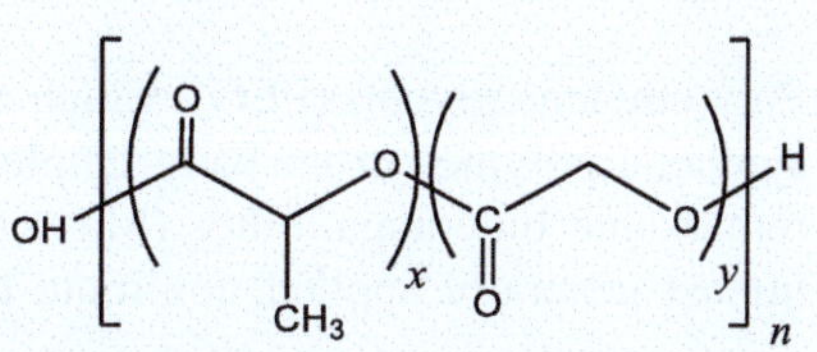

Fig. 4.11 Repeating unit of Poly(lactic-co-glycolic acid)

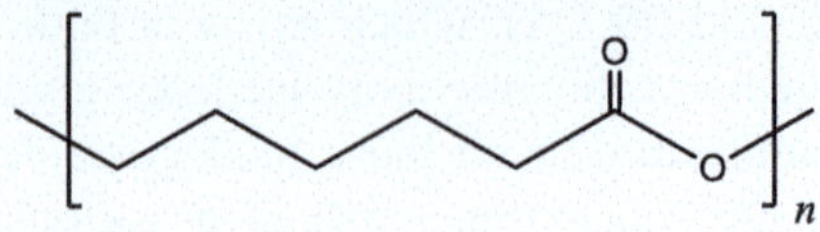

Fig. 4.12 Polycaprolactone unit

4.3.2 Polycaprolactone (PCL)

Polycaprolactone (PCL) is an FDA-approved biodegradable polymer (Danesin et al. 2012) (Fig. 4.12). It is a hydrophobic, semi-crystalline polymer, and its crystallinity tends to reduce with increasing molecular weight (Pan et al. 2012). Moreover, its good solubility, low melting point (59–64 °C), and excellent blend compatibility have made PCL a focus in the biomedical engineering area (Pan et al. 2012).

PCL is a polyester with a lower degradation profile, and it supports various cell types like skeletal muscle, smooth muscle, fibroblasts, chondrocytes, endothelial cells, and human mesenchymal stem cells (Danesin et al. 2012). Due to its viscoelastic properties, it has been used as the tissue-engineering scaffold for various organs or tissues, including bone, cartilage, tendon and ligament, blood vessels, skin, and nerve (Pan et al. 2012). For instance, PCL scaffolds manufactured by selective laser sintering (SLS) surface modified through immersion coating with Collagen are feasible for cartilage tissue engineering in craniofacial reconstruction (Chen et al. 2014). It is usually mixed with other compounds, such as MWNTs/PCL mixture composite scaffolds, that have the potential for bone TE (tissue engineering), and the relatively low concentration of MWNTs (0.5 wt%) is preferred (Pan et al. 2012). Creating more environmentally friendly solutions with long-lasting benefits is possible by utilizing sustainable materials such as PCL in composite scaffolds for tissue engineering. Incorporating growth factors further enhances the sustainability of these scaffolds by promoting efficient tissue regeneration. In addition, the use of 3D bioprinting technology not only allows for the precise fabrication of complex structures but minimizes waste, contributing to a more sustainable approach to tissue engineering. By incorporating MWNTs into PCL, environmentally friendly solutions that promote efficient tissue regeneration can be developed. The use of growth factors and 3D bioprinting technology further enhances the sustainability of these scaffolds, making them a promising approach in tissue engineering (Yilmaz et al. 2020).

4.3.3 Polyethylene Glycol (PEG)

Poly(ethylene glycol) (PEG), which arose in scientific literature in the 1980s, is a synthetic polymer extensively employed in biomedical applications owing to its remarkable biocompatibility (Masson et al. 1982; Dai et al. 2011). PEG is the utmost generally applied non-ionic hydrophilic polymer (Fig. 4.13) with stealth

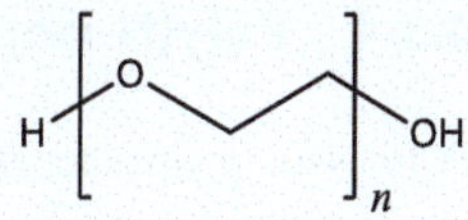

Fig. 4.13 Poly(ethylene glycol) repeating structure

behaviour and has been the most widely used polymer for antifouling applications, such that it has often been termed the "gold standard" of antifouling polymers (Knop et al. 2010; Konradi et al. 2012). PEGylation is a promising method for enhancing the properties of therapeutic compounds in drug delivery systems. It increases solubility and stability, reduces side effects, and improves drug circulation time, leading to more targeted treatment outcomes. PEGylation can tailor delivery systems to patients' specific needs, reducing the need for frequent dosing and improving treatment outcomes. Its ability to mask antigens on the surface also decreases immune response likelihood, making drugs suitable for a broader range of patients. The PEGylation approach contributes to: (i) raising the aqueous solubility and stability, (ii) decreasing immunogenicity, (iii) reducing intermolecular aggregation, and (iv) prolonging the systemic circulation time of a compound (Sah et al. 2013).

PEG can be produced with a diverse range of molar mass. It is used in a wide range of medical and pharmaceutical applications, fluctuating its molar mass from approximately 400 Da to 50 kDa. PEG, having a molar mass of 20 kDa to 50 kDa, is mainly used to conjugate low-molar-mass drugs as small molecules, oligonucleotides, and siRNA. PEGs with lower molar masses (1 kDa to 5 kDa) are frequently applied to conjugate larger drugs, such as antibodies or nanoparticle systems (Knop et al. 2010).

PEG macromonomers can be polymerized using mechanisms such as anionic, cationic, ring-opening metathesis, or free-radical polymerization, typically with acrylate and methacrylate groups (Bencherif et al. 2009; Dai et al. 2011; Kinard et al. 2012; Micic et al. 2000). PEG's biocompatibility and low immunogenicity make it an environmentally friendly choice for drug conjugation and delivery in various therapeutic settings. By utilizing PEG macromonomers in hydrogels, nanoparticles, and micelles, we can enhance the circulation time of drugs in the body while minimizing environmental impact. Ultimately, incorporating sustainable PEG-based materials into pharmaceutical applications aligns with efforts to promote eco-friendly practices within the healthcare industry.

The scaffolds made from PEG can also be chemically functionalized to contain bioactive molecules, including peptides and heparin. Together with stem cells and growth factors, these scaffolds have been evaluated for their suitability and showed promise as therapy for cartilage tissue regeneration (Hutanu et al. 2014; Ferretti et al. 2006).

4.3.4 Poly(N-isopropylacrylamide)

Poly(N-isopropylacrylamide) is a thermos-responsive polymer with 32 °C as the lower critical solution temperature (LCST), in aqueous solutions, making it suitable for biomedical applications. Its LCST can be removed by copolymerizing it with hydrophilic or hydrophobic monomers (da Silva et al. 2008; Constantin et al. 2011; Shen et al. 2006; Schilli et al. 2004). However, as the temperature is increased above its LCST, the polymer becomes hydrophobic by exposing the hydrophobic isopropyl groups to the water interface and becomes insoluble, experiencing a collapse into gel form (Bearat et al. 2011). Drug release can be controlled by adding them to a polymer matrix, which changes from hydrophilic to hydrophobic. It has been shown that this transition may involve the breakage of intermolecular hydrogen bonds with the water molecules, which are substituted by intramolecular hydrogen bonds amongst the dehydrated amide groups (Xu et al. 2020). The hydrophobic methyl groups on poly(NIPAAm) then break down, allowing entanglements of the polymer chains, resulting in a gel (Bearat et al. 2011). This polymer could also be used in tissue engineering, allowing cells to be encapsulated and released at specific temperatures. Poly(NIPAAm) is a commercially available polymer derived from N-isopropylacrylamide (Fig. 4.14).

It can be polymerized using various methods, including radical polymerization for high molecular weight polymers and controlled methods like nitroxide-mediated polymerization, anionic polymerization, adjustable addition-fragmentation chain transfer, and transfer radical polymerization (Spasojevic et al. 2014). Modifications of poly(NIPAAm) were reported to show a great interest in tailoring the LCST of poly(NIPAAm)-based systems. For example, N-isopropylacrylamide (NIPAAm) was copolymerized with N-acryloxysuccinimide (NASI) via free radical polymerization. For example, for *in vivo* applications poly(NIPAAm-co-NASI) was adapted towards poly(NIPAAm-co-cysteamine) over a nucleophilic attack on the carbonyl group of the NASI by the amine group of the cysteamine to create *in situ* physically and chemically crosslinking hydrogel (Robb et al. 2007).

Hydrogels using poly(NIPAAm)-based systems are being developed, reducing the need for single-use materials and promoting environmentally friendly medical treatments. That approach, using nucleophilic attacks, highlights the importance of

Fig. 4.14 Poly(N-isopropylacrylamide) repeating structure

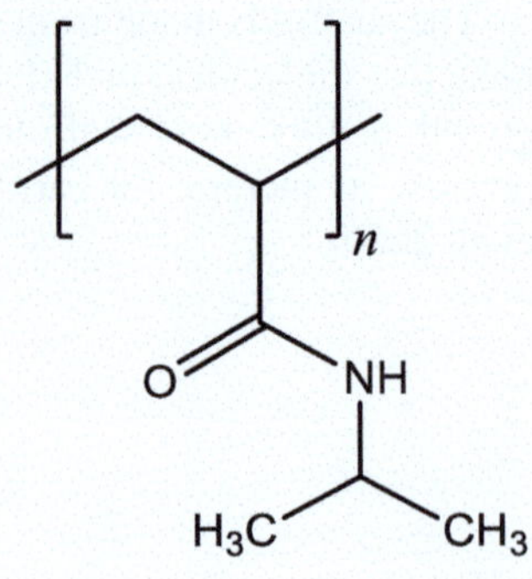

sustainable chemistry in developing innovative materials for various applications. It can offer cost-effective solutions and reduces healthcare's environmental impact, thus promoting a more sustainable future in biomedical fields. Such type of sustainable approach is crucial for advancing research and improving patient outcomes. The hydrophobic monomer is soluble in surfactant micelles, whereas the hydrophilic monomer is soluble in an aqueous media. Commercially accessible triblock copolymers, including PEO-PPO sequences, exhibit sol-gel transitions below physiological temperature, gel-sol transitions at 50 °C, and a lower critical solution temperature (LCST). Poly(NIPAAm) is thoroughly investigated for its applications in controlled drug delivery, cell-sheet engineering, biosensors, and tissue engineering (Spasojevic et al. 2014; Aguilar et al. 2007).

4.4 Sustainable Materials-Fabrication Techniques

Fabrication techniques for sustainable materials, including natural, synthetic, or modified bio-based polymeric materials, reduce manufacturing processes' environmental footprint and enhance the sustainability of these developed products (Arif et al. 2023). These procedures frequently employ renewable resources, reducing energy consumption and minimizing waste generation. Industries could contribute to more eco-friendly and resource-efficient future by implementing sustainable fabrication techniques.

4.4.1 Conventional Manufacturing Techniques

Controlling pore parameters and preserving architectural details while ensuring reproducibility is challenging with conventional manufacturing techniques.

There are several conventional scaffold fabrication methods, but they are mainly divided into 4 categories: (i) electrospinning, (ii) gas foaming, (iii) solvent casting/particulate leaching, and (iv) freeze drying. Other methods, such as electrospinning, sol-gel technique, and thermally induced phase separation, were considered conventional manufacturing techniques. These techniques face limitations in producing scaffolds with pores that are both fully interconnected and uniform in size and distribution. Moreover, it is difficult to completely prevent inconsistencies and variations during the fabrication process, which possibly causes the tissue constructs to be compromised (Krishani et al. 2023).

4.4.2 Additive Manufacturing (AM)

To better control the porosity and the distribution of the scaffolds, 3D printing technology has enabled the implementation of additive manufacturing (AM) techniques. This technology has been widely utilized in the field of tissue engineering to create personalized products for medical purposes. In fact, this technology focuses on producing medical devices customized for individual patients, thereby reducing material waste and allowing for biodegradable materials (Ullah et al. 2023; Patel and Taufik 2024).

Sustainable materials used in 3D printing should possess specific properties like biocompatibility, mechanical strength, thermal and structural stability, excellent processability, and printability. Indeed, these materials must preserve their exact shape accurately and facilitate exact 3D printing (Antezana et al. 2022). Among the several techniques for 3D printing sustainable polymeric materials, we can find inkjet printing (IJP) or binder jetting (BJ). This additive manufacturing process selectively deposits ink or a liquid binder material, layer-by-layer, to create 3D objects with precise control over their structure and composition. Another method is digital light processing (DLP), a photopolymerization-based technology that uses light to cure photopolymer resin layer by layer, creating 3D devices. Stereolithography (SLA) is a widely utilized printing technology that fabricating devices by curing photopolymer resin with a UV laser layer. It is recognized for its ability to produce high-resolution materials. Additionally, extrusion-based printing techniques (EB-AM) fall under a category of 3D printing methods where the material is heat up and extruded via a nozzle, layer by layer. This approach includes two leading technologies: filament extrusion and pellet extrusion, both known for their versatility, affordability, and ease of use.

The benefits and drawbacks of these advanced fabrication techniques for sustainable materials vary according to their application-specific requirements, collectively contributing to a more sustainable manufacturing paradigm aligning industrial practices with environmental stewardship and resource conservation (Arif et al. 2023).

4.4.3 Final Remarks and Future Perspective

The field of tissue engineering is progressing rapidly, and it's truly exciting to see the emphasis placed on incorporating sustainable biomaterials, both natural and synthetic, for its future development. The increasing focus on sustainability in medical applications is driven by the essential need for environmentally friendly, biocompatible, and functional materials that can be efficiently utilized in clinical settings. Natural biomaterials such as collagen, gellan gum, chitosan, and silk fibroin, among others, offer an array of unique benefits, including biodegradability and enhanced cell compatibility, turning them ideal for an extensive range of tissue engineering applications. Additionally, synthetic polymers like PLLA, PLGA, PCL, PEG, and poly(N-isopropylacrylamide) bring versatility and controllable mechanical properties, complementing natural biomaterials by providing structural stability and tunable degradation rates. This progressive approach holds great promise for the future of tissue engineering.

Biomaterials are utilized as artificial scaffolds to create a 3D environment that enhances cellular attachment, migration, proliferation, and differentiation. Working on a unique and sustainable approach to fabricate complex devices for tissue engineering applications is crucial. Conventional methods have been adopted to create biomaterials for tissue regeneration. However, these technologies are limited by their inability to construct highly complex structures. Due to these limitations, 3D printing has gained interest and grown as an attractive alternative. This technology fabricates 3D structures, producing highly complex, personalized structures that can fine-tune the properties of biomaterial-based devices. Natural and synthetic biopolymers have exceptional utilization as sustainable materials for tissue engineering applications due to their unique properties, which are biocompatible, renewable, and biodegradable. These biomaterials can be used to repair and regenerate tissues and organs and can be developed into medical devices. In the long term, adopting sustainable materials in tissue engineering can potentially revolutionize the medical field. It can lead to the development of new therapies that are not only highly effective but also environmentally responsible. As the global community continues emphasizing sustainability, the demand for green biomaterials will likely increase, encouraging further research and investment in this critical area. Ultimately, the future of sustainable materials in tissue engineering promises to create a healthier planet while advancing medical science and improving patient care.

Acknowledgements H. Radhouani and C. Gonçalves were supported by FCT (Foundation for Science and Technology) from Portugal, with references CEECIND/00111/2017 and SFRH/BPD/94277/2013, respectively. The authors acknowledge the financial support provided under the projects "TERM RES Hub – Scientific Infrastructure for Tissue Engineering and Regenerative Medicine" and "ICVS/3 B's – Associate Laboratory, Life and Health Sciences Research Institute / Biomaterials, Biodegradables and Biomimetics Research Group, LA/P/0050/2020". The authors thank ONCOSCREEN project funded by the European Union's Horizon Europe research and innovation programme under grant agreement No. 101097036.

References

Aberoumand A (2012) Comparative study between different methods of Collagen extraction from fish and its properties. World Appl Sci J 16(3):316–319

Aguilar MR et al (2007) Smart polymers and their applications as biomaterials. In: Ashammakhi N, Reis R, Chiellini E (eds) Topics in tissue engineering

Al Mahmud MZ, Mobarak MH, Hossain N (2024) Emerging trends in biomaterials for sustainable food packaging: A comprehensive review. Heliyon 10:e24122

Andersen T et al (2012) Alginates as biomaterials in tissue engineering. J Carbohydr Chem 37:227–258

Antezana PE et al (2022) The 3D bioprinted scaffolds for wound healing. Pharmaceutics 14(2):464

Aranaz I et al (2021) Chitosan: an overview of its properties and applications. Polymers 13(19):3256

Aranda FL, Zúñiga M, Rivas BL (2023) Polymers in circular economy: a comprehensive approach to sustainability. An overview. J Chil Chem Soc 68(3):5950–5962

Arif ZU et al (2023) Additive manufacturing of sustainable biomaterials for biomedical applications. Asian J Pharm Sci 18(3):100812

Baran ET et al (2012) Enzymatic degradation behavior and cytocompatibility of silk fibroin-starch-chitosan conjugate membranes. Mater Sci Eng C Mater Biol Appl 32(6):1314–1322

Bearat HH et al (2011) Synthesis, characterization and properties of a physically and chemically gelling polymer system using Poly(NIPAAm-co-HEMA-acrylate) and Poly(NIPAAm-co-cysteamine). J Biomater Sci 22:1299–1318

Bell AD et al (2012) Bone-induced Chondroinduction in Sheep Jamshidi biopsy defects with and without treatment by subchondral chitosan-blood implant: 1-day, 3-week, and 3-month repair. Cartilage 4(2):131–143

Bencherif SA et al (2009) End-group effects on the properties of PEG-co-PGA hydrogels. Acta Biomater 5(6):1872–1883

Bhardwaj N, Kundu SC (2011) Silk fibroin protein and chitosan polyelectrolyte complex porous scaffolds for tissue engineering applications. Carbohydr Polym 85(2):325–333

Bhardwaj N et al (2011) Potential of 3-D tissue constructs engineered from bovine chondrocytes/silk fibroin-chitosan for in vitro cartilage tissue engineering. Biomaterials 32(25):5773–5781

Biswal T, BadJena SK, Pradhan D (2020) Sustainable biomaterials and their applications: a short review. Mater Today: Proc 30:274–282

Boeriu CG et al (2013) Production methods for hyaluronan. Int J Carbohydr Chem 2013:14

Borsig L et al (2007) Selectin blocking activity of a fucosylated chondroitin sulfate glycosaminoglycan from sea cucumber – effect on tumor metastasis and neutrophil recruitment. J Biol Chem 282(20):14984–14991

Burke KE et al (1983) Bovine collagen implant: histologic chronology in pig dermis. J Dermatol Surg Oncol 9(11):889–895

Cao D, Ding J (2022) Recent advances in regenerative biomaterials. Regen Biomater 9:rbac098

Capuana E et al (2022) Poly-l-lactic acid (PLLA)-based biomaterials for regenerative medicine: a review on processing and applications. Polymers 14(6):1153

Chang NJ et al (2012) The combined effects of continuous passive motion treatment and acellular PLGA implants on osteochondral regeneration in the rabbit. Biomaterials 33(11):3153–3163

Chen JS et al (2000) Shark cartilage extract interferes with cell adhesion and induces reorganization of focal adhesions in cultured endothelial cells. J Cell Biochem 78(3):417–428

Chen C-H et al (2014) Cartilage tissue engineering with silk fibroin scaffolds fabricated by indirect additive manufacturing technology. Materials 7(3):2104–2119

Cole AG, Hall BK (2004) The nature and significance of invertebrate cartilages revisited: distribution and histology of cartilage and cartilage-like tissues within the Metazoa. Zoology 107(4):261–273

Collins MN, Birkinshaw C (2008) Physical properties of crosslinked hyaluronic acid hydrogels. J Mater Sci Mater Med 19(11):3335–3343

Collins MN, Birkinshaw C (2013) Hyaluronic acid based scaffolds for tissue engineering—a review. Carbohydr Polym 92(2):1262–1279

Constantin M et al (2011) Lower critical solution temperature versus volume phase transition temperature in thermoresponsive drug delivery systems. eXPRESS. Polym Lett 5(10):839–848

Coutinho DF et al (2010) Modified Gellan gum hydrogels with tunable physical and mechanical properties. Biomaterials 31(29):7494–7502

da Silva RMP et al (2008) Poly(N-Isopropylacrylamide) surface-grafted chitosan membranes as a new substrate for cell sheet engineering and manipulation. Biotechnol Bioeng 101(6):1321–1331

da Silva LP et al (2014) Engineering cell-adhesive gellan gum spongy-like hydrogels for regenerative medicine purposes. Acta Biomater 10(11):4787–4797

Dai X et al (2011) Free radical polymerization of poly(ethylene glycol) diacrylate macromers: impact of macromer hydrophobicity and initiator chemistry on polymerization efficiency. Acta Biomater 7(5):1965–1972

Danesin R et al (2012) Self-assembling peptide-enriched electrospun polycaprolactone scaffolds promote the h-osteoblast adhesion and modulate differentiation-associated gene expression. Bone 51(5):851–859

Djukić-Vuković A et al (2019) Towards sustainability of lactic acid and poly-lactic acid polymers production. Renew Sustain Energy Rev 108:238–252

Draget KI, Smidsrød O, Skjåk-Bræk G (2005) Alginates from algae, in biopolymers online. Wiley Online Libray

Dunne LW et al (2014) Characterization of dielectrophoresis-aligned nanofibrous silk fibroin-chitosan scaffold and its interactions with endothelial cells for tissue engineering applications. Acta Biomater 10(8):3630–3640

Eswaramoorthy R et al (2012) Sustained release of PTH (1–34) from PLGA microspheres suppresses osteoarthritis progression in rats. Acta biomaterialia 8(6):2254–2262

Fang J et al (2014) Poly(L-glutamic acid)/chitosan polyelectrolyte complex porous microspheres as cell microcarriers for cartilage regeneration. Acta Biomater 10(1):276–288

Ferretti M et al (2006) Controlled in vivo degradation of genipin crosslinked polyethylene glycol hydrogels within osteochondral defects. Tissue Eng 12(9):2657–2663

Fertah M et al (2015) Extraction and characterization of sodium alginate from Moroccan Laminaria digitata brown seaweed. Arab J Chem 8(1):1–142

Filippi M et al (2020) Use of nanoparticles in skeletal tissue regeneration and engineering

Foss C et al (2013) Silk fibroin/hyaluronic acid 3D matrices for cartilage tissue engineering. Biomacromolecules 14(1):38–47

Gong X et al (2014) Physiological pulsatile flow culture conditions to generate functional endothelium on a sulfated silk fibroin nanofibrous scaffold. Biomaterials 35(17):4782–4791

Gorgieva S, Kokol V (2011) Collagen- vs. Gelatine-based biomaterials and their biocompatibility: review and perspectives. In: Pignatello R (ed) Biomaterials applications for Nanomedicine. INTECH Open Access Publisher

Harris AF, Lacombe J, Zenhausern F (2021) The emerging role of decellularized plant-based scaffolds as a new biomaterial. Int J Mol Sci 22(22):12347

Hashimoto T et al (2015) Changes in the properties and protein structure of silk fibroin molecules in autoclaved fabrics. Polym Degrad Stab 112:20–26

Haug A (1964) Composition and properties of alginates. Norwegian Institute of Technology, Trondheim

Haug A, Larsen B (1966) A study on the constitution of alginic acid by partial acid hydrolysis. Proc Int Seaweed Symp 5:271–277

Haug A, Larsen B, Smidsrød O (1966) A study of the constitution of alginic acid by partial hydrolysis. Acta Chem Scand 20:183–190

Hutanu D et al (2014) Recent applications of polyethylene glycols (PEGs) and PEG derivatives. Mod Chem Appl 2(12)

Ibrahim H, El-Zairy EJC (2015) Chitosan as a biomaterial—structure, properties, and electrospun nanofibers. 1(1):81–101

Jerosch J (2011) Effects of glucosamine and chondroitin sulfate on cartilage metabolism in OA: outlook on other nutrient partners especially Omega-3 fatty acids. Int J Rheumatol 2011:17

Jin SH et al (2014a) The effects of tetracycline-loaded silk fibroin membrane on proliferation and osteogenic potential of mesenchymal stem cells. J Surg Res 192(2):e1–e9

Jin J et al (2014b) Transplantation of human placenta-derived mesenchymal stem cells in a silk fibroin/hydroxyapatite scaffold improves bone repair in rabbits. J Biosci Bioeng 118(5):593–598

Jongjareonrak A (2006) Characterization and functional properties of collagen and gelatin from Bigeye Snapper (Priacanthus macracanthus) and Brownstripe Red Snapper (Lutjanus vitta) skins. Prince of Songkla University

Joyce K et al (2021) Bioactive potential of natural biomaterials: Identification, retention and assessment of biological properties. Signal Transduct Target Ther 6(1):122

Kang JY et al (2009) Novel porous matrix of hyaluronic acid for the three-dimensional culture of chondrocytes. Int J Pharm 369(1–2):114–120

Kang D, Zhang F, Zhang H (2015) Fabrication of stable aqueous dispersions of graphene using gellan gum as a reducing and stabilizing agent and its nanohybrids. Mater Chem Phys 149-150:129–139

Karamanos NK et al (1988) Extraction and fractionation of proteoglycans from squid skin. Biochim Biophys Acta 966(1):36–43

Khanarian NT et al (2012) A functional agarose-hydroxyapatite scaffold for osteochondral interface regeneration. Biomaterials 33(21):5247–5258

Kim S-K (2015) In: Kim S-K (ed) Springer handbook of marine biotechnology. Springer, London

Kim IL, Mauck RL, Burdick JA (2011) Hydrogel design for cartilage tissue engineering: a case study with hyaluronic acid. Biomaterials 32(34):8771–8782
Kinard LA, Kasper FK, Mikos AG (2012) Synthesis of oligo(poly(ethylene glycol) fumarate). Nat Protoc 7(6):1219–1227
Kloareg B, Quatrano RS (1988) Structure of the cell-walls of marine-algae and ecophysiological functions of the matrix polysaccharides. Oceanogr Mar Biol 26:259–315
Knop K et al (2010) Poly(ethylene glycol) in drug delivery: pros and cons as well as potential alternatives. Angew Chem 49(36):6288–6308
Kock L, van Donkelaar CC, Ito K (2012) Tissue engineering of functional articular cartilage: the current status. Cell Tissue Res 347(3):613–627
Konradi R, Acikgoz C, Textor M (2012) Polyoxazolines for nonfouling surface coatings—a direct comparison to the gold standard PEG. Macromol Rapid Commun 33(19):1663–1676
Krishani M et al (2023) Development of scaffolds from bio-based natural materials for tissue regeneration applications: a review. Gels 9(2):100
Lafantaisie-Favreau CH et al (2013) Subchondral pre-solidified chitosan/blood implants elicit reproducible early osteochondral wound-repair responses including neutrophil and stromal cell chemotaxis, bone resorption and repair, enhanced repair tissue integration and delayed matrix deposition. BMC Musculoskelet Disord 14:27
Lai JY et al (2012) Nanoscale modification of porous gelatin scaffolds with chondroitin sulfate for corneal stromal tissue engineering. Int J Nanomedicine 7:1101–1114
Lai GJ et al (2014) Composite chitosan/silk fibroin nanofibers for modulation of osteogenic differentiation and proliferation of human mesenchymal stem cells. Carbohydr Polym 111:288–297
Lebbar S et al (2018) Agar extraction by-products from Gelidium sesquipedale as a source of glycerol-galactosides. Molecules 23(12):3364
Li H et al (2004) Studies on bullfrog skin collagen. Food Chem 84(1):65–69
Li C et al (2023) Green production and green technology for sustainability: the mediating role of waste reduction and energy use. Heliyon 9(12):e22496
Liu L et al (2011) Microbial production of hyaluronic acid: current state, challenges, and perspectives. Microb Cell Factories 10:99
Ma PX (2008) Biomimetic materials for tissue engineering. Adv Drug Deliv Rev 60(2):184–198
Mahmud MZA, Islam MD, Mobarak MH (2023) The development of eco-friendly biopolymers for use in tissue engineering and drug delivery. J Nanomater 2023(1):9270064
Mano JF (2013) Biomimetic approaches for biomaterials development. John Wiley & Sons
Masson P et al (1982) Synthesis of polyethylene oxide macromers. Polym Bull 7(1):17–22
Mathieu C et al (2013) Stereological analysis of subchondral angiogenesis induced by chitosan and coagulation factors in microdrilled articular cartilage defects. Osteoarthr Cartil 21(6):849–859
Meyer K, Palmer JW (1934a) The polysaccharide of the vitreous humor. J Biol Chem 107(3):629–634
Meyer K, Palmer JW (1934b) The polysaccharide of the vitreous humor. J Biol Chem 107:629–634
Michelacci YM, Dietrich CP (1976) Structure of chondroitin sulfates. Analyses of the products formed from chondroitin sulfates A and C by the action of the chondroitinases C and AC from Flavobacterium heparinum. Biochim Biophys Acta 451(2):436–443
Micic M et al (2000) A comparative study of enzymatically and photochemically polymerized artificial lignin supramolecular structures using environmental scanning electron microscopy. J Colloid Interface Sci 231(1):190–194
Mirahmadi F et al (2013) Enhanced mechanical properties of thermosensitive chitosan hydrogel by silk fibers for cartilage tissue engineering. Mater Sci Eng C Mater Biol Appl 33(8):4786–4794
Morille M et al (2013) New PLGA-P188-PLGA matrix enhances TGF-beta3 release from pharmacologically active microcarriers and promotes chondrogenesis of mesenchymal stem cells. J Control Release 170(1):99–110
Muller FA et al (2006) Cellulose-based scaffold materials for cartilage tissue engineering. Biomaterials 27(21):3955–3963
Murado MA et al (2012) Optimization of extraction and purification process of hyaluronic acid from fish eyeball. Food Bioprod Process 90(C3):491–498

Naeimi M et al (2014) Silk fibroin-chondroitin sulfate-alginate porous scaffolds structural properties and in vitro studies. J Appl Polym Sci 131

Nagai T, Suzuki N (2000) Isolation of collagen from fish waste material – skin, bone and fins. Food Chem 68(3):277–281

Nalamothu N, Potluri A, Muppalla MB (2014) Review on marine alginates and its applications. Indo Am J Pharm Res 4(10):4006–4015

Noitup P, Garnjanagoonchorn W, Morrissey MT (2005) Fish skin type I Collagen characteristic comparison of albacore tuna (Thunnus alalunga) and silver-line grunt (Pomadasys kaakan). J Aquat Food Prod Technol 14(1):17–27

Noro J et al (2024) Extracellular matrix-derived materials for tissue engineering and regenerative medicine: a journey from isolation to characterization and application. Bioact Mater 34:494–519

Novac O et al (2014) Antibacterial quaternized gellan gum based particles for controlled release of ciprofloxacin with potential dermal applications. Mater Sci Eng C Mater Biol Appl 35:291–299

Ogawa M et al (2003) Biochemical properties of black drum and sheepshead seabream skin collagen. J Agric Food Chem 51(27):8088–8092

Oliveira JT et al (2010) Gellan gum: a new biomaterial for cartilage tissue engineering applications. J Biomed Mater Res A 93(3):852–863

Ong KL, Lovald S, Black J (2015) In: L. Taylor and Francis Group (ed) Orthopaedic biomaterials in research and practice, 2nd edn. CRC Press, Boca Raton, p 476

Oprenyeszk F et al (2013) Protective effect of a new biomaterial against the development of experimental osteoarthritis lesions in rabbit: a pilot study evaluating the intra-articular injection of alginate-chitosan beads dispersed in an hydrogel. Osteoarthr Cartil 21(8):1099–1107

Orellana J (2013) Advanced biomaterials from renewable resources: an investigation on cellulose nanocrystal composites and CO2 extraction of rendered materials in Graduate School of Clemson University. Clemson University, Clemson

Osmalek T, Froelich A, Tasarek S (2014) Application of gellan gum in pharmacy and medicine. Int J Pharm 466(1–2):328–340

Owczarzy A et al (2020) Collagen-structure, properties and application. Eng Biomater 23(156)

Pan L et al (2012) Multiwall carbon nanotubes/polycaprolactone composites for bone tissue engineering application. Colloids Surf B Biointerfaces 93:226–234

Parenteau-Bareil R, Gauvin R, Berthod F (2010) Collagen-based biomaterials for tissue engineering applications. Materials 3(3):1863–1887

Patel A, Taufik M (2024) Extrusion-based technology in additive manufacturing: a comprehensive review. Arab J Sci Eng 49(2):1309–1342

Potaros T et al (2009) Characteristics of Collagen from Nile tilapia (Oreochromis niloticus) skin isolated by two different methods. Kasetsart J 43:584–593

Prajapati VD et al (2013) An insight into the emerging exopolysaccharide gellan gum as a novel polymer. Carbohydr Polym 93(2):670–678

Priks H et al (2020) Physical confinement impacts cellular phenotypes within living materials. ACS Appl Bio Mater 3(7):4273–4281

Rajabimashhadi Z et al (2023) Collagen derived from fish industry waste: progresses and challenges. Polymers (Basel) 15(3):544

Robb SA et al (2007) Simultaneously physically and chemically gelling polymer system utilizing a poly(NIPAAm-co-cysteamine)-based copolymer. Biomacromolecules 8(7):2294–2300

Sah H et al (2013) Concepts and practices used to develop functional PLGA-based nanoparticulate systems. Int J Nanomedicine 8:747–765

Saha S et al (2013) Osteochondral tissue engineering in vivo: a comparative study using layered silk fibroin scaffolds from mulberry and nonmulberry silkworms. PLoS One 8(11):e80004

Schilli CM et al (2004) A new double-responsive block copolymer synthesized via RAFT polymerization: poly(N-isopropylacrylamide)-block-poly(acrylic acid). Macromolecules 37(21):7861–7866

Seno N, Meyer K (1963) Comparative biochemistry of skin; the mucopolysaccharides of shark skin. Biochim Biophys Acta 78:258–264

Shen ZY et al (2006) Synthesis and phase behavior of aqueous poly(N-isopropylacrylamide-co-acrylamide), poly(N-isopropylacrylamide-co-N,N-dimethylacrylamide) and poly (N-isopropylacrylamide-co-2-hydroxyethyl methacrylate). Colloid Polym Sci 284(9):1001–1007

Shen B et al (2010) Hyaluronan: its potential application in intervertebral disc regeneration. Orthop Res Rev 2:17–26

Shi YG et al (2014) Chondroitin sulfate: extraction, purification, microbial and chemical synthesis. J Chem Technol Biotechnol 89(10):1445–1465

Shogren R et al (2019) Plant-based materials and transitioning to a circular economy. Sustain Prod Consump 19:194–215

Silva SS et al (2008) Novel Genipin-cross-linked chitosan silk fibroin sponges for cartilage engineering strategies novel Genipin-cross. Biomacromolecules 9:2764–2774

Silva TH et al (2012) Materials of marine origin: a review on polymers and ceramics of biomedical interest. Int Mater Rev 57(5):276–306

Sionkowska A, Płanecka A (2013) Surface properties of thin films based on the mixtures of chitosan and silk fibroin. J Mol Liq 186:157–162

Sionkowska A et al (2014) The influence of UV-irradiation on thermal and mechanical properties of chitosan and silk fibroin mixtures. J Photochem Photobiol B 140:301–305

Spasojevic M et al (2014) Synthesis and phase behavior of Poly(N-isopropylacrylamide)-b-Poly(L-Lysine Hydrochloride) and Poly(N-Isopropylacrylamide-co-Acrylamide)-b-Poly(L-Lysine Hydrochloride). Materials 7(7):5305–5326

Srinivasan SR et al (1969) Glycosaminoglycans from squid skin. Comp Biochem Physiol 28(1):169–176

Sugahara K et al (1996) Novel sulfated oligosaccharides containing 3-O-sulfated glucuronic acid from king crab cartilage chondroitin sulfate K. Unexpected degradation by chondroitinase ABC. J Biol Chem 271(43):26745–26754

Suzuki Y (2016) Structures of silk fibroin before and after spinning and biomedical applications. Polym J 48(11):1039–1044

Tabatabai AP, Kaplan DL, Blair DL (2015) Rheology of reconstituted silk fibroin protein gels: the epitome of extreme mechanics. Soft Matter 11(4):756–761

Tang Y et al (2012) An improved complex gel of modified gellan gum and carboxymethyl chitosan for chondrocytes encapsulation. Carbohydr Polym 88(1):46–53

Ullah M et al (2023) 3D printing technology: a new approach for the fabrication of personalized and customized pharmaceuticals. Eur Polym J 195:112240

Vauchel P et al (2009) Kinetics modeling of alginate alkaline extraction from Laminaria digitata. Bioresour Technol 100(3):1291–1296

Vazquez JA et al (2013) Chondroitin sulfate, hyaluronic acid and chitin/chitosan production using marine waste sources: characteristics, applications and eco-friendly processes: a review. Mar Drugs 11(3):747–774

Vinatier C et al (2009) Cartilage tissue engineering: towards a biomaterial-assisted mesenchymal stem cell therapy. Curr Stem Cell Res Ther 4(4):318–329

Vu B et al (2009) Bacterial extracellular polysaccharides involved in biofilm formation. Molecules 14(7):2535–2554

Xu X et al (2020) Poly (N-isopropylacrylamide)-based thermoresponsive composite hydrogels for biomedical applications. Polymers 12(3):580

Yan LP et al (2012) Macro/microporous silk fibroin scaffolds with potential for articular cartilage and meniscus tissue engineering applications. Acta Biomater 8(1):289–301

Yilmaz B, Tahmasebifar A, Baran ET (2020) Bioprinting technologies in tissue engineering. In: Current applications of pharmaceutical biotechnology, pp 279–319

Yodmuang S et al (2015) Silk microfiber-reinforced silk hydrogel composites for functional cartilage tissue repair. Acta Biomater 11:27–36

Yudoh K, Karasawa R (2012) A novel biomaterial for cartilage repair generated by self-assembly: creation of a self-organized articular cartilage-like tissue. J Biomater Nanobiotechnol 3:125–129

Zhang Y-Q et al (2007) Formation of silk fibroin nanoparticles in water-miscible organic solvent and their characterization. J Nanopart Res 9:885–900
Zhang L, Hu J, Athanasiou KA (2009) The role of tissue engineering in articular cartilage repair and regeneration. Crit Rev Biomed Eng 37(1–2):1–57
Zhang K et al (2013) Repair of an articular cartilage defect using adipose-derived stem cells loaded on a polyelectrolyte complex scaffold based on poly(l-glutamic acid) and chitosan. Acta Biomater 9(7):7276–7288
Zhao F et al (2014) The application of polysaccharide biocomposites to repair cartilage defects. Int J Polym Sci 2014:9
Zhu Y et al (2014) Manufacture of layered collagen/chitosan-polycaprolactone scaffolds with biomimetic microarchitecture. Colloids Surf B Biointerfaces 113:352–360
Zignego DL et al (2014) The mechanical microenvironment of high concentration agarose for applying deformation to primary chondrocytes. J Biomech 47(9):2143–2148

Advancements in Lignin-Based Binders in Medical Application: From Extraction to Applications

5

Anass Ait Benhamou, Hamza Daoudi,
Abdelghani Boussetta, Mehdi Mennani, Amine Moubarik,
and Véronic Landry

Abstract

Lignin, a renewable and abundant biopolyphenol, promises to revolutionize biomedical applications, particularly in the field of nanomedicine. Its inherent adaptability, functionalization capabilities, and nanoparticle production potential make it an attractive candidate for tackling crucial healthcare challenges. Ongoing research continues to reveal lignin's vast potential in nanomedicine, offering opportunities to develop safer, more effective, and environmentally sustainable therapeutic solutions. Lignin is used in a variety of biomedical applications, including drug delivery systems, scaffolds for tissue engineering, wound healing dressings, and diagnostic imaging agents, among others. However, realizing lignin's full potential is impeded by several challenges and obstacles that need to be overcome. These include biocompatibility with biological systems, scalability of production processes, stability of lignin-based materials, controlled release kinetics of therapeutic agents, regulatory hurdles, and cost-effectiveness. Overcoming these challenges requires interdisciplinary collaboration and

A. A. Benhamou (✉) · V. Landry
Department of Wood and Forest Sciences, Renewable Materials Research Centre (CRMR), Laval University, Quebec, QC, Canada
e-mail: anass.ait-benhamou.1@ulaval.ca

H. Daoudi
Institut national de la recherche scientifique – Centre Eau Terre Environnement, Université du Québec, Quebec, QC, Canada

A. Boussetta · M. Mennani
Materials Science, Energy and Nanoengineering Department (MSN), Mohammed VI Polytechnic University (UM6P), Benguerir, Morocco

A. Moubarik
Chemical Processes and Applied Materials Laboratory, Polydisciplinary Faculty, Sultan Moulay Slimane University (USMS), Beni Mellal, Morocco

M. N. Collins, M. Culebras (eds.), *Sustainable Biopolymers and Composites for Biomedical Applications*, Biomaterials, Bioengineering and Sustainability 5,
https://doi.org/10.1007/978-3-031-91972-5_5

innovative approaches to optimize lignin-based formulations for biomedical use. This work provides an up-to-date survey of the role of lignin in biomedical applications, highlights the challenges that need to be addressed, and outlines the promising prospects for lignin-based innovations in healthcare.

Keywords

Lignin · Adhesive · Hydrogel · Healthcare · Medical applications · Drug delivery · Nanoparticles

5.1 Introduction

The over-reliance on materials and chemicals derived from petroleum and petrochemicals has become a critical issue impacting waste management, environmental integrity, and global energy sustainability. The intensive use of fossil fuels such as coal, oil, and natural gas for power generation, transportation, and industrial operations is one of the main factors behind this problem. These activities release considerable volumes of CO_2 and other pollutants, amplifying the greenhouse effect and accelerating climate change (Imlimthan et al. 2021; Mennani et al. 2024). In addition, conventional processes for converting fossil resources into chemicals are particularly resource-intensive and costly, while generating potentially hazardous by-products (Lopez et al. 2023; Serrano-Ruiz 2020). In response, concerted efforts have been made to explore alternative resources that can replace non-renewable materials, reduce environmental waste streams, and support the transition to a circular economy model. Renewable resources, including biomass, solar, wind, and hydroelectric power, offer sustainable substitutes for fossil fuels by taking advantage of natural energy cycles (Chen et al. 2015; Yang et al. 2024). Among these resources, biomass stands out as a highly promising renewable raw material for a variety of applications covering power generation, transportation fuels, and the production of various bioproducts. Derived from a multitude of sustainable sources such as plants, trees, agricultural residues and organic waste, biomass constitutes a vast and renewable reservoir of organic matter (Kasbaji et al. 2023; Kassab et al. 2020; El Achaby et al. 2018). Biomass is a sustainable and ecologically beneficial resource since it can be organically renewed via processes like photosynthesis, unlike limited, non-renewable fossil fuels. In addition, biomass offers the potential to foster economic growth in rural areas through the development of the bioenergy and bioproducts sectors.

Lignin, which accounts for around 15–35% of lignocellulosic biomass, is a dominant component derived from the wood and paper industries and is the world's second most abundant natural polymer (Mennani et al. 2023; Zhang et al. 2021; Moubarik et al. 2013). Its complex structure is made up of crosslinked polyphenolic compounds, serving as a crucial element in plant cell walls to ensure structural integrity and support. Despite its ubiquity and inherent properties, the use of industrial lignin waste remains surprisingly low, with around 2% currently exploited commercially (Stanisz et al. 2022; Sugiarto et al. 2022). The main application for used lignins is to convert them into lignosulfonates, mainly used as additives in building materials. Most of the residual lignin is relegated to the status of low-grade fuel or, unfortunately, discarded as waste. Global lignin production has reached significant volumes, reflecting an estimated market size of 954.5 million USD in 2019. Projections point to a modest annual growth rate of 2% by 2027, underlining the potential for exploration and exploitation of this abundant, under-utilized resource (Beaucamp et al. 2022; Liao et al. 2020).

In the biomedical field, natural polymers such as cellulose, alginate, chitosan, and chitin are some of the most commonly used materials in the development of drug delivery and tissue engineering due to their unique mechanical properties, availability, biodegradability, and biosafety (Gheorghita Puscaselu et al. 2020; Seddiqi et al. 2021; Anitha et al. 2014). Interestingly, biopolymers are often derived from natural sources, such as plants, animals, or microorganisms, which renders them inherently biocompatible. This means they are well-tolerated by living organisms and are less likely to cause adverse reactions or trigger immune responses when implanted or used in medical devices. Furthermore, the bio-degradability of biopolymers is particularly beneficial for temporary implants or drug delivery systems, as it reduces the risk of long-term complications and eliminates the need for additional surgical procedures to remove the material (Rebelo et al. 2017; Jeevanandam et al. 2022; Baranwal et al. 2022). In this regard, lignin is emerging as a binder, copolymer and support for a variety of medical applications. Lignin exhibits inherent antimicrobial properties, making it effective against a broad spectrum of bacteria, fungi, and other microorganisms (Imlimthan et al. 2021; Luzi et al. 2021). Lignin can be modified to enhance its biocompatibility, allowing it to interact favorably with biological systems without eliciting adverse reactions. This property makes lignin-based materials suitable for use in various biomedical applications, including tissue engineering, drug delivery, and regenerative medicine. Besides, lignin contains phenolic compounds that possess antioxidant and anti-inflammatory properties, which can help mitigate oxidative stress and inflammation in biological tissues (Imlimthan et al. 2021; Sugiarto et al. 2022).

Ongoing research efforts aim to further explore the potential of lignin in biomedical applications, to address pressing healthcare challenges and improve clinical outcomes. This comprehensive exploration elucidates the current status and progress of lignin as an emerging and sustainable biomaterial with diverse medical applications. From wound healing and tissue engineering to drug delivery systems and implantable devices, lignin shows promise as a versatile and environmentally friendly alternative to conventional materials. This work offers valuable insight into the utilization of lignin in the development of bio-binders for medical applications, highlighting its unique properties such as antimicrobial activity, biocompatibility, and durability. By emphasizing lignin's multifaceted role in healthcare, this research contributes to ongoing efforts to develop innovative and sustainable solutions to medical challenges, ultimately benefiting patients and healthcare systems worldwide.

5.2 Fundamentals of Lignin

5.2.1 Lignin: Structure-Property Connections

Wood, much like cellulose and hemicellulose, harbors lignin within its composition (Vaezi and Asadpour 2022; Miao and Hamad 2019; Rybarczyk et al. 2019; Kallel et al. 2016). The proportion of lignin in lignocellulosic raw materials can range from 10% to 35%, depending on the source, as shown in Table 5.1 (Zevallos Torres et al. 2020; García et al. 2014; Van Den Bosch et al. 2015). The cellulose fibers are organized cylindrically inside wood cells and are covered in lignin. Lignin is mostly made up of aromatic alcohols like p-coumaryl, coniferyl, and sinapyl (Gellerstedt et al. 2009). What makes lignin unique is how many methoxy groups it has; more methoxy groups make crosslinking procedures easier. Monolignols, or hydroxyl cinnamyl alcohol monomers (p-coumaryl, coniferyl, and sinapyl alcohol), are dehydrogenatively polymerized to produce lignin (Zevallos Torres et al. 2020; García et al. 2014; Ralph et al. 2023). Technical lignin is mostly a byproduct of the pulp and paper industries and is mostly used in low-cost energy applications. The lignin is classified according to the industrial pulping processes (such as kraft, sulfite, soda, and organosolv techniques) that were used to remove it (Mboowa 2024; Erdocia et al. 2021; José et al. 2020).

Building models for different kinds of lignin is possible, but it requires meticulous execution in accordance with strict mechanistic guidelines. The lignin structures for the three main plant types are depicted in Fig. 5.1.

- *Class (a) – Gymnosperm/Softwood lignin* (Fig. 5.1a): A total of 20 monomeric units, all G-units derived from coniferyl alcohol; two cinnamyl alcohol end group units X from the chain-starting dimerization reactions, both phenylcoumarans B; one respinol C, which is also a starting point for the monolignol dimerization chain; this means that the 20-mer lignin chain has three starting points due to the oligomer-oligomer coupling in the D and E structures; one spirodienone F, emphasizing the reason why one phenolic group in lignin is never etherified – it is actually a conjugated ketone; one biphenyl ether E; and 12 β-ether units A (Sun and Cheng 2002).
- *Class (b) – Angiosperm/Hardwood lignin* (Fig. 5.1b): 13 S and 7 G monomeric units; one phenolic alcohol endgroup unit X from a chain-starting dimerization reaction; one phenylcoumaran B; one resinol C, which is also a starting point for the monolignol dimerization chain; the 20-mer lignin chain has two starting points due to the oligomer-oligomer coupling in the E structure; 1 biphenyl ether

Table 5.1 Cellulose, hemicellulose, and lignin contents in different plant types (Sun and Cheng 2002)

Plant type	Cellulose (%)	Hemicellulose (%)	Lignin (%)
Hardwood	40–55	24–40	18–25
Softwood	45–50	25–35	25–35
Grass	25–40	35–50	10–30

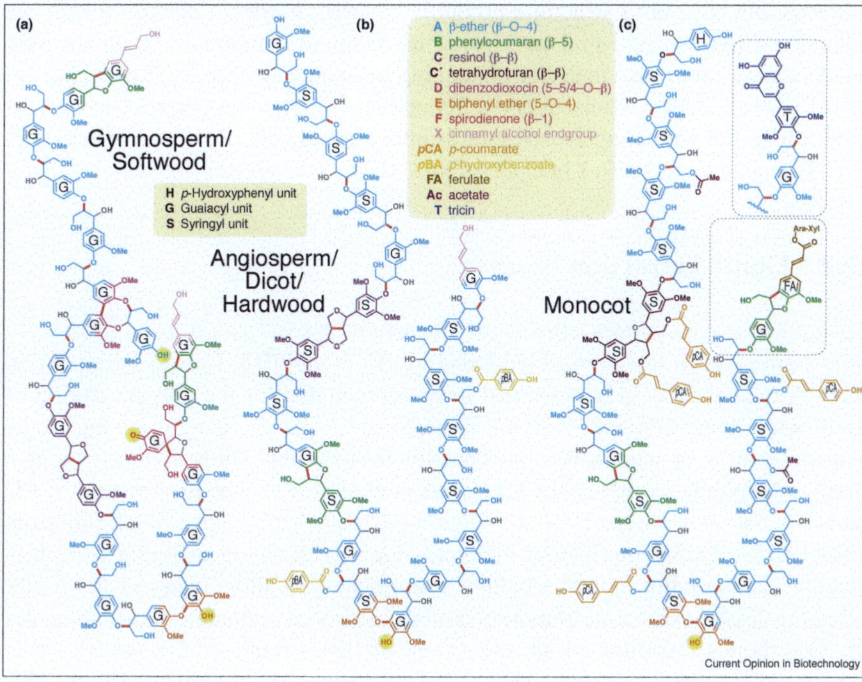

Fig. 5.1 Lignin categories up to the chemical structure. (**a**) A gymnosperm/softwood, (**b**) An angiosperm/hardwood, and (**c**) A monocot/Grass. (Reproduced with permission from Sen et al. (2015))

E, 0 dibenzodioxocins D, 16 β-ether units A, and 0 spirodienones F (Sun et al. 2012; Del Río et al. 2020).

- *Class (c)—Monocot/ Grass lignin* (Fig. 5.1c): 0 Cinnamyl alcohol endgroup units X from a chain-starting dimerization reaction, even though there probably should be one; it has been chosen to be illustrated the chain initiation via either ferulate FA or tricin T, features specific to commelinid monocots, in either case first coupled with coniferyl alcohol to give a G unit; 20 Monomeric units, 13 S and 6 G with one ferulate FA or tricin T unit; 2 phenylcoumarans B; 1 tetrahydrofuran C′, which is also the beginning of a monolignol dimerization chain; however, it originates from the dimerization of two sinapyl p-coumarate conjugates; when the γ-OH is acylated, the rearomatization route is different from that of the dicot's resinol C. 0 β-ether units A; 1 biphenyl ether E; 0 dibenzodioxocins D; 0 spirodienones F (Sen et al. 2015).

One of the biosynthetic processes that requires the greatest energy is the lignin macromolecule synthesis process in plant cells (Boerjan et al. 2003; Amthor 2003). Known as the 'phenylpropanoid pathway,' the enzymatic polymerization and synthesis of monolignols have been studied in great detail over the years by several research organizations (Amthor 2003). Despite these efforts, a comprehensive understanding of lignin's structural properties remains elusive. Recent research has underscored lignin's potential as a valuable chemical compound, being the sole abundant renewable raw material containing aromatic monomers (Erdocia et al. 2021; Liu et al. 2018b). Consequently, lignin depolymerization emerges as a promising avenue for producing an array of aromatic chemicals (Zevallos Torres et al. 2020; Puangsin et al. 2017; Liu et al. 2020).

5.2.2 Lignin Extraction Process

Lignocellulose necessitates efficacious extraction or segregation to procure high-purity lignin with a less compacted structure (Li et al. 2018; Lobato-Peralta et al. 2021). A radical process is presumed to be accountable for the polymerization of lignin, while the extraction of lignin is perceived to be challenging owing to the covalent bonding of specific reactive constituents to hemicelluloses, thus forming a lignin-carbohydrate complex (LCC) (Renders et al. 2019). The disruption of LCC bonds and partial depolymerization of lignin are requisite for separating lignin from carbohydrates. Depolymerization facilitates the solubilization of lignin from biomass by disintegrating it into smaller constituents (Zevallos Torres et al. 2020). Following lignin extraction, polymerization occurrences (condensation) engender new C–C bonds, resulting in an assortment of lignin intermediates with diverse characteristics, attributed to the heightened reactivity of lignin. Isolated lignin frequently exhibits a variable configuration owing to disparities in raw materials, extraction methodologies, and intensity (Kallel et al. 2016; Sun et al. 2012; Kargarzadeh et al. 2012; Szymanska-Chargot et al. 2017). Lignin is mostly produced on an industrial scale by the pulp and paper industry using several biorefinery processes, such as hot water, diluted acid, alkaline, or enzymes for hydrolysis/fractionation, or Kraft pulping, sulfite pulping, soda pulping, or other processes (Table 5.2). The pulp and paper sector employs advanced technologies and represents a firmly established industry (Gellerstedt et al. 2009; Treimanis 1996). Contemporary research predominantly concentrates on lignin extraction from biorefinery processes, owing to antecedent examinations of lignins derived from these technologies (Erdocia et al. 2021; Yoo et al. 2020; Mankar et al. 2021).

5.2.3 Techniques for Lignin Structural Characterization

Over recent decades, the characterization of lignin has advanced significantly, encompassing both destructive and nondestructive techniques (Liao et al. 2020; Lupoi et al. 2015; Rodrigues et al. 2022). Destructive methods such as thioacidolysis, ozonation, and acidolysis have been utilized, albeit with limitations due to their selective breakage of β-O-4 linkages (Reale et al. 2004). Consequently, these techniques offer only partial insights into lignin's structural complexities. Conversely, nondestructive approaches, including NMR spectroscopy, FTIR spectroscopy (see Fig. 5.2d), and Raman spectroscopy (see Fig. 5.2b), provide avenues for

Table 5.2 Main lignin extraction methods

Extraction method	Conditions and reactive	References
New processes		
Ionic solution extraction	50–170 °C, imidazolium-based ionic liquids, nonimidazolium-based ionic liquids	(Martins et al. 2014)
Deep eutectic solvents	80–180 °C, choline chloride, carboxylic acids, polyols	(Chen et al. 2020)
Industrial processes		
Kraft pulping	150–180 °C, H_2O, NaOH, Na_2S	(Deng and Ragauskas 2012)
Sulfite pulping	140–170 °C, H_2O, sulfites (e.g. Na_2SO3, NaHSO3, $(NH_4)2SO_3$, $MgSO_3$, $CaSO_3$)	(Deng and Ragauskas 2012)
Soda pulping	160–170 °C, H_2O, NaOH, (Anthraquinone)	(Deng and Ragauskas 2012)
Biorefinery processes		
Organosolv pulping	100–200 °C, H_2O, alcohol, or alcohol/water mixtures. Formic acid, acetic acid, H_2SO_4	(Lancefield et al. 2017)
Dilute acid hydrolysis	120 °C–300 °C, H_2O, 0–5 wt% HCl, H_2SO_4, H_3PO_4, or HF	(Bhagia et al. 2016)
Concentrated acid hydrolysis	Two-step: 1) 20 °C–30 °C, H_2O, concentrated mineral acid, e.g. 72% H_2SO_4; 2) 121 °C, diluted H_2SO_4	(Ibáñez and Bauer 2014)
Alkaline hydrolysis	40 °C–160 °C, H_2O, NaOH, $ca(OH)_2$, ammonia	(Kim et al. 2016)
Enzymatic hydrolysis	30 °C–60 °C, H_2O, cellulase, hemicellulase, additional pretreatments (e.g., dilute acid, steam explosion, ammonia fiber explosion)	(Hassan et al. 2018)
Reductive or oxidative fractionation	150 °C–250 °C, H_2O or organic solvents, H_2 or H_2-donating solvents or oxidants (e.g., O_2, O_3, H_2O_2)	(Van Den Bosch et al. 2015)
Combined pretreatment methods	25 °C–200 °C, H_2O or organic solvents, e.g., mechanical milling combined with acid catalytic fractionation, deacetylation with mechanical refining	(Calvaruso et al. 2017)
Structure analysis processes		
Mechanical pretreatment	Room temperature, extensive ball milling, solvent extraction	(Björkman 1954)
Ball-milling, cellulolytic enzyme hydrolysis	2-steps: (1) ball-milling; (2) hydrolysis by cellulase and hemicellulase, 40 °C–60 °C, H_2O buffer (pH: 4–5)	(Adler et al. 1975)
Ball-milling, cellulolytic enzyme hydrolysis, and mild acidolysis	3-steps: (1) ball-milling; (2) hydrolysis by cellulase and hemicellulase, 40 °C–60 °C, H_2O, buffer (pH: 4–5); (3) mild acidolysis by HCl, dioxane/H_2O, 80 °C–90 °C	(Deng and Ragauskas 2012)

comprehensive analysis without altering the lignin's integrity (Liao et al. 2020; Lupoi et al. 2015).

Among these techniques, advanced NMR technologies stand out as particularly potent tools for analysing isolated lignin fractions. Notably, 2D-HSQC NMR

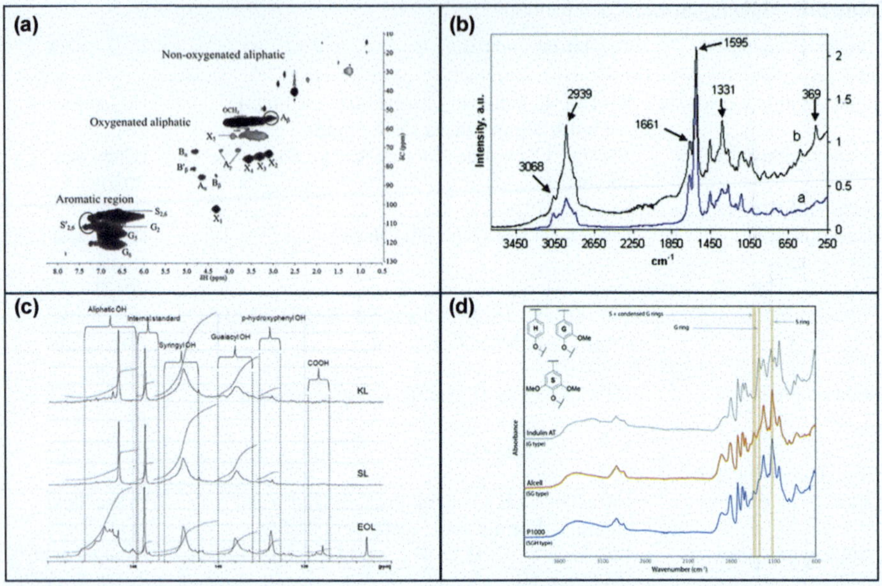

Fig. 5.2 Key structural characteristics of lignin evaluation methodology. The lignin's undissolved portion after dissolving in a methanol/water solution is shown in (**a**) the 2D-HSQC spectrum (Zhang et al. 2017). (**b**) FT-Raman spectra of milled wood lignins from black spruce and aspen. (Reprinted in Rodrigues et al. (2022)). (**c**) Ethanosolv lignin (EOL), soda (SL), and kraft (KL) ^{31}P NMR spectra. (Reprinted with permission from Liao et al. (2020)). (**d**) FTIR spectra of soda lignin (P1000), organosolv lignin (Alcell), and kraft lignin (Indulin AT). (Reprinted with permission from Lancefield et al. (2019))

spectroscopy offers a comprehensive view of lignin's structure, facilitating the identification of specific linkages and substructures (see Fig. 5.2a) (Yuan et al. 2013; Sun 2020). The technique's ability to provide direct C – H correlations in two dimensions enhances its utility in structural elucidation. Furthermore, quantitative determination of various linkages, including β-O-4, β-β, and β-5, can be achieved through computational methods, enriching the characterization process. In addition to elucidating linkages, 2D-HSQC NMR spectroscopy enables the differentiation of lignin units such as H, S, and G and the identification of minor components like p-coumarate and ferulate (Lu et al. 2017). This capability extends to lignin from different sources and processing methods, enhancing our understanding of structural variations. Furthermore, multidimensional NMR techniques aid in the identification of new and minor lignin units, facilitating in-depth structural analysis.

Complementing the insights provided by NMR spectroscopy, ^{31}P NMR spectroscopy offers valuable information on lignin's hydroxyl groups (see Fig. 5.2c) (Lu et al. 2017). This technique enables the quantitative analysis of various hydroxyl groups, including phenolic, aliphatic, and carboxyl groups, which are crucial for assessing lignin's chemical reactivity. Moreover, the high resolution and accuracy of ^{31}P NMR spectroscopy simplify the determination of these functional groups, expediting chemical modification processes (Lu et al. 2017; Nguyen et al. 2015; Lagier et al. 1996). Ultimately, the combined application of advanced NMR techniques enables comprehensive characterization of lignin, from identifying native substructures to evaluating chemical reactivity. Such insights are invaluable for developing lignin-based materials with tailored properties, paving the way for innovative applications in biorefineries and beyond.

5.3 Lignin-Based Formulation for Medical Purposes

In the past three decades, significant advancements in medical technologies have led to the development of diverse bio-based hydrogels formulations. Researchers have focused on factors such as biocompatibility, strength, flexibility, and ease of application when formulating bio-adhesives. Additionally, the combination of different materials, such as polymers, proteins, or nanoparticles, have been utilized to improve adhesive properties and enable targeted drug delivery. These revolutionary developments in bio-based hydrogels have the potential to transform medical treatments by providing effective adhesion to biological tissues and surfaces, as well as controlled release of therapeutic agents. Biobased polymers have gained significant attention in biomedical applications due to their biocompatibility, biodegradability, reduced immune response, minimal toxicity, and the ability to support cell adhesion and growth Fig. 5.3a.

The unique structural properties of lignin make it a promising material for various applications in the biomaterial field. Lignin contains several key functional

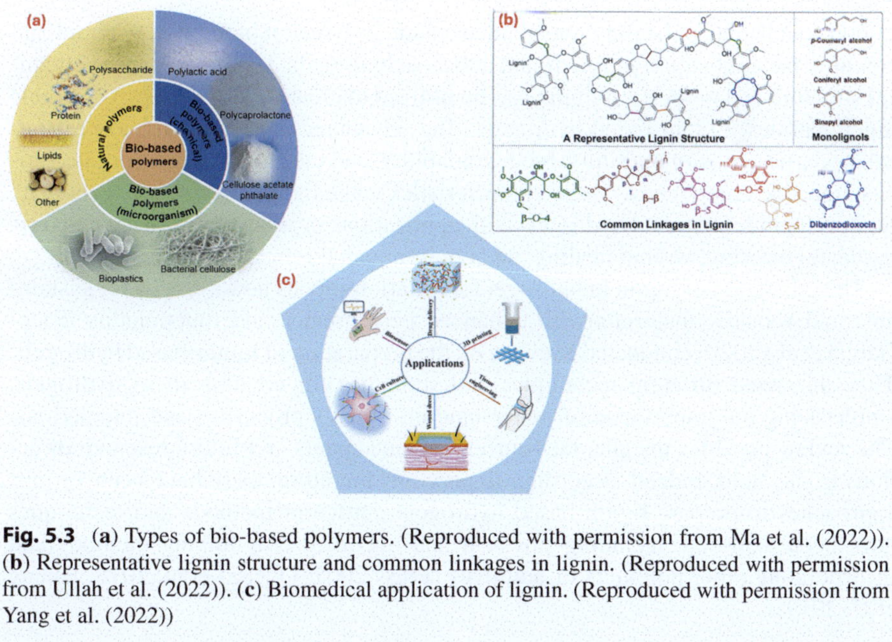

Fig. 5.3 (**a**) Types of bio-based polymers. (Reproduced with permission from Ma et al. (2022)). (**b**) Representative lignin structure and common linkages in lignin. (Reproduced with permission from Ullah et al. (2022)). (**c**) Biomedical application of lignin. (Reproduced with permission from Yang et al. (2022))

groups, including phenolic and aliphatic hydroxyl, carboxylic, carbonyl, and methoxyl groups. As mentioned in Fig. 5.3b. These functional groups contribute to lignin's reactivity and versatility in biomedical applications (Ullah et al. 2022). The phenolic hydroxyl groups in lignin provide antioxidant and UV-absorbing properties, making it suitable for use in materials that require protection against degradation caused by environmental factors. The aliphatic hydroxyl groups offer the potential for chemical modification and crosslinking reactions, allowing for the development of tailored lignin-based biomaterials with desired properties (Agustiany et al. 2022). However, the presence of carboxylic groups in lignin enables its interaction with other biomaterials, facilitating compatibility and adhesion in composite systems. The carbonyl groups contribute to lignin's ability to undergo chemical reactions, forming crosslinked networks and improving mechanical strength in biomaterial applications. Furthermore, the methoxyl groups in lignin provide hydrophobicity, influencing its water resistance and barrier properties. This makes lignin suitable for applications requiring moisture resistance or as an additive in hydrophobic biomaterial formulations. By leveraging the diverse functional groups present in lignin, researchers can explore its potential for various biomaterial applications, including tissue engineering, drug delivery systems, and bioactive coatings (Meng et al. 2019). The utilization of lignin in biomaterials holds promise for developing sustainable and functional materials that can contribute to advancements in the field of biomedicine. Several studies have tried to improve the bio-adhesive properties of the lignin by conjugating different adhesive agents to lignin network.

5.3.1 Lignin in Hydrogels

Lignin stands out as the only abundant aromatic polymer, which gives it significant potential for application in functional adhesive hydrogels. Due to its unique chemical structure and properties, lignin can be utilized to create hydrogels with desirable functionalities. Lignin-based hydrogels offer advantages such as tunable mechanical properties, biocompatibility, biodegradability, and the ability to incorporate various bioactive compounds. These characteristics make lignin an attractive candidate for developing functional hydrogels with applications in areas such as drug delivery, tissue engineering, wound healing, and environmental remediation Fig. 5.3c.

The utilization of lignin in hydrogel formulations opens new avenues for sustainable and versatile materials with enhanced performance and functionality. Rico-García et al. (2020) conducted a review on the preparation of lignin-based hydrogels. They discussed different techniques and strategies for creating these hydrogels, emphasizing the importance of understanding lignin's properties and interactions. The review provides insights into current advancements and future research directions in this field. Indeed, according to previous literature, there have been various approaches to prepare lignin-based hydrogels. Different methods and techniques have been explored, including physical and chemical crosslinking methods and incorporating other polymers or additives (Press 2007; Oveissi et al. 2018; Huang et al. 2019).

In 2021, Yonghao Ni's team unveiled a novel hydrogel characterized by consistent adhesion, firmly adhering to human skin while effectively blocking waste (Wang et al. 2021). Notably, this hydrogel, equipped with a built-in pressure sensor, exhibits remarkable resistance to interference and ensures wearable comfort (Fig. 5.4). To achieve this, the researchers employed lignosulfonate sodium (LS), a water-soluble salt containing catechol structures, as both an adhesive and a conductive agent, along with a softener for the highly stretchable P(AA-co-LS) hydrogel (Fig. 5.4a). Subsequently, a Fe^{3+} solution was applied to the hydrogel's upper surface to neutralize its adhesive properties, rendering it non-adhesive (Fig. 5.4b). Remarkably, this targeted Fe^{3+} treatment did not compromise the adhesive nature of the hydrogel's base, ensuring strong adherence to the skin. Experimental findings demonstrated that LS-doped PAA hydrogels exhibit uniform adhesion (with an adhesive strength of approximately ~30.5 kPa), conductivity (~0.45 S/m), remarkable stretchability (up to ~2250%), and a low compressive modulus (~20 kPa). Following the addition of the Fe^{3+} solution, the hydrogel displayed asymmetric adhesion characteristics between its upper and lower surfaces, with virtually no adhesive strength on the upper surface and strong adhesion (~27 kPa) on the bottom surface.

The same team employed functionalized lignin nanoparticles (LNP) as enhancers in hydrogel formulation (Cui et al. 2021). Initially, they synthesized lignin

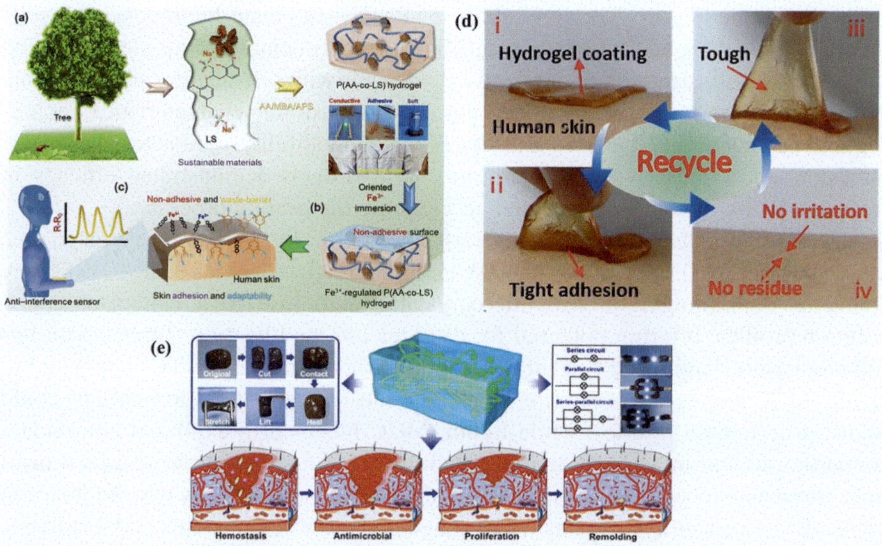

Fig. 5.4 (**a–c**) The preparation process of plant-derived LS-doped P(AA-co-LS) hydrogel from extraction to application. (Reproduced with permission from Wang et al. (2021)). (**d**) Photo demonstrating the LNP@Ag–Fe-PAA hydrogel repeatedly adhered to the author's skin. No irritation or residue on author's skin was observed after peeling off several times. (Reproduced with permission from Cui et al. (2021)). (**e**) Schematic illustrations of wound healing by hydrogel therapy. (Reproduced with permission from Deng et al. (2021))

nanoparticles with a narrow size distribution ranging from 250 to 350 nm, which were subsequently adorned with Ag nanoparticles (~10 nm) on their surfaces. The gelation process involved the utilization of LNP@Ag, Fe^{3+}, ammonium persulfate (APS), and acrylic acid (AA), resulting in an ultrafast PAA polymerization at room temperature, completed in just a few minutes. Moreover, owing to the dynamic catechol redox-Fe^{3+} system, the hydrogel incorporating LNP@Ag–Fe^{3+} (Fig. 5.4d) exhibited remarkable mechanical properties, particularly outstanding durability, sustained adhesion over an extended period, and swift and efficient self-healing capabilities. As nanofillers, LNP@Ag further fortified the hydrogels, displaying an impressive compression strength of approximately ~810 kPa and exceptional elasticity (able to stretch up to 13 times its original length). Additionally, the composite hydrogel showcased superb conductivity, ultraviolet-blocking characteristics, and potent antibacterial activity attributed to the presence of metal ions, lignin, and Ag nanoparticles. This study introduces a novel approach utilizing lignin nanofillers in hydrogel fabrication, and the resulting multifunctional hydrogel, facile to produce, holds promising prospects for applications in human-machine electronics.

In a separate study, research.ers utilized alkali lignin/hydroxymethyl cellulose/Ag nanoparticles to develop a versatile hydrogel capable of promoting wound healing and resisting bacteria such as *E. coli*, *Staphylococcus aureus*, *C. albicans*, and drug-resistant MRSA (Deng et al. 2021). Figure 5.4e illustrates some of the key properties of these hydrogels and their healing mechanism. The authors proposed that Ag nanoparticles, reduced by lignin in situ, could be combined with phenylboric acid-modified hydroxypropyl cellulose (PAHC) to create hydrogels with self-healing, conductive, and antibacterial attributes. Experimental findings demonstrated the successful construction of conductive hydrogels with self-healing and injectable properties. These hydrogels exhibited a myriad of desirable characteristics, including self-healing ability, biocompatibility, blood compatibility, antibacterial efficacy, adhesion, and conductivity. Furthermore, the hydrogels demonstrated efficacy in treating MRSA-infected wounds and accelerating the healing process.

In a study conducted by Domínguez-Robles et al., lignin was investigated as a tablet excipient, a field with limited research (Domínguez-Robles et al. 2019). They found that combining lignin with microcrystalline cellulose (MCC) alters tablet dissolution profiles, offering potential for drug release modification. Tablets with lignin alone were fragile and less effective in releasing tetracycline (TC) compared to lignin /MCC blends. Incorporating small amounts of lignin into formulations could adjust drug release profiles, while lignin /MCC blends also exhibited antioxidant properties, aiding in active ingredient stability. Lignin shows promise as a renewable alternative to synthetic excipients, with potential applications beyond pharmaceuticals. Its versatility suggests wider usage in dietary supplements and fertilizers. Exploiting lignin's properties as a pharmaceutical excipient offers promising avenues for various applications.

Culebras et al., have demonstrated the potential of lignin-based hydrogels as sustainable platforms for drug delivery systems (Culebras et al. 2021). These hydrogels, characterized by a porous structure post-freeze drying, exhibit increased swelling capacity with higher lignin and poly(ethylene) glycol diglycidyl ether (PEGDGE) contents. Their study underscores the importance of understanding the structural, chemical, and mechanical behavior of organosolv lignin for developing efficient drug release platforms. By crosslinking lignin with PEGDGE, the researchers produced hydrogels with tunable properties, influenced by the crosslinker ratio. Paracetamol release studies revealed higher release rates for hydrogels with a lignin:PEGDGE ratio of 1:1, attributed to reduced H-bonding interactions within the hydrogel network. These findings highlight the potential of lignin-based hydrogels as next-generation sustainable platforms for drug delivery applications.

Gan et al. developed a novel adhesive hydrogel inspired by plants, utilizing Ag-lignin core-shell nanoparticles to trigger a dynamic catechol-based redox system in poly(acrylic acid)/pectin hydrogels (*see* Fig. 5.5b) (Gan et al. 2019). This innovative approach resulted in a continuous reductive/oxidative environment within the hydrogel network, enabling self-gelation at ambient conditions and providing long-term adhesiveness. The adhesive mechanism is attributed to hydrogen bonding or hydrophobic interactions with different surfaces, validated by adhesion and stripping tests on skin tissue. Notably, the hydrogel exhibited high antibacterial activity due to the presence of catechol groups and the bactericidal properties of Ag-Lignin nanoparticles. This study introduces a promising strategy for designing tough and adhesive hydrogels based on dynamic plant catechol chemistry.

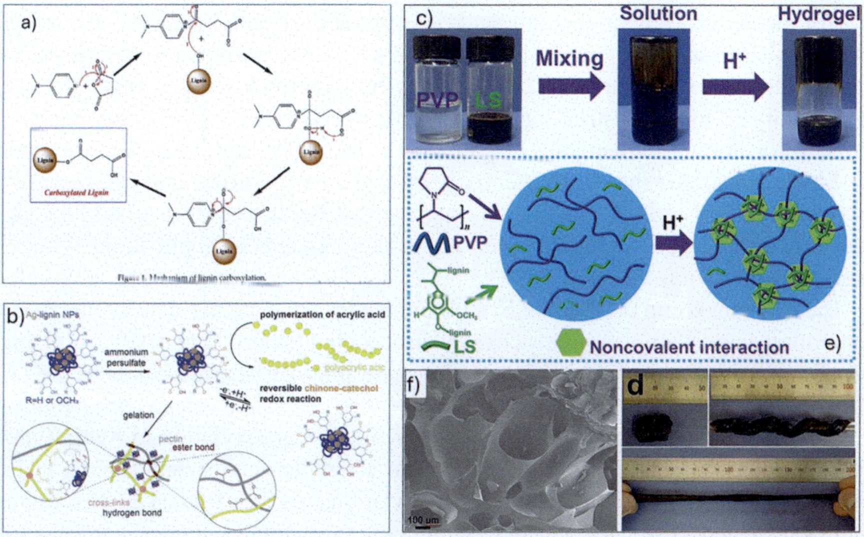

Fig. 5.5 (**a**) Mechanism of lignin carboxylation. (Reproduced from Pishnamazi et al. (2019)). (**b**) Multi-component adhesion system comprising pectin and polyacrylic acid macromolecules combined with plant-inspired, DOPA-modified Ag-lignin nanoparticles (NPs). These particles trigger the gelation process of the mixture based on the redox reaction of chinones. (Reproduced with permission from Lutz et al. (2022)). (**c**) Photographs showing the formation process of the LPC hydrogel. (**e**) Schematic illustration and structure of the LPC hydrogel. (**f**) SEM image of the LPC-3 hydrogel. (**d**) Photographs of the LPC hydrogel. (Reproduced with permission from Cao et al. (2022))

In a different study, Jinfeng Cao introduced a novel approach to creating flexible and adhesive hydrogels with self-healing capabilities, leveraging noncovalent interactions such as hydrogen bonds and hydrophobic interactions (*see* Fig. 5.5c–f) (Cao et al. 2022). By mixing lignosulfonate (LS) and polyvinylpyrrolidone (PVP) in water and adjusting the pH to neutral, Cao achieved the formation of rigid noncovalent junctions from LS and a flexible network from PVP. Variations in LS and PVP concentrations yielded a range of hydrogel formulations with unique properties. The resulting hydrogel demonstrated remarkable toughness and self-healing ability, attributed to its dynamic and reversible gelation mechanism. Moreover, the abundance of active groups and improved cohesion endowed the LS/PVP composite (LPC) hydrogel with excellent adhesive properties to diverse substrates. Additionally, the LPC hydrogel exhibited outstanding biocompatibility, making it suitable for biomedical applications. Notably, hydrogel was successfully utilized as a hemostatic agent for treating organ injuries, highlighting its potential in biomaterials. Overall, this study presents a promising platform for multifunctional lignin-based hydrogels, offering versatility and applicability in various fields.

5.3.2 Lignin in Drug Delivery

Drug delivery systems are advanced technologies that aim to improve the effectiveness of medicines or natural compounds by targeting specific locations, like tumor sites, while reducing potential side effects. One of the notable characteristics of lignin is its lack of cytotoxicity. In the study by Ugartondo et al. (2008), the cell cytotoxicity of four industrial lignins was investigated, and it was found that they are safe for normal human cells (Ugartondo et al. 2008). Similarly, Tortora et al. (2014) demonstrated that lignin microcapsules are not cytotoxic and can be easily incorporated into cells. These findings suggest that lignin possesses good biocompatibility and can be potentially used in various biomedical applications without causing harm to normal cells.

The research group of Maurice N. Collins also investigated pH-dependent tablets containing paracetamol as the active pharmaceutical ingredient (API), utilizing Alcell and carboxylated Alcell *lignin* alongside microcrystalline cellulose (MCC 101) (Pishnamazi et al. 2019). The study aimed to assess the release behaviour of modified lignin and its impact on drug release rates. Carboxylation of lignin functional groups was conducted to modify lignin, which was confirmed through FTIR analysis. Results indicated successful carboxylation (*see* Fig. 5.5a). The dissolution studies revealed that carboxylated lignin tablets exhibited higher paracetamol release rates, attributed to reduced interaction between lignin and the API due to deprotonation of –COOH groups from modified lignin. Furthermore, controlled release properties of carboxylated lignin were demonstrated at both gastric (pH 1.2) and intestinal (pH 7.2) conditions. Tablet disintegration tests indicated faster disintegration times for carboxylated lignin tablets compared to pure lignin tablets, owing to lower tablet hardness. These findings showcase the effective use of carboxylated lignin as a natural biopolymer excipient in oral dosage forms, offering desirable controlled-release properties.

Lignin-based nanoparticles (LNPs) are being explored as a promising drug delivery system. They enhance therapeutic compounds' bioavailability, absorption, and solubility, ultimately improving their therapeutic efficacy. Various methods have been investigated for the preparation of lignin-based nanoparticles (LNPs). These methods include self-assembly, ultrasonication, nanoprecipitation, emulsion-based techniques, and coacervation. In this context, Gilca et al. (Andrei et al. 2015) synthesized lignin nanoparticles from commercially available lignin using ultrasonication. The nanoparticles were spherical and ranged in size from 0.01 to 0.05 µmThe acoustic irradiation during ultrasonication led to the degradation of phenylcoumaran and pinoresinol subunits, resulting in a reduction in particle size, as depicted in Fig. 5.6a. LNPs have been investigated for their potential applications in drug delivery, including cancer drug delivery.In this aspect, Siddiqui et al. (2020) fabricated LNPs from kraft lignin that demonstrated low hemolytic activity and no toxicity to normal cells. They exhibited significant cytotoxicity against folate receptor-positive cancer cells, indicating their potential for targeted drug delivery. The LNPs efficiently loaded and sustained the release of the anticancer drug irinotecan. These

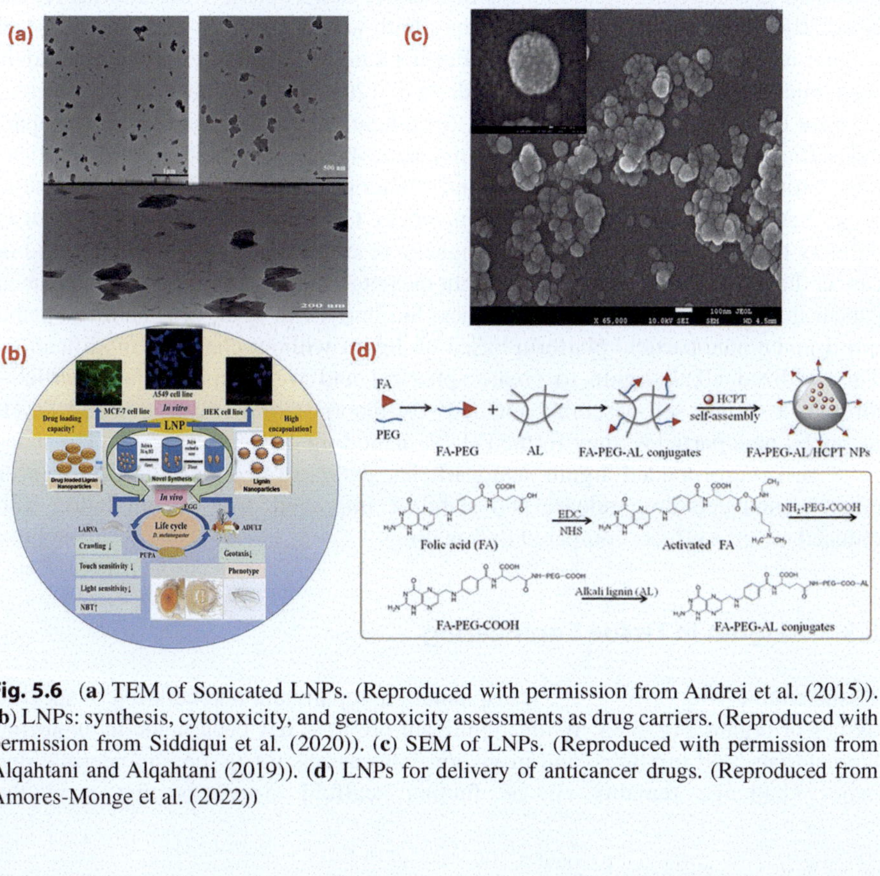

Fig. 5.6 (**a**) TEM of Sonicated LNPs. (Reproduced with permission from Andrei et al. (2015)). (**b**) LNPs: synthesis, cytotoxicity, and genotoxicity assessments as drug carriers. (Reproduced with permission from Siddiqui et al. (2020)). (**c**) SEM of LNPs. (Reproduced with permission from Alqahtani and Alqahtani (2019)). (**d**) LNPs for delivery of anticancer drugs. (Reproduced from Amores-Monge et al. (2022))

findings suggest that LNPs have promise as safe and effective drug carriers, but more research is needed for clinical applications Fig. 5.6b. Alqahtani et al. developed LNPs with high curcumin entrapment efficiency and particle size Fig. 5.6c (Alqahtani and Alqahtani 2019). The LNPs showed prolonged drug release, stability in gastric fluids, and improved permeability compared to the free drug. The bioavailability of curcumin was enhanced tenfold with LNPs. These results suggest the potential of LNPs for cancer treatment. Frangville et al. (2012) investigated the use of nontoxic LNPs for entrapping Rhodamine 6G. The study found that lignin nanoparticles exhibited a high drug loading capacity, making them promising carriers for drug delivery applications. Liu et al. (2018a) developed LNPs for efficient delivery of the anticancer drug HCPT Fig. 5.6d. The NPs showed high binding affinity to tumor cells, prolonged circulation time, and demonstrated in vitro cytotoxicity against LLC and L929 cells. In an LLC-tumor mouse model, the NPs exhibited promising in vivo anticancer effects.

However, magnetic nanocarriers, including lignin nanoparticles combined with metal nanocarriers, offer targeted drug delivery, site control, and therapeutic concentration maintenance. This combination shows promise in cancer drug delivery, enhancing treatment efficacy and reducing off-target effects. In this context, Zahou et al., prepared hollow lignin nanoparticles filled with magnetic nanoparticles and folic acid as a targeting ligand for the delivery of doxorubicin hydrochloride (Zhou et al. 2019). These folic acid-metal lignin hollow nanoparticles showed enhanced cellular uptake of drugs in HeLa cells. Further studies are required before considering clinical trials. Figure 5.7a Figueiredo et al. (2017a) prove that LNPs hold great promise for drug delivery applications. Specifically, Fe_3O_4-infused lignin nanoparticles (Fe_3O_4-LNPs) exhibit superparamagnetic behaviour, making them particularly promising for cancer therapy and diagnosis. Figure 5.7b Their magnetic properties enable applications, such as magnetic targeting, which can enhance drug delivery to specific tumor sites, and magnetic resonance imaging, which can aid in cancer diagnosis. These features highlight the potential of Fe_3O_4-LNPs for advanced cancer treatment and imaging techniques. Similarly, Dai et al. (2017) developed a novel green nanoparticle platform based on lignin without chemical modification. They utilized alkali lignin to create spherical and well-dispersed nanoparticles through a simple self-assembly method. By incorporating resveratrol and Fe_3O_4 magnetic nanoparticles, they formed stable nanodrug carriers Fig. 5.7c. The magnetic resveratrol-loaded lignin nanoparticles demonstrated excellent anticancer effects, enhanced drug release and stability, improved drug accumulation, and reduced adverse effects compared to free drugs.

5.3.3 Lignin in Tissue Engineering

Tissue engineering involves the transplantation, repair, and regeneration of specific tissues or organs Fig. 5.8a. While significant progress has been made in exploring biomaterials, cell mixtures, and in vivo/in vitro assays for tissue engineering, one major challenge remains i.e. as finding scaffold structures that meet the

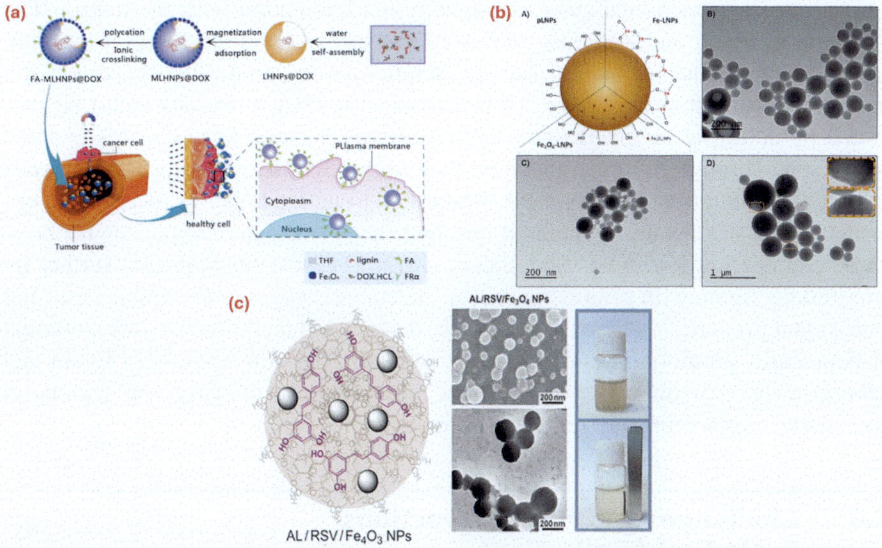

Fig. 5.7 (**a**) Magnetic LNPs for the delivery of doxorubicin. (Reproduced with permission from Garg et al. (2022)). (**b**) TEM images of magnetic LNPs. (Reproduced with permission from Mohammadinejad et al. (2019)). (**c**) Magnetic resveratrol loaded LNPs. (Reproduced from Liu et al. (2022a))

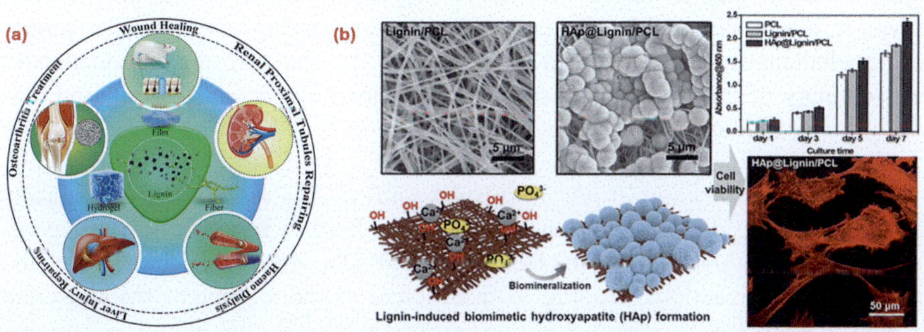

Fig. 5.8 (**a**) Application of lignin and lignin-based composites in different tissue engineering fields. (Reproduced with permission from Liu et al. (2022b)). (**b**) Lignin/polycaprolactone nanofibers for hydroxyapatite biomineralization. (Reproduced with permission from Wang et al. (2019))

requirements of cell affinity, non-cytotoxicity, and biodegradability (Figueiredo et al. 2017b). Lignin has emerged as a potential tissue-engineering agent due to its ability to serve as a platform for cell attachment and proliferation. Lignin-based composites have gained attention in the biomedical field due to their biocompatibility and excellent technical properties (Rico-García et al. 2020). In the context of bone tissue engineering, the development of scaffolds combining polymers, such as lignin, and active compounds is crucial for promoting bone regeneration and healing. Luzi et al. (2020) found that a film made of PLA and lignin/ZnO enhanced human bone mesenchymal stem cell growth and interaction with the matrix. The inclusion of lignin and ZnO also improved the stiffness and elasticity of the film, making it promising for bone tissue regeneration. Wang et al. (2019) conducted a study suggesting that the growth of hydroxyapatite (HAp) crystals could be promoted by culturing an electrospun lignin/polycaprolactone matrix in a simulated body fluid. Through multiple analyses, they found that the resulting HAp crystals exhibited structural and mechanical similarities to native bone. In recent developments, lignin has been incorporated into hydrogels to create composites for bone tissue engineering Fig. 5.8b. Abdullah et al. (2021) took this approach further by crosslinking lignin with gelatin to produce injectable cryogels with antibacterial and antioxidant properties. These cryogels were designed to facilitate the differentiation of bone cells, promoting bone tissue regeneration. The combination of lignin and gelatin in the crosslinked cryogels offers promising potential for applications in bone tissue engineering and regenerative medicine.

5.4 Challenges and Future Directions in Medical Applications

Developing lignin-based bio-adhesives for medical applications presents a promising avenue for addressing the growing demand for biocompatible and sustainable adhesive materials. These bio-adhesives, derived from renewable sources such as lignin, offer potential advantages such as biodegradability, abundance, and low cost. However, their successful implementation in medical settings requires overcoming several challenges (Stanisz et al. 2022). Based on the search results provided, here is a summary of the key challenges and future directions facing lignin-based bio-adhesives for medical applications; this includes:

- *Inadequate absorption of phenolic compounds during modification processes:* The search results note that one of the major hurdles in using phenolic compounds to modify biomacromolecules for bio-adhesion is the low yield of the modification reactions, leading to insufficient phenolic content (Montazerian et al. 2023).
- *Compatibility with crosslinking mechanisms:* The research findings emphasize the importance of ensuring that the crosslinking mechanisms employed for bio-adhesive gelation are compatible with polyphenolic components. This is crucial because the presence of phenolic compounds can interfere with free-radical polymerization due to their scavenging effects on free radicals (Montazerian et al. 2023).
- *Attaining specific material characteristics:* Lignin-derived polyurethanes (PUs) have been explored, but the search results indicate that the special properties of lignosulfonates, such as water solubility and hydrophilicity, lead to different material properties compared to conventional lignin-derived Pus (Vieira et al. 2022).

It is important to note that the lignin-based PUs discussed in this context contain isocyanates, which are known for their potential toxicity concerns. However, progress has been made in developing safer lignin-based PUs by using aliphatic isocyanates that are less toxic than the commonly used aromatic isocyanates. The unique properties of lignosulfonate-based PUs, such as water solubility and hydrophilicity, could make them interesting candidates for various biomedical applications, including:

- Wound dressings due to their water absorption capacity
- Controlled drug delivery systems owing to their water solubility
- Tissue engineering scaffolds by leveraging their potential biocompatibility

Nevertheless, further studies are necessary to thoroughly evaluate the biocompatibility and toxicity of these materials before considering any medical applications. We have mentioned these potential applications only to highlight the interest in the particular properties of lignosulfonate-derived PUs compared to conventional PUs.

Addressing these challenges will require interdisciplinary research efforts spanning material science, bioengineering, and biomedical applications. Moreover, collaboration between researchers, industry partners, and regulatory agencies is essential to advance the development and translation of lignin-based bio-adhesives into clinically viable products that can improve patient outcomes and contribute to sustainable healthcare solutions."

5.5 Conclusions

The exploration of lignin-based binders in the medical field represents a significant advance toward the use of sustainable biomaterials for innovative healthcare solutions. Throughout this chapter, we have explored the multifaceted potential of lignin formulations in various medical contexts, ranging from drug delivery systems to tissue engineering scaffolds. The development of lignin hydrogels illustrates the versatility and adaptability of lignin-based materials for biomedical applications. Furthermore, by exploiting lignin's inherent properties, such as its biocompatibility and ability to encapsulate drugs, new drug delivery platforms can be designed for targeted and sustained release of therapeutics, thereby improving patient compliance and outcomes. In recent decades, there has been increasing demand for the development of various nanomedicines, particularly for biomedical applications such as cancer therapy, oral delivery, and regenerative medicine (e.g. liver regeneration and cardiovascular disease). Lignin as a bio-polyphenol offers great potential for adaptability, functionalization and applicability to reproduce nanoparticles and nanospheres, thus promoting the use of desirable, high-performance biomaterials in the aforementioned medical systems. This potential still faces challenges and hurdles to overcome to ensure compatibility with biological systems and minimize the risk of adverse reactions or toxicity when used in medical applications.

Overall, advances in lignin-based biocompatible binders for medical applications represent a fundamental shift towards sustainable and environmentally-friendly solutions in healthcare. In the future, continued research and innovation in this field promise to address crucial healthcare challenges and improve patient care through the development of lignin-based formulations with improved efficacy and safety profiles.

References

Abdullah T, Colombani T, Alade T, Bencherif SA, Memić A (2021) Injectable lignin-co-gelatin cryogels with antioxidant and antibacterial properties for biomedical applications. Biomacromolecules 22:4110–4121. https://doi.org/10.1021/acs.biomac.1c00575

Adler E, Miksche G, Brown W (1975) Comparative studies on cellulolytic enzyme lignin and milled wood lignin of sweetgum and spruce. Holzforschung 29:153–159. https://doi.org/10.1515/HFSG.1975.29.5.153/MACHINEREADABLECITATION/RIS

Agustiany EA, Rasyidur Ridho M, Rahmi DNM, Madyaratri EW, Falah F, Lubis MAR et al (2022) Recent developments in lignin modification and its application in lignin-based green composites: a review. Polym Compos 43:4848–4865. https://doi.org/10.1002/pc.26824

Alqahtani MS, Alqahtani A (2019) Novel lignin nanoparticles for oral drug delivery. J Mater Chem B:4461–4473. https://doi.org/10.1039/c9tb00594c

Amores-Monge V, Goyanes S, Ribba L, Lopretti M, Sandoval-Barrantes M, Camacho M et al (2022) Pineapple agro-industrial biomass to produce biomedical applications in a circular economy context in Costa Rica. Polymers (Basel):14. https://doi.org/10.3390/polym14224864

Amthor JS (2003) Efficiency of lignin biosynthesis: a quantitative analysis. Ann Bot 91:673–695. https://doi.org/10.1093/AOB/MCG073

Andrei I, Popa VI, Crestini C (2015) Obtaining lignin nanoparticles by sonication. Ultrason Sonochem 23:369–375. https://doi.org/10.1016/j.ultsonch.2014.08.021

Anitha A, Sowmya S, Kumar PTS, Deepthi S, Chennazhi KP, Ehrlich H et al (2014) Chitin and chitosan in selected biomedical applications. Prog Polym Sci 39:1644–1667. https://doi.org/10.1016/j.progpolymsci.2014.02.008

Baranwal J, Barse B, Fais A, Delogu GL, Kumar A (2022) Biopolymer: a sustainable material for food and medical applications. Polymers (Basel):14. https://doi.org/10.3390/polym14050983

Beaucamp A, Muddasar M, Amiinu IS, Moraes Leite M, Culebras M, Latha K et al (2022) Lignin for energy applications – state of the art, life cycle, technoeconomic analysis and future trends. Green Chem:8193–8226. https://doi.org/10.1039/d2gc02724k

Behr M, Jaziri M El, Baucher M. Lignin-Based Materials for Biomedical Applications. Lignin-Based Mater Biomed Appl 2021:35–60. https://doi.org/10.1016/c2019-0-01345-3

Bhagia S, Li H, Gao X, Kumar R, Wyman CE (2016) Flowthrough pretreatment with very dilute acid provides insights into high lignin contribution to biomass recalcitrance. Biotechnol Biofuels 9:1–15. https://doi.org/10.1186/S13068-016-0660-5/FIGURES/6

Björkman A (1954) Isolation of lignin from finely divided wood with neutral solvents. Nature 174(4440):1057–1058. https://doi.org/10.1038/1741057a0

Boerjan W, Ralph J, Baucher M (2003) Lignin biosynthesis. Annu Rev Plant Biol 54:519–546. https://doi.org/10.1146/ANNUREV.ARPLANT.54.031902.134938/1

Calvaruso G, Clough MT, Rinaldi R (2017) Biphasic extraction of mechanocatalytically-depolymerized lignin from water-soluble wood and its catalytic downstream processing. Green Chem 19:2803–2811. https://doi.org/10.1039/C6GC03191A

Cao J, Zhao Y, Jin S, Li J, Wu P, Luo Z (2022) Flexible lignin-based hydrogels with self-healing and adhesive ability driven by noncovalent interactions. Chem Eng J 429:132252. https://doi.org/10.1016/j.cej.2021.132252

Chen W-H, Lin B-J, Huang M-Y, Chang J-S (2015) Thermochemical conversion of microalgal biomass into biofuels: a review. Bioresour Technol 184:314–327. https://doi.org/10.1016/j.biortech.2014.11.050

Chen Z, Ragauskas A, Wan C (2020) Lignin extraction and upgrading using deep eutectic solvents. Ind Crop Prod 147:112241. https://doi.org/10.1016/J.INDCROP.2020.112241

Cui H, Jiang W, Wang C, Ji X, Liu Y, Yang G et al (2021) Lignin nanofiller-reinforced composites hydrogels with long-lasting adhesiveness, toughness, excellent self-healing, conducting, ultraviolet-blocking and antibacterial properties. Compos Part B Eng 225:109316. https://doi.org/10.1016/j.compositesb.2021.109316

Culebras M, Pishnamazi M, Walker GM, Collins MN (2021) Facile tailoring of structures for controlled release of paracetamol from sustainable lignin derived platforms. Molecules 26:1–9. https://doi.org/10.3390/molecules26061593

Dai L, Liu R, Hu L, Zou Z, Si C, Dai L et al (2017) Lignin nanoparticle as a novel green carrier for the efficient delivery of resveratrol Lignin nanoparticle as a novel green carrier for the efficient delivery of resveratrol, ACS Sustain Chem Eng. https://doi.org/10.1021/acssuschemeng.7b01903

Del Río JC, Rencoret J, Gutiérrez A, Elder T, Kim H, Ralph J (2020) Lignin monomers from beyond the canonical Monolignol biosynthetic pathway: another brick in the wall. ACS Sustain Chem Eng 8:4997–5012. https://doi.org/10.1021/ACSSUSCHEMENG.0C01109/ASSET/IMAGES/LARGE/SC0C01109_0006.JPEG

Deng Y, Ragauskas A (2012) Dry Kraft pulping at ambient pressure for cost effective energy saving and pollution deduction. https://doi.org/10.2172/1049310

Deng P, Chen F, Zhang H, Chen Y, Zhou J (2021) Conductive, self-healing, adhesive, and antibacterial hydrogels based on lignin/cellulose for rapid mrsa-infected wound repairing. ACS Appl Mater Interfaces 13:52333–52345. https://doi.org/10.1021/acsami.1c14608

Domínguez-Robles J, Stewart SA, Rendl A, González Z, Donnelly RF, Larrañeta E (2019) Lignin and cellulose blends as pharmaceutical excipient for tablet manufacturing via direct compression. Biomol Ther:9. https://doi.org/10.3390/biom9090423

El Achaby M, Kassab Z, Barakat A, Aboulkas A (2018) Alfa fibers as viable sustainable source for cellulose nanocrystals extraction: application for improving the tensile properties of biopolymer nanocomposite films. Ind Crop Prod 112:499–510. https://doi.org/10.1016/j.indcrop.2017.12.049

Erdocia X, Hernández-Ramos F, Morales A, Izaguirre N, de Hoyos-Martínez PL, Labidi J (2021) Lignin extraction and isolation methods. Lignin-Based Mater Biomed Appl Prep Charact Implement:61–104. https://doi.org/10.1016/B978-0-12-820303-3.00004-7

Figueiredo P, Lintinen K, Kiriazis A, Hynninen V, Liu Z (2017a) In vitro evaluation of biodegradable lignin-based nanoparticles for drug delivery and enhanced antiproliferation effect in cancer cells. Biomaterials 121:97–108. https://doi.org/10.1016/j.biomaterials.2016.12.034

Figueiredo P, Ferro C, Kemell M, Liu Z, Kiriazis A, Lintinen K et al (2017b) Functionalization of carboxylated lignin nanoparticles for targeted and pH-responsive delivery of anticancer drugs. Nanomedicine 12:2581–2596. https://doi.org/10.2217/nnm-2017-0219

Frangville C, Rutkevičius M, Richter AP, Velev OD, Stoyanov SD, Paunov VN (2012) Fabrication of environmentally biodegradable lignin nanoparticles. ChemPhysChem 13:4235–4243. https://doi.org/10.1002/cphc.201200537

Gan D, Xing W, Jiang L, Fang J, Zhao C, Ren F et al (2019) Plant-inspired adhesive and tough hydrogel based on Ag-Lignin nanoparticles-triggered dynamic redox catechol chemistry. Nat Commun 10:1–10. https://doi.org/10.1038/s41467-019-09351-2

García A, González Alriols M, Labidi J (2014) Evaluation of different lignocellulosic raw materials as potential alternative feedstocks in biorefinery processes. Ind Crop Prod 53:102–110. https://doi.org/10.1016/J.INDCROP.2013.12.019

Garg J, Nee Chiu M, Krishnan S, Kumar Tripathi L, Pandit S, Farasati Far B et al (2022) Applications of lignin nanoparticles for cancer drug delivery: an update. Mater Lett 311:131573. https://doi.org/10.1016/j.matlet.2021.131573

Gellerstedt G, Ek M, Henriksson G (2009) Wood chemistry and biotechnology. https://doi.org/10.1515/9783110213409/HTML
Gheorghita Puscaselu R, Lobiuc A, Dimian M, Covasa M (2020) Alginate: from food industry to biomedical applications and management of metabolic disorders. Polymers (Basel):12. https://doi.org/10.3390/polym12102417
Hassan SS, Williams GA, Jaiswal AK (2018) Emerging technologies for the pretreatment of lignocellulosic biomass. Bioresour Technol 262:310–318. https://doi.org/10.1016/J.BIORTECH.2018.04.099
Huang S, Su S, Gan H, Wu L, Lin C, Xu D et al (2019) Facile fabrication and characterization of highly stretchable lignin-based hydroxyethyl cellulose self-healing hydrogel. Carbohydr Polym 223. https://doi.org/10.1016/j.carbpol.2019.115080
Ibáñez AB, Bauer S (2014) Downscaled method using glass microfiber filters for the determination of Klason lignin and structural carbohydrates. Biomass Bioenergy 68:75–81. https://doi.org/10.1016/J.BIOMBIOE.2014.06.013
Imlimthan S, Figueiredo P, Santos HA, Sarparanta M (2021) Introduction to lignocellulosic materials. Lignin-Based Mater Biomed Appl:1–34. https://doi.org/10.1016/c2019-0-01345-3
Jeevanandam J, Pan S, Rodrigues J, Elkodous MA, Danquah MK (2022) Medical applications of biopolymer nanofibers. Biomater Sci 10:4107–4118. https://doi.org/10.1039/D2BM00701K
José F, Gomes B, Eloy De Souza R, Lelis R (2020) A review on lignin sources and uses. https://doi.org/10.15406/jabb.2020.07.00222
Kallel F, Bettaieb F, Khiari R, García A, Bras J, Chaabouni SE (2016) Isolation and structural characterization of cellulose nanocrystals extracted from garlic straw residues. Ind Crop Prod. https://doi.org/10.1016/j.indcrop.2016.04.060
Kargarzadeh H, Ahmad I, Abdullah I, Dufresne A, Zainudin SY, Sheltami RM (2012) Effects of hydrolysis conditions on the morphology, crystallinity, and thermal stability of cellulose nanocrystals extracted from kenaf bast fibers. Cellulose 19:855–866. https://doi.org/10.1007/s10570-012-9684-6
Kasbaji M, Mennani M, Oubenali M, Ait Benhamou A, Boussetta A, Ablouh EH et al (2023) Bio-based functionalized adsorptive polymers for sustainable water decontamination: a systematic review of challenges and real-world implementation. Environ Pollut 335:122349. https://doi.org/10.1016/j.envpol.2023.122349
Kassab Z, Abdellaoui Y, Salim MH, Bouhfid R, Qaiss AEK, El Achaby M (2020) Micro- and nano-celluloses derived from hemp stalks and their effect as polymer reinforcing materials. Carbohydr Polym 245:116506. https://doi.org/10.1016/j.carbpol.2020.116506
Kim JS, Lee YY, Kim TH (2016) A review on alkaline pretreatment technology for bioconversion of lignocellulosic biomass. Bioresour Technol 199:42–48. https://doi.org/10.1016/j.biortech.2015.08.085
Lagier CM, Zuriaga M, Monti G, Olivieri AC (1996) Urea-phosphoric acid complex studied by variable temperature 31P NMR spectroscopy and semiempirical calculations. J Phys Chem Solids 57:1183–1190. https://doi.org/10.1016/0022-3697(95)00294-4
Lancefield CS, Panovic I, Deuss PJ, Barta K, Westwood NJ (2017) Pre-treatment of lignocellulosic feedstocks using biorenewable alcohols: towards complete biomass valorisation. Green Chem 19:202–214. https://doi.org/10.1039/C6GC02739C
Lancefield CS, Constant S, de Peinder P, Bruijnincx PCA (2019) Linkage abundance and molecular weight characteristics of technical lignins by attenuated total reflection-FTIR spectroscopy combined with multivariate analysis. ChemSusChem 12:1139–1146. https://doi.org/10.1002/cssc.201802809
Li W, Amos K, Li M, Pu Y, DeBolt S, Ragauskas AJ et al (2018) Fractionation and characterization of lignin streams from unique high-lignin content endocarp feedstocks. Biotechnol Biofuels 11:1–14. https://doi.org/10.1186/S13068-018-1305-7/FIGURES/6
Liao JJ, Latif NHA, Trache D, Brosse N, Hussin MH (2020) Current advancement on the isolation, characterization and application of lignin. Int J Biol Macromol 162:985–1024. https://doi.org/10.1016/j.ijbiomac.2020.06.168

Liu K et al (2018a) Development of novel lignin-based targeted polymeric nanoparticle platform for efficient delivery of anticancer drugs. ACS Biomater Sci Eng. https://doi.org/10.1021/acsbiomaterials.8b00260

Liu W, Chen W, Hou Q, Wang S, Liu F (2018b) Effects of combined pretreatment of dilute acid pre-extraction and chemical-assisted mechanical refining on enzymatic hydrolysis of lignocellulosic biomass. RSC Adv 8:10207–10214. https://doi.org/10.1039/c7ra12732d

Liu X, Bouxin FP, Fan J, Budarin VL, Hu C, Clark JH (2020) Recent advances in the catalytic depolymerization of lignin towards phenolic chemicals: a review. ChemSusChem 13:4296–4317. https://doi.org/10.1002/cssc.202001213

Liu K, Zhuang Y, Chen J, Yang G, Dai L (2022a) Research progress on the preparation and high-value utilization of lignin nanoparticles. Int J Mol Sci:23. https://doi.org/10.3390/ijms23137254

Liu Y, Wang X, Wu Q, Pei W, Teo MJ, Chen ZS et al (2022b) Application of lignin and lignin-based composites in different tissue engineering fields. Int J Biol Macromol 222:994–1006. https://doi.org/10.1016/j.ijbiomac.2022.09.267

Lobato-Peralta DR, Duque-Brito E, Villafán-Vidales HI, Longoria A, Sebastian PJ, Cuentas-Gallegos AK et al (2021) A review on trends in lignin extraction and valorization of lignocellulosic biomass for energy applications. J Clean Prod:293. https://doi.org/10.1016/j.jclepro.2021.126123

Lopez G, Keiner D, Fasihi M, Koiranen T, Breyer C (2023) From fossil to green chemicals: sustainable pathways and new carbon feedstocks for the global chemical industry. Energy Environ Sci 16:2879–2909. https://doi.org/10.1039/D3EE00478C

Lu Y, Lu YC, Hu HQ, Xie FJ, Wei XY, Fan X (2017) Structural characterization of lignin and its degradation products with spectroscopic methods. J Spectrosc 2017. https://doi.org/10.1155/2017/8951658

Lupoi JS, Singh S, Parthasarathi R, Simmons BA, Henry RJ (2015) Recent innovations in analytical methods for the qualitative and quantitative assessment of lignin. Renew Sust Energ Rev 49:871–906. https://doi.org/10.1016/J.RSER.2015.04.091

Lutz TM, Kimna C, Casini A, Lieleg O (2022) Bio-based and bio-inspired adhesives from animals and plants for biomedical applications. Mater Today Bio 13:100203. https://doi.org/10.1016/j.mtbio.2022.100203

Luzi F, Tortorella I, Di Michele A, Dominici F, Argentati C, Morena F et al (2020) Novel nanocomposite PLA films with lignin/zinc oxide hybrids: design, characterization, interaction with mesenchymal stem cells. Nano 10:1–21. https://doi.org/10.3390/nano10112176

Luzi F, Yang W, Ma P, Torre L, Puglia D (2021) Lignin-based materials with antioxidant and antimicrobial properties, 1st edn. Elsevier. https://doi.org/10.1016/B978-0-12-820303-3.00003-5

Ma W, Hua D, Xiong R, Huang C (2022) Bio-based stimuli-responsive materials for biomedical applications. Mater Adv 4:458–475. https://doi.org/10.1039/d2ma01011a

Mankar AR, Pandey A, Modak A, Pant KK (2021) Pretreatment of lignocellulosic biomass: a review on recent advances. Bioresour Technol 334:125235. https://doi.org/10.1016/j.biortech.2021.125235

Martins MAP, Frizzo CP, Tier AZ, Moreira DN, Zanatta N, Bonacorso HG (2014) Update 1 of: ionic liquids in heterocyclic synthesis. Chem Rev 114:PR1–70. https://doi.org/10.1021/CR500106X/ASSET/IMAGES/MEDIUM/CR-2014-00106X_0050.GIF

Mboowa D (2024) A review of the traditional pulping methods and the recent improvements in the pulping processes. Biomass Convers Biorefinery 14:1–12. https://doi.org/10.1007/S13399-020-01243-6/TABLES/1

Meng Y, Lu J, Cheng Y, Li Q, Wang H (2019) Lignin-based hydrogels: a review of preparation, properties, and application. Int J Biol Macromol 135:1006–1019. https://doi.org/10.1016/j.ijbiomac.2019.05.198

Mennani M, Kasbaji M, Ait Benhamou A, Boussetta A, Mekkaoui AA, Grimi N et al (2023) Current approaches, emerging developments and functional prospects for lignin-based catalysts—review. Green Chem 25:2896–2929. https://doi.org/10.1039/D3GC00072A

Mennani M, Kasbaji M, Ait Benhamou A, Boussetta A, Kassab Z, El Achaby M et al (2024) The potential of lignin-functionalized metal catalysts – a systematic review. Renew Sust Energ Rev 189:113936. https://doi.org/10.1016/j.rser.2023.113936

Miao C, Hamad WY (2019) Critical insights into the reinforcement potential of cellulose nanocrystals in polymer nanocomposites. Curr Opin Solid State Mater Sci 23:100761. https://doi.org/10.1016/j.cossms.2019.06.005

Mohammadinejad R, Maleki H, Larrañeta E, Fajardo AR, Nik AB, Shavandi A et al (2019) Status and future scope of plant-based green hydrogels in biomedical engineering. Appl Mater Today 16:213–246. https://doi.org/10.1016/j.apmt.2019.04.010

Montazerian H, Sampath RR, Annabi N, Khademhosseini A, Weiss PS (2023) Polyphenolic gelatin-based bioadhesives. Accounts Mater Res 4:627–640. https://doi.org/10.1021/accountsmr.3c00055

Moubarik A, Grimi N, Boussetta N, Pizzi A (2013) Isolation and characterization of lignin from Moroccan sugar cane bagasse: production of lignin-phenol-formaldehyde wood adhesive. Ind Crop Prod 45:296–302. https://doi.org/10.1016/j.indcrop.2012.12.040

Nguyen MM, Al-Abdul-Wahid MS, Fontenot KR, Graves EE, Chang SC, Condon BD et al (2015) Understanding the mechanism of action of triazine-phosphonate derivatives as flame retardants for cotton fabric. Molecules 20:11236–11256. https://doi.org/10.3390/MOLECULES200611236

Oveissi F, Naficy S, Le TYL, Fletcher DF, Dehghani F (2018) Tough and processable hydrogels based on lignin and hydrophilic polyurethane. ACS Appl Bio Mater 1(6):2073–2081. https://doi.org/10.1021/acsabm.8b00546

Pishnamazi M, Hafizi H, Shirazian S, Culebras M, Walker GM, Collins MN (2019) Design of controlled release system for paracetamol based on modified lignin. Polymers (Basel) 11:1–10. https://doi.org/10.3390/POLYM11061059

Press AIN (2007) Hydrogel biomaterials: a smart future? Biomaterials 28:5185–5192. https://doi.org/10.1016/j.biomaterials.2007.07.044

Puangsin B, Soeta H, Saito T, Isogai A (2017) Characterization of cellulose nanofibrils prepared by direct TEMPO-mediated oxidation of hemp bast. Cellulose 24:3767–3775. https://doi.org/10.1007/S10570-017-1390-Y/FIGURES/5

Ralph J, Kim H, Lu F, Smith RA, Karlen SD, Nuoendagula et al (2023) Lignins and lignification. Recent. Adv Polyphen Res:1–50. https://doi.org/10.1002/9781119844792.CH1

Reale S, Di Tullio A, Spreti N, De Angelis F (2004) Mass spectrometry in the biosynthetic and structural investigation of lignins. Mass Spectrom Rev 23:87–126. https://doi.org/10.1002/MAS.10072

Rebelo R, Fernandes M, Fangueiro R (2017) Biopolymers in medical implants: a brief review. Procedia Eng 200:236–243. https://doi.org/10.1016/j.proeng.2017.07.034

Renders T, Van den Bossche G, Vangeel T, Van Aelst K, Sels B (2019) Reductive catalytic fractionation: state of the art of the lignin-first biorefinery. Curr Opin Biotechnol 56:193–201. https://doi.org/10.1016/j.copbio.2018.12.005

Rico-García D, Ruiz-Rubio L, Pérez-Alvarez L, Hernández-Olmos SL, Guerrero-Ramírez GL, Vilas-Vilela JL (2020) Lignin-based hydrogels: synthesis and applications. Polymers (Basel) 12:1–23. https://doi.org/10.3390/polym12010081

Rodrigues RCLB, Green Rodrigues B, Vieira Canettieri E, Acosta Martinez E, Palladino F, Wisniewski A et al (2022) Comprehensive approach of methods for microstructural analysis and analytical tools in lignocellulosic biomass assessment—a review. Bioresour Technol 348:126627. https://doi.org/10.1016/J.BIORTECH.2021.126627

Rybarczyk MK, Li Y, Qiao M, Hu YS, Titirici MM, Lieder M (2019) Hard carbon derived from rice husk as low cost negative electrodes in Na-ion batteries. J Energy Chem:17–22. https://doi.org/10.1016/j.jechem.2018.01.025

Seddiqi H, Oliaei E, Honarkar H, Jin J, Geonzon LC, Bacabac RG et al (2021) Cellulose and its derivatives: towards biomedical applications. Cellulose 28:1893–1931. https://doi.org/10.1007/s10570-020-03674-w

Sen S, Patil S, Argyropoulos DS (2015) Thermal properties of lignin in copolymers, blends, and composites: a review. Green Chem 17:4862–4887. https://doi.org/10.1039/c5gc01066g

Serrano-Ruiz JC (2020) Biomass: a renewable source of fuels, chemicals and carbon materials. Molecules:25. https://doi.org/10.3390/molecules25215217

Siddiqui L, Bag J, Mittal D, Leekha A, Mishra H, Mishra M (2020) Assessing the potential of lignin nanoparticles as drug carrier: synthesis , cytotoxicity and genotoxicity studies. Int J Biol Macromol 152:786–802. https://doi.org/10.1016/j.ijbiomac.2020.02.311

Stanisz M, Klapiszewski, Collins MN, Jesionowski T (2022) Recent progress in biomedical and biotechnological applications of lignin-based spherical nano- and microstructures: a comprehensive review. Mater Today Chem 26:101198. https://doi.org/10.1016/j.mtchem.2022.101198

Sugiarto S, Leow Y, Tan CL, Wang G, Kai D (2022) How far is lignin from being a biomedical material? Bioact Mater 8:71–94. https://doi.org/10.1016/j.bioactmat.2021.06.023

Sun RC (2020) Lignin source and structural characterization. ChemSusChem 13:4385–4393. https://doi.org/10.1002/CSSC.202001324

Sun Y, Cheng J (2002) Hydrolysis of lignocellulosic materials for ethanol production: a review. Bioresour Technol 83:1–11. https://doi.org/10.1016/S0960-8524(01)00212-7

Sun SN, Li MF, Yuan TQ, Xu F, Sun RC (2012) Sequential extractions and structural characterization of lignin with ethanol and alkali from bamboo (Neosinocalamus affinis). Ind Crop Prod 37:51–60. https://doi.org/10.1016/J.INDCROP.2011.11.033

Szymanska-Chargot M, Chylinska M, Gdula K, Koziol A, Zdunek A (2017) Isolation and characterization of cellulose from different fruit and vegetable pomaces. Polymers (Basel):9. https://doi.org/10.3390/polym9100495

Tortora M, Cavalieri F, Mosesso P, Ciaffardini F, Melone F, Crestini C (2014) Ultrasound driven assembly of lignin into microcapsules for storage and delivery of hydrophobic molecules. Biomacromolecules 15:1634–1643. https://doi.org/10.1021/bm500015j

Treimanis A (1996) Wood pulp fiber structure and chemical composition, their influence on technological processes. Nord Pulp Pap Res J 11:146–151. https://doi.org/10.3183/npprj-1996-11-03-p146-151

Ugartondo V, Mitjans M, Vinardell MP (2008) Comparative antioxidant and cytotoxic effects of lignins from different sources. Bioresour Technol 99:6683–6687. https://doi.org/10.1016/j.biortech.2007.11.038

Ullah I, Chen Z, Xie Y, Khan SS, Singh S, Yu C et al (2022) Recent advances in biological activities of lignin and emerging biomedical applications: a short review. Int J Biol Macromol 208:819–832. https://doi.org/10.1016/j.ijbiomac.2022.03.182

Vaezi K, Asadpour G (2022) Effects of HCl hydrolyzed cellulose nanocrystals from waste papers on the hydroxypropyl methylcellulose/cationic starch biofilms. Waste Biomass Valoriz 13:2035–2051. https://doi.org/10.1007/S12649-021-01651-3/FIGURES/9

Van Den Bosch S, Schutyser W, Vanholme R, Driessen T, Koelewijn SF, Renders T et al (2015) Reductive lignocellulose fractionation into soluble lignin-derived phenolic monomers and dimers and processable carbohydrate pulps. Energy Environ Sci 8:1748–1763. https://doi.org/10.1039/C5EE00204D

Vieira FR, Magina S, Evtuguin DV, Barros-Timmons A (2022) Lignin as a renewable building block for sustainable polyurethanes. Materials (Basel):15. https://doi.org/10.3390/ma15176182

Wang D, Jang J, Kim K, Kim J, Park CB (2019) "Tree to bone": lignin/polycaprolactone nanofibers for hydroxyapatite biomineralization. Biomacromolecules 20:2684–2693. https://doi.org/10.1021/acs.biomac.9b00451

Wang Q, Lan J, Hua Z, Ma X, Chen L, Pan X et al (2021) An oriented Fe3+-regulated lignin-based hydrogel with desired softness, conductivity, stretchability, and asymmetric adhesiveness towards anti-interference pressure sensors. Int J Biol Macromol 184:282–288. https://doi.org/10.1016/j.ijbiomac.2021.05.203

Yang Y, Xu L, Wang J, Meng Q, Zhong S, Gao Y et al (2022) Recent advances in polysaccharide-based self-healing hydrogels for biomedical applications. Carbohydr Polym 283:119161. https://doi.org/10.1016/j.carbpol.2022.119161

Yang Y, Zhou T, Cheng M, Xie M, Shi N, Liu T et al (2024) Recent advances in organic waste pyrolysis and gasification in a CO2 environment to value-added products. J Environ Manag 356:120666. https://doi.org/10.1016/j.jenvman.2024.120666

Yoo CG, Meng X, Pu Y, Ragauskas AJ (2020) The critical role of lignin in lignocellulosic biomass conversion and recent pretreatment strategies: a comprehensive review. Bioresour Technol 301:122784. https://doi.org/10.1016/j.biortech.2020.122784

Yuan TQ, Xu F, Sun RC (2013) Role of lignin in a biorefinery: separation characterization and valorization. J Chem Technol Biotechnol 88:346–352. https://doi.org/10.1002/JCTB.3996

Zevallos Torres LA, Lorenci Woiciechowski A, de Andrade Tanobe VO, Karp SG, Guimarães Lorenci LC, Faulds C et al (2020) Lignin as a potential source of high-added value compounds: a review. J Clean Prod 263:121499. https://doi.org/10.1016/j.jclepro.2020.121499

Zhang H, Bai Y, Yu B, Liu X, Chen F (2017) A practicable process for lignin color reduction: fractionation of lignin using methanol/water as a solvent. Green Chem 19:5152–5162. https://doi.org/10.1039/c7gc01974b

Zhang W, Ma Y, Wang C, Li S, Zhang M, Chu F et al (2021) Development and characterization of a wood adhesive using bagasse lignin. Int J Adhes Adhes 65:7996–8004. https://doi.org/10.3390/molecules26092533

Zhou Y, Han Y, Li G, Yang S, Xiong F, Chu F (2019) Preparation of targeted lignin-based hollow nanoparticles for the delivery of doxorubicin. Nanomaterials (Basel). https://doi.org/10.3390/nano9020188

6 Polysaccharide-Based Encapsulation of Active Ingredients for Biomedical Applications: From Macroscale to Nanoscale

Asmaa M. Elzayat, Luis Fernando Jiménez-Hernández, and Rafael Muñoz-Espí

Abstract

This chapter explores the design and synthesis of polysaccharide-based organic–inorganic hybrid systems for the encapsulation and controlled release of hydrophilic active ingredients in biomedical applications. By integrating biopolymers such as chitosan and alginate with silica nanostructures, the resulting materials achieve enhanced mechanical stability, biocompatibility, and tunable release profiles. Three main encapsulation strategies are detailed: (1) macroscopic hydrogel beads and scaffolds formed via ionotropic gelation, (2) microparticles prepared through spray drying, and (3) nanocapsules generated using inverse nanoemulsions. Each technique enables size-controlled encapsulation, with potential applications ranging from drug delivery to tissue engineering and catalysis. The incorporation of silica contributes to sustained release behavior and structural integrity across all scales. The chapter highlights the versatility and scalability of these hybrid systems, advocating for future developments such as hydrophobic drug loading and targeted delivery via surface functionalization.

Keywords

Sustainable materials · Polysaccharides · Alginate · Silica nanoparticles · Encapsulation · Biomedical applications

---

A. M. Elzayat (✉)
Institute of Materials Science (ICMUV), University of Valencia, Paterna, Spain

Physics Department, Faculty of Science, Mansoura University, Mansoura, Egypt
e-mail: am_elzayat@mans.edu.eg

L. F. Jiménez-Hernández · R. Muñoz-Espí (✉)
Institute of Materials Science (ICMUV), University of Valencia, Paterna, Spain
e-mail: rafael.munoz@uv.es

M. N. Collins, M. Culebras (eds.), *Sustainable Biopolymers and Composites for Biomedical Applications*, Biomaterials, Bioengineering and Sustainability 5,
https://doi.org/10.1007/978-3-031-91972-5_6

6.1 Introduction

Controlling the release of active ingredients to target specific sites of action, while enhancing therapeutic bioavailability and reducing side effects or toxicity, has attracted significant attention in recent years (Zamani et al. 2017; Vong et al. 2017). Among other strategies, researchers have been looking to increase the therapeutic performance and minimize the side effects of such ingredients by incorporating them into polymer matrices. The encapsulation of active substances can enhance their availability, stability, and biological activity, additionally providing protection against degradation in harsh physiological environments. Specifically, polysaccharide/inorganic hybrid materials are attractive due to the synergistic combination of the chemical properties of the biopolymers and the physical properties of the inorganic matter (Couvreur and Vauthier 2006; Prabaharan and Mano 2004).

Common strategies for preparing polysaccharide-based delivery systems include the formation of hydrogels, microparticles, nanoparticles, nanogels, micelles, and dendrimers (Farasati Far et al. 2022). For those purposes, cross-linking significantly affects the biocompatibility, biodegradability, safety, and cost-effectivity of the final system (Farrugia and Groves 1999). Polysaccharides, such as pectin, agarose, agar, cellulose, dextran, alginate, or chitosan, can form hydrogels upon physical or chemical cross-linking to create three-dimensional hydrophilic networks that swell without dissolving when brought into contact with water or other biological fluids (Nair and Laurencin 2007; Wen and Oh 2014).

Although biobased hydrogels are ideal biomaterials, incorporating biocompatible inorganic moieties can enhance their properties, giving them advantages for specific applications, such as delivery carriers, scaffolds, implants, and more (Baishya et al. 2024). The incorporation of silica, recognized as safe by the US Food and Drug Administration (FDA), can help to address important challenges in the design of targeted and controlled release systems (Ehlerding et al. 2016). Silica has emerged as a component for promising drug vehicles because it is nearly nontoxic, biocompatible, and easy to be surface-modified (Wang et al. 2016). Silica nanoparticles in suspension can be formed by sol–gel processes in the presence of polysaccharides, yielding the formation of a hybrid polymer structure with potential use in the delivery of therapeutic agents (Zhang et al. 2015; Doan-Nguyen et al. 2019; Blin et al. 2016; Fan et al. 2018; Ilhan-Ayisigi and Yesil-Celiktas 2018; Niyom et al. 2019; Pramanik et al. 2018). Organic/inorganic hybrid structures can protect the encapsulated payloads from the surrounding environment and allow their release in a controlled manner (De Koker et al. 2012; Gaitzsch et al. 2016; Behzadi et al. 2016; Hood et al. 2014).

The development of new soft encapsulation techniques has enabled the use of biopolymers, especially polysaccharides, for encapsulating active ingredients with pharmaceutical applications. Some versatile techniques, such as electrospinning, microfluidics, and layer-by-layer assembly, allow for a relatively straightforward preparation of polysaccharide–inorganic hybrid hydrogels. However, despite the successful integration of the polymer and inorganic moieties, controlling their structure remains a challenge (Hamedi et al. 2018). To address this issue, innovative

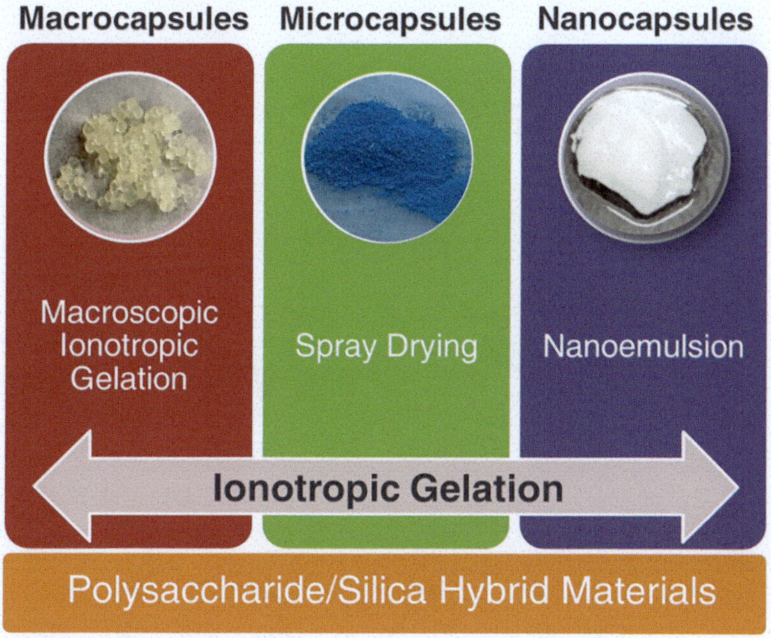

Fig. 6.1 Infographic of selected techniques used to prepare polysaccharide/silica hybrid hydrogels from macro- to nanosized scale

synthetic strategies must be properly designed to ensure a controlled and reproducible structure with homogeneous properties. In this respect, this chapter presents the preparation of polysaccharide–inorganic hybrid hydrogels by different techniques involving ionotropic gelation. As shown in Fig. 6.1, the preparation of these hybrid hydrogel materials can be approached through different methods, resulting in a variety of materials ranging from the macro- to the nanoscale. The materials described herein are specifically designed for the encapsulation and entrapment of hydrophilic substances, so that their release behavior can be controlled in different media.

Ionotropic gelation via polyelectrolyte complexation provides an eco-friendly strategy that minimizes the use of toxic organic solvents or cross-linking agents. Chitosan and alginate are two widely used, non-toxic, and biocompatible hydrophilic polysaccharides that readily swell in aqueous media. Figure 6.2 illustrates the mechanism of ionotropic gelation of chitosan and alginate, which involves electrostatic interactions between the polysaccharides functional groups and opposite-charged ions resulting in the hydrogel formation (Fernando et al. 2019; Boi et al. 2020; Silva et al. 2020). Specifically, as a representative example, chitosan can interact with triphosphate in acidic media via electrostatic forces to create ionically cross-linked networks. Alginate, on the other hand, demonstrates excellent performance as a gel when physically cross-linked with $CaCl_2$.

Unlike the simple interaction between monomeric ions, where the electroneutrality principle typically applies, the interaction between a polyanion and

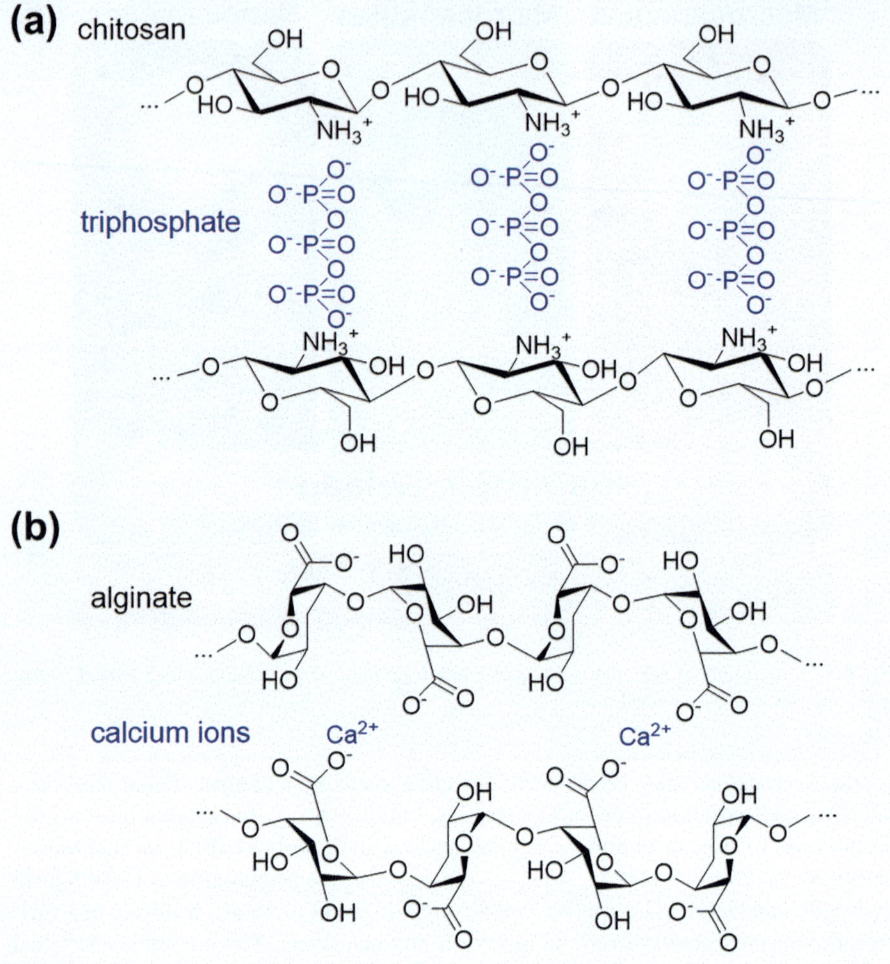

Fig. 6.2 Physical cross-linking of (**a**) chitosan with triphosphate ions and (**b**) alginate with calcium ions.

cations (or a polycation and anions) is more complex. The three-dimensional structure of the polymer, along with the presence of functional groups, influences how well the ions bind to the polymer. This means that the formation of the cross-linked network is not merely about charge neutrality but is also shaped by the overall molecular architecture of the materials involved.

In the following sections, we describe how the ionotropic gelation of chitosan and alginate, as representative examples of polysaccharides, leads to the formation of hydrogels at the macro, micro, and nanoscale. Carrying out ionotropic gelation in bulk is a simple process that rapidly forms hydrogels by extrusion of an aqueous solution in the form of droplets into the cross-linking agent receptor, yielding sub-millimetric hydrogel beads (Elzayat et al. 2021a). Such beads can also be assembled in larger scaffolds for biomedical applications (Elzayat et al. 2022).

The combination of ionotropic gelation with spray drying allows for the formation of microsized hydrogels. It is a fast and continuous process based on the transformation of liquid feed into dry particles in three steps: atomization, mixing of fine droplets with a gas stream, and separation and collection of dried microparticles (Elzayat et al. 2023).

On the nanoscale, the preparation of hybrid polymer–inorganic nanoparticles can take place by using the nanoemulsion (or miniemulsion) technique through two different protocols: a "one-nanoemulsion" process, in which the cross-linking occurs during the ionotropic gelation; and a "two-nanoemulsion" process, in which the ionically cross-linking mechanism is allowed to take place during the mixing and fusion process of two separated nanoemulsions with a polycationic biopolymer and a polyanionic cross-linker in the disperse phase (Elzayat et al. 2025). In both cases, hydrophilic compounds are entrapped in situ within a polymer matrix.

6.2 Polysaccharide-Based Macrocapsules: Preparation by Macroscopic Ionotropic Gelation

Many polysaccharides can be used as polymer matrices to encapsulate hydrophilic model drugs. Particularly, the bulk preparation of submillimetric hybrid chitosan and alginate-based hydrogels can be easily achieved via ionotropic gelation. Chitosan, a cationic polyelectrolyte, interacts with anionic cross-linkers such as sodium triphosphate ($P_3O_{10}{}^{5-}$), leading to the formation of hydrogel beads (Fig. 6.2a). On the other hand, alginate, a polyanion that contains carboxylate groups (COO^-), cross-links with divalent calcium ions (Ca^{2+}) (Fig. 6.2b), forming a stable gel. During this process, silica nanostructures can also be incorporated into the polymer matrices through an in-situ sol–gel method, which involves the hydrolysis and condensation of tetraethyl orthosilicate (TEOS), as schematically represented in Fig. 6.3. TEOS is added to a polysaccharide solution, and the mixture is stirred while a suspension of silica nanoparticles is formed. The resulting chitosan/silica mixture is then added dropwise to a solution of the cross-linking agent ($P_3O_{10}{}^{5-}$ or Ca^{2+}, for chitosan and alginate, respectively). Polysaccharide/silica sub-millimetric beads with encapsulated erioglaucine disodium salt and ephedrine hydrochloride were prepared following this methodology (Elzayat et al. 2021a). The silica nanostructures were homogeneously distributed throughout the polymer network during cross-linking, providing additional structural integrity. The inclusion of these inorganic nanostructures enhanced the mechanical stability of the resulting hydrogel beads and helped in controlling the release of the encapsulated drug. This effect was particularly notable in both neutral and acidic environments, in which the nanostructures slowed down the drug release rate. An advantage of ionotropic gelation is that it uses aqueous solvents, reducing the need for toxic organic solvents commonly used in other encapsulation methods. Such an approach is safer and more environmentally friendly for drug delivery systems (Tığlı Aydın and Pulat 2012;

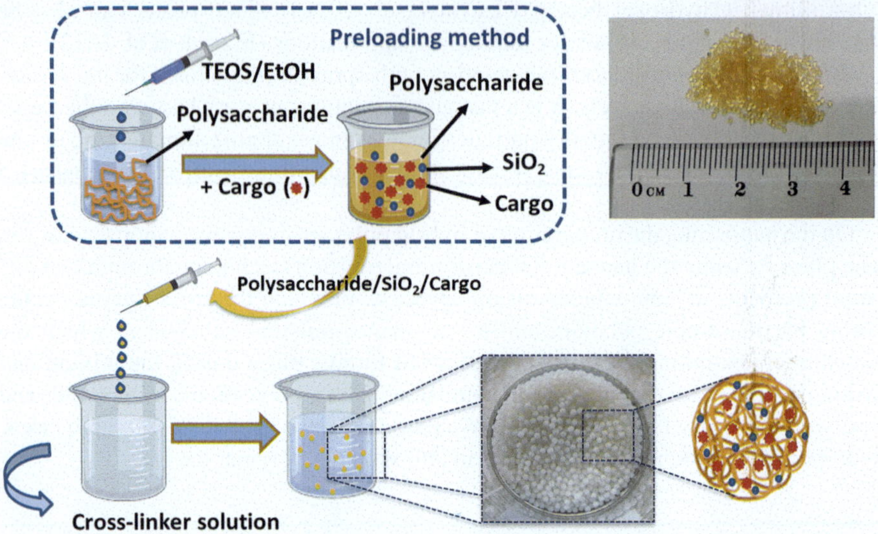

Fig. 6.3 Schematic representation of the formation of cross-linked polysaccharide/silica hybrid submillispheres encapsulating active hydrophilic molecules. The color of the spheres changes from white to yellow (upper photograph) after the drying process. (Copyright (2021) Wiley. Reproduced with permission from Elzayat et al. (2021a))

Alam et al. 2012; Meng et al. 2011; Nanjwade et al. 2010; Bhattarai et al. 2006; Pan et al. 2002).

The assembly of particles can lead to the formation of scaffolds. Therefore, the method was expanded to develop a 3D chitosan/silica hybrid scaffold, prepared in two key steps, as illustrated in Fig. 6.4 (Elzayat et al. 2022). Two different hydrophilic molecules were encapsulated in each of the steps. First, ibuprofen disodium salt was encapsulated within the chitosan submillispheres in a process analogous to the previously described. Second, these hydrogel spheres were assembled into a 3D scaffold by binding them with a chitosan solution. During this step, a post-loading technique was employed to encapsulate a second hydrophilic molecule, erioglaucine disodium salt, within the scaffold. Different scaffold compositions were prepared based on this strategy, allowing for the development of advanced materials with potential applications in drug delivery and tissue engineering.

As also observed for the unassembled particles, the presence of silica was found to retard the release of both entrapped substances compared to samples containing only chitosan. The release mechanism for erioglaucine was primarily diffusion-based, following a Korsmeyer–Peppas kinetics. In contrast, ibuprofen was released through a mixed mechanism, requiring passage through a "double barrier": the release of the beads during the swelling process and subsequent diffusion from the scaffold into the release medium. While swelling influenced the release of ibuprofen, it had little effect on the release of erioglaucine, which was entrapped outside during the scaffold formation.

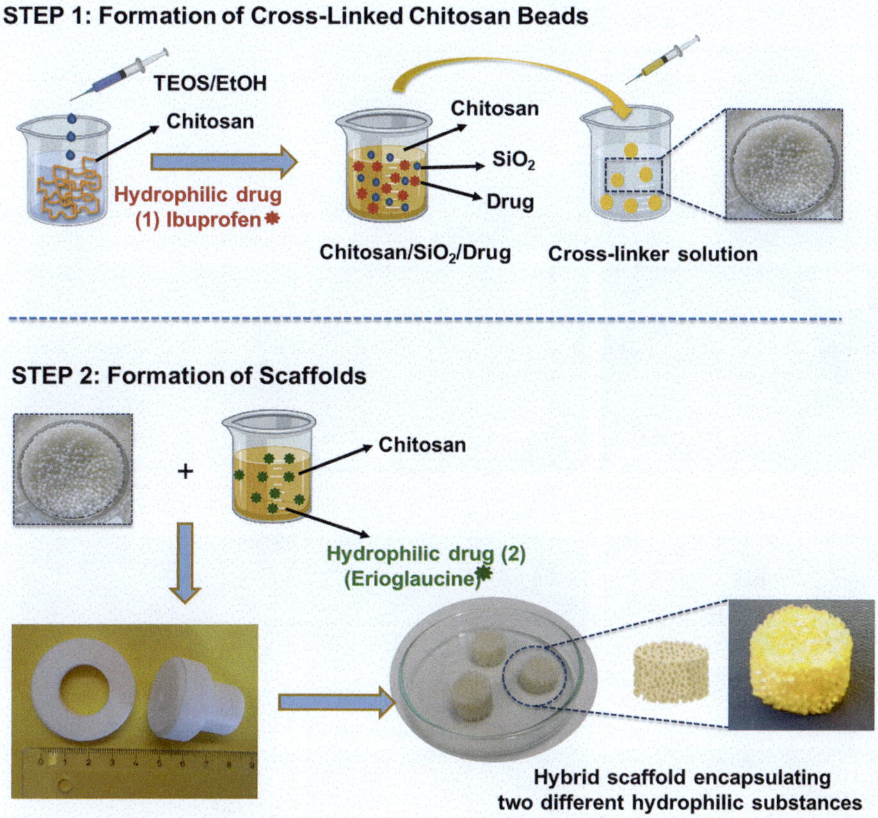

Fig. 6.4 Formation of chitosan/silica scaffolds in two steps: first, preparation of cross-linked chitosan/silica hydrogels encapsulating a first hydrophilic substance by in situ loading; and second, collecting and adhesion process of hydrogel beads to form the hybrid scaffold. (Adapted from Elzayat et al. (2022). Creative Commons CC BY-NC-ND license)

The morphology of the prepared pristine chitosan scaffolds was compared to the hybrid chitosan/silica ones by optical microscopy and scanning electron microscopy (SEM). The corresponding micrographs are shown in Fig. 6.5. The pure chitosan scaffold (labeled as sample SF1) presents a regular structure with a smooth surface, while chitosan/silica hybrid samples (labeled as sample SF2) show a certain roughness, attributed to the presence of silica nanostructures, that homogeneously embedded within the chitosan matrix during the formation process. The silica plays a significant role in both increasing the structural stability of the scaffold and retarding the release behavior in neutral environments.

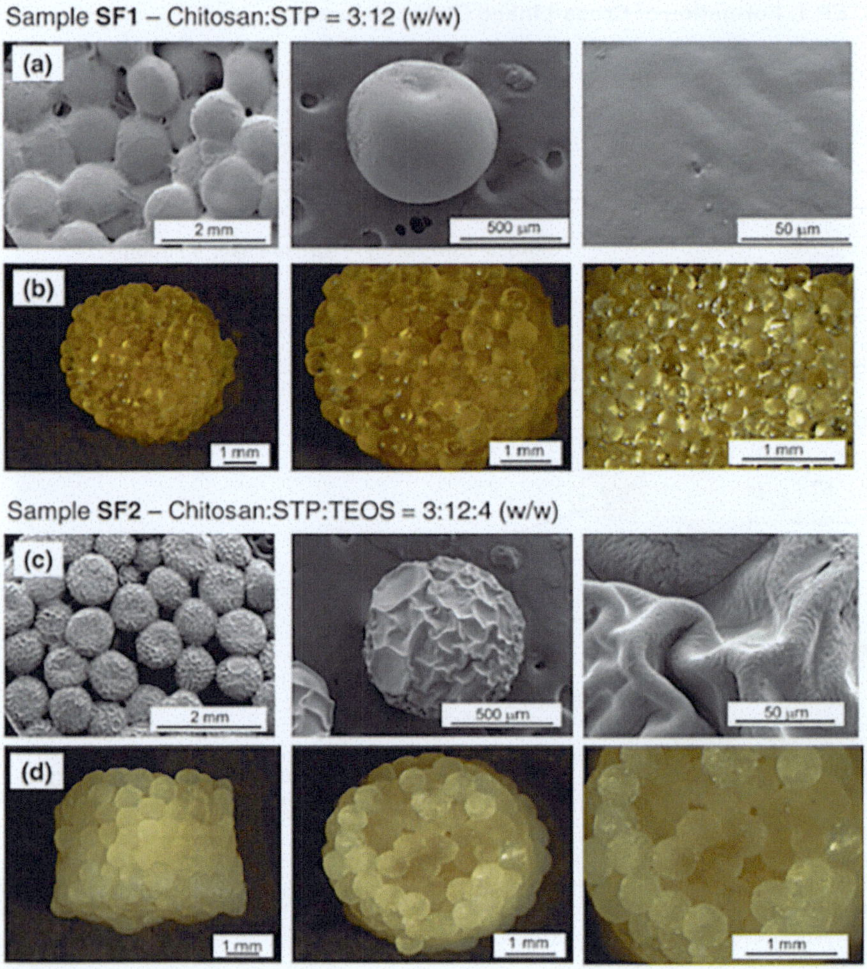

Fig. 6.5 Micrographs of a chitosan and a chitosan/silica scaffold by SEM (**a** and **c**) and optical microscopy (**b** and **d**). (Reproduced from Elzayat et al. (2022). Creative Commons CC BY-NC-ND license)

6.3 Polysaccharide-Based Microcapsules: Preparation by Spray Drying

Spray drying is a rapid and reproducible method for producing dry microparticles, very especially in the pharmaceutical and food industries. This method is effective due to its continuous nature, ease of scalability, and relatively low processing costs. The process begins with the preparation of an aqueous polysaccharide solution, which is atomized to form small droplets. These droplets are then mixed with a drying gas, causing the liquid phase to evaporate and resulting in the formation of polymeric microparticles (Ngan et al. 2014; Sinsuebpol et al. 2013).

In our work, spray drying was employed to prepare microparticles, extending the previously described strategies for chitosan/silica hybrid macroparticles and macroscaffolds (Elzayat et al. 2023). Polysaccharide/silica hybrid microcapsules were produced through ionic gelation followed by spray-drying. Chitosan and alginate served as the biopolymer matrices, with in-situ prepared silica acting as a structuring additive. As for the macrocapsules, the microparticles were employed for the encapsulation of a model hydrophilic molecule, erioglaucine disodium salt. In parallel, as an additional alternative application, the microparticles were also applied as supports for palladium nanoparticles used as catalysts in the reduction of *p*-nitrophenol by sodium borohydride. In this latter case, chloropalladate was complexed on the surface of chitosan microparticles, followed by the reduction of palladium(II) to palladium(0), resulting in highly effective heterogeneous catalysts.

A specific amount of the hydrophilic cargo was mixed with the polysaccharide solution, both with and without TEOS. After dissolution of the dye dissolved, a cross-linker solution was added to these mixtures, followed by spray-drying to produce dye-loaded microparticles. The morphology of the resulting microparticles, shown in Fig. 6.6a–b, was similar to those produced without erioglaucine. The release behavior was investigated through dissolution studies in a phosphate-buffered solution (pH 7.4) at 37 °C. Figure 6.6c illustrates the release process of spray-dried chitosan–STP microparticles. The majority of the release occurred rapidly within the first 3 h (approximately 40–60%), likely due to the substantial

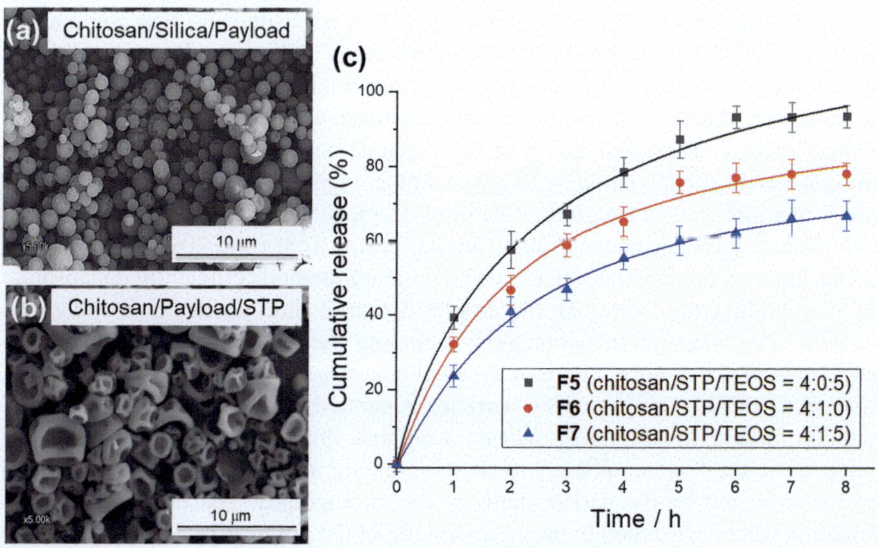

Fig. 6.6 (**a** and **b**) SEM images of spray-dried polysaccharide microparticles loaded with erioglaucine in the presence and absence of silica with a polymer/TEOS ratio of 3:4. (**c**) Cumulative release of erioglaucine loaded samples with (samples F5 and F7) and without (sample F6) silica. The solid lines represent the theoretical fitting according to the Hill equation. (Adapted from Elzayat et al. (2023). Creative Commons CC-BY license).

amount of erioglaucine adhering to the microcapsule surface during the drying steps. Overall, the release was governed by diffusion, influenced by the swelling process.

6.4 Polysaccharide-Based Nanocapsules: Preparation from Nanoemulsions

Direct nanoemulsions (oil-in-water) are ideal for encapsulating hydrophobic components, while inverse nanoemulsions (water-in-oil) efficiently encapsulate hydrophilic substances. The application of nanoemulsions for biomedical nanocarriers has been reviewed in detail elsewhere in a previous work of our group (Elzayat et al. 2021b). This approach was employed to produce nanohydrogels by utilizing a nanoemulsion in which the biopolymer was dissolved in the dispersed phase. Physically cross-linked chitosan and chitosan/silica hybrid nanocapsules were synthesized using an inverse water-in-oil nanoemulsion combined with ionotropic gelation to encapsulate hydrophilic molecules (Elzayat et al. 2025). This nanoemulsion-based approach further complements the previously described microcapsule systems, offering additional flexibility and control over particle size and encapsulation efficiency, and expanding the potential for biomedical applications, such as controlled drug release and targeted delivery.

Two different methods utilizing nanoemulsions, illustrated in Fig. 6.7, were implemented. The first approach, referred to as the "one-emulsion" method, involves the direct addition of the cross-linking agent to a nanoemulsion that contains an aqueous solution of chitosan in the dispersed phase. Following this, an additional ultrasonication step facilitates the physical cross-linking, resulting in gelation and the formation of nanoparticles. The second approach, termed as the "two-emulsion" method, involves the combination of two separate nanoemulsions: one containing chitosan and the other containing the cross-linker. In this case, gelation and nanoparticle formation occur through the fusion of droplets from the two nanoemulsions. Both methods produce nanocapsules ranging in size from 50 to 200 nm.

Our findings demonstrate that both preparation methods efficiently encapsulate the hydrophilic cargo, although the droplet-fusion method yields more stable suspensions. The preparation parameters, including the chitosan/STP ratio, significantly influence the morphology of the final nanostructures. Transmission electron microscopy (TEM) images of the particles generated through the "two-emulsion" method, presented in Fig. 6.8, indicate a notably smaller size compared to those obtained via the "one-emulsion" method, revealing a clear capsule-like morphology, as indicated by the darker shells in the micrographs. The observed capsule formation can be attributed to the cross-linking of the polymer by STP occurring at the water/oil interface of the inverse nanoemulsion. These structures are significantly smaller (<50 nm) than the dimensions measured by dynamic light scattering (DLS); however, it is essential to note that the sizes captured by electron microscopy correspond to the dry particles, while DLS measures the hydrodynamic diameters of the swollen capsules.

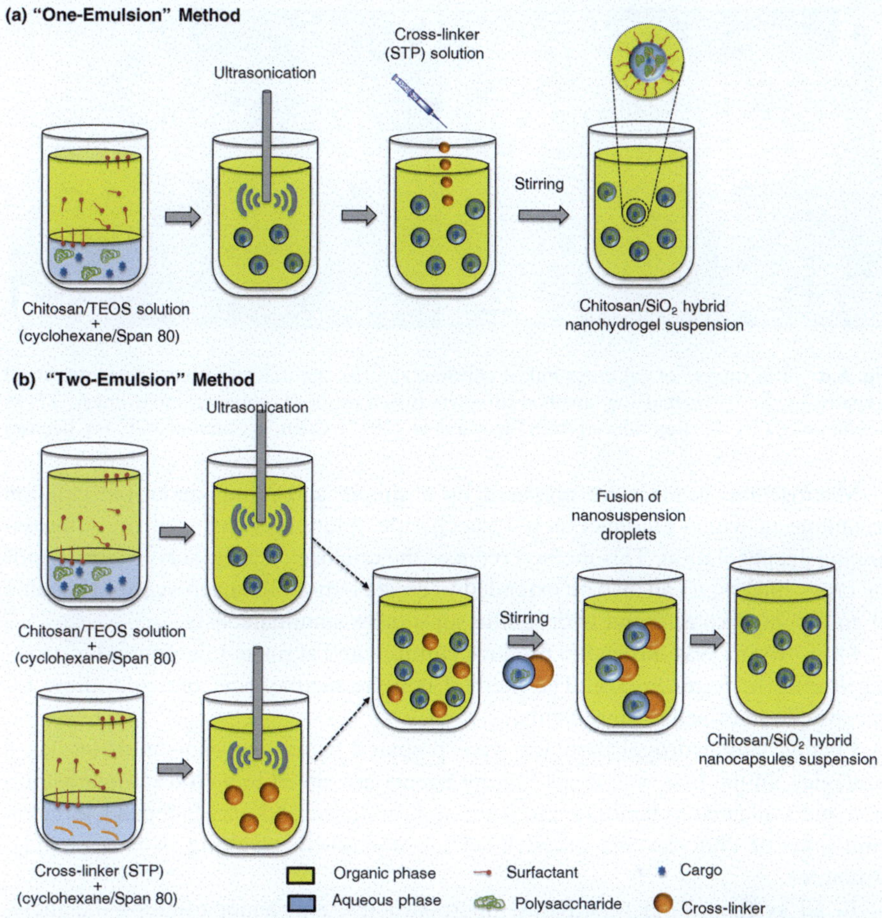

Fig. 6.7 Schematic representation of the formation of cross-linked chitosan nanohydrogels encapsulating an active hydrophilic molecule through two (**a**) a "one-emulsion" method and (**b**) a "two-emulsion" method (droplet-fusion method). (Reproduced from Elzayat et al. (2025). Creative Commons CC-BY license)

6.5 Conclusions and Outlook

This chapter has discussed the fabrication of organic–inorganic polysaccharide-based hydrogel carriers using three distinct methods that yield materials of varying size scales: submillimetric beads via ionotropic gelation, microparticles through spray drying, and nanoparticles using the nanoemulsion (or miniemulsion) technique. Chitosan and alginate were employed as the primary polysaccharides, while silica was integrated as a structuring additive to enhance stability and function. The research highlights the capacity of these systems to efficiently encapsulate hydrophilic molecules.

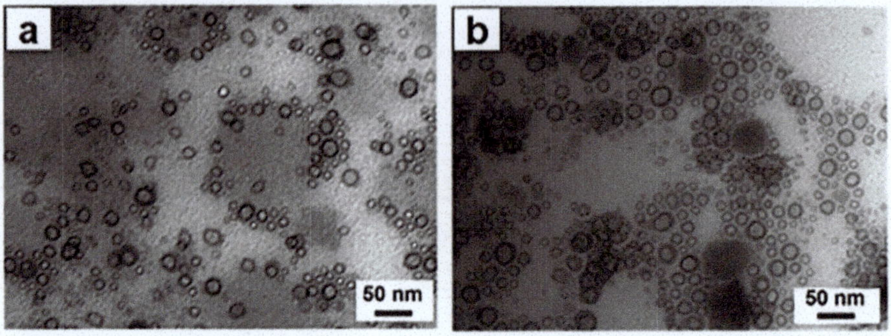

Fig. 6.8 TEM images of (**a**) cross-linked chitosan and (**b**) chitosan/silica hybrid nanohydrogel prepared by the "two-emulsion" method (droplets fusion method) (polymer: cross-linker: TEOS weight ratios (3:1:4). (Reproduced from Elzayat et al. (2025). Creative Commons CC-BY license)

Macroscopic beads were prepared by a simple and rapid ionotropic gelation technique in which an aqueous polysaccharide solution is extruded into a cross-linking agent solution. This method reduces the reliance on toxic solvents or chemical cross-linkers; it can also be extended to create hybrid 3D macroscaffold capable of entrapping two different hydrophilic substances simultaneously.

Spray drying was utilized to produce chitosan and alginate microparticles, ranging from 1 to 5 μm in size. The method is reproducible, scalable, and allow for encapsulation of active ingredients.

Finally, nanohydrogel particles were prepared using two nanoemulsion-based strategies. In the first one, cross-linking agents are added to a chitosan nanoemulsion and sonicated to facilitate cross-linking. In the second one, independent nanoemulsions of chitosan and cross-linker are combined, resulting in nanocapsular structures.

In all systems—macroparticles, microparticles, and nanoparticles—the inclusion of silica nanostructures enhance the structural stability, modulating the swelling behavior and delaying the release of encapsulated molecules.

The versatility of polysaccharide chemistry opens up opportunities for creating diverse biopolymer/inorganic hybrid particles tailored to specific applications, with size scales from macroscopic to nanometric. Future research could explore the use of hydrophobized polysaccharides to encapsulate hydrophobic drugs, enabling the design of hierarchical, multifunctional materials for various therapeutic applications. Additionally, surface functionalization with specific ligands could enhance targeted delivery of the carriers to specific biological sites.

References

Alam S, Khan ZI, Mustafa G, Kumar M, Islam F, Bhatnagar A et al (2012) Development and evaluation of thymoquinone-encapsulated chitosan nanoparticles for nose-to-brain targeting: a pharmacoscintigraphic study. Int J Nanomedicine 7:5705–5718. https://doi.org/10.2147/IJN.S35329

Baishya G, Parasar B, Limboo M, Kumar R, Dutta A, Hussain A et al (2024) Advancements in nanocomposite hydrogels: a comprehensive review of biomedical applications. Discov Mater 4(1):40. https://doi.org/10.1007/s43939-024-00111-8

Behzadi S, Steinmann M, Estupiñán D, Landfester K, Crespy D (2016) The pro-active payload strategy significantly increases selective release from mesoporous nanocapsules. J Control Release 242:119–125. https://doi.org/10.1016/j.jconrel.2016.08.040

Bhattarai N, Ramay HR, Chou S-H, Zhang M (2006) Chitosan and lactic acid-grafted chitosan nanoparticles as carriers for prolonged drug delivery. Int J Nanomedicine 1(2):181–187. https://doi.org/10.2147/nano.2006.1.2.181

Blin J-L, Stébé M-J, Lebeau B (2016) Hybrid/porous materials obtained from nano-emulsions. Curr Opin Colloid Interface Sci 25:75–82. https://doi.org/10.1016/j.cocis.2016.07.002

Boi S, Rouatbi N, Dellacasa E, Di Lisa D, Bianchini P, Monticelli O et al (2020) Alginate microbeads with internal microvoids for the sustained release of drugs. Int J Biol Macromol 156:454–461. https://doi.org/10.1016/j.ijbiomac.2020.04.083

Couvreur P, Vauthier C (2006) Nanotechnology: intelligent design to treat complex disease. Pharm Res 23(7):1417–1450. https://doi.org/10.1007/s11095-006-0284-8

De Koker S, Hoogenboom R, De Geest BG (2012) Polymeric multilayer capsules for drug delivery. Chem Soc Rev 41(7):2867–2884. https://doi.org/10.1039/C2CS15296G

Doan-Nguyen TP, Natsathaporn P, Jenjob R, Niyom Y, Ittisanronnachai S, Flood A et al (2019) Regulating payload release from hybrid nanocapsules with dual silica/polycaprolactone shells. Langmuir 35(35):11389–11396. https://doi.org/10.1021/acs.langmuir.9b01176

Ehlerding EB, Chen F, Cai W (2016) Biodegradable and renal clearable inorganic nanoparticles. Adv Sci 3(2):1500223. https://doi.org/10.1002/advs.201500223

Elzayat A, Tolba E, Pérez-Pla FF, Oraby A, Muñoz-Espí R (2021a) Increased stability of polysaccharide/silica hybrid sub-millicarriers for retarded release of hydrophilic substances. Macromol Chem Phys 222(9):2100027. https://doi.org/10.1002/macp.202100027

Elzayat A, Adam-Cervera I, Álvarez-Bermúdez O, Muñoz-Espí R (2021b) Nanoemulsions for synthesis of biomedical nanocarriers. Colloids Surf B: Biointerfaces 203:111764. https://doi.org/10.1016/j.colsurfb.2021.111764

Elzayat AM, Pérez-Pla FF, Muñoz-Espí R (2022) A chitosan/silica hybrid 3D scaffold for simultaneous entrapment of two different hydrophilic substances. Mater Lett 326:132941. https://doi.org/10.1016/j.matlet.2022.132941

Elzayat AM, Adam-Cervera I, Albus M, Cháfer A, Badia JD, Pérez-Pla FF et al (2023) Polysaccharide/silica microcapsules prepared via ionic gelation combined with spray drying: application in the release of hydrophilic substances and catalysis. Polymers 15(20):4116. https://doi.org/10.3390/polym15204116

Elzayat AM, Landfester K, Muñoz-Espí R (2025) Chitosan/silica hybrid nanogels by inverse nanoemulsion for encapsulating hydrophilic substances. Macromol Mater Eng 310:2400151. https://doi.org/10.1002/mame.202400151

Fan J, Wang S, Sun W, Guo S, Kang Y, Du J et al (2018) Anticancer drug delivery systems based on inorganic nanocarriers with fluorescent tracers. AIChE J 64(3):835–859. https://doi.org/10.1002/aic.15976

Farasati Far B, Naimi-Jamal MR, Safaei M, Zarei K, Moradi M, Yazdani NH (2022) A review on biomedical application of polysaccharide-based hydrogels with a focus on drug delivery systems. Polymers 14(24):5432. https://doi.org/10.3390/polym14245432

Farrugia CA, Groves MJ (1999) Gelatin behaviour in dilute aqueous solution: designing a nanoparticulate formulation. J Pharm Pharmacol 51(6):643–649. https://doi.org/10.1211/0022357991772925

Fernando IPS, Lee W, Han EJ, Ahn G (2019) Alginate-based nanomaterials: fabrication techniques, properties, and applications. Chem Eng J 391:123823. https://doi.org/10.1016/j.cej.2019.123823

Gaitzsch J, Huang X, Voit B (2016) Engineering functional polymer capsules toward smart nanoreactors. Chem Rev 116(3):1053–1093. https://doi.org/10.1021/acs.chemrev.5b00241

Hamedi H, Moradi S, Hudson SM, Tonelli AE (2018) Chitosan based hydrogels and their applications for drug delivery in wound dressings: a review. Carbohydr Polym 199:445–460. https://doi.org/10.1016/j.carbpol.2018.06.114

Hood MA, Mari M, Muñoz-Espí R (2014) Synthetic strategies in the preparation of polymer/inorganic hybrid nanoparticles. Materials 7(5):4057–4087. https://doi.org/10.3390/ma7054057

Ilhan-Ayisigi E, Yesil-Celiktas O (2018) Silica-based organic-inorganic hybrid nanoparticles and nanoconjugates for improved anticancer drug delivery. Eng Life Sci 18(12):882–892. https://doi.org/10.1002/elsc.201800038

Meng J, Sturgis TF, Youan B-BC (2011) Engineering tenofovir loaded chitosan nanoparticles to maximize microbicide mucoadhesion. Eur J Pharm Sci 44(1):57–67. https://doi.org/10.1016/j.ejps.2011.06.007

Nair LS, Laurencin CT (2007) Biodegradable polymers as biomaterials. Prog Polym Sci 32(8):762–798. https://doi.org/10.1016/j.progpolymsci.2007.05.017

Nanjwade BK, Singh J, Parikh KA, Manvi FV (2010) Preparation and evaluation of carboplatin biodegradable polymeric nanoparticles. Int J Pharm 385(1):176–180. https://doi.org/10.1016/j.ijpharm.2009.10.030

Ngan LTK, Wang S-L, Hiep ĐM, Luong PM, Vui NT, Đinh TM et al (2014) Preparation of chitosan nanoparticles by spray drying, and their antibacterial activity. Res Chem Intermed 40(6):2165–2175. https://doi.org/10.1007/s11164-014-1594-9

Niyom Y, Phakkeeree T, Flood A, Crespy D (2019) Synergy between polymer crystallinity and nanoparticles size for payloads release. J Colloid Interface Sci 550:139–146. https://doi.org/10.1016/j.jcis.2019.04.085

Pan Y, Li Y-j, Zhao H-y, Zheng J-m, Xu H, Wei G et al (2002) Bioadhesive polysaccharide in protein delivery system: chitosan nanoparticles improve the intestinal absorption of insulin in vivo. Int J Pharm 249(1):139–147. https://doi.org/10.1016/S0378-5173(02)00486-6

Prabaharan M, Mano J (2004) Chitosan-based particles as controlled drug delivery systems. Drug Deliv 12(1):41–57. https://doi.org/10.1080/10717540590889781

Pramanik SK, Seneca S, Peters M, D'Olieslaeger L, Reekmans G, Vanderzande D et al (2018) Morphology-dependent pH-responsive release of hydrophilic payloads using biodegradable nanocarriers. RSC Adv 8(64):36869–36878. https://doi.org/10.1039/C8RA07066K

Silva B, Marto J, Braz BS, Delgado E, Almeida AJ, Gonçalves L (2020) New nanoparticles for topical ocular delivery of erythropoietin. Int J Pharm 576:119020. https://doi.org/10.1016/j.ijpharm.2020.119020

Sinsuebpol C, Chatchawalsaisin J, Kulvanich P (2013) Preparation and in vivo absorption evaluation of spray dried powders containing salmon calcitonin loaded chitosan nanoparticles for pulmonary delivery. Drug Des Devel Ther 7:861–873. https://doi.org/10.2147/DDDT.S47681

Tığlı Aydın RS, Pulat M (2012) 5-fluorouracil encapsulated chitosan nanoparticles for pH-stimulated drug delivery: evaluation of controlled release kinetics. J Nanomater 2012:313961. https://doi.org/10.1155/2012/313961

Vong LB, Kimura S, Nagasaki Y (2017) Newly designed silica-containing redox nanoparticles for oral delivery of novel TOP2 catalytic inhibitor for treating colon cancer. Adv Healthc Mater 6(20):1700428. https://doi.org/10.1002/adhm.201700428

Wang S, Chen M, Wu L (2016) One-step synthesis of cagelike hollow silica spheres with large through-holes for macromolecule delivery. ACS Appl Mater Interfaces 8(48):33316–33325. https://doi.org/10.1021/acsami.6b11639

Wen Y, Oh JK (2014) Recent strategies to develop polysaccharide-based nanomaterials for biomedical applications. Macromol Rapid Commun 35(21):1819–1832. https://doi.org/10.1002/marc.201400406

Zamani F, Jahanmard F, Ghasemkhah F, Amjad-Iranagh S, Bagherzadeh R, Amani-Tehran M et al (2017) Nanofibrous and nanoparticle materials as drug-delivery systems. In: Nanostructures for drug delivery. Elsevier, pp 239–270

Zhang Y, Hsu BYW, Ren C, Li X, Wang J (2015) Silica-based nanocapsules: synthesis, structure control and biomedical applications. Chem Soc Rev 44(1):315–335. https://doi.org/10.1039/C4CS00199K

Lignin Chemistry and Functionalization for Potential Medical Applications 7

Mehdi Mennani, Meriem Kasbaji, Yassine El Khayat Driaa, Anass Ait Benhamou, Zineb Ouahouah, Mounir El Achaby, Amine Moubarik, and Zineb Kassab

Abstract

Lignin is considered one of the most abundant yet under-exploited biomass materials globally. Lignin is a versatile lignocellulosic biopolymer with many desirable properties, including antioxidant, antibacterial, UV protection and biocompatibility. The functionalization of lignin as a complex aromatic polymer has attracted considerable attention due to its potential to unlock diverse applications in various fields, including materials science, biotechnology and environmental engineering. This chapter explores the multifaceted strategies employed for lignin functionalization, which inherently offer precise control over lignin structure and properties, enabling improved solubility, reactivity and compatibility with other materials. In addition, the chapter explores the wide range of potential medical applications for functionalized lignin, from the development of lignin-based biomaterials and drug delivery systems to tissue engineering scaffolds, wound healing dressings and materials with intrinsic antibacterial properties.

M. Mennani (✉) · M. Kasbaji
Materials Science, Energy and Nanoengineering (MSN) Department, Mohammed VI Polytechnic University, Ben Guerir, Morocco

Chemical Processes and Applied Materials Laboratory, Polydisciplinary Faculty, Sultan Moulay Slimane University, Beni Mellal, Morocco
e-mail: mehdi.mennani@um6p.ma

Y. E. K. Driaa
Chemical Processes and Applied Materials Laboratory, Polydisciplinary Faculty, Sultan Moulay Slimane University, Beni Mellal, Morocco

Sorbonne Université, Université de Technologie de Compiègne, Laboratoire Transformations Intégrées de la Matière Renouvelable (UTC/ESCOM, EA 4297 TIMR), Centre de recherches Royallieu, Compiègne Cedex, France

M. N. Collins, M. Culebras (eds.), *Sustainable Biopolymers and Composites for Biomedical Applications*, Biomaterials, Bioengineering and Sustainability 5,
https://doi.org/10.1007/978-3-031-91972-5_7

The challenges and regulatory considerations associated with lignin functionalization are also discussed, as are the emerging trends and opportunities that could shape its future in the medical field.

Keywords

Lignin · Medical applications · Biomedical · Tissue engineering · Drug delivery · Biocompatibility

7.1 Introduction

Biomass is one of the renewable energy sources obtained from organic matters such as plants, animals and microorganisms which has gained popularity because of its role in tackling greenhouse emissions and relying on fossil fuels (Pei et al. 2024; Hunter et al. 2022). The constituents of biomass, such as cellulose, hemicellulose, and lignin, hold significant importance individually. Examination of the impact of different sources of lignin and extraction processes on its characteristics and attributes is crucial for optimizing lignin utilization techniques. Lignin, constituting approximately 20–30% of the weight of biomass, presents challenges in degradation due to its intricate composition and resistance properties (Sugiarto et al. 2022; Mennani et al. 2024a; Ait Benhamou et al. 2024).

Lignin is the second most abundant natural substance on earth. It accounts for between 15% and 35% of lignocellulosic biomass from wood and paper production processes (Tsegaye et al. 2019; Kasbaji et al. 2024). Lignin contains a series of cross-linked polyphenolic structures providing structural support for plants and making a major contribution to the creation of cell walls (Khadem et al. 2024; Mennani et al. 2023; Mennani et al. 2022). Lignin is the product of phenylpropane lignols such as coniferyl alcohol (G), sinapyl alcohol (S), and paracoumaryl alcohol (H), which are known to be heterogeneous. The S/G ratio is used to classify lignin, gymnosperms having predominantly G lignin and angiosperms having both G and S lignin (Yuan et al. 2021; Mennani et al. 2024b). The molecular weight of lignin is more than 10,000 u and it is hydrophobic because of its aromatic substructure. At present, it is estimated that only less than 2% of lignin residues used industrially are

A. A. Benhamou
Department of Wood and Forest Sciences, Renewable Materials Research Centre (CRMR), Université Laval, Quebec, QC G1V 0A6, Canada

Z. Ouahouah · A. Moubarik
Chemical Processes and Applied Materials Laboratory, Polydisciplinary Faculty, Sultan Moulay Slimane University, Beni Mellal, Morocco

M. El Achaby · Z. Kassab (✉)
Materials Science, Energy and Nanoengineering (MSN) Department, Mohammed VI Polytechnic University, Ben Guerir, Morocco
e-mail: zineb.kassab@um6p.ma

commercially viable (Ullah et al. 2022; Schoenherr et al. 2018). In fact, the majority of recovered lignin is in the form of lignosulfonates for use as additives in building materials, while the remaining lignin is mainly converted into low-grade fuels or disposed of as residues (Cao et al. 2018). Currently, lignin is produced in large quantities worldwide, with an estimated market of 954.5 million USD in 2019 and an expected annual growth rate of 2% by 2027 (Sugiarto et al. 2022).

Large-scale production, combined with growing awareness of sustainable development, has led to a growing interest in the valorization of lignin in various fields, such as materials and chemicals. In the biomedical field, natural polymers such as cellulose, alginate, chitosan and chitin are among the materials that have contributed to the development of drug-delivery techniques and tissue engineering (Seddiqi et al. 2021; Ndaba et al. 2020). Biomaterial demands and properties for application in biomedical devices, implants, and tissue-engineered scaffolds are the key factors in biomedical engineering (Khadem et al. 2024; Vasile and Baican 2023). Biomaterials destined for biomedical purposes must have a certain set of qualities for them to be biocompatible, mechanically strong, and durable in a biological environment. Key features include biocompatibility to minimize unwanted reactions, bioactivity to support tissue absorption, mechanically engineered properties that fit the application, degradation kinetics that match the healing rate of the tissue, and ease of sterilization that ensures sterile conditions (Sugiarto et al. 2022; Zare et al. 2021). As well, factors like surface topography, porosity, and surface chemistry are the cornerstones of cell adhesion, proliferation, and differentiation, and therefore, they are the predominant factors affecting biomaterials functionality and efficiency in biomedical applications. Identifying and applying these characteristics and specifications are pivotal for the successful development and use of biomaterials in different areas of biomedical applications (Trucillo 2024).

Lignin, a rather multi-talented biomass, in recent times, has been recognized for its functional applications in different industries such as medical science. Its specific characteristics, which comprise antioxidant, antibacterial, and anti-UV properties, make it a fine material for biomedical applications (Sugiarto et al. 2022; Vasile and Baican 2023). Specifically, the construction branch has been researching the use of lignin-derived materials for green construction since they provide better thermal insulation, less energy consumption, and more durability (Jędrzejczak et al. 2021). In biomedicine, lignin has been investigated for its usefulness when it comes to the development of biomedical materials that can be used to construct different implantable devices, tissue engineering scaffolds, and wound dressings. Its biocompatibility, mechanical strength, and degradation rate also make it a great choice for use in biomedical applications. In addition, lignin acting as an antioxidant and antimicrobial can improve the lifetime of medical treatment materials and diminish the risk of infections (Sugiarto et al. 2022; Vasile and Baican 2023). However, lignin remains a relatively unknown product in the biomedical sector. Due to the heterogeneity of natural lignin, its development for biomedical applications is relatively difficult. Indeed, the heterogeneous nature of lignin is due to the multiplicity of resources and extraction processes employed for this purpose. Furthermore, in recent research and applications of lignin-based biomaterials, no particular attention

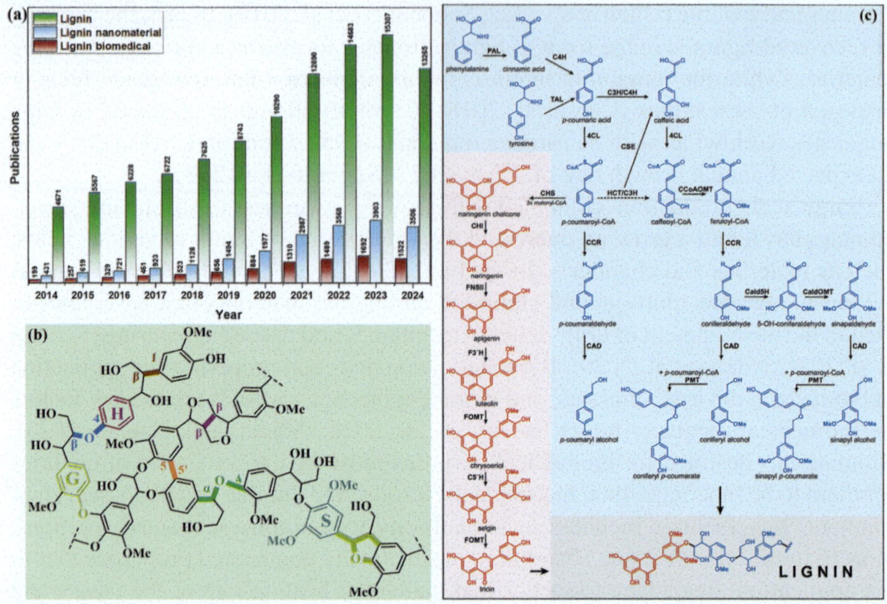

Fig. 7.1 (**a**) Illustration of the number of scientific publications in the last 10 years of lignin in biomedical and lignin functional materials, using the search terms "lignin", "lignin biomedical" and lignin nanomaterials." Data analysis was completed using *ScienceDirect* platform on July 15, 2024. (**b**) Structures of the three canonical monolignols, p-coumaryl alcohol, coniferyl alcohol, and sinapyl alcohol. (**c**) Lignin biosynthetic route in grasses illustrating the interconnections of monolignol and flavonoid biosynthetic pathways (Del Río et al. 2020)

has been paid to in vivo biocompatibility and biodegradability. Today, a thorough understanding of the mechanism by which lignin is broken down by the human body is one of the greatest challenges facing the valorization of this substance as a biomaterial. Despite these disadvantages, lignin is also endowed with several exceptional characteristics (antioxidant and anti-UV properties, as well as strong antimicrobial activities), which are crucial for biomedical applications (Witzler et al. 2018; Liu et al. 2020a; Stanisz et al. 2022). With such advantages, lignin has the potential to act as a bioactive compound complementing commonly used biomaterials such as cellulose. Over the last few years, lignin has attracted increasing interest as a functional material and its biomedical applications have grown, as shown in Fig. 7.1a, demonstrating lignin's potential as a great candidate for the development of innovative and sustainable biomaterials. In recent years, several researchers have come to demonstrate the value of using lignins with antioxidant, anti-UV and antimicrobial properties in biomedical applications, such as drug and gene delivery, and bio-imaging (Liu et al. 2020a; Siddiqui et al. 2020).

This chapter provides an in-depth overview of the current status and evolution of lignin as a biomaterial. We have described advanced methods for the production, modification and functionalization of lignin and highlighted lignin's unique characteristics for biomedical activities, including its antioxidant, antimicrobial, anti-UV and biocompatibility properties. In addition, this study provided a detailed analysis of the potential uses of lignin in several biomedical applications, including tumor treatment, bio-imaging/biosensors, tissue engineering and 3D printing. Besides, providing insights into the prospects and challenges associated with the utilization of lignin in biomedical fields.

7.2 Chemistry of Lignin

7.2.1 Biosynthesis and Structure of Lignin

7.2.1.1 Monolignol Precursors and their Linkages

Monolignol precursors, including p-coumarates, ferulates, and tricin, play a crucial role in the formation of lignin structures (Gao and Mortimer 2022; Wang et al. 2018a) (Fig. 7.1b). These precursors undergo radical coupling reactions, leading to the creation of various linkages within lignin, such as β-O-4, β-β, β-5, β-1, 5–5, and 4-O-5 linkages (Li et al. 2022a) (Fig. 7.1c). The composition and prevalence of these linkages vary based on plant species, tissue type, and developmental stage (Chen et al. 2023a). For example, guaiacyl (G) lignin is enriched in the water-conducting cells of the xylem, providing structural support essential for fluid transport, whereas syringyl (S) lignin is more predominant in structural fibers, enhancing the plant's rigidity and strength.

The biosynthesis of hydroxyphenyl (H), guaiacyl (G), and syringyl (S) units requires specific enzymatic activities, with enzymes such as laccases and peroxidases playing critical roles in lignin polymerization (Behr et al. 2018). These enzymes facilitate the coupling of monolignol precursors into complex lignin polymers, highlighting the intricate biochemical pathways that result in the diverse structural configurations of lignin in plants. This detailed understanding of monolignol precursors and their linkages not only sheds light on the complexity of lignin biosynthesis but also emphasizes the structural diversity and functional properties of lignin across different plant species and tissues.

7.2.1.2 Heterogeneity of Native Lignin

Native lignin exhibits significant heterogeneity in its structure and properties, influenced by a variety of factors. The composition of native lignin can differ markedly depending on the plant source, with notable distinctions between softwood and hardwood lignins (Ma et al. 2023). Structural analyses of native lignins reveal variability in inter-monomer bonding and functional groups, highlighting differences in lignin composition within various parts of the plant cell wall (Otromke et al. 2019). These differences are crucial for understanding the functional roles of lignin in different plant tissues.

Furthermore, the process of isolating lignin introduces additional variability into its structure. Industrial extraction methods can significantly alter the molecular characteristics of lignin, leading to deviations from its native form (Lizundia et al. 2021). Despite these alterations, lignins obtained from chemical pulps under controlled conditions can closely mimic the structure of native wood lignins (Serrano et al. 2019). This underscores the complexity and diversity of native lignin structures, which are shaped by both inherent biological factors and external processing techniques. Understanding this heterogeneity is essential for leveraging lignin's properties in various applications, from materials science to biomedicine.

7.2.2 Isolation and Characterization of Lignin

7.2.2.1 Major Types of Technical Lignins

Technical lignins can be classified into various types based on their sources and processes. Some major types include Kraft lignin, lignosulfonate lignin, soda and alkali lignin, organosolv lignin, and steam explosion lignin (Otromke et al. 2019; Mastrolitti et al. 2021). These technical lignins are derived from different industrial processes like the Kraft process, sulfite process, and organosolv pulping, each with unique characteristics and applications. Additionally, the functional heterogeneity of technical lignins plays a crucial role in their material use, with different lignins exhibiting varying functional group distributions along their molar mass profiles (Musl et al. 2022). Furthermore, lignin functionalization techniques such as amination and methylation contribute to enhancing the properties and applications of technical lignins, making them suitable for a wide range of value-added products (Suota et al. 2021).

Kraft lignin is a type of lignin obtained through the Kraft pulping process, where lignin is extracted from lignocellulosic materials using an alkaline solution containing Na_2S and NaOH. This process leads to the formation of Kraft lignin with unique properties, including the presence of hydrophobic thiol groups and a low sulfur content. Kraft lignin is recovered from the black liquor formed during the pulping process and can be isolated through acidification. It is characterized by its potential for chemical modification and utilization in various industrial applications. Additionally, Kraft lignin is a renewable and sustainable resource that holds promise for the synthesis of bio-aromatic chemicals and bio-based polymeric materials, contributing to greener and more sustainable practices in different industries (Karthäuser et al. 2021; Luo and Abu-Omar 2017; Isaac et al. 2019). Organosolv lignin is a type of lignin extracted using organic solvents in the organosolv process. It is known for its high purity, sulfur-free composition, and excellent solubility in alkaline solutions and various organic solvents (Serrano et al. 2019; Zhu et al. 2020). The organosolv process involves treating biomass with polar organic solvents like methanol, acetone, ethanol, acetic acid, and formic acid to isolate lignin, resulting in lignin with limited carbohydrate contamination and a narrow polydispersity (Luo and Abu-Omar 2017; Lu et al. 2017). This type of lignin is attractive for biomaterial synthesis due to its uniform molecular distribution and less need for modification, making it a valuable resource for various industries, including energy storage and conversion applications like rechargeable batteries and supercapacitors (Yue and Lu 2019). Soda lignin is a type of lignin obtained through the soda pulping process, which involves the use of sodium hydroxide to separate lignin from biomass like agricultural residues (Isaac et al. 2019; Phan and Lee 2020). This method is preferred for its sulfur-free nature and the lignin's close resemblance to natural lignin, making it suitable for various applications without the need for additional purification steps (Kun and Pukánszky 2017). Soda lignin is commonly derived from non-woody sources like straws and bagasse, offering a sustainable alternative for lignin extraction (Chen et al. 2023a). The extracted soda lignin possesses a molecular weight ranging from 1000 to 3000 g/mol and is utilized in various industries for producing phenolic resins, polymers, and low molecular weight substances (Domínguez-Robles et al. 2017).

7.2.2.2 Methods for Lignin Isolation and Purification

Several methods were utilized for the isolation of lignin, each offering distinct advantages and suited to different types of biomasses (Fig. 7.2). One common method is the isolation of milled wood lignin (MWL) using the Björkman method, which has been widely applied to various plant materials (Serrano et al. 2019; Kärkäs 2017; Katahira et al. 2018; Shi et al. 2019). For example, MWL isolation from bamboo has revealed the presence of syringyl (S), guaiacyl (G), and p-hydroxyphenyl (H) units, which are characteristic of grass-type lignin structures (Kumar et al. 2020). This method is particularly effective in maintaining the native structure of lignin. Organosolv processes are another widely used method, involving the heating of biomass with organic solvents such as methanol or acetone to extract lignin. This method is advantageous for its ability to produce high-purity lignin. Additionally, chemical methods like acid hydrolysis and the kraft process are commonly employed. Acid hydrolysis involves the reflux of wood pulp under acidic conditions, which solubilizes lignin, making it easier to extract. The kraft process, a

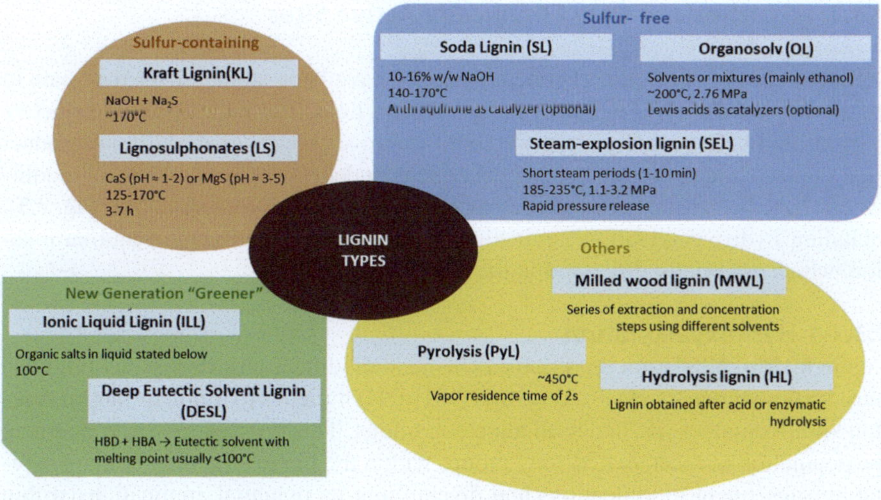

Fig. 7.2 Different sources of lignin and the corresponding isolation processes (Zevallos Torres et al. 2020)

well-established industrial method, also facilitates the breakdown and extraction of lignin from plant materials. These diverse methods of lignin isolation are essential for extracting lignin from various sources, each method providing unique benefits depending on the desired application. Whether maintaining the native structure of lignin for detailed studies or producing high-purity lignin for industrial applications, these techniques play a crucial role in the effective utilization of lignin in numerous fields.

Various techniques are utilized for the purification of lignin, each with its own advantages. Chemical methods such as acid hydrolysis, the kraft process, the lignosulfonate process, and organosolv processes are widely employed for lignin extraction (Wang et al. 2020). These methods are effective in breaking down complex plant materials to isolate lignin. Additionally, physical methods, including steam-assisted processes and extraction from bio-oils, are also used to purify lignin (Kim and Um 2020). These approaches often complement chemical methods by enhancing the efficiency of lignin recovery and purity. Moreover, specialized techniques like the FastPrep method are employed to isolate lignin while preserving its native structure and purity (Bajwa et al. 2019). This method is particularly valuable for obtaining lignin samples that are suitable for precise structural determination and sensitive functional assays. By enabling the extraction of pure lignin from plant tissues and specific cell wall regions, these methods facilitate a deeper understanding of lignin's properties and potential applications. Overall, an integrated approach that combines both chemical and physical methods is essential for effectively purifying lignin for diverse applications in research and industry.

7.3 Functionalization Strategies for Lignin

7.3.1 Synthesis of New Chemically Active Sites

Different changes in lignin chemical structure have been studied over the years to increase its reactivity to increase the application field. The inclusion of new active sites in the lignin complex network could improve properties in the final product such as mechanical, thermal, physicochemical, and so on. Several chemical modifications have been used to introduce new chemical sites in lignin structure (Fig. 7.3), including hydroxyalkylation, amination, nitration, sulfomethylation and sulfonation, which are briefly discussed in the next subsections.

7.3.1.1 Hydroxyalkylation

Lignin hydrox-alkylation represents a chemical modification strategy involving the introduction of reactive hydroxymethyl (-CH_2OH) moieties to lignin through a reaction with formaldehyde under alkaline conditions. This process serves to augment the population of reactive hydroxyl groups within the lignin structure, thereby facilitating subsequent modifications and diversifying its potential applications within the realm of materials science and biotechnology (Londono-Zuluaga et al. 2018). This modification enhances lignin's reactivity and thermal stability, rendering it

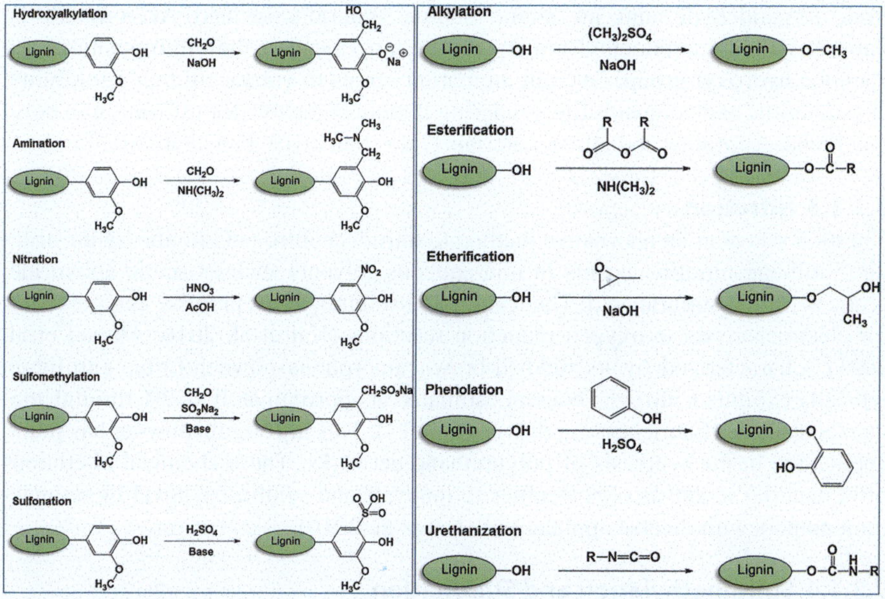

Fig. 7.3 Overview of the chemical modifications of lignin structure: different types and synthesis of new chemically active sites (Figueiredo et al. 2018)

valuable in applications such as polymer synthesis and composites (Eraghi Kazzaz et al. 2019).

Hydroxyalkylation of lignin encompasses demethylation, and methylolation as integral components of its modification pathway: Demethylation transforms methoxyl groups into hydroxyl groups, thereby enhancing the reactivity of lignin-derived aromatic compounds. This process can be efficiently executed using acidic concentrated lithium bromide (ACLB) under moderate conditions (Chen et al. 2023b). While methylolation, also referred to as hydroxymethylation, entails the introduction of reactive hydroxymethyl (-CH_2OH) groups to lignin via a reaction with formaldehyde under alkaline conditions. This augmentation amplifies the quantity of reactive hydroxyl groups on lignin, facilitating subsequent modifications (Laurichesse and Avérous 2014).

7.3.1.2 Amination

Amination techniques facilitate the integration of amine functional groups into the lignin matrix, imparting ionizable properties that render them positively charged under acidic environments. Various chemical methodologies are employed for this purpose, with the Mannich reaction emerging as a straightforward approach (Figueiredo et al. 2018). Recent investigations have commonly involved lignin amination in conjunction with diethylamine and formaldehyde, employing diverse reaction conditions. The Mannich reaction ensues through the interaction between a carbon site possessing elevated electron density and an immonium ion originating from formaldehyde and an amine source (Laurichesse and Avérous 2014). Subsequently, an aminoethyl moiety can be introduced at the ortho position of a phenolic hydroxyl group. Overall, amination serves to enhance lignin's solubility, dispersibility, and compatibility, rendering it more amenable for utilization in polymer blends, coatings, and allied materials (Jiao et al. 2019; Pan et al. 2013).

7.3.1.3 Nitration

Nitration serves as an alternative method to introduce nitrogen into the lignin structure, utilizing nitrating agents in non-aqueous solvents such as acetic anhydride, acetic acid, and sulfuric acid. The resulting nitrolignin holds promise as a precursor for electrocatalysts in oxygen reduction reactions (Kai et al. 2016; Ahmad et al. 2021). Characterized by its reddish-brown amorphous powder form, nitrolignin typically exhibits a nitrogen content estimated at approximately 6–7% through elemental analysis (Laurichesse and Avérous 2014). This nitrolignin powder has found application in the synthesis of polyurethane networks. These chemical alterations offer material scientists opportunities to innovate and synthesize novel lignin macromonomers with diverse applications (Kai et al. 2016).

7.3.1.4 Sulfomethylation and Sulfonation

Sulfomethylation facilitates the incorporation of methylene sulfonate groups onto the aromatic ring, a process achieved through the reaction of formaldehyde and an alkali metal sulfite salt in an aqueous medium under alkaline conditions (Hopa and Fatehi 2020). In this sequence, formaldehyde introduces the hydroxymethyl group into the lignin, subsequently substituted by the sulfite, leading to the formation of methylene sulfonate groups (Chandna et al. 2024). This chemical alteration has been employed in the fabrication of adsorption materials intended for the removal of cationic dyes (Lopez-Camas et al. 2020).

Instead, Sulfonation introduces sulfonate groups to lignin through treatment with sulfuric acid or sodium sulfite (Hopa and Fatehi 2020). This process involves the formation of covalent bonds between the sulfating agent and the aromatic rings of lignin, as depicted in. Sodium sulfite assists in lignin degradation within the sulfite process, forming aliphatic C–S bonds (Chandna et al. 2024). The resulting lignosulfonates find applications as dispersants in concrete and as binding agents.

7.3.2 Functionalization of Hydroxyl Groups

Functionalizing hydroxyl groups represents a promising approach for the synthesis of versatile lignin copolymers. Among these, phenolic hydroxyl groups exhibit heightened reactivity, significantly influencing the chemical properties of resultant materials. Alterations to hydroxyl groups can result in the production of lignin polyol derivatives. To achieve this, various reactions have been investigated for introducing diverse functional groups onto lignin.

7.3.2.1 Alkylation/Dealkylation

Alkylation is the process of introducing an alkyl group into an organic compound through substitution or addition, while dealkylation involves the removal of an alkyl group (Lopez-Camas et al. 2020). Lignin provides various sites for alkylation, including the oxygen atoms of hydroxyl, carbonyl, and carboxyl groups. Several methods exist for alkylating lignin, such as reacting with diazoalkanes, and alcohol in the presence of a catalyst like hydrochloric acid, or using alkylsulfates and sodium hydroxide (Figueiredo et al. 2018). Among these techniques, demethylation stands out, as demethylated lignins are significant byproducts of dimethyl sulfoxide (DMSO) production (Laurichesse and Avérous 2014). DMSO, a polar aprotic solvent, plays a crucial role in polymer synthesis and processing. The synthesis of DMSO begins with the reaction between lignin and molten sulfur in alkaline media, where two methyl groups are transferred from lignin to sulfur, forming dimethyl sulfide (DMS). Subsequently, DMS is oxidized with nitrogen dioxide to yield DMSO. This process underscores the versatility of lignin in generating valuable chemical intermediates for various industrial applications.

7.3.2.2 Esterification

Esterification stands out as a straightforward method for modifying lignin's hydroxyl groups. Various esterifying agents, including acidic compounds, acid anhydrides, and acid chlorides, have been employed for this purpose (Kai et al. 2016). In esterification, the hydroxyl groups of lignin react with an activated acid, such as an acid anhydride or acid chloride, often catalyzed by substances like pyridine or imidazole (Chandna et al. 2024). These bifunctional reagents enable the synthesis of lignin-based polyester networks through condensation reactions or ring-opening polymerization. Depending on the reagent used, by-products such as water, hydrochloric acid, and carboxylic acid are generated (Lopez-Camas et al. 2020). For instance, the reaction between e-caprolactone and hydroxypropylated lignin yields lignin-based polyesters with a star-like structure, where hydroxypropylated lignin constitutes the core, while polycaprolactones form the arm segments (Figueiredo et al. 2018). Additionally, lactide can serve as a copolymerization agent with lignin to produce lignin-polylactide polyester, facilitated by triazabicyclodecene as a catalyst in metal and solvent-free systems (Laurichesse and Avérous 2014).

7.3.2.3 Etherification

Etherification, a chemical modification process applicable to lignin, introduces ether linkages into its structure by reacting hydroxyl groups (both phenolic and aliphatic) with compounds containing reactive groups like epoxides or alkyl halides (Figueiredo et al. 2018). This incorporation of new ether linkages can significantly modify lignin's properties and reactivity. One prominent method within etherification is oxypropylation, widely studied and esteemed for its effectiveness in generating novel macropolyols from lignin (Sadeghifar et al. 2012). Oxypropylation transforms solid, insoluble lignin into highly soluble polyols, readily dispersible in common organic solvents. The mechanism of oxypropylation involves the reaction of oxianions generated from lignin's hydroxyl groups, facilitated by a basic catalyst, with propylene oxide. Typically, KOH catalyzes oxyalkylation involving hydroxyl groups (Laurichesse and Avérous 2014).

7.3.2.4 Phenolation

Phenolation of lignin involves the condensation of phenol with lignin's aromatic rings and side chains in an acidic environment, leading to the introduction of additional phenolic hydroxyl groups onto lignin. This enrichment in phenolic hydroxyl content enhances lignin's chemical reactivity, particularly in the synthesis of lignin-based phenol resins (Kai et al. 2016; Peng et al. 2023). This modification process also includes reacting lignin with phenol or its derivatives to introduce phenol groups at the α position of the side chain, further boosting the abundance of phenolic hydroxyl groups and augmenting lignin's reactivity. This reaction can take place under either acidic or alkaline conditions (Peng et al. 2023). Furthermore, phenolation serves as a modification technique that activates aliphatic hydroxyls, increasing the presence of phenol groups within the lignin structure through C-C bond formation (Chandna et al. 2024).

Various reaction conditions have been investigated to determine the optimal parameters for the effective phenolation of lignin. In the wood-based composites industry, adhesive plays a crucial role in determining the final product properties. Phenol-formaldehyde resins are commonly used adhesives, typically in concentrations ranging from 5 to 15% w/w. Given that the resin cost significantly impacts the overall price of wood products, wood industries are inclined towards more cost-effective options. Lignin-based resins have demonstrated the ability to substitute up to 30% of phenol in phenol-formaldehyde resins, serving as viable adhesives for particle board production (Lopez-Camas et al. 2020).

7.3.2.5 Urethanization

Another reaction with hydroxyl groups involves combining them with isocyanate groups like 4,4′-diphenyl methane diisocyanate (MDI), forming a urethane link (active RNC=O sites) through a heat-releasing reaction (Chandna et al. 2024). This process, known as Urethanization, enables the conversion of lignin into an alternative source for making polyurethanes. Traditionally, polyurethanes are made from polyols and diisocyanates, offering versatile products (Lopez-Camas et al. 2020). Research indicates that lignin can replace up to 30% of the materials in polyurethane synthesis, although excessive amounts can make the material brittle (Lopez-Camas et al. 2020). There are two main methods for creating lignin-based polyurethane: one involves a single-step reaction with diisocyanate, and the other entails a two-step process, starting with the production of a prepolymer using isocyanate and a polyol, followed by polymerizing lignin with the prepolymer serving as a chain extender (Figueiredo et al. 2018). Urethanized lignin products often demonstrate enhanced properties and reactivity compared to untreated lignin, rendering them useful for various applications (Laurichesse and Avérous 2014; Antonino et al. 2021).

7.3.3 Enzymatic Approaches

Utilizing enzymes to modify lignins represents a promising strategy aimed at enhancing their properties and expanding their potential applications. Different types of enzymes, like laccases, peroxidases, hydrolases, and some lipases, are involved in this process (Mayr et al. 2021). Laccases are especially promising because they only need simple things like oxygen to work well compared to other enzymes (Chandna et al. 2024). They can work with lots of different biopolymers including lignin, and they are mainly found in plants, fungi, insects, and bacteria (Chandna et al. 2024; Mayr et al. 2021). Enzyme-based methods have some advantages over chemical ones, like needing gentler conditions (lower temperature and pH), using fewer harmful chemicals, and making less waste (Mayr et al. 2021; Fabbri et al. 2023). An interesting study used a laccase from a fungus called T. hirsuta to attach different types of fluorophenols onto lignin. This made the material more water-repellent, showing how useful enzyme changes can be (Kudanga et al. 2010). Generally, using enzymes to transform lignins is a good way of making valuable products without harming the environment. However, there is still work to be done to ensure that this process works well for all types of lignin. Convincingly, the functionalization of lignin plays a crucial role in improving its properties for biomedical applications. By modifying lignin's phenolic and aliphatic hydroxyl groups, its solubility can be improved, enabling better structural characterization and use in the medical field. These functionalization strategies improve lignin's biocompatibility, antimicrobial and antioxidant properties, making it a promising candidate for advanced healthcare engineering purposes.

7.4 Potential Medical Applications of Functionalized Lignin

7.4.1 Antibacterial and Antimicrobial Properties

Lignin exhibits antibacterial and antimicrobial properties due to its phenolic components, such as p-coumaric and ferulic acids, which play a role in its effectiveness against various microorganisms. Studies have shown that lignin extracts can hinder the growth of bacteria like Escherichia coli and Staphylococcus aureus (Sugiarto et al. 2022; Chao et al. 2023). The antimicrobial efficacy of lignin can differ based on extraction methods, plant sources, and chemical compositions. Various materials based on lignin, including nanoparticles and composites, have been developed for use in drug delivery, gene delivery, wound healing, and tissue engineering, demonstrating the range of biological functions of lignin (Tran et al. 2021; Das et al. 2024). Research has indicated that phenolic elements in lignin can inhibit enzyme activities and the proliferation of microorganisms such as Escherichia coli, Saccharomyces cerevisiae, Bacillus licheniformis, and Aspergillus niger. The antimicrobial effects of phenolic compounds in lignin are determined by their side chain structure and functional groups. Phenolics with oxygen-containing groups are less inhibitory, while those with double bonds and methyl groups have increased biocidal effects

(Luzi et al. 2021). Interestingly, the purity, surface area, and size of lignin impact its antimicrobial properties. Higher purity, larger surface area, and smaller size enhance its effectiveness against microorganisms. Additionally, the extraction process of lignin influences its chemical structure, purity, and molecular weight, which are essential factors in its antioxidant and antimicrobial properties. Two potential mechanisms are involved in elucidating the antibacterial properties of extracted lignin, which are associated with both its chemical composition and structural configuration. Initially, the action of polyphenols leads to cell wall disruption through lysis, consequently facilitating the leakage of intracellular contents. It was postulated that the high antioxidative behavior of nanolignin, attributed to the aggregation of reactive oxygen species (ROS) by polyphenolic compounds on its surface, could trigger oxidative stress upon interaction with bacteria, thereby perturbing the normal redox processes. This observation underscores the correlation between the antioxidant capabilities of lignin and its antibacterial efficacy, primarily driven by ROS generation (Luzi et al. 2021; Yang et al. 2018). Lignin nanoparticles possess an enlarged surface area, leading to the enhancement of their antioxidant properties, with research focusing on depolymerization as a means to augment their activity. The antioxidative potential of lignin is intricately connected to the steadiness of phenoxy radicals, which can be influenced by variables such as dissociation enthalpy and the presence of ortho groups. In general, the antioxidative capacity of lignin can be impacted by the content of phenolic hydroxyl and methoxyl groups, as well as factors like molecular weight and polydispersity. The antioxidative efficacy of monophenolic compounds is closely associated with the stability of phenoxy radicals (Ar-O•). Furthermore, a decrease in the dissociation enthalpy of the phenolic hydroxyl bond (Ar-O•••H) facilitates the cleavage of Ar-O•••H and the release of hydrogen protons to generate structurally robust Ar-O• radicals, thereby displaying antioxidant properties (Sugiarto et al. 2022; Das et al. 2024).

Liu and Sipponen (2023) formulated a bio-derived nanocomposite film consisting of chitosan (~60 wt %), lignin nanoparticles (LNPs, ~40 wt %), glutaraldehyde (1.5 wt %), and AgNPs (0.072 wt %) (Fig. 7.4a). The synthesized LNPs were utilized as a reducing agent and stabilizer for the conversion of Ag^+ ions to AgNPs under the influence of UV light. Subsequently, the Ag@LNP dispersion was amalgamated with chitosan in the presence of glutaraldehyde as a cross-linker and casted into films. Chitosan was selected as the polymer matrix due to its biodegradability and electrostatic affinity with lignin (Fig. 7.4b). The CC-AgLNP film exhibited remarkable solar absorption capabilities throughout the spectrum, capturing 89% of radiation within the range of 200–2500 nm, thereby positioning it as a promising candidate for photothermal applications. Notably, the control samples displayed a negligible reduction in bacterial colonies, suggesting that light exposure alone did not possess sterilization properties. Conversely, the CC-Ag@LNP films showcased impressive antibacterial efficacy, achieving a reduction in E. coli viability of over 99.9% despite containing a minimal silver content of merely 0.072 wt%. This exceptional sterilization capacity is likely attributed to the extensive surface area of the silver nanoparticles in conjunction with the broad solar light absorption exhibited by the photothermal CC-Ag@LNP material. While marginal decreases in

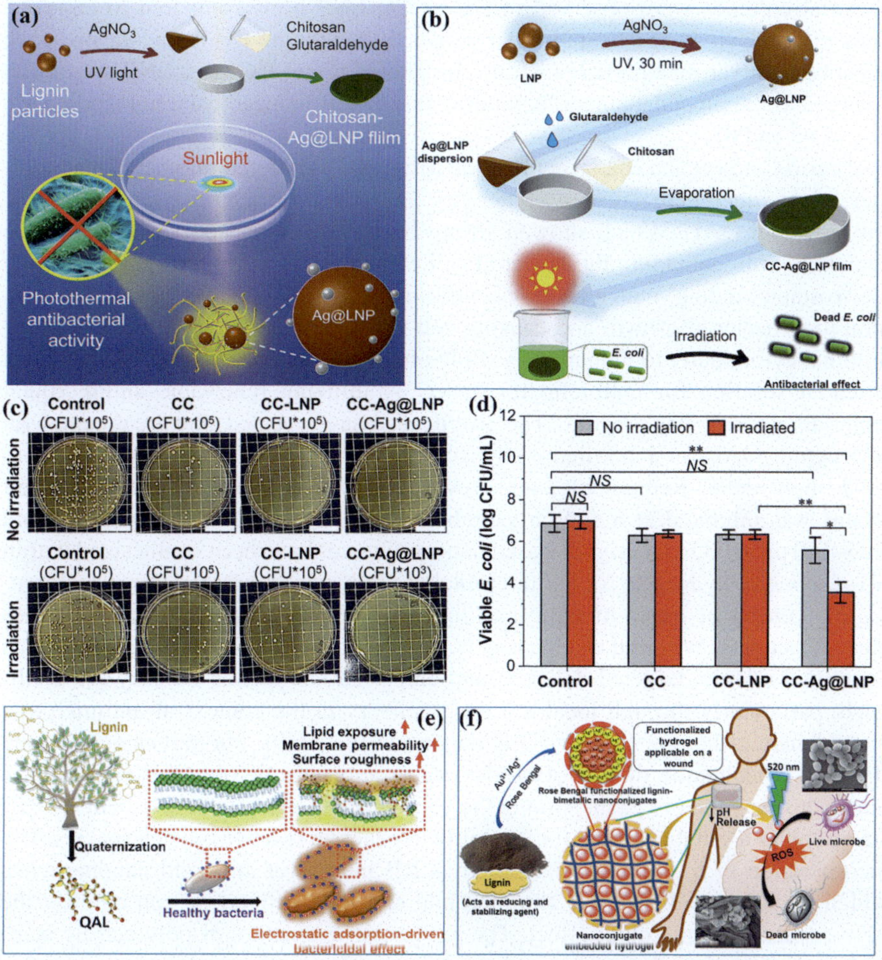

Fig. 7.4 (**a**) Chitosan films with increased wet mechanical strength and photothermal performance. (**b**) Preparation method of Ag@LNP and CC-Ag@LNP film and demonstration of phtothermal antibacterial application. The antibacterial efficacy of the cross-linked chitosan and nanocomposite films, featuring a consistent lignin content of 40 wt%: (**c**) digital representations of bacterial colonies of E. coli subsequent to various treatment regimens (scale bar of 3 cm). (**d**) E. coli samples were subjected to treatments involving CC, CC-LNP, and CC-Ag@LNP films for a duration of 15 minutes, both with and without exposure to simulated solar irradiation at an intensity of 0.1 W/cm^2. The error bars displayed in the results correspond to the standard deviation calculated across the entire sample population (n = 3). The statistical significance levels were denoted as $*p < 0.05$ and $**p < 0.01$, while outcomes with $p > 0.05$ were considered non-significant (NS) (Liu and Sipponen 2023). (**e**) development of quaternary ammonium lignin QAL with electrostatic adsorption-driven effect (Acurio Cerda et al. 2023). (**f**) The development of nanocomposite hydrogels incorporating lignin-based photodynamic nanoconjugates is crucial for the stabilization and reduction of silver and gold nanoparticles (Chandna et al. 2020)

bacterial colonies were observed in CC or CC-LNP films compared to controls, these effects were insignificant from a statistical standpoint. Evidently, the presence of metallic silver nanoparticles within the photothermal CC-Ag@LNP composite emerged as the pivotal element facilitating rapid light-induced bacterial eradication (Fig. 7.4c and d).

Acurio Cerda et al. (2023) reported the beneficial use of naturally abundant polymer lignin functionalized with quaternary ammonium groups to yield a cationic antimicrobial QAL. Which showed strong bacteriostatic and bacteriolytic effects against E. coli, damaging the bacterial cell envelope and inner membrane through electrostatic binding, with a low concentration of 25–150 μg/mL being effective in inhibiting bacterial growth and causing cell death (Fig. 7.4e). QAL demonstrated minimal cytotoxicity to human cells while effectively killing bacteria, suggesting a potential solution for antibiotic resistance by utilizing renewable antimicrobial materials derived from lignin. The live/dead assay revealed that treatment with >25 μg/mL QAL for 1 h killed ~90% of the bacteria cells and caused damage to ~4% more cells. Remarkably, the growth of wild-type and antibiotic-resistant strains was inhibited at a similarly high level (~90–100% CFU reduction using ~25–150 μg/mL QAL). Lignin-based nanoconjugates have been synthesized within pH-responsive hydrogels for antimicrobial photodynamic therapy. These nanoconjugates consist of lignin-metallic and lignin-bimetallic structures decorated with photosensitizers. Within these hydrogels containing antimicrobial nano-agents, the controlled release, targeted delivery, and enhanced therapeutic efficacy are facilitated, particularly through localized drug delivery in the context of antimicrobial photodynamic therapy (Fig. 7.4f) (Chandna et al. 2020). Photodynamic therapy (PDT) is a technique that involves the deactivation of microbes utilizing light, a photosensitizer, and oxygen. Among the various photosensitizers, rose bengal (RB) stands out as a suitable option for its ability to generate reactive oxygen species. The incorporation of a photosensitizer such as RB into silver and gold nanoparticles, which are renowned for their antimicrobial and PDT properties, can amplify the light-assisted antimicrobial effect. The pH-responsive nature of poly(acrylic acid) hydrogels is evident through their degradation under acidic conditions, suggesting the potential for pH-triggered release of antimicrobial agents. By introducing photosensitizer nanoconjugates into the hydrogel matrix, the lifetime of the triplet state is prolonged, a critical factor for the production of reactive oxygen species in antimicrobial photodynamic therapy. Altogether, the developed antimicrobial photodynamic hydrogels exhibit significant potential as targeted therapeutic agents for wound healing and other biomedical applications, including the creation of nanocoatings for stimuli-responsive antimicrobial effects.

7.4.2 Targeted Drug and Gene Delivery Systems

Drug and gene delivery systems are pivotal components in contemporary medicine, facilitating precise and regulated administration of therapeutic substances to specific anatomical locations. These systems employ diverse methodologies and substances to ensure effective delivery while minimizing undesired effects (Stanisz et al. 2022; Mukheja et al. 2023). Biomaterials and biopolymers sourced from natural origins have attracted considerable attention in this domain owing to their compatibility with biological systems, degradability, and adaptability (Sugiarto et al. 2022; Liu et al. 2020b). The advancement of drug and gene delivery techniques encompasses the utilization of nanoparticles, encapsulation, and microspheres to achieve targeted and controlled release of therapeutic agents. Issues like the toxic nature of existing carriers, for instance, polyethylenimine (PEI), have prompted the investigation of substitute materials such as lignin-based substances, recognized for their limited toxicity and potential as gene delivery vectors. Nanoparticles like liposomes, polymeric nanoparticles, and dendrimers are widely employed for drug and gene conveyance purposes. These minute particles can enclose drugs or genetic material, shielding them from deterioration and enabling regulated discharge at the intended location. Additionally, hydrogels, which are intricate structures of hydrophilic polymers, can be tailored to dispense drugs or genes in reaction to specific stimuli, like pH variations, temperature fluctuations, or enzymatic actions, thereby providing precise management of release kinetics (Stanisz et al. 2022; Chen et al. 2021; Paudel et al. 2021). Naturally sourced biomaterials inherently possess biocompatibility and are less inclined to trigger adverse immune responses, rendering them suitable for medical applications. Furthermore, they can undergo enzymatic breakdown within the body, ensuring safe elimination and minimal long-term accumulation (Ali and Mehanna 2022). Figure 7.5a succinctly summarizes the fundamental aspects of drug and gene delivery technologies, the associated challenges, and the crucial role of biomaterials and naturally derived biopolymers in overcoming these challenges. An in-depth analysis of the illustrated components facilitates a deeper comprehension of the intricate relationship among technology, obstacles, and biomaterial remedies. The highlighted challenges, encompassing biocompatibility, targeting accuracy, sustainability, and efficacy, represent significant hurdles that necessitate resolution to unlock the complete potential of drug and gene delivery systems (Stanisz et al. 2022; Mukheja et al. 2023). In tackling these obstacles, biomaterials and naturally derived biopolymers emerge as promising solutions due to their intrinsic biocompatibility, degradability, adaptability, and sustainability. Lignin-based nanoparticles have shown promise in drug loading, sustained release, and gene transfection, with studies demonstrating their effectiveness in entering cells and delivering DNA. The need for enhanced natural and biocompatible materials in drug and gene delivery systems has driven the interest in lignin-derived biomaterials, leveraging their antimicrobial, antioxidant, and biocompatible properties for improved therapeutic outcomes. Lignin is commonly used in gene delivery applications due to its low cytotoxicity and potential as a gene carrier. Studies have shown that lignin-based materials, such as lignin nanotubes (LNTs) and lignin copolymers, exhibit promising gene transfection capabilities. Additionally, lignin-based particles have been explored for targeted drug delivery systems, showing high sensitivity to pH changes and efficient drug release properties. Furthermore, lignin has been incorporated into composites for potential biomedical applications,

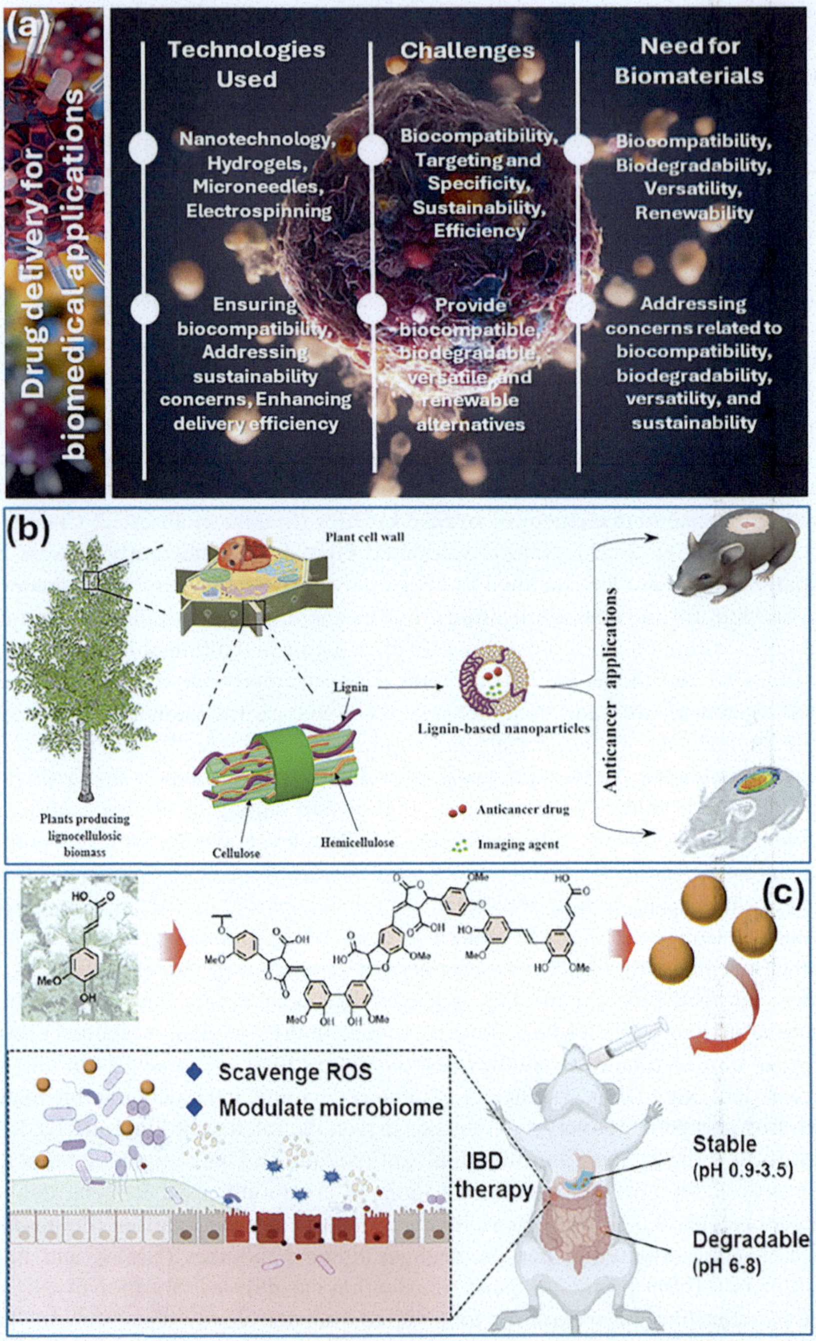

Fig. 7.5 (**a**) Summary of the main aspects of drug delivery, technologies challenges, and the benefits of included biomaterials. (**b**) Lignin nanoparticles promoted anticancer drug delivery and controlled release (Ali and Mehanna 2022). (**c**) The functions of FALNP as an orally administered

demonstrating resistance to bacterial adherence and significant antioxidant properties (Sugiarto et al. 2022; Liu et al. 2020b; Chaudhary and Sinha 2023).

Lignin-encapsulated porous silicon nanoparticles were utilized in the enhancement of oral insulin delivery, with the ability to bypass biological barriers that contribute to suboptimal drug absorption and bioavailability following oral intake. This innovation has the potential to revolutionize the management of diabetes for a large population of patients, providing an efficient, secure, user-friendly, and cost-effective substitute for insulin injections (Martins et al. 2022). The nanosystem comprises an insulin-laden porous silicon NP enclosed within a pH-responsive lignin framework and modified on the surface with the Fc fragment of immunoglobulin G, serving as a targeting ligand for the neonatal Fc receptor (FcRn) (Fig. 7.5c). Under gastric and intestinal pH conditions, the NPs remained structurally sound, selectively releasing the drug at pH 7.4, which replicates the environment of blood circulation. This particular formulation exhibited significant cytocompatibility, and investigations utilizing surface plasmon resonance indicated that FcRn-targeted NPs possess an increased ability to interact with and be internalized by Caco-2 cells, expressing FcRn, as confirmed through Western blot analysis. Ultimately, permeability studies conducted in vitro revealed that Fc-functionalized NPs prompted a rise in the quantity of insulin permeating through a Caco-2/HT29-MTX co-culture model, displaying apparent permeability coefficients (Papp) of 2.37×10^{-6} cm/s. Zhao et al. (2023) conducted a study utilizing ferulic acid-derived lignin nanoparticles (FALNP) known for their advantageous antioxidant properties in the management of inflammatory bowel disease (IBD). The pH-responsive degradability of FALNP within the intestinal environment enables it to withstand the rigorous conditions of gastric acidity, overcome physiological obstacles, and effectively target the gastrointestinal tract for drug delivery. Ferulic acid (FA), sourced from natural plants such as corn and angelica, undergoes oxidation via a horse radish peroxidase/hydrogen peroxide (HRP/H_2O_2) system, producing electron-delocalized intermediates. The coupling of these intermediates leads to the creation of FA-derived lignin (FAL), which further self-assembles to form FALNP. Experimental trials on animals using a dextran sulfate sodium (DSS)-induced acute colitis mouse model were carried out to assess the therapeutic potential of FALNP. Remarkably, FALNP exhibited notable therapeutic effects in the acute colitis mouse model by mitigating oxidative stress, regulating the gut microbiome, and thereby alleviating pathological symptoms. Furthermore, the strong antioxidant properties of FALNP stem from the presence of phenolic hydroxyl groups and conjugated substructures, enabling effective neutralization of free radicals like DPPH, ABTS, and HO. Moreover, FALNP displayed versatile capabilities for loading various drugs such as paclitaxel, linezolid, rifampin, dexamethasone, cyclosporin A, and meso-tetraphenylporphine-4,4′,4″,4″‘-tetracarboxylic acid, positioning it as a promising candidate for facilitating oral drug delivery.

Fig. 7.5 (continued) therapeutic nano-agent for the treatment of IBD are twofold: (i) FALNP is resistant to the acidic gastric environment but degrades efficiently in the alkaline conditions of the intestines within the gastrointestinal tract; (ii) FALNP degradation results in the dispersion of FAL polymers, which can attenuate inflammation in the intestines by decreasing levels of reactive oxygen species (ROS) and regulating inflammatory cytokines and the gut microbiota (Zhao et al. 2023)

The data depicted in Table 7.1 functions as evidence of the pivotal role of biomaterials, specifically emphasizing lignin, in addressing significant obstacles and driving progress in drug delivery technologies, ultimately resulting in improved therapeutic results (Sugiarto et al. 2022; Stanisz et al. 2022). The highlighted discoveries illustrate the diverse capabilities of lignin-based materials as promising options for drug delivery applications. Demonstrating exceptional biocompatibility of lignin is crucial for ensuring the safety and harmony of drug delivery systems with biological systems. By illustrating the positive interactions between lignin-based materials and biological contexts, the table emphasizes lignin's potential to reduce adverse effects and facilitate biocompatible drug delivery. Notably, through various formulation approaches and adjustments, carriers based on lignin can attain precise control over drug release kinetics, enabling customized therapeutic interventions and optimized dosing schedules. These capabilities play a key role in enhancing therapeutic effectiveness, reducing side effects, and enhancing patient adherence.

7.4.3 Tissue Engineering and Regenerative Medicine

In the domain of regenerative medicine, tissue engineering involves the advancement of biocompatible functional materials by integrating various interdisciplinary principles. Tissue engineering serves as a clever method for the restoration, substitution, enhancement, or conservation of specific biological tissues or organs. Depending on the specific application areas, tissue engineering can be categorized into bone tissue engineering, nerve tissue engineering, muscle tissue engineering, and so on. Distinct requirements are essential for diverse tissue-engineering materials, such as the necessity for robust mechanical stability in bone transplant scaffolds. In comparison to existing commercially accessible materials, lignin is preferred due to its relatively high biocompatibility, lack of cytotoxicity, suitable biodegradability, and cost-effectiveness. Incorporating lignin into polymer composite matrices can enhance their mechanical characteristics and cellular compatibility. Lignin possesses structural attributes that make it a desirable option for constructing scaffolds in tissue engineering. Being a natural biopolymer, lignin provides inherent biocompatibility and degradability, rendering it suitable for fostering cell proliferation and tissue rejuvenation. The exceptional biological properties make lignin a highly promising bioactive option for various biomedical applications, including tissue engineering. Typically, lignin bears structural resemblances to the extracellular matrix (ECM) present in natural tissues, positioning it as a superb biomimetic material for tissue engineering purposes. Through emulating the composition and layout of native ECM, lignin-based scaffolds can enhance cell-matrix interactions, regulate cellular responses, and facilitate tissue regeneration mechanisms. Additionally, lignin-based composites like hydrogels and scaffolds have been investigated for their biocompatibility and technical attributes in tissue engineering, supporting cell growth and rejuvenation (Fig. 7.6) (Liu et al. 2022). By integrating bioactive agents such as growth factors, peptides, or nanoparticles onto lignin-based

Table 7.1 Summary of Lignin-based particles with drug release efficiencies

Material	Model drug	Particle size/ shape	Lignin source/extraction method	pH	Time (h)	Release rate (%)	References
Enzymatic hydrolysis lignin/chitosan oligosaccharide nanoparticles (EHL/COS-x)	Cytarabine (Ara-C)	176–790 nm (spherical)	Enzymatic hydrolysis lignin extracted from corncobs	6	5	97	(Chen et al. 2021)
MT_SLS-MCs	Methylated thymol	2.9 mm (spherical)				24.8	(Piombino et al. 2020)
LNP(Enflx)	Enrofloxacin	117 nm (spherical)	Alkaline lignin	7.4	70	100	(Paudel et al. 2021)
Acryloyl alkali lignin-g-polymethacrylate (AAL-g-PMAA)	Ibuprofen	100 nm (spherical)	Alkali lignin	1.5	72	15.64	(Cheng et al. 2020)
QC/LS LBL coated nanoparticles	Quinacrine	138 nm (spherical)	Lignosulfonate	5.5	48	65	(Etman et al. 2020)
Lignosulfonate- cetyltrimethylammonium bromide (LS-CTAB)	Ibuprofen	50 nm (spherical)	Sodium lignosulfonate	1.2	48	15	(Liu et al. 2020b)
Lignin-based nanosphere (LN)	Ibuprofen	100–400 nm (spherical)	Industrial alkali lignin (AL) – Kraft lignin	1.2	2–6	18	(Wang et al. 2021)
BT_SLS-MCs	4-bromothymol	3.4 mm (spherical)				37.1	(Piombino et al. 2020)
Acetone soluble fraction Kraft lignin and cholesterol particles (ASLK-Chol)	Folic acid	320 nm	Softwood Kraft lignin	5.5	40	39	(Piombino et al. 2020)
Aminated lignin-histidine conjugate and 10-Hydroxy-camptothecin nanoparticles (AL-His/HCPT NPs)	10- hydroxy-camptothecin	40 nm (spherical)	Kraft lignin	4.5	19	72.5	(Zhao et al. 2020)

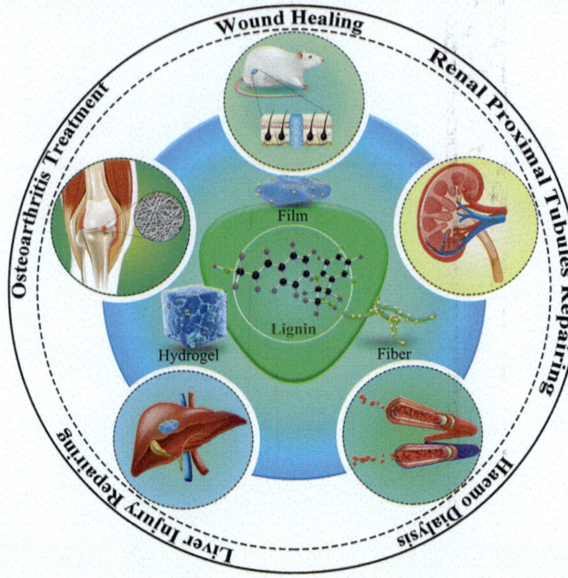

Fig. 7.6 Elucidating the biological roles of lignin in the context of its utilization in diverse areas of tissue engineering, including bone and organ regeneration, as well as wound management (Liu et al. 2022)

scaffolds, their characteristics can be customized to encourage specific cellular behaviors like adhesion, migration, and differentiation. Recent research has spotlighted the immunomodulatory impacts of lignin, hinting at its potential usefulness in modulating immune reactions within tissue engineering contexts. Lignin-based scaffolds have demonstrated the ability to control inflammatory processes, stimulate tissue restructuring, and boost vascularization, thereby establishing a conducive microenvironment for tissue regeneration.

Researchers have been exploring novel scaffold designs and fabrication techniques to enhance the properties and functionality of lignin-based scaffolds. This includes the development of hierarchical structures, surface patterning techniques, and the incorporation of bioactive molecules to promote cell adhesion, proliferation, and differentiation. The concept of utilizing lignin/polycaprolactone (PCL) nanofibers as a scaffold for hydroxyapatite biomineralization was introduced, aiming to mimic the natural process of bone formation (Wang et al. 2019). Interestingly, lignin facilitates the formation of human bone-like hydroxyapatite (HAp) by providing reactive sites for chelation with Ca^{2+} and $PO4^{3-}$, resulting in structurally and mechanically similar HAp crystals to native bone. The mineralized PCL nanofibrous films, created through incubation in simulated body fluid, promote adhesion and proliferation of osteoblasts by directing filopodial extension, showing potential for future applications in bio-interfaces and hard-tissue engineering. (Fig. 7.7a). Lignin/PCL nanofibrous film was prepared using electrospinning with a rotating drum collector. A solution of chloroform/DMF containing PCL and lignin was electrospun at 18 kV with a feeding rate of 10 μL/min onto a grounded wheel. HAp crystals were formed using lignin as a template in a simulated body fluid (SBF) with specific ion concentrations. Substrates were soaked in 1.5 × SBF and incubated at

37 °C to allow HAp crystal formation before characterization. Cell colonization and proliferation were significantly higher on HAp@lignin/PCL nanofibers compared to PCL and lignin/PCL scaffolds. HAp@lignin/PCL nanofibers induced elongated cell morphology with filopodia formation, promoting cell migration and adhesion. The nanofibers also provided good osteoblast adhesion in a 3D nanotopography matrix, enhancing cell viability and osteoconductivity.

Engineered biomaterials like functionalized lignin are being used for wound healing to provide antioxidation and deliver oxygen for enhanced vascularization without causing inflammation. Lignin composites with oxygen-releasing nanoparticles showed increased calcium quantity and released oxygen for at least 7 days, promoting tissue granulation, blood vessel formation, and collagen remodeling. By adjusting methacrylated gelatin concentration, injectability and stiffness of lignin composites suitable for wound healing were maintained, showing potential for balanced antioxidation and controlled oxygen release in wound healing applications (Fig. 7.7b) (Balaji et al. 2023). Injectable lignin composites were developed to provide antioxidation and locoregional oxygenation by combining lignosulfonate with thiolation, unmodified sodium lignosulfonate, and methacrylated gelatin to modulate mechanical properties for injectability. Wound healing studies were carried out in wild-type (WT) C57BL/6 N mice (8–10 weeks old, female and male).

Wounds that received treatment with a composite containing CPO lignin (consisting of a GelMA matrix and TLS and SLS-PLGA/CaO_2 NPs) displayed notable improvements in the healing process, demonstrating minimal scarring and the formation of a mature collagen structure within 28 days following the injury. Scar tissue, which typically lacks the distinct layers found in normal skin such as the epidermis, dermis with appendages, adipose layer, and muscle layer, showed a different outcome after the application of CPO treatment. This treatment resulted in the development of smaller scars with the reconstruction of dermal appendages and muscle layers. The collagen structure observed in wounds treated with CPO exhibited a unique intertwined network, contrasting with the linear fibers seen in other treatment cohorts. In-depth examinations of scars in mice focused on various factors including collagen fiber density, arrangement, and the presence of dermal appendages, which are essential for evaluating the strength of skin repair. Moreover, the treatment with lignin composite demonstrated promising outcomes in reducing fibrotic markers in human dermal fibroblasts, suggesting its potential to promote wound healing. Notably, the use of lignin composites also impacted the expression of fibrotic genes in fibroblasts with both high and low scarring tendencies, indicating a potential adjustment in fibroblast characteristics during the process of tissue repair. The incorporation of lignosulfonate into the wound environment could potentially further diminish fibrotic responses by influencing the characteristics of fibroblasts (Fig. 7.7c–e).

The diverse range of lignin types and their respective composites offer unique characteristics and functionalities that contribute to the advancement of tissue engineering strategies. From nerve tissue engineering to wound dressing and soft-tissue regeneration, lignin-derived materials have demonstrated significant potential across various applications (Table 7.2). These materials exhibit a wide range of

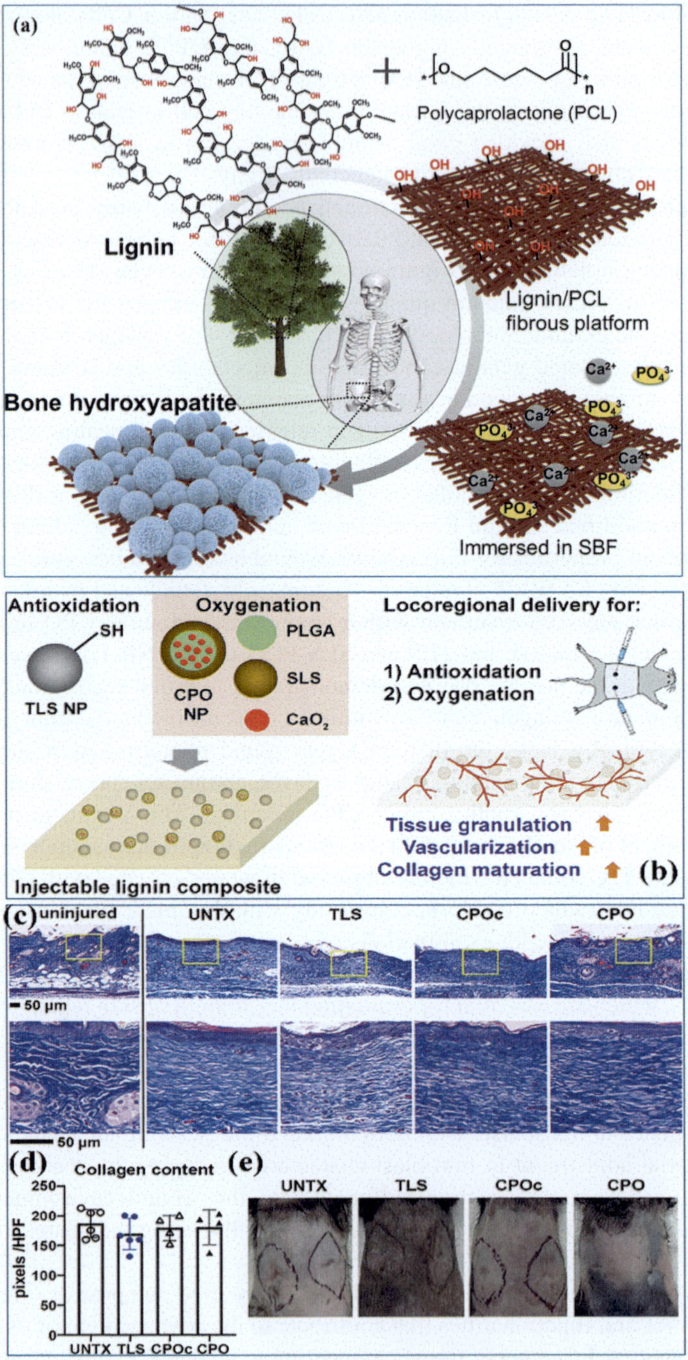

Fig. 7.7 (**a**) Schematic description for the biomineralization of bone HAp induced by lignin. Lignin/PCL fibrous platform was prepared by electrospinning, followed by incubation in an SBF. Lignin contains many OH groups, which can donate adequate reactive sites to bind with

Table 7.2 Overview of the utilization of lignin-derived composites in various facets of tissue engineering (Liu et al. 2022)

Lignin types	Materials used	Characteristics	Potential applications	References
Alkali lignin	PCL	Mechanical and antioxidant properties; cell viability	Nerve tissue engineering	(Wang et al. 2018b)
Laccase-polymerized lignin	Methacrylated O-acetyl-galactoglucomannan (GGMMA) and silver nanoparticles	Antioxidant; cell viability	Wound dressing	(Wang et al. 2022)
Softwood Kraft lignin	Cellulose nanofibril (CNF) and alginate	117 nm (spherical)	Soft-tissue engineering and regenerative-medicine applications.	(Zhang et al. 2020)
Lignin obtained from wheat straw	Alginate	Non-cytotoxic and cell adhesion	Tissue engineering and regenerative medicine	(Quraishi et al. 2015)
Klason lignin and acid soluble lignin	Nanocellulose	Non-cytotoxicity	Lung and kidney tissue therapy	(Kim et al. 2020)
Macelignan		Anti-inflammation, antioxidant	Renal tissue repairing	(Long et al. 1995)
Sugarcane bagasse lignin	Silica gel and iron/silica	Biodegradable and drug slow-releasing	Drug vehicles for arthritis disease	(Zhang et al. 2012)
Lignin from poplar tree	Polysaccharide	Biocompatible	Human hepatocyte culture	(Zhao et al. 2018)
Lignin from sulfite papermaking pulp	Chitosan and PVA	Biocompatibility, antibacterial and mechanical strength	Wound healing	(Huang et al. 2020)
Sulfonated lignin	Polyoxazoline	Anti-inflammatory and antimicrobial	Wound healing	(Li et al. 2022b)

Fig. 7.7 (continued) metal ions and facilitate the nucleation and growth of HAp through coprecipitation of Ca^{2+} and PO_4^{3-} (Wang et al. 2019). (**b**) Preparation and application of lignin-based composites for wound healing. Scar evaluation was conducted on wounds that received treatment with lignin composites 28 days post-surgery. Wound samples taken from WT C57BL/6 N mice that were subjected to lignin composite treatment underwent staining with trichrome, with a focus on assessing the amount of collagen present. The trichrome images displayed are representative of the wounds at both low (top row) and high magnification (bottom row) of the specified region highlighted in yellow boxes (**c**). The quantification of collagen content was performed per high-power field (HPF) through the application of color thresholding in ImageJ (**d**). Images of the wounds at the 28-day mark after surgery were captured. In preparation for scar evaluation, photographs were taken from each of the four treatment groups before the final analysis (**e**). The scale bar for reference in the images is set at 50 μm, with a sample size ranging from 3 to 6. Bar graphs have been utilized to present the mean ± standard deviation values for each mouse wound (Balaji et al. 2023)

characteristics, including mechanical strength, antioxidant properties, biocompatibility, and drug release capabilities, making them suitable for addressing diverse tissue engineering challenges. Furthermore, the biodegradability and bioactivity of lignin-derived materials enhance their suitability for in vivo applications, paving the way for the development of biocompatible and sustainable tissue-engineered constructs. In all, further investigations into the optimization of fabrication techniques, characterization methods, and in vivo performance are warranted to fully realize the potential of lignin-based materials in regenerative medicine and tissue engineering.

7.4.4 Biocompatibility Enhancement: Regulatory Aspects and AI Integration

Biocompatibility represents a critical factor in the advancement of materials for applications in the biomedical field, such as carriers for drugs and genes at the nanoscale. Biocompatible polymers, particularly polysaccharides, polyphenols, and proteins, have attracted considerable interest among researchers due to their potential utility in these specific domains. The primary distinguishing characteristic of biomaterials, as opposed to other types of materials, lies in their capacity to interact harmoniously with the human body, prompting an appropriate response from the host in a given context (Sugiarto et al. 2022; Stanisz et al. 2022; Larrañeta et al. 2018). Biomaterials sourced from natural reservoirs, such as vegetation, typically demonstrate favorable biocompatibility. Although extensive research has been devoted to plant-based polymers like cellulose and pectin, there has been relatively minimal exploration of the biocompatibility of lignin. Nevertheless, it is imperative to acknowledge that inherent lignin and extracted lignin exhibit variances in their attributes owing to the chemical processes utilized for extraction. These extraction procedures have the potential to modify the physical and chemical properties of lignin, encompassing aspects like its molecular weight, solubility, chemical alterations, aromatic composition, and the presence of contaminants like sulfur and ash (Chaudhary and Sinha 2023; Balaji et al. 2023; Wang et al. 2019). Elevated temperatures and rigorous chemical treatments, as observed in the kraft process, often lead to irreversible deterioration of the densely packed lignin structure, primarily by reducing ether bond connections, notably β-O-4 bonds. This deterioration can lower the chemical responsiveness of the processed lignin relative to its original state (Sugiarto et al. 2022). Consequently, it is indispensable to undertake comprehensive investigations into the biocompatibility and degradability of each distinct form of lignin, given that the extraction methodologies and resultant alterations can significantly influence these characteristics. Moreover, the consideration of biocompatibility holds utmost importance in the validation procedures for medical equipment and commodities. Regulatory entities, such as the U.S. Food and Drug Administration (FDA) and the European Medicines Agency (EMA), have established criteria and benchmarks for appraising biocompatibility. Typically, these standards encompass a sequence of evaluations, including cytotoxicity assessments, sensitization tests, irritation analyses, acute systemic toxicity examinations, and implantation studies, aimed at evaluating the physiological reaction to the material or apparatus. Progress in research and development within this domain is propelling the advancement of biocompatible materials tailored for diverse medical applications.

Advanced biomaterials, such as biodegradable polymers, hydrogels, and nanomaterials, have been designed to replicate the characteristics of natural tissues, thereby enhancing biocompatibility and facilitating tissue integration. Furthermore, Artificial Intelligence (AI), a burgeoning and fascinating tool that is being incorporated into biomedical approaches, can make a profound impact on the field of biocompatibility enhancement. The integration of AI methodologies, including machine learning and deep learning, opens up promising avenues for research. Specifically, within the realm of material design and refinement, AI algorithms can be trained on vast datasets containing material properties, biological reactions, and experimental findings to predict and improve material compositions or surface attributes to enhance biocompatibility. Furthermore, AI-driven image analysis and pattern recognition can assist in evaluating and quantifying cellular responses, protein absorption patterns, and tissue integration, thereby providing valuable insights for biocompatibility assessments. By combining diverse data sources such as material properties, biological data, and clinical results, AI can create predictive models for the biocompatibility of materials and guide the development of innovative materials or devices. Ultimately, AI-powered virtual screening and simulation techniques can be utilized to evaluate potential biocompatibility issues, predict biological responses, and guide experimental design before physical experimentation (Garza-Ulloa 2022; Shokrani et al. 2023).

7.5 Conclusions

The current chapter has presented a synopsis of the significance of biocompatibility in the progression of materials for biomedical purposes, especially in the realm of carriers for pharmaceuticals and genetic material at the nanoscale. Biocompatible polymers, such as polysaccharides, polyphenols, and proteins, have arisen as prominent candidates owing to their potential efficacy in these specialized fields. The distinguishing characteristic of biomaterials resides in their capacity to seamlessly engage with the human body, eliciting a suitable reaction from the host in particular circumstances. Although natural biomaterials derived from plants typically exhibit advantageous biocompatibility, the investigation of lignin, a plant-derived polymer with less extensive research, introduces both obstacles and prospects. Additionally, this chapter has illuminated the processes of extraction and chemical modifications that lignin experiences, influencing its biocompatibility and appropriateness for medical uses.

The exploitation of lignin's distinct attributes, encompassing its antioxidant and antimicrobial features, shows potential for furthering medical therapies and enhancing patient results. Overall, this work functions as an exhaustive reference, furnishing an elaborate overview of the most recent developments and progressions in the utilization of lignin as a biomaterial, particularly within the biomedical field. It accentuates the unique characteristics of lignin and delves into its potential applications in various facets of biomedicine, such as cancer therapy, diagnostics, tissue regeneration, and additive manufacturing.

References

Acurio Cerda K, Kathol M, Purohit G, Zamani E, Morton MD, Khalimonchuk O, Saha R, Dishari SK (2023) Cationic lignin as an efficient and biorenewable antimicrobial material. ACS Sustain Chem Eng 11:10364–10379. https://doi.org/10.1021/acssuschemeng.3c01414

Ahmad Z, Paleologou M, Xu CC (2021) Oxidative depolymerization of lignin using nitric acid under ambient conditions. Ind Crop Prod 170:113757. https://doi.org/10.1016/j.indcrop.2021.113757

Ait Benhamou A, Boussetta A, Salim MH, Mennani M, Kasbaji M, Kassab Z, Landry V, Tardy BL, Pizzi A, El Achaby M, Moubarik A (2024) How can cellulosic fibers enhance adhesion in engineered wood? Mater Sci Eng R Rep 161:100852. https://doi.org/10.1016/j.mser.2024.100852

Ali DA, Mehanna MM (2022) Role of lignin-based nanoparticles in anticancer drug delivery and bioimaging: an up-to-date review. Int J Biol Macromol 221:934–953. https://doi.org/10.1016/j.ijbiomac.2022.09.007

Antonino LD, Gouveia JR, de Sousa Júnior RR, Garcia GES, Gobbo LC, Tavares LB, Dos Santos DJ (2021) Reactivity of aliphatic and phenolic hydroxyl groups in Kraft lignin towards 4,4′ mdi. Molecules 26:1–12. https://doi.org/10.3390/molecules26082131

Bajwa DS, Pourhashem G, Ullah AH, Bajwa SG (2019) A concise review of current lignin production, applications, products and their environment impact. Ind Crop Prod 139:111526. https://doi.org/10.1016/j.indcrop.2019.111526

Balaji S, Short WD, Padon BW, Belgodere JA, Jimenez SE, Deoli NT, Guidry AC, Green JC, Prajapati TJ, Farouk F, Kaul A, Son D, Jung OS, Astete CE, Kim M, Jung JP (2023) Injectable antioxidant and oxygen-releasing lignin composites to promote wound healing. ACS Appl Mater Interfaces 15:18639–18652. https://doi.org/10.1021/acsami.2c22982

Behr M, Sergeant K, Leclercq CC, Planchon S, Guignard C, Lenouvel A, Renaut J, Hausman JF, Lutts S, Guerriero G (2018) Insights into the molecular regulation of monolignol-derived product biosynthesis in the growing hemp hypocotyl. BMC Plant Biol 18:1–18. https://doi.org/10.1186/s12870-017-1213-1

Cao L, Yu IKM, Liu Y, Ruan X, Tsang DCW, Hunt AJ, Ok YS, Song H, Zhang S (2018) Lignin valorization for the production of renewable chemicals: state-of-the-art review and future prospects. Bioresour Technol 269:465–475. https://doi.org/10.1016/j.biortech.2018.08.065

Chandna S, Thakur NS, Kaur R, Bhaumik J (2020) Lignin-bimetallic nanoconjugate doped pH-responsive hydrogels for laser-assisted antimicrobial photodynamic therapy. Biomacromolecules 21:3216–3230. https://doi.org/10.1021/acs.biomac.0c00695

Chandna S, Olivares MCA, Baranovskii E, Engelmann G, Böker A, Tzschucke CC, Haag R (2024) Lignin upconversion by functionalization and network formation. Angew Chemie Int Ed 63:e202313945. https://doi.org/10.1002/anie.202313945

Chao Y, Yu S, Zhang H, Gong D, Li J, Wang F, Chen J, Zhu J, Chen J (2023) Architecting lignin/poly(vinyl alcohol) hydrogel with carbon nanotubes for photothermal antibacterial therapy. ACS Appl Bio Mater 6:1525–1535. https://doi.org/10.1021/acsabm.2c01061

Chaudhary M, Sinha VR (2023) Lignin-based carriers for drug delivery applications: from an industrial waste to a pharmaceutical aid. Eur Polym J 195:112206. https://doi.org/10.1016/j.eurpolymj.2023.112206

Chen K, Qian Y, Wang C, Yang D, Qiu X, Binks BP (2021) Tumor microenvironment-responsive, high internal phase Pickering emulsions stabilized by lignin/chitosan oligosaccharide particles for synergistic cancer therapy. J Colloid Interface Sci 591:352–362. https://doi.org/10.1016/j.jcis.2021.02.012

Chen M, Li Y, Liu H, Zhang D, Shi QS, Zhong XQ, Guo Y, Xie XB (2023a) High value valorization of lignin as environmental benign antimicrobial. Mater Today Bio 18:100520. https://doi.org/10.1016/j.mtbio.2022.100520

Chen Y, Shen J, Wang W, Lin L, Lv R, Zhang S, Ma J (2023b) Demethylation of lignin with mild conditions and preparation of green adhesives to reduce formaldehyde emissions and health risks. Int J Biol Macromol 242:124462. https://doi.org/10.1016/j.ijbiomac.2023.124462

Cheng L, Deng B, Luo W, Nie S, Liu X, Yin Y, Liu S, Wu Z, Zhan P, Zhang L, Chen J (2020) pH-responsive lignin-based nanomicelles for oral drug delivery. J Agric Food Chem 68:5249–5258. https://doi.org/10.1021/acs.jafc.9b08171

Das AK, Mitra K, Conte AJ, Sarker A, Chowdhury A, Ragauskas AJ (2024) Lignin – a green material for antibacterial application — a review. Int J Biol Macromol 261:129753. https://doi.org/10.1016/j.ijbiomac.2024.129753

Del Río JC, Rencoret J, Gutiérrez A, Elder T, Kim H, Ralph J (2020) Lignin monomers from beyond the canonical Monolignol biosynthetic pathway: another brick in the wall. ACS Sustain Chem Eng 8:4997–5012. https://doi.org/10.1021/ACSSUSCHEMENG.0C01109/ASSET/IMAGES/LARGE/SC0C01109_0006.JPEG

Domínguez-Robles J, Sánchez R, Espinosa E, Savy D, Mazzei P, Piccolo A, Rodríguez A (2017) Isolation and characterization of Gramineae and Fabaceae soda lignins. Int J Mol Sci 18. https://doi.org/10.3390/ijms18020327

Eraghi Kazzaz A, Hosseinpour Feizi Z, Fatehi P (2019) Grafting strategies for hydroxy groups of lignin for producing materials. Green Chem 21:5714–5752. https://doi.org/10.1039/c9gc02598g

Etman SM, Abdallah OY, Mehanna RA, Elnaggar YSR (2020) Lactoferrin/hyaluronic acid double-coated lignosulfonate nanoparticles of quinacrine as a controlled release biodegradable nanomedicine targeting pancreatic cancer. Int J Pharm 578:119097. https://doi.org/10.1016/j.ijpharm.2020.119097

Fabbri F, Bischof S, Mayr S, Gritsch S, Jimenez Bartolome M, Schwaiger N, Guebitz GM, Weiss R (2023) The biomodified lignin platform: a review. Polymers (Basel) 15. https://doi.org/10.3390/polym15071694

Figueiredo P, Lintinen K, Hirvonen JT, Kostiainen MA, Santos HA (2018) Properties and chemical modifications of lignin: towards lignin-based nanomaterials for biomedical applications. Prog Mater Sci 93:233–269. https://doi.org/10.1016/j.pmatsci.2017.12.001

Gao Y, Mortimer JC (2022) Reimagining lignin for the biorefinery. Plant Cell Physiol 63:734–736. https://doi.org/10.1093/pcp/pcac051

Garza-Ulloa J (2022) Chapter 3 – Artificial intelligence models applied to biomedical engineering. In: Garza-Ulloa CM (ed) Applied biomechatronics using mathematical models. Academic Press, pp 113–173. https://doi.org/10.1016/B978-0-12-820718-5.00004-0

Hopa DY, Fatehi P (2020) Using sulfobutylated and sulfomethylated lignin as dispersant for kaolin suspension. Polymers (Basel) 12:11–14. https://doi.org/10.3390/POLYM12092046

Huang C, Dong H, Zhang Z, Bian H, Yong Q (2020) Procuring the nano-scale lignin in prehydrolyzate as ingredient to prepare cellulose nanofibril composite film with multiple functions. Cellulose 27:9355–9370. https://doi.org/10.1007/s10570-020-03427-9

Hunter RD, Ramírez-Rico J, Schnepp Z (2022) Iron-catalyzed graphitization for the synthesis of nanostructured graphitic carbons. J Mater Chem A 10:4489–4516. https://doi.org/10.1039/d1ta09654k

Isaac E, Samson A, Adeosun O (2019) Sustainable lignin for carbon fibers: principles, techniques, and applications. https://doi.org/10.1007/978-3-030-18792-7

Jędrzejczak P, Collins MN, Jesionowski T, Klapiszewski Ł (2021) The role of lignin and lignin-based materials in sustainable construction—a comprehensive review. Int J Biol Macromol 187:624–650. https://doi.org/10.1016/j.ijbiomac.2021.07.125

Jiao GJ, Peng P, Sun SL, Geng ZC, She D (2019) Amination of biorefinery technical lignin by Mannich reaction for preparing highly efficient nitrogen fertilizer. Int J Biol Macromol 127:544–554. https://doi.org/10.1016/j.ijbiomac.2019.01.076

Kai D, Tan MJ, Chee PL, Chua YK, Yap YL, Loh XJ (2016) Towards lignin-based functional materials in a sustainable world. Green Chem 18:1175–1200. https://doi.org/10.1039/c5gc02616d

Kärkäs MD (2017) Lignin hydrogenolysis: improving lignin disassembly through formaldehyde stabilization. ChemSusChem 10:2111–2115. https://doi.org/10.1002/cssc.201700436

Karthäuser J, Biziks V, Mai C, Militz H (2021) Lignin and lignin-derived compounds for wood applications—a review. Molecules 26. https://doi.org/10.3390/molecules26092533

Kasbaji M, Mennani M, Barhoumi S, Esshouba Y, Oubenali M (2024) Synergy of magnetic nanoparticles and sodium alginate-coated lignin for effective pollutant remediation, simple recovery, and cost-effective regeneration. Langmuir 40:20657–20678. https://doi.org/10.1021/acs.langmuir.4c02734

Katahira R, Elder TJ, Beckham GT (2018) Chapter 1: A brief introduction to lignin structure. In: Lignin valorization, RSC energy and environment series, pp 1–20. https://doi.org/10.1039/9781788010351-00001

Khadem E, Ghafarzadeh M, Kharaziha M, Sun F, Zhang X (2024) Lignin derivatives-based hydrogels for biomedical applications. Int J Biol Macromol 261:129877. https://doi.org/10.1016/j.ijbiomac.2024.129877

Kim GH, Um BH (2020) Fractionation and characterization of lignins from Miscanthus via organosolv and soda pulping for biorefinery applications. Int J Biol Macromol 158:443–451. https://doi.org/10.1016/j.ijbiomac.2020.04.229

Kim D, Jeong J, Ryu J-A, Choi SR, Lee JM, Bunch H (2020) In vitro evaluation of lignin-containing nanocellulose. Materials (Basel) 13. https://doi.org/10.3390/ma13153365

Kudanga T, Prasetyo EN, Widsten P, Kandelbauer A, Jury S, Heathcote C, Sipilä J, Weber H, Nyanhongo GS, Guebitz GM (2010) Laccase catalyzed covalent coupling of fluorophenols increases lignocellulose surface hydrophobicity. Bioresour Technol 101:2793–2799. https://doi.org/10.1016/j.biortech.2009.12.002

Kumar R, Gupta A, Chawla M, Aadil KR, Dutt S, Kumar VB, Chaudhary A (2020) Advances in nanotechnology based strategies for synthesis of nanoparticles of lignin. In: Lignin. https://doi.org/10.1007/978-3-030-40663-9_7

Kun D, Pukánszky B (2017) Polymer/lignin blends: interactions, properties, applications. Eur Polym J 93:618–641. https://doi.org/10.1016/j.eurpolymj.2017.04.035

Larrañeta E, Imízcoz M, Toh JX, Irwin NJ, Ripolin A, Perminova A, Domínguez-Robles J, Rodríguez A, Donnelly RF (2018) Synthesis and characterization of lignin hydrogels for potential applications as drug eluting antimicrobial coatings for medical materials. ACS Sustain Chem Eng 6:9037–9046. https://doi.org/10.1021/acssuschemeng.8b01371

Laurichesse S, Avérous L (2014) Chemical modification of lignins: towards biobased polymers. Prog Polym Sci 39:1266–1290. https://doi.org/10.1016/j.progpolymsci.2013.11.004

Li M, Pu Y, Meng X, Chen F, Dixon RA, Ragauskas AJ (2022a) Strikingly high amount of tricin-lignin observed from vanilla (Vanilla planifolia) aerial roots. Green Chem 24:259–270. https://doi.org/10.1039/d1gc03625d

Li S, Zhang Y, Ma X, Qiu S, Chen J, Lu G, Jia Z, Zhu J, Yang Q, Chen J, Wei Y (2022b) Antimicrobial lignin-based polyurethane/ag composite foams for improving wound healing. Biomacromolecules 23:1622–1632. https://doi.org/10.1021/acs.biomac.1c01465

Liu J, Sipponen MH (2023) Ag-lignin hybrid nanoparticles for high-performance solar absorption in photothermal antibacterial chitosan films. IScience 26:108058. https://doi.org/10.1016/j.isci.2023.108058

Liu R, Dai L, Xu C, Wang K, Zheng C, Si C (2020a) Lignin-based micro- and nanomaterials and their composites in biomedical applications. ChemSusChem 13:4266–4283. https://doi.org/10.1002/cssc.202000783

Liu D, Liu J, Zhou Y, Chen J, Zhan P, Yang G, Wu Z (2020b) Assembly of lignin-based colloidal particles: effects of cationic surfactants, molecular weight, and solvent on morphology. RSC Adv 10:18594–18600. https://doi.org/10.1039/D0RA01444C

Liu Y, Wang X, Wu Q, Pei W, Teo MJ, Chen ZS, Huang C (2022) Application of lignin and lignin-based composites in different tissue engineering fields. Int J Biol Macromol 222:994–1006. https://doi.org/10.1016/j.ijbiomac.2022.09.267

Lizundia E, Sipponen MH, Greca LG, Balakshin M, Tardy BL, Rojas OJ, Puglia D (2021) Multifunctional lignin-based nanocomposites and nanohybrids. Green Chem 23:6698–6760. https://doi.org/10.1039/d1gc01684a

Londono-Zuluaga C, Du J, Chang HM, Jameel H, Gonzalez R (2018) Lignin modifications and perspectives towards applications of phenolic foams: a review. Bioresources 13:9158–9179. https://doi.org/10.15376/biores.13.4.londono-zuluaga

Long J, Qian K, Tan S, Liu J, Li J (1995) Macelignan protects against renal ischemia-reperfusion injuryvia inhibition of inflammation and apoptosis of renal epithelial cells. Cell Mol Biol Res 41:207–216

Lopez-Camas K, Arshad M, Ullah A (2020) Chemical modification of lignin by polymerization and depolymerization. In: Springer Ser Polym Compos Mater. Springer, Cham, pp 203–229. https://doi.org/10.1007/978-3-030-40663-9_5

Lu Y, Lu YC, Hu HQ, Xie FJ, Wei XY, Fan X (2017) Structural characterization of lignin and its degradation products with spectroscopic methods. J Spectrosc 2017:1–15. https://doi.org/10.1155/2017/8951658

Luo H, Abu-Omar MM (2017) Chemicals from lignin. Encycl Sustain Technol:573–585. https://doi.org/10.1016/B978-0-12-409548-9.10235-0

Luzi F, Yang W, Ma P, Torre L, Puglia D (2021) Lignin-based materials with antioxidant and antimicrobial properties, 1st edn. Elsevier. https://doi.org/10.1016/B978-0-12-820303-3.00003-5

Ma CY, Luo XT, Xu LH, Sun Q, Wen JL, Liang XF, Liu HZ, Yuan TQ (2023) Structural elucidation and targeted valorization of untractable lignin from pre-hydrolysis liquor of xylose production via a simple and robust separation approach. Int J Biol Macromol 253:127029. https://doi.org/10.1016/j.ijbiomac.2023.127029

Martins JP, Figueiredo P, Wang S, Espo E, Celi E, Martins B, Kemell M, Moslova K, Mäkilä E, Salonen J, Kostiainen MA, Celia C, Cerullo V, Viitala T, Sarmento B, Hirvonen J, Santos HA (2022) Neonatal Fc receptor-targeted lignin-encapsulated porous silicon nanoparticles for enhanced cellular interactions and insulin permeation across the intestinal epithelium. Bioact Mater 9:299–315. https://doi.org/10.1016/j.bioactmat.2021.08.007

Mastrolitti S, Borsella E, Guiliano A, Petrone MT, De Bari I, Gosselink R, Van Erven G, Annevelink E, Triantafyllidis KS, Stichnothe H (2021) Sustainable lignin valorization. IEA Bioenergy 2:1–193

Mayr SA, Subagia R, Weiss R, Schwaiger N, Weber HK, Leitner J, Ribitsch D, Nyanhongo GS, Guebitz GM (2021) Oxidation of various Kraft lignins with a bacterial laccase enzyme. Int J Mol Sci 22. https://doi.org/10.3390/ijms222313161

Mennani M, Ait Benhamou A, Kasbaji M, Boussetta A, Ablouh E, Boussetta N, Kassab Z, El Achaby M, Moubarik A (2022) Insights on the physico chemical properties of alkali lignins from different agro-industrial residues and their use in phenol-formaldehyde wood adhesive formulation. Int J Biol Macromol 221:149–162. https://doi.org/10.1016/j.ijbiomac.2022.08.191

Mennani M, Kasbaji M, Ait Benhamou A, Boussetta A, Mekkaoui AA, Grimi N, Moubarik A (2023) Current approaches, emerging developments and functional prospects for lignin-based catalysts—review. Green Chem 25:2896–2929. https://doi.org/10.1039/D3GC00072A

Mennani M, Benhamou A, Mekkaoui A (2024a) Probing the evolution in catalytic graphitization of biomass-based materials for enduring energetic applications. J Mater Chem A 12:6797–6825. https://doi.org/10.1039/d3ta07449h

Mennani M, Kasbaji M, Ait Benhamou A, Boussetta A, Kassab Z, El Achaby M, Grimi N, Moubarik A (2024b) The potential of lignin-functionalized metal catalysts – a systematic review. Renew Sustain Energy Rev 189:113936. https://doi.org/10.1016/j.rser.2023.113936

Mukheja Y, Kaur J, Pathania K, Sah SP, Salunke DB, Sangamwar AT, Pawar SV (2023) Recent advances in pharmaceutical and biotechnological applications of lignin-based materials. Int J Biol Macromol 241:124601. https://doi.org/10.1016/j.ijbiomac.2023.124601

Musl O, Galler S, Wurzer G, Bacher M, Sulaeva I, Sumerskii I, Mahler AK, Rosenau T, Potthast A (2022) High-resolution profiling of the functional heterogeneity of technical lignins. Biomacromolecules 23:1413–1422. https://doi.org/10.1021/acs.biomac.1c01630

Ndaba B, Roopnarain A, Daramola MO, Adeleke R (2020) Influence of extraction methods on antimicrobial activities of lignin-based materials: a review. Sustain Chem Pharm 18:100342. https://doi.org/10.1016/j.scp.2020.100342

Otromke M, White RJ, Sauer J (2019) Hydrothermal base catalyzed depolymerization and conversion of technical lignin—an introductory review. Carbon Resour Convers 2:59–71. https://doi.org/10.1016/j.crcon.2019.01.002

Pan H, Sun G, Zhao T (2013) Synthesis and characterization of aminated lignin. Int J Biol Macromol 59:221–226. https://doi.org/10.1016/j.ijbiomac.2013.04.049

Paudel S, Peña-Bahamonde J, Shakiba S, Astete CE, Louie SM, Sabliov CM, Rodrigues DF (2021) Prevention of infection caused by enteropathogenic E. coli O157:H7 in intestinal cells using enrofloxacin entrapped in polymer based nanocarriers. J Hazard Mater 414:125454. https://doi.org/10.1016/j.jhazmat.2021.125454

Pei W, Yu Y, Wang P, Zheng L, Lan K, Jin Y, Yong Q, Huang C (2024) Research trends of bio-application of major components in lignocellulosic biomass (cellulose, hemicellulose and lignin) in orthopedics fields based on the bibliometric analysis: a review. Int J Biol Macromol 267:131505. https://doi.org/10.1016/j.ijbiomac.2024.131505

Peng Z, Jiang X, Si C, Joao Cárdenas-Oscanoa A, Huang C (2023) Advances of modified lignin as substitute to develop lignin-based phenol-formaldehyde resin adhesives. ChemSusChem 16:e202300174. https://doi.org/10.1002/cssc.202300174

Phan DP, Lee EY (2020) Controlled hydrogenolysis over heterogeneous catalysts for lignin valorization. Catal Rev Sci Eng 62:607–630. https://doi.org/10.1080/01614940.2020.1770401

Piombino C, Lange H, Sabuzi F, Galloni P, Conte V, Crestini C (2020) Lignosulfonate microcapsules for delivery and controlled release of thymol and derivatives. Molecules 25. https://doi.org/10.3390/molecules25040866

Quraishi S, Martins M, Barros AA, Gurikov P, Raman SP, Smirnova I, Duarte ARC, Reis RL (2015) Novel non-cytotoxic alginate–lignin hybrid aerogels as scaffolds for tissue engineering. J Supercrit Fluids 105:1–8. https://doi.org/10.1016/j.supflu.2014.12.026

Sadeghifar H, Cui C, Argyropoulos DS (2012) Toward thermoplastic lignin polymers. Part 1. Selective masking of phenolic hydroxyl groups in Kraft lignins via methylation and oxypropylation chemistries. Ind Eng Chem Res 51:16713–16720. https://doi.org/10.1021/ie301848j

Schoenherr S, Ebrahimi M, Czermak P (2018) Lignin degradation processes and the purification of valuable products. Lignin Trends Appl. https://doi.org/10.5772/intechopen.71210

Seddiqi H, Oliaei E, Honarkar H, Jin J, Geonzon LC, Bacabac RG, Klein-Nulend J (2021) Cellulose and its derivatives: towards biomedical applications. Cellulose 28:1893–1931. https://doi.org/10.1007/s10570-020-03674-w

Serrano L, Luque R, Sels BF (2019) Lignin chemistry. https://doi.org/10.1038/237054a0

Shi Z, Xu G, Deng J, Dong M, Murugadoss V, Liu C, Shao Q, Wu S, Guo Z (2019) Structural characterization of lignin from D. sinicus by FTIR and NMR techniques. Green Chem Lett Rev 12:235–243. https://doi.org/10.1080/17518253.2019.1627428

Shokrani H, Shokrani A, Seidi F, Kucińska-Lipka J, Makurat-Kasprolewicz B, Saeb MR, Ramakrishna S (2023) Artificial intelligence for biomedical engineering of polysaccharides: a short overview. Curr Opin Biomed Eng 27:100463. https://doi.org/10.1016/j.cobme.2023.100463

Siddiqui L, Bag J, Seetha D, Mittal A, Leekha H, Mishra M, Mishra AK, Verma PK, Mishra A, Ekielski Z, Iqbal ST (2020) Assessing the potential of lignin nanoparticles as drug carrier: synthesis, cytotoxicity and genotoxicity studies. Int J Biol Macromol 152:786–802. https://doi.org/10.1016/j.ijbiomac.2020.02.311

Stanisz M, Klapiszewski MN, Collins TJ (2022) Recent progress in biomedical and biotechnological applications of lignin-based spherical nano- and microstructures: a comprehensive review. Mater Today Chem 26:101198. https://doi.org/10.1016/j.mtchem.2022.101198

Sugiarto S, Leow Y, Tan CL, Wang G, Kai D (2022) How far is lignin from being a biomedical material? Bioact Mater 8:71–94. https://doi.org/10.1016/j.bioactmat.2021.06.023

Suota MJ, Kochepka DM, Moura MGG, Pirich CL, Matos M, Magalhaes WLE, Ramos LP (2021) Lignin functionalization strategies and the potential applications of its derivatives – a review. Bioresources 16:6471–6511. https://doi.org/10.15376/BIORES.16.3.SUOTA

Tran NT, Nguyen TTT, Ha D, Nguyen TH, Nguyen NN, Baek K, Nguyen NT, Tran CK, Van Tran TT, Van Le H, Nguyen DM, Hoang D (2021) Highly functional materials based on nano-lignin, lignin, and lignin/silica hybrid capped silver nanoparticles with antibacterial activities. Biomacromolecules 22:5327–5338. https://doi.org/10.1021/acs.biomac.1c01250

Trucillo P (2024) Biomaterials for drug delivery and human applications. Materials (Basel) 17. https://doi.org/10.3390/ma17020456

Tsegaye B, Balomajumder C, Roy P (2019) Microbial delignification and hydrolysis of lignocellulosic biomass to enhance biofuel production: an overview and future prospect. Bull Natl Res Cent 43. https://doi.org/10.1186/s42269-019-0094-x

Ullah I, Chen Z, Xie Y, Khan SS, Singh S, Yu C, Cheng G (2022) Recent advances in biological activities of lignin and emerging biomedical applications: a short review. Int J Biol Macromol 208:819–832. https://doi.org/10.1016/j.ijbiomac.2022.03.182

Vasile C, Baican M (2023) Lignins as promising renewable biopolymers and bioactive compounds for high-performance materials. Polymers (Basel) 15:1–52. https://doi.org/10.3390/polym15153177

Wang JP, Matthews ML, Williams CM, Shi R, Yang C, Tunlaya-Anukit S, Chen HC, Li Q, Liu J, Lin CY, Naik P, Sun YH, Loziuk PL, Yeh TF, Kim H, Gjersing E, Shollenberger T, Shuford CM, Song J, Miller Z, Huang YY, Edmunds CW, Liu B, Sun Y, Lin YCJ, Li W, Chen H, Peszlen I, Ducoste JJ, Ralph J, Chang HM, Muddiman DC, Davis MF, Smith C, Isik F, Sederoff R, Chiang VL (2018a) Improving wood properties for wood utilization through multi-omics integration in lignin biosynthesis. Nat Commun 9:1579. https://doi.org/10.1038/s41467-018-03863-z

Wang J, Tian L, Luo B, Ramakrishna S, Kai D, Loh XJ, Yang IH, Deen GR, Mo X (2018b) Engineering PCL/lignin nanofibers as an antioxidant scaffold for the growth of neuron and Schwann cell. Colloids Surf B Biointerfaces 169:356–365. https://doi.org/10.1016/j.colsurfb.2018.05.021

Wang D, Jang J, Kim K, Kim J, Park CB (2019) “Tree to bone”: lignin/polycaprolactone nanofibers for hydroxyapatite biomineralization. Biomacromolecules 20:2684–2693. https://doi.org/10.1021/acs.biomac.9b00451

Wang YY, Meng X, Pu Y, Ragauskas AJ (2020) Recent advances in the application of functionalized lignin in value-added polymeric materials. Polymers (Basel) 12:1–24. https://doi.org/10.3390/polym12102277

Wang M, Yang D, Xu Q, Li P, Yi C, Qian Y, Qiu X (2021) Highly efficient evaporation method to prepare pH-responsive lignin-hollow-nanosphere with controllable size and its application in oral drug delivery. Ind Crop Prod 162:113230. https://doi.org/10.1016/j.indcrop.2020.113230

Wang L, Wang Q, Slita A, Backman O, Gounani Z, Rosqvist E, Peltonen J, Willför S, Xu C, Rosenholm JM, Wang X (2022) Digital light processing (DLP) 3D-fabricated antimicrobial hydrogel with a sustainable resin of methacrylated woody polysaccharides and hybrid silver-lignin nanospheres†. Green Chem 24:2129–2145. https://doi.org/10.1039/d1gc03841a

Witzler M, Alzagameem A, Bergs M, El Khaldi-Hansen B, Klein SE, Hielscher D, Kamm B, Kreyenschmidt J, Tobiasch E, Schulze M (2018) Lignin-derived biomaterials for drug release and tissue engineering. Molecules 23:1–22. https://doi.org/10.3390/molecules23081885

Yang W, Fortunati E, Gao D, Balestra GM, Giovanale G, He X, Torre L, Kenny JM, Puglia D (2018) Valorization of acid isolated high yield lignin nanoparticles as innovative antioxidant/antimicrobial organic materials. ACS Sustain Chem Eng 6:3502–3514. https://doi.org/10.1021/acssuschemeng.7b03782

Yuan Y, Jiang B, Chen H, Wu W, Wu S, Jin Y, Xiao H (2021) Recent advances in understanding the effects of lignin structural characteristics on enzymatic hydrolysis. Biotechnol Biofuels 14:1–21. https://doi.org/10.1186/s13068-021-02054-1

Yue F, Lu F (2019) Monolignol acylation in lignin biosynthesis, lignin biosynthesis. Funct Econ Significance:25–49

Zare M, Bigham A, Zare M, Luo H, Rezvani Ghomi E, Ramakrishna S (2021) pHEMA: an overview for biomedical applications. Int J Mol Sci 22. https://doi.org/10.3390/ijms22126376

Zevallos Torres LA, Lorenci Woiciechowski A, de Andrade Tanobe VO, Karp SG, Guimarães Lorenci LC, Faulds C, Soccol CR (2020) Lignin as a potential source of high-added value compounds: a review. J Clean Prod 263:121499. https://doi.org/10.1016/j.jclepro.2020.121499

Zhang Y, Khan D, Delling J, Tobiasch E (2012) Mechanisms underlying the osteo- and adipo-differentiation of human mesenchymal stem cells. Sci World J 2012:1–14. https://doi.org/10.1100/2012/793823

Zhang X, Morits M, Jonkergouw C, Ora A, Valle-Delgado JJ, Farooq M, Ajdary R, Huan S, Linder M, Rojas O, Sipponen MH, Österberg M (2020) Three-dimensional printed cell culture model based on spherical colloidal lignin particles and cellulose nanofibril-alginate hydrogel. Biomacromolecules 21:1875–1885. https://doi.org/10.1021/acs.biomac.9b01745

Zhao HK, Chen XK, Wu HF, Li JL, Xie YM (2018) Preparation of degradable biological carrier with LCC and its application in culture of hepatocytes. IOP Conf Ser Mater Sci Eng 359:012036. https://doi.org/10.1088/1757-899X/359/1/012036

Zhao J, Zheng D, Tao Y, Li Y, Wang L, Liu J, He J, Lei J (2020) Self-assembled pH-responsive polymeric nanoparticles based on lignin-histidine conjugate with small particle size for efficient delivery of anti-tumor drugs. Biochem Eng J 156:107526. https://doi.org/10.1016/j.bej.2020.107526

Zhao C, Yang J, Chen M, Chen W, Yang X, Ye H, Wang L, Wang Y, Shi J, Yue F, Ma X (2023) Synthetic lignin-derived therapeutic nano reagent as intestinal pH-sensitive drug carriers capable of bypassing the gastric acid environment for colitis treatment. ACS Nano 17:811–824. https://doi.org/10.1021/acsnano.2c11188

Zhu J, Yan C, Zhang X, Yang C, Jiang M, Zhang X (2020) A sustainable platform of lignin: from bioresources to materials and their applications in rechargeable batteries and supercapacitors. Prog Energy Combust Sci 76:100788. https://doi.org/10.1016/j.pecs.2019.100788

8 Lignin as an Emerging Sustainable Biosensing Platform for Medical Applications

Anne Beaucamp, Aashrith Dayanand,
and Maurice N. Collins

Abstract

The aging of the population amplifies the need for both early detection and continuous monitoring of biomarkers of disease. Biosensing is the determination of the amount of a biomarker using a measurable signal. Over the last decade, there has been extensive studies on the development of biosensors that allow real time monitoring, miniaturized implantable devices or handheld testing kits. Lignin has shown increasing potential as the precursor for biosensor materials. This chapter focuses on this new and exciting field where the development of lignin for biosensing applications offers a sustainable biomedical advance. While this field is still in its infancy, the influence of lignin chemical structure on the performance of the sensors shows promising results and places this natural polymer at the forefront of the next generation of biosensors.

Keywords

Lignin · Nanocomposites · Sensors · Electrodes · Sustainability

A. Beaucamp (✉) · A. Dayanand
Stokes Labs, Bernal Institute, School of Engineering, University of Limerick, Limerick, Ireland
e-mail: anne.mcloughlin@ul.ie

M. N. Collins
School of Engineering, Health Research Institute and Bernal Institute, University of Limerick, Limerick, Ireland

AMBER and BiOrbic SFI Center, University of Limerick, Limerick, Ireland

M. N. Collins, M. Culebras (eds.), *Sustainable Biopolymers and Composites for Biomedical Applications*, Biomaterials, Bioengineering and Sustainability 5,
https://doi.org/10.1007/978-3-031-91972-5_8

8.1 Introduction

A biosensor uses a transducing system to produce a signal (electrochemical, optical, piezoelectric or thermal) in presence of a given analyte. The strength of the signal is dependent on the amount of analyte in a given sample. Biosensors are of high interest in the biomedical field thanks to their high sensitivity, high selectivity, low cost and fast detection time when in contact with a biological analyte. They are used for various biomedical applications, early disease detection, contrast imaging, heart diagnosis and general health monitoring (Haleem et al. 2021).

Lignin is an aromatic polymer naturally present in the cell-wall of plants. It is derived from the polymerisation by biosynthesis of three monolignols, p-coumaryl alcohol (H), coniferyl alcohol (G) and sinapyl alcohol (S). Lignin is the second most abundant biopolymer found in nature and contains over 60% carbon. The extraction of cellulose for the pulp industry produces lignin as a by-product, as much as an estimated 140 million tonnes yearly, in 2019 (Becker and Wittmann 2019). The properties of lignin are greatly impacted by the method used to extract it. The kraft and the lignosulfonate processes partially cleave α and β-ether as well as adding sulfur to the structure. Purer lignin can be obtained via the organosolv and soda processes, however their yield is poor (25–50% for the organosolv) and production volume low due to non-existent deployment at industrial scale (Beaucamp et al. 2022a). The industrial use of lignin is currently limited to energy cogeneration in the pulp industry and low value products (dispersant and adhesives) (Becker and Wittmann 2019). However, recent research has shown that lignin can be used in a wide range of applications, including energy harvesting (Muddasar et al. 2024a; Dalton et al. 2019), energy storage (Beaucamp et al. 2022b; Culebras et al. 2019; Muddasar et al. 2024b, c), carbon fibres (Beaucamp et al. 2019; Culebras et al. 2018), composite materials (Beaucamp et al. 2024).

The present chapter details the use of lignin for biosensing applications as reported in literature.

8.2 Types of Lignin-Based Biosensors

Biosensors can detect different signal types, for example mechanical, optical and electrochemical signals. The different types of biosensors derived from lignin reported in the last three years are shown in Table 8.1.

Lignin based carbons are responsive to various stimuli such as light, strain and chemical compounds. The nature of the stimuli sensed is dependent on the preparation of the lignin-based material.

8.2.1 Optical Sensors from Lignin

Recent research on lignin for sensing applications has focused on the green synthesis of quantum carbon dots (QCD). These carbon-based nanomaterials have a size below 10 nm, conferring them fluorescent optical properties due to quantum

Table 8.1 Compilation of literature on lignin-based biosensors over the last three years

Sensor Type	Analyte	Signal	Sensitivity	Limit of detection	Lignin type	Material	Ref
Electrochemical	Dopamine		0.12–100 µM	0.035 µM	Lignosulfonate	Lignosulfonate in situ-modified reduced graphene oxide	Yuan et al. (2022)
	Troponin I	Change in Impedance	1 fM – 1 nM	1 fM or 30 fg/mL	Oil palm lignin	Lignin-scribed graphene (LSG) conjugated with nitrogen-doped graphene quantum dots (N-GQDs) and ligninderived silver nanoparticles	Vasudevan et al. (2023a)
			100 aM – 100 pM	100 aM	Oil palm lignin	LSG/MoS_2/N-GQDs/L-Ag NPs	Vasudevan et al. (2023b)
	Glucose	Enzyomatic	0.5–9 mM	145 µM	Kraft lignin	SiO_2/Lig hybrid	Jędrzak et al. (2018)
			10–80 mM	–	Kraft lignin	PE/Fe_3O_4/Lig/PDA/GOx/Fc	Jędrzak et al. (2019)
		Enzyomatic	0.15–2.7 mmol. L^{-1}	89 µmol L^{-1}	Organosolv Hardwood Lignin	PLA-Lignin based Carbon nanofibres	Beaucamp et al. (2021)

(continued)

Table 8.1 (continued)

Sensor Type	Analyte	Signal	Sensitivity	Limit of detection	Lignin type	Material	Ref
Optical	Fe^{3+}	Fluorometric	0–300 μM	0.77 μM	Alkali lignin (sigma)	Carbon Quantum Dots by acidolysis and hydrothermal	Zhu et al. (2021)
		Fluorometric with pH monitoring	50–500 μM	0.15 μM	Enzymatic Hydrolysis Lignin	Lignin based carbon dots	Lin et al. (2023)
	Xanthine Oxidase	Fluorometric	0.5–120 $U.L^{-1}$	0.13 $U.L^{-1}$	Sodium Lignosulfonate	Modified Carbon dots	Yin et al. (2024)
	H_2O_2	Fluorometric	10^{-1} – 10^{-6} M	–	Alkali Lignin from Acacia	Acacia lignin stabilized silver nanoparticles	Aadil et al. (2016)
	Fe^{3+}, Al^{3+} and Cu^{2+}	Fluorometric	0–500 μM	0.45–3.90 μM	Alkali lignin from corncob	Heteroatom-engineered multicolor lignin carbon dots	Zhou et al. (2023)
	Formaldehyde	Fluorometric	0–500 μM	500 nM	Sodium Lignosulfonate	Ag^{+}-mediated nitrogen-sulfur co-doped carbon dots	Zhou et al. (2022)
		Fluorometric	0–1 $mg.L^{-1}$	7.40 $\mu g.L^{-1}$	Unspecified Lignin	Lignin derived multicolor carbon dots	Li et al. (2023)
	Ascorbic Acid	Fluorometric	0–1000 μM	1.62 μM	Alkali lignin (Sigma)	Lignin based carbon dots	Zhu et al. (2022a)
	Hexavalent Chromium	Fluorometric	–	–		Nitrogen and boron co-doped carbon quantum dots	Zhu et al. (2022b)

Mechanical	Piezoresistance	Strain			Lignosulfonate (Sigma)	Lignosulfonate composite conductive hydrogels	Wang et al. (2024)
		Strain and pressure		0.27–14.1 kPa	Lignosulfonate	Activated carbon loaded in a polyvinyl alcohol, carboxymethyl chitosan, cellulose nanofibrils hydrogel	Li et al. (2021)
		Strain				Lignin / Single Walled Carbon Nanotubes / Graphene oxyde aerogel	Peng et al. (2022)
		Strain				Lignocellulose nanofiber-decorated graphite-flake nanocomposites	Lin et al. (2022)

confinement effect, where the excitation wavelength is dependent on the size of the QCD (Bhattacharya et al. 2015). In addition, QCD present extensive properties such as hydrophilicity, biocompatibility, high conductivity, low toxicity and controllable fluorescent properties (Zhu et al. 2021). Since the first report of their synthesis in 2004 (Xu et al. 2004), there has been over 26,000 research articles published on the subject (Clarivate 2024). The QCD can be synthetised from organic molecules such as carbohydrates (glucose, fructose, starch, etc.…) or citric acid via chemical, electrochemical, physical or hydrothermal routes, as reviewed in Wang and Hu (2014), Ozyurt et al. (2023). The quality of the QCD produced is determined by their size, excitation and emission wavelength as well as by the quantum yield (QY), ratio of the number of photons emitted vs that of the number of photons absorbed by the QCD. Heteroatoms (S, N, B or F) doping enhances the QY, photoluminescence intensity and emission wavelength (Ozyurt et al. 2023).

Lignin has placed itself as a promising QCD precursor due to its high carbon content (>60%) and conjugated aromatic structure, rendering it chromophoric properties (Sheridan et al. 2024). Hydrothermal synthesis is the method of choice for deriving QCD from lignin despite a low QY (reportedly 1.5–14%) and low reaction yield (0.8–12 wt%). Chu et al. (2024) have improved the hydrothermal reaction yield by modifying the lignin chemistry via the Mannich reaction, increasing its solubility in water and introducing covalently-bonded N-dopants. As the hydrothermal reaction starts by the decomposition of the lignin ether bonds into lignin trimers, dimers and monomers (Zhao et al. 2022), improving the solubility of lignin in water improves both the decomposition reaction yield and the QY of the CD produced, up to 68 wt% and to 42.7% respectively (Chu et al. 2024). Interestingly, Chu has reported the high dependency of the QY on the plant source of lignin, as the π-conjugation of lignin is more likely to take place in grass-based lignin due to the presence of monolignol p-coumarates and ferulate conjugates (Chu et al. 2024). In a second step, the formed lignin small particles re-polymerise under high temperature and pressure conditions to form QCDs (Zhao et al. 2022). Parameters such as temperature, solvent or acidic conditions were found to influence the excitation and emission wavelengths of the QCDs (Li et al. 2023). Li et al. tuned the emission wavelength of the QCD by adjusting the amount of hydrochloric acid in the hydrothermal reaction medium. Blue-emitting QCDs were produced without HCL while green-emitting QCDs were produced with HCl introduced in excess (Li et al. 2023). Zhu et al. studied the effect of the acid additive concentration, retention time and reaction temperature. All parameters influenced the properties of the synthesised QCD, i.e. their size, wavelength of emission and QY. The optimisation of these parameters allowed to produce a green emitting QCD (λ_{em} = 476 nm) with a QY of 23.7%. The acid used, o-amino benzenesulfonic acid, was reported to form oxygen-, nitrogen- and sulphur- functional groups as well as breaking ether and C-C linkages from lignin (Zhu et al. 2021).

QCD have been reported to show a very high selectivity to Fe^{3+} in comparison to other metal anions (Pb^{2+}, K^+, Na^+, Mg^{2+}, Ni^{2+}, Co^{2+}, Cu^{2+}, Ca^{2+}, Cd^{2+}, Zn^{2+}) (Lin et al. 2023; Zhu et al. 2022a). When in presence of Fe^{3+}, the QCD fluorescence is quenched by up to 90% (Zhu et al. 2021). This quenching effect is both linearly dependent on the concentration of Fe^{3+} (Zhu et al. 2021, 2022a; Lin et al. 2023) and independent of the amount of QCD in the solution (Zhu et al. 2022a). The quenching effect is speculated to be due to the formation of a QCD-Fe^{3+} complex, stopping the luminescence (Zhu et al. 2021, 2022a). Zhu et al. demonstrated that this effect can be reversed by the addition of ascorbic acid in the solution, reducing Fe^{3+} to Fe^{2+} and therefore restoring fluorescence. This effect is limited to solutions where both species are present (Zhu et al. 2022a).

Other species can also be detected using QCD, using different approaches. Yin et al. used the catalytic activity of ligno-sulfonates-based CD on hydrogen peroxyde to detect xanthine oxidase, an enzyme associated with liver injuries and gout disease. The detection of hydrogen peroxide was possible through the presence of O-phenylenediamine groups at the surface of modified QCD, enhancing yellow luminescence (Yin et al. 2024). Other strategies use silver nanoparticules (AGNP) to detect H_2O_2. In this case, lignin acts as a stabilising and reducing agent, with UV-absorption bands centered at 410–430 nm. When in presence of H_2O_2, Ag is reduced to Ag^+, leading to a loss of absorbance intensity as the concentration of H_2O_2 increases in the solution (Aadil et al. 2016). Zhou et al. used silver ions as a mediator for the sensing of formaldehyde (FA). They prepared N and S doped QCDs (NSCD) by hydrothermal treatment of lignosulfonate in acidic conditions before adding silver nitrate to the solution. The NSCD produces display fluorescence with an excitation peak at 360 nm and an emission peak at 455 nm with a QY of 17.7%. When in presence of Ag^+, fluorescence is quenched with a drop of the QY down to 4.4%. The addition of FA leads to the formation of Ag nanoparticles by reduction of the Ag + ions. In response, the fluorescence of the NSCD increases as FA concentration increases, leading to a highly linear sensor with low detection range (Zhou et al. 2022). Vasudevan et al. used AGNP coupled with N_2-doped graphene quantum dots for the sensing of troponin I. AGNP act as a binder, immobilising the protein thiol-branches on the sensing platform (Vasudevan et al. 2023b).

While doping with N or S atoms are the most common approaches for QY enhancing, other elements such as boron can be used. Zhu et al. induced triple-emission fluorescence at 300, 330 and 490 nm by doping the CQD with boron and nitrogen functional groups, enhancing intramolecular charge transfer and improving emission efficiency (Zhu et al. 2022b).

8.2.2 Strain and Pressure Sensors

Strain and pressure sensors are based on a change in electric signal as a function of the pressure or the strain applied on the material. Li et al. used lignin-based activated carbon as a conductive filler to induce conductivity in carboxymethyl chitosan-PVA hydrogels. When under mechanical pressure, the three-dimensional hydrogel framework had a reduced electrical resistance. This effect could be used to measure the pressure applied on the materials (Li et al. 2021).

Peng et al. showed that channels aligned within a conductive lignosulfonate-based aerogel allowed for wide detection region and high sensitivity. They used single walled carbon nanotubes (SWCNT) as the conductive filler within the aerogel. As the material is compressed., the adjacent conductive channels come in contact, decreasing the materials electric resistance and increasing the current going through. This effect takes place within the linear elastic deformation region of the material (Peng et al. 2022). Wang et al. developed a conductive hydrogel from lignosulfonate, which demonstrated excellent piezoresistant properties when subjective to strain of flexion. The effect was attributed to the narrowing of the ionic path as the material is deformed. The effect was sensitive enough to be applied to the detection of body motion during sleep as well as voice recognition (Wang et al. 2024). The same approach was taken by Lin et al., using lignocellulose-based nanofibres decorated graphite-flake as conductive fillers in a PVA-borax matrix (Lin et al. 2022).

8.3 Electrochemical Sensors

- Electrochemical sensors are based on the change of current intensity as a function of an analyte concentration, at a given potential. The electric signal can be mediated by the redox reaction between the analyte and the sensing platform. This approach is widely used to detect glucose using immobilised glucose oxidase (GOX) (Jędrzak et al. 2018, 2019; Beaucamp et al. 2021). In each case, the nanomaterial formed from lignin is used to immobilise GOX at the surface of the electrode and collect the electric signal from the redox of the enzyme. Electrospinning has been reported as a versatile technique to prepare electrochemical platform (Beaucamp et al. 2021). Electrospinning works on the principle of electro-thermodynamics, where a drop of liquid ideally possesses electrical conductivity. The process begins with charging the droplet which gives rise to Taylor cone, and a collector plate where solid fibers are deposited is grounded. Optimization of the voltage and the feed rate to produce the droplet will lead to a jet of stretched and extended fine solid fibers. Thinning of these fibers occurs in the presence of applied electric field and phenomenon known as whipping instability. The solid fibers are deposited on the collector plate due to the potential difference. The processing parameters are governed by mathematical that enables one to estimate the voltage to generate the Taylor cone considering the (a) solution properties such as conductivity, surface tension, (b) the distance of the collector, type of collector (flat plate or cylinder), polymer flowrate and, (c) environmental factor such as solution temperature or humidity (Sun et al. 2014). The parameters influence the processability of the fibres such as:
- Solution flowrate beyond the critical value will result in beads, increase in pore size and generally, flowrate and voltage are directly related.
- Polymer concentrations and its viscosity have an impact on the process parameters. Low viscosity- applied field and surface tension causes entanglement and breakage of chains into fragments. High concentrations- overcomes the above effects to produce fibres and concentration beyond CV dries the solution at the tip.

- Solution conductivity influences Taylor cone formation. Largely governed by electrostatic force of surface charges created by electric field. Increase in conductivity will increase surface charging and decrease in diameter. Solvents ideally must complete soluble in the polymer and must have moderate boiling point. Generally volatile solvents are preferred as high evaporation rate encourages fibre formation (phase separation/porous nanofibers). Humidity and temperature play an important role in the fibre formation (Haider et al. 2018).

The critical value of the voltage is majorly material dependent, increase in voltage beyond that value will result in beads due to decrease in Taylor cone and increase in fibre diameter (Haider et al. 2018).

After electrospinning, the nanofibers obtained can be heat treated and carbonized. The surface of the sensor is then functionalized, either by immobilising enzymes or metallic nanoparticles. There are various ways of depositing the metallic nanoparticles, such as chemical vapor deposition, physical vapor deposition or other chemical reduction methodologies to utilize the mesoporous sites on the surface. This can be termed as a way of functionalizing the CNFs to have additional or boosting functionality.

It is good to investigate the various sensing methodologies, to start off with the amperometric biosensors is one that was developed in 1956 to sense oxygen (Lupu et al. 2013).

Cyclic voltammetry (CV) produces a sweeping potential that is applied between the electrodes that are near to the redox reaction of the analyte. This generates a double peak one for oxidation and the other for reductio correlating to the concentration of the analyte and quantitatively assessing the amount of glucose. In this methodology it has also seen that the intensity of the peaks will naturally reduce thereby indicating the levels of glucose in the analyte, thereby allowing first hand qualitative assessment. The eventual outcome of the CV analysis is that we can plot calibration curves to quantify the compound, this is done using the intensity of the peaks of either oxidation or reduction depending on the dominant response or the reaction that is being quantified to detect the presence (Elgrishi et al. 2018).

When a pulsed potentials are applied within a linear potential scanning this technique is called differential pulse voltammetry. It is highly sensitive and capable of detecting low concentrations even when the electron kinetics of electron transfer is slow (Prete et al. 2022). The procedure behind the plot is that the base potential is chosen where there is no faradaic reaction, then this potential is increased in equal steps and before each increment the current is measured. The difference in current is plotted on the graph against the applied potential. Also, DPV is much preferred techniques as oxidation peaks in the voltammogram it is more useful to incorporate such a technique as it helps in discriminating amongst other oxidation prone interferants as they all provide a unique peak for each of them.

All these nanofibers can be implemented on an electrode, and the current generation of electrodes have been miniaturized. For the experiment screen printed electrodes that can be functionalised with various materials depending on the type of analyte being sensed. The active compound that will sense the compound is formulated in the form of a paste or liquid viscous enough to be incorporated on the electrode.

The electrospinning of lignin necessitates the use of a polymer binder to reach appropriate viscosity, such as PEO (Dallmeyer et al. 2010), PAN (Seo et al. 2011) or PVA (Lai et al. 2014) Dimethylformamide (DMF) is generally the solvent of choice for electrospinning, at concentrations varying between 10–50 wt.% of polymer. After electrospinning, the nanofibres produced can be heat treated to produce carbon based nanofibres. This heat treatment is typically performant in two steps, with an oxidative, low ramp rate stabilisation first, to stop the fibres from melting, followed with a carbonisation in inert atmosphere up to 1000degC or above (Poursorkhabi et al. 2020). Zheng et al. developed a sensor for uric acid using phosphated lignin electrospun with cellulose acetate (Zheng et al. 2022). Beaucamp et al. used poly(Lactic acid) as a sacrificial polymer binder, which in a first step allowed for easy electrospinning of hardwood organosolv lignin before being fully degraded during carbonisation. After carbonisation, the removed PLA left behind a 3 D structure with voids, opening up the porosity inherent to lignin. The pores created were used as sites for the redox centres of glucose oxidase for selectivity, high sensitivity, a linear range and a detection limit that are suitable for detecting glucose in human saliva samples (Beaucamp et al. 2021).

8.4 Conclusion

Due to the aromatic structure and the multiple active sites within lignin can be used as precursor material for QCD, conductive hydrogels and nanofibres. The diversity of lignin sources and extraction methods, which allows the inclusion of heteroatoms within its structure, is usually detrimental to its valorisation. However, for sensing applications heteroatom doping is beneficial, making lignin a very interesting low-cost candidate for biosensing applications.

References

Aadil KR et al (2016) Hydrogen peroxide sensing and cytotoxicity activity of Acacia lignin stabilized silver nanoparticles. Int J Biol Macromol 82:39–47

Beaucamp A et al (2019) Carbon fibres from renewable resources: the role of the lignin molecular structure in its blendability with biobased poly(ethylene terephthalate). Green Chem 21(18):5063–5072

Beaucamp A, Culebras M, Collins MN (2021) Sustainable mesoporous carbon nanostructures derived from lignin for early detection of glucose. Green Chem 23(15):5696–5705

Beaucamp A et al (2022a) Lignin for energy applications—state of the art, life cycle, technoeconomic analysis and future trends. Green Chem 24(21):8193–8226

Beaucamp A et al (2022b) Sustainable lignin precursors for tailored porous carbon-based supercapacitor electrodes. Int J Biol Macromol 221:1142–1149

Beaucamp A et al (2024) Sustainable lignin-based carbon fibre reinforced polyamide composites: production, characterisation and life cycle analysis. Composit Commun 45:101782

Becker J, Wittmann C (2019) A field of dreams: lignin valorization into chemicals, materials, fuels, and health-care products. Biotechnol Adv 37(6):107360

Bhattacharya A et al (2015) Size-dependent penetration of carbon dots inside the ferritin nanocages: evidence for the quantum confinement effect in carbon dots. Phys Chem Chem Phys 17(19):12833–12840

Chu T et al (2024) Improving the revenue of lignin conversion into carbon dots by prior amino modification. Green Chem 26(5):2773–2782

Clarivate (2024) Web of Science. Clarivate

Culebras M et al (2018) Biobased structurally compatible polymer blends based on lignin and thermoplastic elastomer polyurethane as carbon fiber precursors. ACS Sustain Chem Eng 6(7):8816–8825

Culebras M et al (2019) Bio-derived carbon nanofibres from lignin as high-performance Li-ion anode materials. ChemSusChem 12(19):4516–4521

Dallmeyer I, Ko F, Kadla JF (2010) Electrospinning of technical lignins for the production of fibrous networks. J Wood Chem Technol 30(4):315–329

Dalton N et al (2019) Thermoelectric properties of electrospun carbon nanofibres derived from lignin. Int J Biol Macromol 121:472–479

Elgrishi N et al (2018) A practical beginner's guide to cyclic voltammetry. J Chem Educ 95(2):197–206

Haider A, Haider S, Kang I-K (2018) A comprehensive review summarizing the effect of electrospinning parameters and potential applications of nanofibers in biomedical and biotechnology. Arab J Chem 11(8):1165–1188

Haleem A et al (2021) Biosensors applications in medical field: a brief review. Sens Int 2:100100

Jędrzak A et al (2018) Carbon paste electrode based on functional GOx/silica-lignin system to prepare an amperometric glucose biosensor. Sensors Actuators B Chem 256:176–185

Jędrzak A et al (2019) Bio-inspired magnetite/lignin/polydopamine-glucose oxidase biosensing nanoplatform. From synthesis, via sensing assays to comparison with others glucose testing techniques. Int J Biol Macromol 127:677–682

Lai C et al (2014) Free-standing and mechanically flexible mats consisting of electrospun carbon nanofibers made from a natural product of alkali lignin as binder-free electrodes for high-performance supercapacitors. J Power Sources 247:134–141

Li M et al (2021) Flexible conductive hydrogel fabricated with polyvinyl alcohol, carboxymethyl chitosan, cellulose nanofibrils, and lignin-based carbon applied as strain and pressure sensor. Int J Biol Macromol 166:1526–1534

Li Y et al (2023) Lignin derived multicolor carbon dots for visual detection of formaldehyde. Ind Crop Prod 192:116006

Lin F et al (2022) One-pot mechanochemical assembly of lignocellulose nanofiber/graphite nanocomposites for wearable electronic devices. Chem Eng J 437:135286

Lin S et al (2023) Sustainable synthesis of lignin-derived carbon dots with visible pH response for Fe3+ detection and bioimaging. Spectrochim Acta A Mol Biomol Spectrosc 302:123111

Lupu S et al (2013) Development of amperometric biosensors based on nanostructured tyrosinase-conducting polymer composite electrodes. Sensors (Basel) 13(5):6759–6774

Muddasar M et al (2024a) Lignin-derived ionic conducting membranes for low-grade thermal energy harvesting. Adv Funct Mater 34(12):2306427

Muddasar M et al (2024b) High performance all lignin derived supercapacitors for energy storage applications. Mater Today Sustain 26:100767

Muddasar M, Culebras M, M.N. (2024c) Collins lignin-derived materials for sustainable development of ionic thermoelectric supercapacitors. Mater Proc 17. https://doi.org/10.3390/materproc2024017025

Ozyurt D et al (2023) Properties, synthesis, and applications of carbon dots: a review. Carbon Trends 12:100276

Peng Z, Yu C, Zhong W (2022) Facile preparation of a 3D porous aligned graphene-based wall network architecture by confined self-assembly with shape memory for artificial muscle, pressure sensor, and flexible supercapacitor. ACS Appl Mater Interfaces 14(15):17739–17753

Poursorkhabi V et al (2020) Processing, carbonization, and characterization of lignin based electrospun carbon fibers: a review. Front Energy Res 8(208)

Prete MC, Rocha LR, Tarley CRT (2022) Chapter 4 - Development of new electroanalytical method based on graphene oxide-modified glassy carbon electrode for mephedrone illicit drug determination. In: Manjunatha JG, Hussain CM (eds) Carbon nanomaterials-based sensors. Elsevier, pp 43–56

Seo DK et al (2011) Preparation and characterization of the carbon nanofiber mat produced from electrospun PAN/lignin precursors by electron beam irradiation. Rev Adv Mater Sci 28(1):31–34

Sheridan E et al (2024) A systematic study on the processes of lignin extraction and nanodispersion to control properties and functionality. Green Chem 26(6):2967–2984

Sun B et al (2014) Advances in three-dimensional nanofibrous macrostructures via electrospinning. Prog Polym Sci 39(5):862–890

Vasudevan M et al (2023a) Lignin derived nanoparticle intercalation on nitrogen-doped graphene quantum dots for electrochemical sensing of cardiac biomarker. Microchem J 195:109405

Vasudevan M et al (2023b) A quadruplet 3-D laser scribed graphene/MoS2, functionalised N2-doped graphene quantum dots and lignin-based ag-nanoparticles for biosensing. Int J Biol Macromol 253:126620

Wang Y, Hu A (2014) Carbon quantum dots: synthesis, properties and applications. J Mater Chem C 2(34):6921–6939

Wang J et al (2024) Rapid preparation of dynamic-crosslinked nanocomposite hydrogel sensors with efficiency self-healing and adhesion properties for elderly health and sleep management. Chem Eng J 480:148324

Xu X et al (2004) Electrophoretic analysis and purification of fluorescent single-walled carbon nanotube fragments. J Am Chem Soc 126(40):12736–12737

Yin C et al (2024) Novel lignin-derived carbon dots nanozyme cascade-amplified for ratiometric fluorescence detection of xanthine oxidase and intracellular imaging. Sensors Actuators B Chem 406:135458

Yuan Y et al (2022) Lignosulfonate in situ-modified reduced graphene oxide biosensors for the electrochemical detection of dopamine. RSC Adv 12(48):31083–31090

Zhao S et al (2022) Interaction of lignin and xylan in the hydrothermal synthesis of lignocellulose-based carbon quantum dots and their application in in-vivo bioimaging. Int J Biol Macromol 222:1876–1887

Zheng H et al (2022) A green flexible and wearable biosensor based on carbon nanofibers for sensitive detection of uric acid in artificial urine. J Mater Chem B 10(41):8450–8461

Zhou X et al (2022) A novel signal-on fluorometric sensor based on metal ion-mediated carbon dots for formaldehyde determination and lysosome-targeted bioimaging. New J Chem 46(36):17540–17547

Zhou P et al (2023) Heteroatom-engineered multicolor lignin carbon dots enabling bimodal fluorescent off-on detection of metal-ions and glutathione. Int J Biol Macromol 253:126714

Zhu L et al (2021) Sustainable synthesis of bright green fluorescent carbon quantum dots from lignin for highly sensitive detection of Fe3+ ions. Appl Surf Sci 565:150526

Zhu L et al (2022a) Lignin-based fluorescence-switchable graphene quantum dots for Fe3+ and ascorbic acid detection. Int J Biol Macromol 194:254–263

Zhu L, Shen D, Hong Luo K (2022b) Triple-emission nitrogen and boron co-doped carbon quantum dots from lignin: highly fluorescent sensing platform for detection of hexavalent chromium ions. J Colloid Interface Sci 617:557–567

Lignin Composites for Biomedical Applications

9

Nazish Jabeen and Clara M. Gómez

Abstract

Lignin, a renewable and abundant biopolymer derived from lignocellulosic biomass, offers a sustainable alternative to conventional synthetic materials. Its complex structure, rich in functional groups, imparts valuable properties such as antioxidant, antimicrobial, and biocompatibility. These attributes, combined with lignin's versatility and potential for cost-effective processing, have stimulated extensive research for biomedical applications. In recent years, lignin composites have emerged as promising candidates for developing innovative medical materials and devices. This chapter provides a comprehensive overview of lignin's composition, properties, and extraction methods while discussing fabrication techniques for lignin composites that highlight their biological activities. The recent advancements in utilizing lignin composites for biomedical applications, particularly in drug delivery, wound healing, and tissue engineering, are thoroughly reviewed. Additionally, the chapter outlines future directions, serving as a valuable resource for promoting the use of lignin composites in the biomedical field.

Keywords

Lignin composites · Antioxidant property · Tissue engineering · Drug delivery · Biomedical application

N. Jabeen (✉) · C. M. Gómez
Institute of Material Science, (ICMUV) University of Valencia, Valencia, Spain
e-mail: Nazish.jabeen@uv.es

M. N. Collins, M. Culebras (eds.), *Sustainable Biopolymers and Composites for Biomedical Applications*, Biomaterials, Bioengineering and Sustainability 5,
https://doi.org/10.1007/978-3-031-91972-5_9

9.1 Introduction

The rapid growth of the global population and industrialization has led to an increasing reliance on fossil fuels, raising significant environmental concerns and highlighting the need for sustainable alternatives. Among the various solutions proposed, biomass resources have emerged as promising candidates to replace fossil fuels, offering a renewable and environmentally friendly energy source (Lobato-Peralta et al. 2021). In particular, lignocellulosic biomass, derived from woody materials in forest ecosystems, has gained attention due to its potential to reduce energy consumption and associated pollution by replacing conventional synthetic materials. Lignocellulosic biomass is composed of three main components: cellulose (38–50%), hemicellulose (23–32%), and lignin (12–25%). The complex structure of lignocellulosic materials is attributed to the ether and ester bonds linking cellulose and hemicellulose to lignin. Lignin, the second most abundant renewable biopolymer after cellulose, is a heterogeneous and amorphous substance that plays a critical role in reinforcing cellulose fibers within plant cell walls, serving as a matrix that provides mechanical support and chemical protection against external stresses (Zhou et al. 2019; Witzler et al. 2018; Wang et al. 2015a, 2021a). Despite its abundant availability, lignin remains significantly underutilized, with much of the approximately 70 million tons produced annually by the paper industry either burned as low-grade fuel or discarded as waste. Few years ago, lignin was widely recognized for its antioxidant properties, which are attributed to its polyphenolic structure containing numerous carboxyl and hydroxyl functional groups. Other structural components such as ortho-substituents, CH_2 groups, and methoxyl groups also affect the potential activity of lignin (Liu et al. 2022). Recently, lignin has gained significant attention as a versatile biomaterial based on multiple biological functions and excellent cellular compatibility, particularly as an antibacterial and anti-inflammatory additive in implant agents. Unlike synthetic chemicals, lignin is a renewable resource with outstanding biodegradability, aligning well with the goals of sustainable development (Terzioğlu et al. 2020; Parham et al. 2020). These unique properties of lignin have sparked growing interest into the high-value product in biomedical sector instead of low-value biofuel. Researchers have explored its use in various applications, including mechanical reinforcement in composites, antioxidant functions, UV protection, and as an antimicrobial additive (Shu et al. 2021). As the search for innovative biomedical materials continues, lignin has emerged as a material of significant interest due to these remarkable properties. It has proven effective in diverse biomedical applications, including tissue engineering scaffolds, antibacterial agents, and drug delivery systems (Nan et al. 2022). The notable characteristics of lignin and its derivatives such as cost efficiency, eco-friendly, strong adhesiveness, desirable mechanical properties, and high thermal stability have further sparked interest in developing lignin composites (Arya et al. 2023). By combining lignin with other polymers, researchers have successfully produced composites with enhanced functionality, making them suitable for a wide range of biomedical applications. This represents a significant step forward in the creation of next-generation biomaterials, as lignin's unique biological properties continue to expand its potential in the biomedical field (Liu et al. 2022; Parham et al. 2020; Nan et al. 2022; Jabeen and Atif 2024).

This chapter offers a thorough exploration of lignin's composition, structural properties, and extraction methods, laying the groundwork for understanding its potential in biomedical applications. In the subsequent sections, we delve into various fabrication techniques for lignin composites, emphasizing their antioxidant, UV-absorbing, and antitumor properties. Recent advancements in the use of lignin composites, particularly in drug delivery, wound healing, and tissue engineering, are comprehensively reviewed. The chapter concludes by highlighting future directions and emphasizing the importance of continued innovation in overcoming current limitations. By advancing the application of lignin composites, especially in tissue engineering and wound healing, this chapter aims to serve as a valuable resource for researchers in the biomedical field, guiding the development of next-generation biomaterials.

9.2 Lignin: Structural and Chemical Characteristics

Lignin is one of the three primary biopolymers found in lignocellulose materials, alongside cellulose and hemicellulose. In plant cell walls, cellulose is tightly bound by hemicellulose and lignin, creating a rigid and robust structure. As a complex aromatic biopolymer, lignin forms strong electrostatic interactions with the polar regions of xylan within plant secondary cell walls, contributing significantly to their overall structural integrity (Kang et al. 2019). It also provides structural support, enhances water resistance, and plays a critical role in the defence against pathogens. Lignin biopolymer composed of phenylpropanoid units such as syringyl (S), guaiacyl (G), and p-hydroxyphenyl (H), derived from the radical coupling of sinapyl, coniferyl, and p-coumaryl alcohols as illustrated in Fig. 9.1. These monolignols are linked together during the lignification process through various interunit bonds, including ether linkages (β–O–4, α–O–4, and 4–O–5) and carbon-carbon linkages (β–β, β–5, β–1, and 5–5). This bonding results in the formation of amorphous lignin macromolecules, which are much more heterogeneous compared to the more regularly structured cellulose and hemicelluloses (Wang et al. 2021a; Shuai et al. 2016; Bertella and Luterbacher 2020).

The chemical diversity in lignin arises from its varied monolignol composition and extensive range of linkages, resulting in functional groups such as aromatic rings, aliphatic and phenolic hydroxyls, carboxyls, carbonyls, and methoxy groups. These functional groups give lignin several beneficial properties, including UV absorption, hydrophobicity, fluorescence, metal ion absorption and chelation, and thermal stability. The abundance of chemical sites and functional groups in lignin allows for extensive chemical modifications, enhancing its applicability in various fields (Srisapoome et al. 2018; Barapatre et al. 2015). The solubility of lignin in many organic solvents also facilitates structural modifications, particularly through the functionalization of aromatic rings and hydroxyl groups, as well as polymerization processes. These properties make lignin an attractive and cost-effective

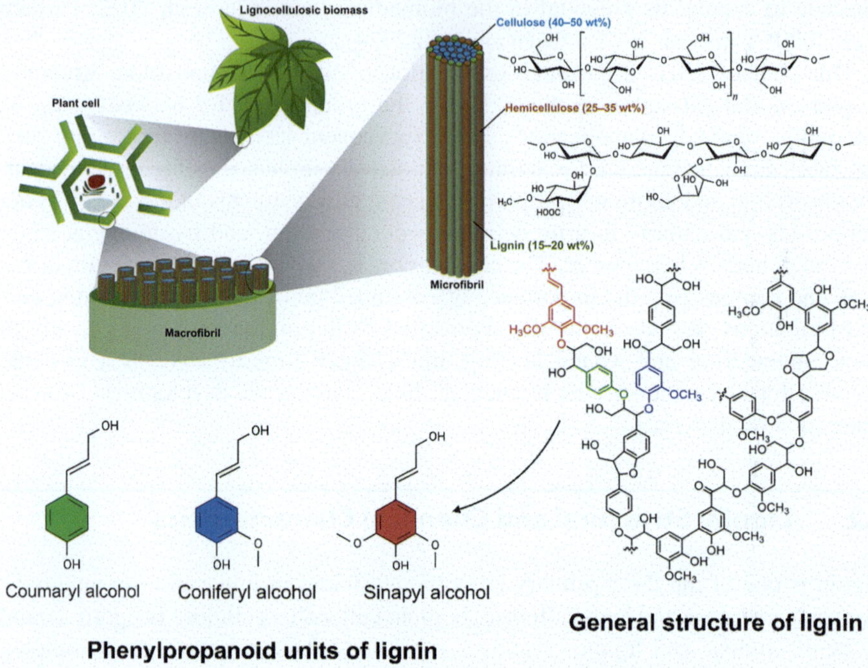

Fig. 9.1 Lignocellulose biomass, structure of lignin and phenylpropanoid units. (Reproduced with permission Bertella and Luterbacher (2020). Copyright 2020, Elsevier)

candidate for the development of functional polymeric materials. In addition to its structural and chemical attributes, lignin has shown potential bioactivities, including antiviral, antimicrobial, antidiabetic, anticancer, and anticoagulant properties, making it a promising material for biomedical applications. Lignin's monomer composition and chemical structure vary significantly based on extraction methods, influencing its overall properties and expanding its potential applications (Wang et al. 2021a; Figueiredo et al. 2017).

9.3 Lignin-Extraction Techniques

Bjökman was the first to extract lignin utilizing a dioxane–water combination in 1956 (Liao et al. 2020). To promote lignin valorization, researchers have developed several techniques for lignin extraction from various biomass sources (Huang et al. 2020). The extraction of lignin from biomass is a pivotal process in utilizing it for producing valuable products across various industries, including biofuels, bioplastics, energy storage and biomedical applications. The choice of extraction method depends on the intended application, as it influences the yield, purity, and structural properties of the extracted lignin (Carvajal et al. 2016). Various industrial lignin extraction techniques have been developed and can be broadly categorized into

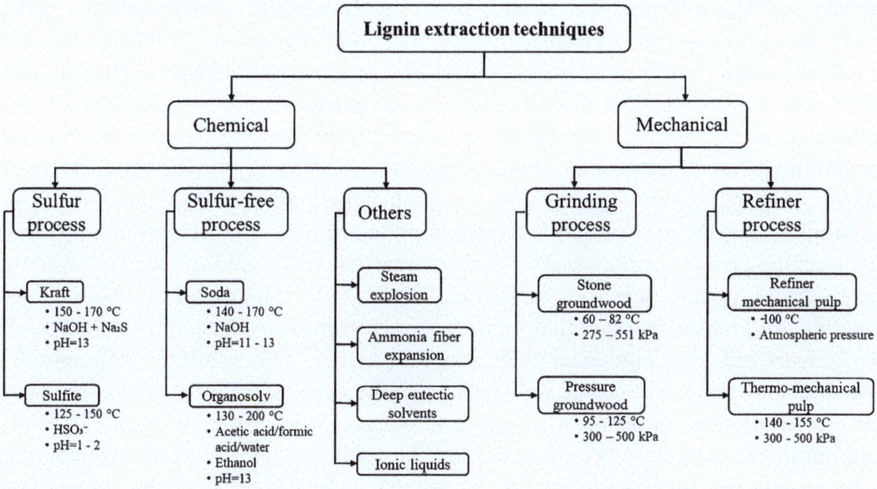

Fig. 9.2 Schematic representation of lignin extraction techniques. (Reproduced with permission Lobato-Peralta et al. (2021). Copyright 2021, Elsevier)

chemical and mechanical techniques as represented in Fig. 9.2. Mechanical methods, such as refining and grinding, are typically employed for ethanol production via fermentation. In contrast, chemical extraction techniques, more prevalent in lignin production, are classified into sulfur-based and sulfur-free processes, each offering different advantages depending on the desired end-use (Lobato-Peralta et al. 2021; Shah et al. 2023).

In addition to these conventional methods, alternative extraction approaches, such as alkaline extraction, have been developed to improve the performance of lignin separation and to expand its applicability. These methods not only enhance the purity of lignin but also allow for the production of intermediate products with diverse applications, including in biocomposites, biofuels, and other high-value products. Despite its beneficial properties, lignin's processability and mechanical tunability present challenges for direct application. However, combining lignin with other materials has effectively addressed these limitations, producing composites with improved functionalities (Shah et al. 2023).

9.4 Lignin Composites and Their Fabrication Techniques

Lignin stands out as a valuable candidate for composite production due to its rich aromatic structure, thermal stability, high carbon content, and inherent rigidity. Lignin-based composites are innovative biomaterials that integrate lignin with conventional polymers (Nan et al. 2022). The presence of functional groups in lignin, such as methoxyl, hydroxyl, carbonyl, and carboxyl groups, provides active sites essential for the composite fabrication process. Recent advancements have expanded the range of lignin composites, leading to the creation of films, hydrogels, aerogels, fibers, nanocomposites, scaffolds, fibrous mats, and membranes with diverse and functional properties. Lignin has been widely utilized to enhance composites by improving mechanical characteristics, increasing material porosity and drug release behaviour, and providing antioxidant and antibacterial benefits. Literature reported lignin/chitosan biocomposites (Jaganathan et al. 2018), lignin/alginate cryogels (Barros et al. 2016), and lignin/gelatin cryogels, which are produced using freezing techniques, have been explored for applications in tissue repair and wound healing. The freezing process promotes ice crystal formation, and rapid freezing followed by freeze-drying results in porous structures. Research by Memic. et al. (Memic and Abudula 2021) demonstrated that lignin not only improved the mechanical strength of cryogels but also enhanced their shape recovery. The resulting microporous structure showed excellent free radical scavenging activity and effectively inhibited the growth of both gram-positive and gram-negative bacteria. Additionally, alginate/lignin aerogels have been investigated for their potential in tissue engineering and regenerative medicine (Quraishi et al. 2015). In the last decade, researchers reported several techniques employed for lignin composite fabrication including such as electrospinning, three-dimensional printing, melt extrusion, hot pressing, blending, solvent casting, and spin coating. By combining lignin with biodegradable polymers, these approaches yield advanced biomaterials with enhanced mechanical strength, and controlled degradation rates. Research indicates that these fabricated lignin composites hold significant promise for applications in wound dressings, drug delivery system, tissue engineering, and regenerative medicine, including nerve, skin, bone, cartilage, and hard tissue repair. This chapter offers a comprehensive overview of fabrication techniques for lignin composites, highlighting its potential to create sustainable and innovative materials for a broad range of biomedical applications (Nan et al. 2022).

9.4.1 Electrospinning

In the past decade, electrospinning has emerged as one of the most versatile manufacturing technologies, particularly for producing lignin composites for potential applications. This technique excels in producing nanofibers and scaffolds with desirable properties, including high aspect ratio, surface area, porosity, flexibility, structural diversity, and capacity for bioactive agent delivery (Yang et al. 2020; Alven et al. 2021). Electrospinning generates ultrafine fibers by applying a high-voltage electric field to a charged polymer solution or melt ejected from a spinneret. This versatile technique offers various process configurations such as blend, coaxial, emulsion, and needleless electrospinning as illustrated in Fig. 9.3a (Parham et al. 2020; Nan et al. 2022). A research study conducted by Abdullah and colleagues (Abdullah et al. 2018), used coaxial electrospinning to encapsulate chitin-lignin gels with polycaprolactone (PCL), resulting in gel fibrous scaffolds that demonstrated controlled drug release capabilities. Furthermore, they fabricated hybrid nanofibrous scaffolds using a blend of chitin/lignin sol-gel and elastomeric

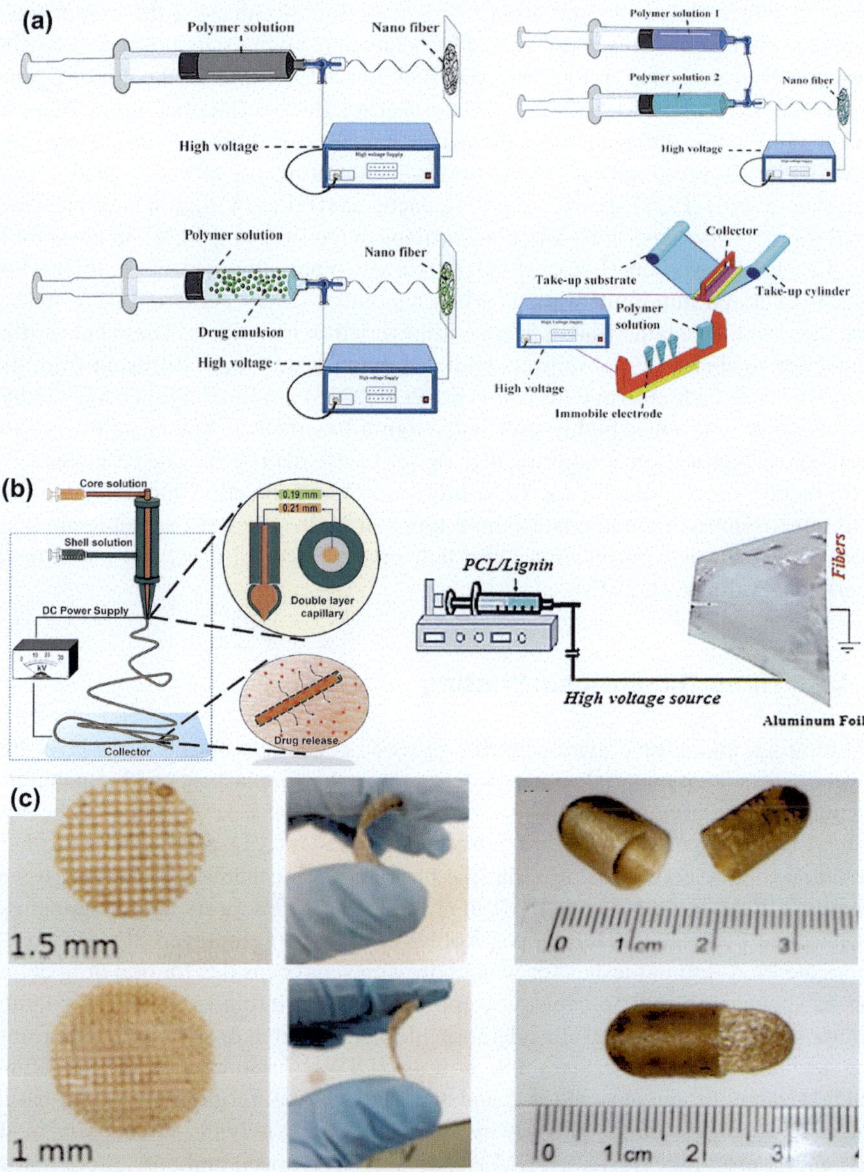

Fig. 9.3 (**a**) Schematic representation of electrospinning technologies, (**b**) coaxial electrospinning and blend electrospinning of PCL–lignin nanocomposite scaffold, (**c**) 3D printed meshes and oral capsules. (Reproduced with permission Nan et al. (2022). Copyright 2022, MDPI)

poly(glycerol sebacate) (PGS) through electrospinning. In another study, Salami et al. (2017) utilized electrospun lignin-PCL scaffolds to increase cellular biological responses through mechanical signals as shown in Fig. 9.3b. The findings of this research indicate that incorporation of 10 wt% lignin enhances the composite's porosity, biodegradability, pore size, fiber diameter, young's modulus and tensile strength (Nan et al. 2022). Recently, Saudi et al. (2019) explored the use of lignin-filled PVA-PGS fibers for nerve tissue engineering, discovering that lignin incorporation (1–5 wt%) reduced fiber diameter, increased modulus of elasticity, and promoted cell proliferation. Furthermore, nanofibrous membranes made from poly(lactic acid) (PLA)-lignin and poly(L-lactic acid) (PLLA)-lignin have been utilized for repairing superficial articular cartilage defects (Zhang 2020). In latest finding, Lee and co-workers (Lee et al. 2018) fabricated nanofibrous webs composed of lignin-decorated thin multi-walled carbon nanotubes (t-MWNTs) and PVA, noting that these webs contained small pores within very thin nanofibers. These pores offer protection against external impacts while enabling water vapor diffusion from the body. In last decade, Kai and his team (Kai et al. 2015) modified lignin using methyl methacrylate to produce highly stretchable lignin-based electrospun nanofibers with biomedical applications. Additionally, lignin-based hydrogels can be created by introducing various chemicals, including poly-2-hydroxyethyl methacrylate and poly-glucosylethyl methacrylate. These types of hydrogels have versatile applications, such as water purification, drug delivery, biomedical uses, and biomimetic scaffolds (Aminzadeh 2018).

9.4.2 Three-Dimensional Printing

3D printing, an additive manufacturing process, constructs objects via a layer-by-layer process from materials like powders, resins, thermoplastics, and biomaterials. Its potential for creating patient-specific medical products is revolutionizing healthcare. Lignin-based materials are prime candidates for 3D printing due to their potential to connect critical criteria like printability, mechanical properties, tissue biomimicry, and non-cytotoxicity (Liu et al. 2019). A few years ago, Domínguez-Robles and colleagues (Domínguez-Robles et al. 2019) employed 3D printing to fabricate PLA–lignin meshes for wound dressings and capsules for oral drug delivery as shown in Fig. 9.3c. However, optimizing 3D printing techniques for lignin composites requires careful consideration of factors related to the appropriate printing technology such as direct ink writing (DIW), fused deposition modelling (FDM), stereolithography (SLA), and bioprinting, and formulating lignin-based inks. FDM and SLA are commonly used for 3D printing polymer-based parts, models, and microfluidic devices. FDM stands out by its speed and cost-effectiveness but produces relatively rough surfaces and lacks of strength. Thermoplastic lignin composites are potentially suitable inks for both SLA and FDM printing. Methacrylate resins reinforced with lignin-coated cellulose nanocrystals are good candidates as SLA printing inks (Fan et al. 2019). Lignin-based hydrogels also hold good potential as innovative bioinks for 3D bioprinting applications in tissue engineering. Inkjet, laser-assisted bioprinting, and micro extrusion techniques could benefit from utilizing these hydrogels. Inkjet bioprinting employs a non-contact method to deposit pico-liter bio-ink droplets onto a substrate, whereas micro-extrusion printing utilizes droplet ejection with three-dimensional movement.

Laser-assisted bioprinting leverages bioink optical properties to direct ink ejection. Recent advancements in 3D printing technology will bring significant innovations for medical and pharmaceutical applications (Nan et al. 2022; Ramiah et al. 2020).

9.4.3 Melt Extrusion

Melt extrusion offers potential advantage over other techniques as it eliminates the need for solvents. However, nanoparticle agglomeration during fabrication needs careful handling. While the equipment is like standard polymer processing, it requires adjustments to accommodate nanoparticles. Researchers must closely monitor the extrusion temperature to ensure the polymer does not degrade, as well as the time required for proper nanoparticle dispersion. Lignin/polymer composite ratios are achieved through thermal extrusion, mechanical mixing, and the use of a single or twin-screw extruder, operating at rotation speeds of 200–250 rpm and a take-up speed of 100 m/min. The extrusion temperatures typically range from 145 °C to 247 °C, depending on the composite's composition (Arya et al. 2023).

9.4.4 Vapor-Induced Phase Separation

Nevárez et al. (2011) developed biopolymer-based composite films using cellulose triacetate (CTA) and lignin. Vapor-induced phase separation was employed to incorporate hydrolytic, organosolv, and kraft lignin into the CTA matrix to fabricate the self-supported films, with careful control over temperature and relative humidity. Ago and their colleagues (Ago et al. 2013) fabricated defect-free electrospun nanofibers and thin films from lignin/poly(vinyl alcohol) dispersions reinforced with cellulose nanocrystals. Their findings revealed that the spin-coated cross-sections of the materials closely resembled the electrospun fiber mats, rather than the surfaces of the as-prepared films. The addition of cellulose nanocrystals further enhanced molecular interactions and improved the stability of the nanocomposites against water absorption (Wang et al. 2015a).

9.4.5 Casting Methods

Chitosan, a versatile polysaccharide renowned for its biocompatibility, and multifunctional properties, has garnered significant research interest in fields such as water treatment, biosensors, and tissue engineering (Kumar 2000). Chen and their colleagues (Chen et al. 2009) fabricated biodegradable lignin/chitosan composite films using a casting/solvent evaporation method. Strong interfacial interactions promoted homogeneous lignin dispersion at concentrations below 20 wt%. These composites exhibited enhanced tensile strength, storage modulus, thermal stability, and glass transition temperature, showcasing their potential for wound dressing applications (Wang et al. 2015a).

9.5 Lignin Composites in Biomedical Applications

Lignin composites are gaining recognition as a versatile biomaterial with extraordinary properties in a variety of biomedical fields. These biological properties include antimicrobial, antioxidant and UV-protective effects, making lignin composites attractive candidates for elevating the performance of biomedical materials. Additionally, lignin composites have exhibited hemostatic properties, influencing blood coagulation, which further broadens its potential uses (Hachimi Alaoui et al. 2023). These attributes collectively position lignin composites as a promising material due to their biological activities for the development of innovative biomedical applications, including tissue engineering, drug delivery systems and wound dressings as reported in Table 9.1 (Liu et al. 2022).

9.5.1 Bioactivities of Lignin Composites

9.5.1.1 Antimicrobial Activity

Recent research has recognized lignin as a promising green substitute to fossil-based antimicrobial agents for combating harmful microorganisms. The antimicrobial properties of lignin are primarily due to its methoxy and epoxy groups, which interact with bacterial cells, leading to membrane disruption and subsequent bacterial lysis. This unique capability has stimulated research to develop antimicrobial biomaterials lignin-based such as hydrogels, nanofibers, films, and nanoparticles (Ndaba et al. 2020). Furthermore, the effectiveness of lignin towards antimicrobial activity is significantly influenced by the specific methods used to prepare these composites. Recently, lignin nanoparticles within a polylactic acid matrix have demonstrated sustained antibacterial properties. Additionally, lignin composites have been engineered to prevent bacterial adhesion. A notable example is a lignin-derived hydrogel with silver nanoparticles that exhibits antimicrobial efficacy against *Staphylococcus aureus* (S. aureus) and *Escherichia coli* (E. coli) (Liu et al. 2022). Lignin composites can be combined with other antimicrobial agents to achieve synergistic effects. However, replacing the core of silver nanoparticles with lignin results in enhanced antibacterial properties while avoiding the release of silver ions, which are known to have harmful ecological impacts (Shu et al. 2021) as shown in Fig. 9.4.

9.5.1.2 Antioxidant Activity

Lignin composites exhibit significant antioxidant properties attributed to the phenolic and methoxy groups within the lignin structure. These groups are essential in disrupting oxidative chain reactions by donating hydrogen atoms, thereby demonstrating strong antioxidant capabilities. This antioxidant property of lignin has been effectively applied across various domains, including medicine, pharmaceuticals such as anticarcinogenic agents and polymer applications where improving thermal stability is crucial. Due to its potent antioxidant potential, lignin is gaining recognition as a sustainable substitute for synthetic antioxidants, such as butylated

Table 9.1 Summary of lignin-based composites, fabrication techniques, and biomedical applications

Lignin	Lignin-Based Biocomposites	Technique	Application	Improved Properties	Ref.
Lignin (*artocarpus heterophyllus* waste)	Lignin-chitosan biocomposites	Freezing technique	Wound healing & dressing	Mechanical stability	Jaganathan et al. (2018)
Enzyme hydrolysis lignin (wheat straw)	Lignin-alginate cryogels porous scaffolds	Freezing technique	Tissue engineering, regenerative medicine	Porous structure	Barros et al. (2016)
Lignin nanoparticles	Lignin-gelatin cryogels	Freezing technique	Wound healing, tissue engineering	Mechanical properties, antibacterial	Memic and Abudula (2021)
Alginate-lignin (wheat straw)	Wet and dry alginate-lignin aerogels	Using CO_2 induced gelation	Tissue engineering, regenerative medicine	Reduce hydrophility of alginate	Quraishi et al. (2015)
Bio-lignin	Chitin nanofibrils and nano lignin complexes loaded with GA	Spray drier	Skin regeneration	Cytocmpatible, anti-inflammatory	Liu et al. (2022)
Alkali lignin	Lignin-chitosan microfibres	Wet-spinning	Tissue repair & regeneration	Mechanical properties	Liu et al. (2022)
Bio-lignin	PLC-chitin-lignin gel fibrous scaffolds	Coaxial electrospinning	Drug release, wound dressing	Controlled drug release, antibacterial	Figueiredo et al. (2017
Bio-lignin	Chitin-lignin sol-gel nanofibrous scaffolds	Electrospinning	Wound care products	Mechanical properties, antibacterial	Abdullah et al. (2018)
Lignin (Mn: 3000; Aldrich)	PCL-lignin nanoscaffold	Electrospinning	Tissue engineering	Biological response of the cells	Salami et al. (2017)
Lignin	Nanofibrous PVA-PGS-lignin scaffolds	Aligned electrospinning	Nerve tissue engineering	Neural cell proliferation, differentiation	Saudi et al. (2019)
Lignin	Lignin-PLA, PLLA-lignin nanofibrous membranes	Electrostatic spinning	Cartilage tissue engineering	Mechanical properties	Zhang (2020)
Lignin (sigma Aldrich, Korea)	Lignin-*t*-MWNT-PVA nanofibers	Electrospinning	Wound healing	Antimicrobial properties	Lee et al. (2018)
Kraft lignin (softwood)	Lignin-PLA nanocomposite	3D printing	Wound dressing	Mechanical & surface properties, antioxidant	Domínguez-Robles et al. (2019)

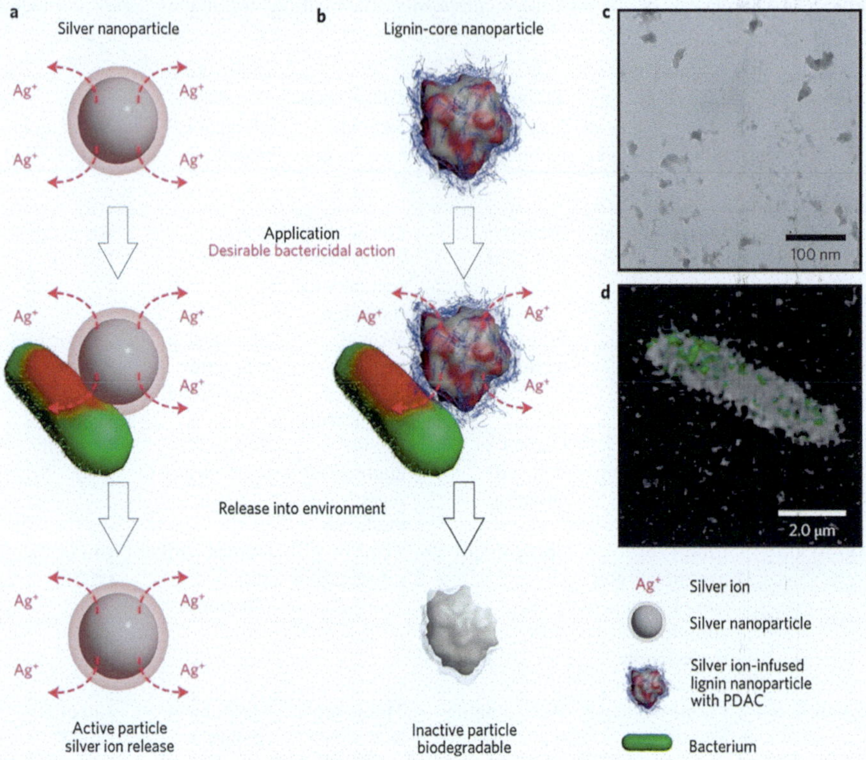

Fig. 9.4 Bactericidal mechanism of nanoparticles with a lignin core and silver nanoparticles. (Reproduced with permission Shu et al. (2021). Copyright 2021, American Chemical Society)

hydroxytoluene and butylated hydroxyanisole, commonly used in pharmaceutical, cosmetic, and food industries (Yang et al. 2016). Several factors influence the effectiveness of lignin as an antioxidant, including the source of biomass, molecular weight, polydispersity, extraction techniques, and subsequent treatment processes. The antioxidant capacity of lignin composites is frequently assessed using the 2,2-diphenyl-1-picrylhydrazyl (DPPH) assay, a standard method for evaluating radical-scavenging activity. The antioxidant capacity of lignin composites has been demonstrated in several studies (Dizhbite et al. 2004). Few years ago, Kaur et al. observed that unmodified lignin from sugarcane bagasse exhibited superior antioxidant properties compared to its chemically modified counterparts (Kaur et al. 2017). Lignin's dual properties of antioxidant and antimicrobial activity make it a promising candidate for a wide range of applications, including drug delivery systems, particularly in cancer therapy (Witzler et al. 2018). A novel research reported that lignin-capped silver nanoparticles exhibited both antibacterial and antifungal properties against pathogens such as *Staphylococcus aureus*, *Escherichia coli*, and *Aspergillus niger*, along with notable antioxidant activity. These nanoparticles also exhibited non-toxic behavior, as they did not cause lysis of red blood cells in hemolytic assays (Shu et al. 2021).

9.5.1.3 Antitumor Activity

The antitumor properties of lignin are attributed to its free phenolic hydroxyl groups, as evidenced by numerous in vitro studies. As far back as 1998, a research suggested that lignin might interact with dietary fiber to combat colon cancer, possibly due to its ability to trap free radicals, thereby enhancing the protective effects of dietary fiber against colon cancer (Lu et al. 1998). Based on these findings, Jeyaraj et al. (2016) enhanced the antitumor activity of lignin through methacrylate modification. In another study, Barapatre et al. (2016) demonstrated the anticancer potential of lignin extracted from *Acacia*, specifically targeting breast cancer cells while exhibiting minimal toxicity to hepatic stellate cells. These findings indicate the great promise of lignin as a natural anticancer agent, particularly in preventing free radical-induced diseases. Furthermore, Figueiredo et al. (2017) studied the anticancer efficacy of pure benzazulene (BZL) and benzazulene-loaded lignin nanoparticles (BZL-PLNPs). While pure BZL showed no significant impact, BZL-PLNPs dramatically reduced cancer cell viability from approximately 90% to 0%. This study suggests that lignin not only enhances drug protection but also amplifies anticancer activity, suggesting a new paradigm for natural anticancer drug development. Lignin/carbohydrate complexes (LCCs) extracted from plants have also shown potent antitumor activity. Recent advancement demonstrated that two LCCs derived from *Inonotus obliquus* inhibited nuclear transcription factor (NF-κB) activation in cancer cells (Wang et al. 2015b). Few years ago, Huang et al. (2018) reported that bamboo-derived LCCs inhibited breast tumor cell (MCF-7) growth while potentially stimulating macrophage activity, suggesting a potential role in reducing breast tumor incidence. In recent years, novel a water-soluble lignin derivative, benzene poly(carboxylic acid) compound (BP-Cx-1), formed from polyphepan, has exhibited diverse pharmacological effects on neurotransmitter receptors, transporters, and ligand ion channels. This derivative may also offer therapeutic potential for complex diseases like type 2 diabetes and cancer (Shu et al. 2021). In last decade, Rai et al. (2021) successfully employed bagasse-based kraft lignin (KL) to develop materials with potential applications in cancer treatment. Dextran aldehyde (Dex-ald) and bovine serum albumin (BSA) were conjugated with kraft lignin (KL) via an ascorbic acid/H_2O_2 redox reaction, resulting in materials such as Dex-ald–KL and BSA–KL with enhanced solubility. These conjugates exhibited significant antitumor activity against colon cancer cells (SW480), reducing cell viability by 55–61% within 48 h. These findings concluded that combining lignin with other biopolymers could enhance its therapeutic effects, positioning it as a potential alternative chemotherapeutic agent for treating malignant tumors.

9.5.1.4 Anti-ultraviolet Capacity

Few years ago, different studies showed that lignin composites exhibit significant UV shielding properties, making them promising candidates for use as natural, broad-spectrum sun blockers. Recent research demonstrated the effectiveness of lignin composites in UV protection, suggesting their potential in developing antimicrobial biomaterials and healthcare products (Terzioğlu et al. 2020). Further research have highlighted the superior UV absorption capabilities of lignin-derived products from various sources. Wang et al. (2021b) found that soda lignin extracted from palm fiber displayed exceptional UV-blocking performance. This effectiveness is attributed to aromatic branched structure of lignin that underlies its enhanced UV shielding properties. These characteristics make lignin a promising material to substitute traditional petroleum-based ones in applications like food packaging and biomedical applications. Recent study by Sadeghifar et al. (2017) emphasized the role of lignin as a biomaterial with UV-absorbing functionalities. They demonstrated that incorporating lignin into renewable cellulose-based films produced UV-resistant material that remained stable under UV exposure and high temperatures. This highlights the potential of lignin as a sustainable component in UV-resistant products. However, lignin can be integrated into commercial sunscreen formulations to enhance their sun protection factor. Qian et al. (2017) developed lignin colloidal spheres through self-assembly and incorporated them into skin creams. These creams demonstrated enhanced UV protection compared to formulations using unmodified lignin. These studies demonstrate that lignin composites offer considerable potential in developing UV-protective materials for various biomedical and healthcare applications (Hachimi Alaoui et al. 2023).

9.5.2 Lignin Composites in Drug Delivery System

Drug delivery systems seek to optimize therapeutic efficacy by precisely targeting diseased tissues while minimizing adverse effects. Lignin has been effectively integrated into composite films for drug delivery applications (Jabeen et al. 2024). Çalgeris et al. (2012) demonstrated the use of alkaline lignin derived from waste hazelnut shells to enhance the mechanical properties of thermoplastic corn starch films. Lignin was incorporated at concentrations ranging from 1.2 to 2.4 wt %, while the antibiotic ciprofloxacin was maintained at a 2 wt % loading. The films, which appeared brown with deeper shades as lignin content increased, were evaluated for drug release. Films having 2 wt % lignin, exhibit enhanced mechanical properties and were employed for drug release. These tests revealed that the films were pH-sensitive, with ciprofloxacin release accelerating at lower pH levels. Composite films demonstrated that the swelling ratio increases as the pH increases. Drug release kinetics were evaluated using the Korsmeyer–Peppas model, indicating Fickian diffusion-controlled release at both pH 5.0 and 7.4 (Terzioğlu et al. 2020). The films showed rapid ciprofloxacin release within the first 60 min, followed by a slower, steady release rate by the tenth day, highlighting the efficiency of ciprofloxacin/starch/lignin biofilms as effective drug delivery carriers. In another study, Liu et al. (2018) developed novel drug-loaded PLLA/lignin–poly-D-lactide (PDLA)stereo-complex composite films using solvent volatilization to improve the stability and controlled release of trans-resveratrol. The integrated lignin–PDLA films enhanced the thermal and mechanical properties, including their strength, strain, and toughness. The PLLA/lignin–PDLA composite films offered superior UV protection, safeguarding the light-sensitive trans-resveratrol from degradation. However, stereo complex films exhibit notable DPPH radical scavenging activity and antitumor effects in CCK-8 assays, enhancing their suitability for biomedical applications (Terzioğlu et al. 2020).

Zhou and colleagues (2019) created a dual-targeted drug delivery system by encapsulating doxorubicin, a hydrophilic drug, within lignin nanoparticles (LNPs). To enhance their functionality, these LNPs were modified with Fe_3O_4 nanoparticles and folic acid using a layer-by-layer self-assembly approach (Fig. 9.5a). The magnetic Fe_3O_4 nanoparticles were evenly distributed within the LNPs, which were then coated with folic acid, forming folic-magnetic functionalized lignin nanoparticles (FA-M–LNPs). Doxorubicin was released from the nanoparticles in a controlled manner over 30 h, effectively killing tumor cells at concentrations exceeding 150 μg/ml. Moreover, the modified LNPs efficiently penetrates the cytoplasm of cells that overexpress folic acid receptors, promoting drug accumulation in the nucleus (Figueiredo et al. 2017; Chaudhary and Sinha 2023). A novel pH-sensitive lignin-based micelle was developed through the acylation of alkali lignin with acryloyl chloride, followed by graft copolymerization with methacrylic acid. In vitro studies demonstrated that the micelles retained over 84% of ibuprofen in simulated gastric fluid (pH 1.5) and gradually released approximately 82% in simulated intestinal fluid (pH 7.4) over 72 h as shown in Fig. 9.5b. The nano micelles exhibited biocompatibility, stimulating proliferation of human bone marrow stromal cells and mouse embryonic fibroblasts. The nano micelles demonstrated remarkable anticancer activity, reducing human colon cancer cell survival to 5.34%. This highlights the potential of lignin-based nano micelles as a novel oral drug delivery system (Cheng et al. 2020; Yuan et al. 2019).

9.5.3 Lignin Composites in Tissue Engineering

Tissue engineering employed the development and design of biological substitutes to replace or restore the function of damaged tissues or organs. This field encompasses various applications, such as bone tissue engineering, nerve tissue engineering, and muscle tissue engineering. Each type of tissue engineering material must meet specific requirements for example strong mechanical stability is expected for bone graft scaffolds. Lignin composites offer good mechanical properties and cell compatibility. This section is focused on recent advancements using lignin composites for tissue repair and regeneration (Liu et al. 2022).

9.5.3.1 Bone Regeneration

Lignin's biological properties make it a promising candidate for developing polymer composites for bone engineering applications. Luzi et al. (2020) investigated the effects of PLA and lignin/ZnO films on human bone regeneration. Their study demonstrated that human bone mesenchymal stem cells (hBMSCs) and adipose stem cells adhered and proliferated on the films, as evidenced by vinculin focal adhesion points. Additionally, incorporation of ZnO into lignin improved the films elasticity and stiffness. Wang et al. (2019) demonstrated that electrospun lignin/polycaprolactone (PCL) matrices cultured in simulated body fluid induced

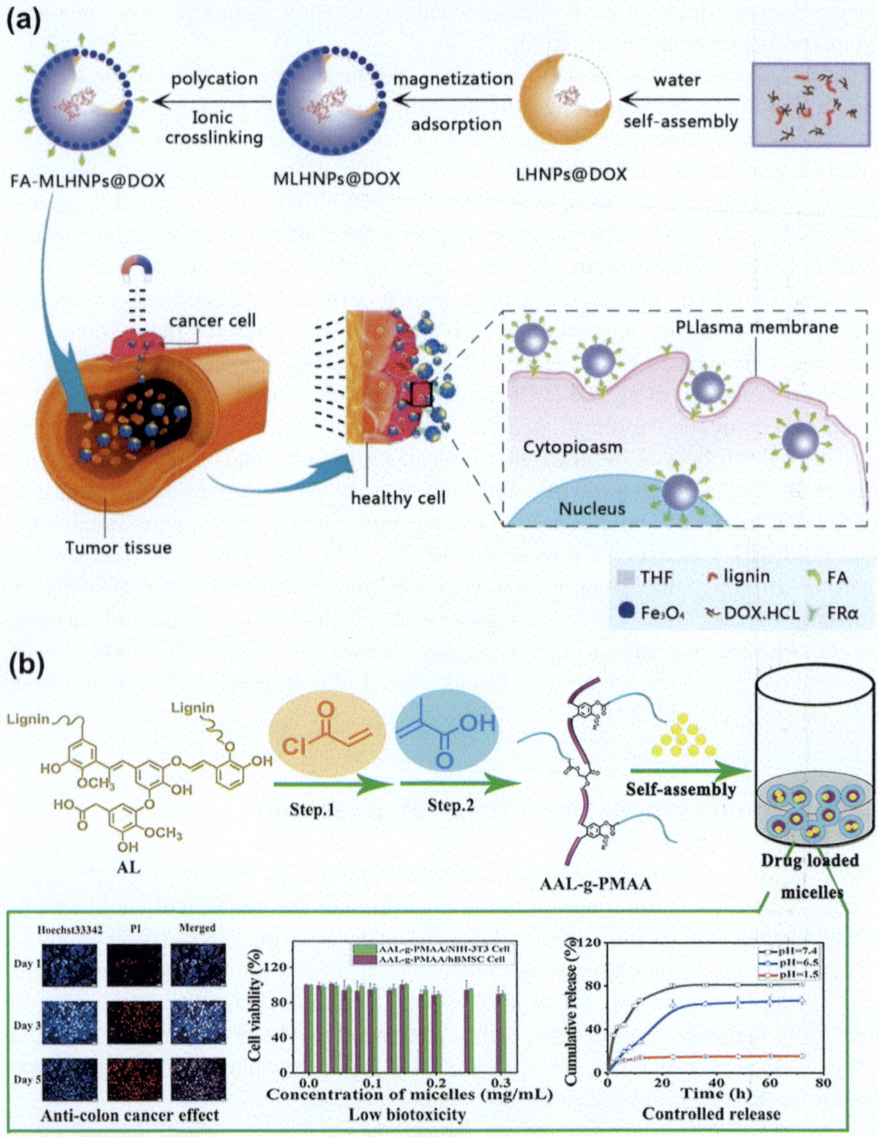

Fig. 9.5 (**a**) Fabrication of folic acid and magnetically functionalized lignin nanoparticles containing a drug. (Reproduced with permission Zhou et al. (2019). Copyright 2019, MDPI) (**b**) pH-responsive lignin-based nanomicelles designed for oral drug delivery. (Reproduced with permission Cheng et al. (2020). Copyright 2020, American Chemical Society)

hydroxyapatite (Hap) crystal formation. The formed hydroxyapatite crystals exhibited structural and mechanical properties resembling native bone. The lignin/containing nanofibrous membrane promoted osteoblast adhesion and proliferation by guiding filopodial extension. Lignin has been integrated into hydrogels for bone tissue engineering applications. Literature reported that Abudula et al. in 2021 developed antibacterial, antioxidant, and injectable cryogels by crosslinking lignin with gelatin (Abdullah et al. 2021). Incorporating 0.2% lignin into gelatin significantly enhanced the compression modulus and stress compared to pure gelatin gels. Cell studies indicated that lignin-based cryogels elicited minimal activation of mouse bone marrow-derived dendritic cells while demonstrating excellent biocompatibility. Figure 9.6 depicts the lignin-induced biomineralization of bone hydroxyapatite (Hap) (Wang et al. 2019). This hybrid system presents novel opportunities for lignin composites in bone therapies and tissue engineering. In vitro studies demonstrated that electrospun nanofibers composed of polycaprolactone-lignin-poly(methyl methacrylate) (PCL-L-PMMA) effectively adhered to and interacted with human dermal fibroblasts (Kumar et al. 2021).

9.5.3.2 Liver Regeneration

Recent advancements in liver tissue engineering have been attained due to the development of innovative scaffold materials and cell engineering strategies (Ghahremanzadeh et al. 2021). Among these, lignin has emerged as a promising

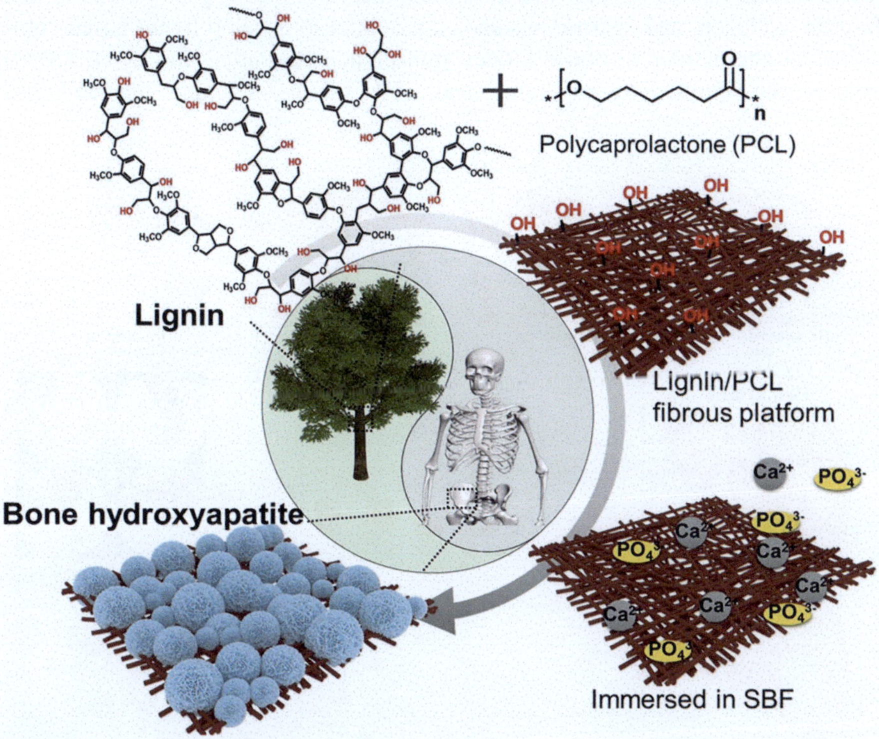

Fig. 9.6 Systemic representation of biomineralization of bone hydroxyapatite (Hap) induced by lignin nanofibers for tissue engineering. (Reproduced with permission Wang et al. (2019). Copyright 2019, American Chemical Society)

material to enhance hepatocyte growth and adhesion. Few years ago, Zhao et al. (2017) investigated the biocompatibility of Ginkgo-derived lignin-carbohydrate complexes (LCCs) by culturing human hepatocytes on LCC-based scaffolds and monitoring cell growth and metabolism over five days. LCC bio-scaffolds demonstrated enhanced cell adhesion and proliferation compared to the control. LCC bio-scaffolds significantly upregulated hepatocyte metabolism, increasing glucose uptake and albumin secretion by 51.7% and 38.6%, respectively. The scaffold's non-cytotoxic nature and metabolic regulatory properties warrant further in vivo investigations. In another study, Wahba et al. (2015) demonstrated the potential of lignin as a methotrexate (MTX) delivery system for treating liver disease in rats. Histological analysis revealed that lignin mitigated MTX-induced liver degeneration and hemorrhage, suggesting its potential as a drug carrier for liver disease management. Researchers developed an injectable and conductive lignin-cellulose hydrogel for treating rat liver injury (Deng et al. 2021). The hydrogel demonstrated accelerated wound healing, reduced blood loss, and exhibited excellent adhesion and biocompatibility with rat liver tissue as shown in Fig. 9.7a–f (Liu et al. 2022).

9.5.3.3 Kidney Regeneration

Recent advancements suggest that tissue engineering, utilizing biopolymers like chitosan, collagen, and agarose has shown potential to develop lignin-based composites as alternatives to donor kidney transplants. Recently, Kim et al. (2020) assessed the cytotoxicity of lignin and 21% lignin-containing nanocellulose

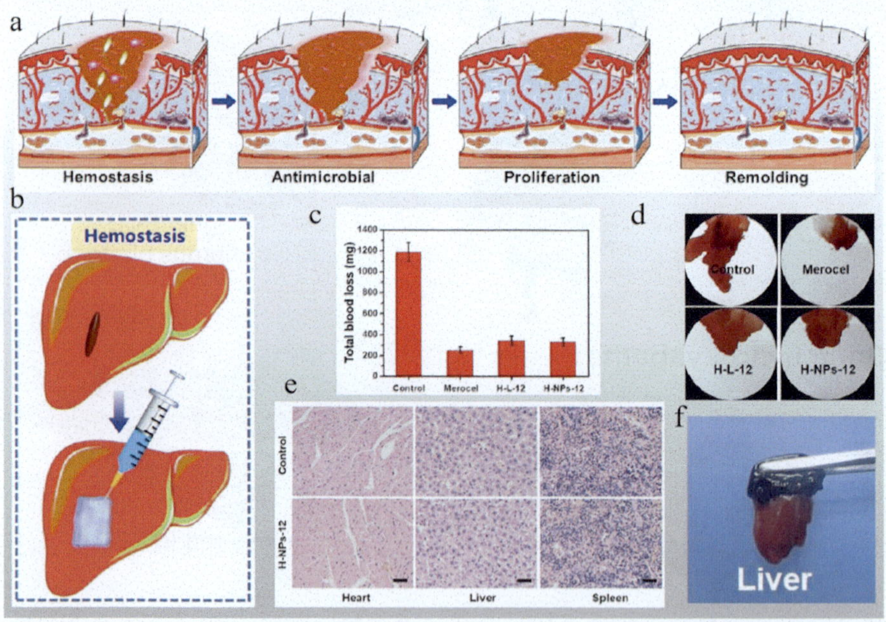

Fig. 9.7 (**a–f**) Schematic representation of tissue engineering in liver tissues mediated by lignin hydrogel therapy. (Reproduced with permission Liu et al. (2022). Copyright 2022, Elsevier)

(L-MFC) on human kidney cells. While both materials exhibited some toxicity, L-MFC demonstrated lower cytotoxicity ($LC_{50} = 0.102\%$). The Klason lignin used in this research was isolated from black liquor and may have contained impurities affecting observed toxicity. Conversely, the L-MFC's high glucose content (above 60%) likely contributed to improved cell viability. Another study investigated lignin-derived lignophenols (LPs) for their anti-inflammatory effects in treating kidney damage in obese mice. LP treatment reduced macrophage infiltration and inflammatory cytokine levels compared to controls (Sato et al. 2020). LP-treated rats exhibited a significant reduction in renal fibrosis, suggesting lignin's protective role against high-fat diet-induced kidney damage. Recently, Long et al. (2020) demonstrated macelignan's renoprotective effects against ischemia-reperfusion injury by suppressing inflammation, apoptosis, and enhancing antioxidant systems. In addition to transplantation, dialysis is a common therapy for chronic kidney diseases. Lignin composites have been investigated for its use in hemodialysis as a binding agent in monoliths. Animal studies in rats have shown that lignin-based binders can improve toxin absorption efficiency during dialysis while maintaining normal blood indices, highlighting the potential of lignin in hemodialysis applications (Liu et al. 2022).

9.5.4 Lignin Composites in Wound Dressing

In the last decade, film and hydrogel technologies have been used to obtain lignin-based wound healing material. A research study conducted by Pérez et al. (2021) created a hydrogel incorporating lignin-capped silver nanoparticles (AgNPs) using nanoparticle-driven techniques. This hydrogel exhibited potent antioxidant and antibacterial properties against *Staphylococcus aureus* and *Pseudomonas aeruginosa*, demonstrating its potential for chronic wound management as represented by Fig. 9.8a. In recent years, Deng et al. (2021) evaluated a lignin-based hydrogel in a rat model of methicillin-resistant *S. aureus* infection. Compared to traditional gauze and commercial ointments, the hydrogel demonstrated superior wound healing, reducing wound area by 74.6% within three days as shown in Fig. 9.8b. In addition to this, Alqahtani et al. (2020) reported that lignin nanoparticles loaded with curcumin effectively inhibited *S. aureus* growth, demonstrating a 95.4% reduction in bacterial count. These findings underscore the potential of lignin-based composites in enhancing wound healing through their antimicrobial properties (Liu et al. 2022; Deng et al. 2021). 3D-printed wound dressings have also been developed using lignin composites. One approach involves incorporating Kraft lignin into poly(lactic acid) (PLA) pellets treated with castor oil, along with tetracycline. The radical scavenging capacity of the resulting 3D-printed filament, assessed using 2,2-diphenyl-1-picrylhydrazyl highlights its potential for wound care applications (Domínguez-Robles et al. 2019). 3D-printed meshes composed of PLA and 2 wt % Kraft lignin. While lignin contributed antioxidant properties, the antimicrobial effect primarily stemmed from the incorporated tetracycline. This customizable approach holds promise for developing patient-specific wound care solutions (Yu and Kim 2020).

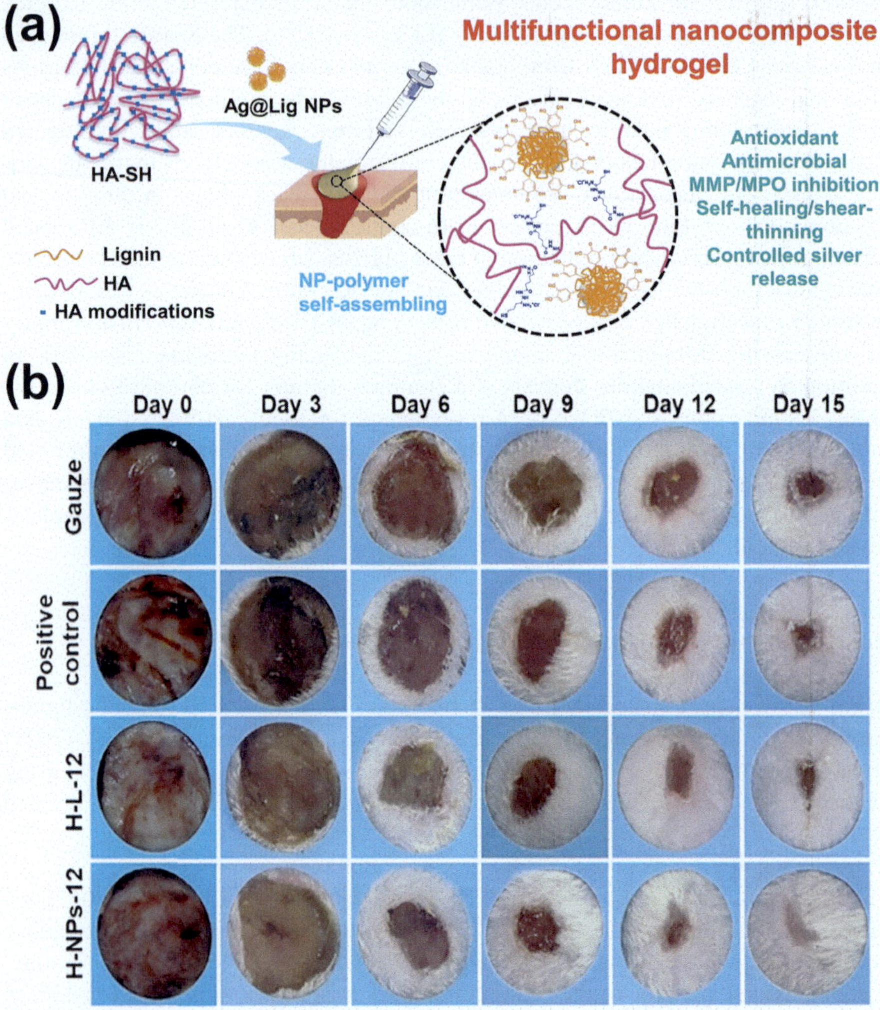

Fig. 9.8 (**a**) Lignin-based multifunctional nanocomposite hydrogel in wound dressing. (Reproduced with permission Pérez-Rafael et al. (2021). Copyright 2021, Elsevier). (**b**) Representation of images of the wound treated with gauze. (Reproduced with permission Deng et al. (2021). Copyright 2021, American Chemical Society)

9.6 Future Advancement in Lignin Composites for Biomedical Applications

Lignin composites offer significant potential for revolutionizing the biomedical field. While significant progress has been made, challenges related to complex and heterogeneous nature of lignin, technical limitations in synthesis processes, and regulatory hurdles persist. Overcoming these obstacles, future research should focus on enhancing material properties, exploring novel fabrication techniques, and addressing regulatory considerations as follows (Nan et al. 2022)

- Research should aim to understand and manipulate lignin's structure to improve its compatibility with various polymers and biological systems (Kaur et al. 2017).
- Exploring innovative methods such as 3D printing and advanced surface modifications to create tailored lignin composites with precise control over structure and properties.
- A comprehensive understanding of lignin's influence on cellular behaviour and tissue response is essential for the incorporation of lignin into polymer-based bone scaffolds during bone regeneration. Future research should focus on elucidating these mechanisms, as well as evaluating the material's biomechanical properties, degradation profile, and potential side effects to facilitate clinical translation.
- The liver's complex cellular composition necessitates the inclusion of multiple cell types in evaluating the toxicity and biocompatibility of lignin composites. Precisely replicating the liver's intricate structure within bio-composites remains a challenge. Moreover, the interplay of various signalling factors governing liver function must be considered when designing lignin-based liver tissue. Elucidating the mechanisms by which lignin interacts with hepatocytes is crucial for developing safe and effective liver disease treatments.
- Research on lignin composites for kidney disease treatments is limited. While initial studies have assessed lignin cytotoxicity on kidney cells, a comprehensive understanding of lignin's impact on kidney function and regeneration is still needed. The kidney's complex structure presents significant challenges for developing effective lignin-based therapies (Liu et al. 2022).

Future research should focus on enhancing lignin composite properties and functionalities to address current challenges. This involves exploring new applications in tissue engineering, drug delivery, and medical devices, while overcoming limitations related to lignin's complex nature and processing challenges. This includes establishing clear guidelines and standards for the safe and effective use of lignin-based materials in biomedical applications, improving their mechanical strength, stability, and biocompatibility, while incorporating controlled drug release capabilities. Furthermore, fundamental research on lignin composites as a growth regulator is still ongoing and needs further exploration to maximize its potential for biomedical applications.

9.7 Conclusion

The development of natural polymer-based composites is increasingly crucial in the biomedical field, driven by the need for materials that are sustainable, biocompatible, and versatile. Lignin, with its inherent low toxicity, biodegradability, biocompatibility, and modifiable chemical structure, stands out as a promising candidate for a wide range of biomedical applications. Recent advances have demonstrated lignin's potential in creating innovative composite materials that could serve as effective drug carriers, wound healing agents, and scaffolds for tissue engineering. However, to fully harness the potential of lignin, more comprehensive research is needed to understand its biological, chemical, and physical properties. While current studies have provided valuable insights, most are at an early stage, emphasizing in vitro findings. To advance lignin's application in the biomedical field, it is essential to conduct in vivo studies and focus on developing lignin composites tailored to specific biomedical needs. Further research in this area will be key to achieve the full potential of lignin in future medical applications.

Acknowledgements This research was supported through the Grant PID2021-124845OA-I00 and PID2023-152347OB-I00 funded by MCIN/AEI/10.13039/501100011033 and by the "European UnionNextGenerationEU/PRTR". NJ acknowledge the SANTIAGO GRISOLIA program CIGRIS/2022/132 funded by the Generalitat Valenciana.

Authors Contribution Nazish Jabeen: writing – original draft preparation, visualization, review & editing. Clara M Gómez: visualization, review & editing. Mario Culebras: supervision, review & editing, funding acquisition.

Conflict of Interest The authors declare that there is no conflict of interest.

References

Abdullah T, Gzara L, Simonetti G, Alshahrie A, Salah N, Morganti P, Chianese A, Fallahi A, Tamayol A, Bencherif SA (2018) The effect of poly (glycerol sebacate) incorporation within hybrid chitin–lignin sol–gel nanofibrous scaffolds. Materials 11(3):451

Abdullah T, Colombani T, Alade T, Bencherif SA, Memic A (2021) Injectable lignin-co-gelatin cryogels with antioxidant and antibacterial properties for biomedical applications. Biomacromolecules 22(10):4110–4121

Ago M, Jakes JE, Rojas OJ (2013) Thermomechanical properties of lignin-based electrospun nanofibers and films reinforced with cellulose nanocrystals: a dynamic mechanical and nanoindentation study. ACS Appl Mater Interfaces 5(22):11768–11776

Alqahtani MS, Alqahtani A, Kazi M, Ahmad MZ, Alahmari A, Alsenaidy MA, Syed R (2020) Wound-healing potential of curcumin loaded lignin nanoparticles. J Drug Deliv Sci Technol 60:102020

Alven S, Buyana B, Feketshane Z, Aderibigbe BA (2021) Electrospun nanofibers/nanofibrous scaffolds loaded with silver nanoparticles as effective antibacterial wound dressing materials. Pharmaceutics 13(7):964

Aminzadeh S (2018) Valorization of Kraft lignin by fractionation and chemical modifications for different applications. KTH Royal Institute of Technology

Arya A, Ahamad A, Kumar P, Chandra A (2023) A review on lignin based nanocomposites: fabrication, characterization and application. Mater Today 78:A10–A15

Barapatre A, Aadil KR, Tiwary BN, Jha H (2015) In vitro antioxidant and antidiabetic activities of biomodified lignin from Acacia nilotica wood. Int J Biol Macromol 75:81–89

Barapatre A, Meena AS, Mekala S, Das A, Jha H (2016) In vitro evaluation of antioxidant and cytotoxic activities of lignin fractions extracted from Acacia nilotica. Int J Biol Macromol 86:443–453

Barros A, Quraishi S, Martins M, Gurikov P, Subrahmanyam R, Smirnova I, Duarte ARC, Reis RL (2016) Hybrid alginate-based cryogels for life science applications. Chemie Ingenieur Technik 88(11):1770–1778

Bertella S, Luterbacher JS (2020) Lignin functionalization for the production of novel materials. Trends Chem 2(5):440–453

Çalgeris İ, Çakmakçı E, Ogan A, Kahraman MV, Kayaman-Apohan N (2012) Preparation and drug release properties of lignin–starch biodegradable films. Starch-Stärke 64(5):399–407

Carvajal JC, Gómez Á, Cardona CA (2016) Comparison of lignin extraction processes: economic and environmental assessment. Bioresour Technol 214:468–476

Chaudhary M, Sinha V (2023) Lignin-based carriers for drug delivery applications: from an industrial waste to a pharmaceutical aid. Eur Polym J 195:112206

Chen L, Tang C-Y, Ning N-Y, Wang C-Y, Fu Q, Zhang Q (2009) Preparation and properties of chitosan/lignin composite films. Chin J Polym Sci 27(05):739–746

Cheng L, Deng B, Luo W, Nie S, Liu X, Yin Y, Liu S, Wu Z, Zhan P, Zhang L (2020) pH-responsive lignin-based nanomicelles for oral drug delivery. J Agric Food Chem 68(18):5249–5258

Deng P, Chen F, Zhang H, Chen Y, Zhou J (2021) Conductive, self-healing, adhesive, and antibacterial hydrogels based on lignin/cellulose for rapid MRSA-infected wound repairing. ACS Appl Mater Interfaces 13(44):52333–52345

Dizhbite T, Telysheva G, Jurkjane V, Viesturs U (2004) Characterization of the radical scavenging activity of lignins—natural antioxidants. Bioresour Technol 95(3):309–317

Domínguez-Robles J, Martin NK, Fong ML, Stewart SA, Irwin NJ, Rial-Hermida MI, Donnelly RF, Larrañeta E (2019) Antioxidant PLA composites containing lignin for 3D printing applications: a potential material for healthcare applications. Pharmaceutics 11(4):165

Fan D, Staufer U, Accardo A (2019) Engineered 3D polymer and hydrogel microenvironments for cell culture applications. Bioengineering 6(4):113

Figueiredo P, Lintinen K, Kiriazis A, Hynninen V, Liu Z, Bauleth-Ramos T, Rahikkala A, Correia A, Kohout T, Sarmento B (2017) In vitro evaluation of biodegradable lignin-based nanoparticles for drug delivery and enhanced antiproliferation effect in cancer cells. Biomaterials 121:97–108

Ghahremanzadeh F, Alihosseini F, Semnani D (2021) Investigation and comparison of new galactosylation methods on PCL/chitosan scaffolds for enhanced liver tissue engineering. Int J Biol Macromol 174:278–288

Hachimi Alaoui C, Réthoré G, Weiss P, Fatimi A (2023) Sustainable biomass lignin-based hydrogels: a review on properties, formulation, and biomedical applications. Int J Mol Sci 24(17):13493

Huang C, Tang S, Zhang W, Tao Y, Lai C, Li X, Yong Q (2018) Unveiling the structural properties of lignin–carbohydrate complexes in bamboo residues and its functionality as antioxidants and immunostimulants. ACS Sustain Chem Eng 6(9):12522–12531

Huang D, Li R, Xu P, Li T, Deng R, Chen S, Zhang Q (2020) The cornerstone of realizing lignin value-addition: exploiting the native structure and properties of lignin by extraction methods. Chem Eng J 402:126237

Jabeen N, Atif M (2024) Polysaccharides based biopolymers for biomedical applications: a review. Polym Adv Technol 35(1):e6203

Jabeen N, Iram F, Atif M, Fatimah NE (2024) Functionalization of arabinoxylan in chitosan based blends by periodate oxidation for drug release study. ChemistrySelect 9(5):e202303496

Jaganathan G, Manivannan K, Lakshmanan S, Sithique MA (2018) Fabrication and characterization of Artocarpus heterophyllus waste derived lignin added chitosan biocomposites for wound dressing application. Sustain Chem Pharm 10:27–32

Jeyaraj M, Praphakar RA, Rajendran C, Ponnamma D, Sadasivuni KK, Munusamy MA, Rajan M (2016) Surface functionalization of natural lignin isolated from Aloe barbadensis miller biomass by atom transfer radical polymerization for enhanced anticancer efficacy. RSC Adv 6(56):51310–51319

Kai D, Jiang S, Low ZW, Loh XJ (2015) Engineering highly stretchable lignin-based electrospun nanofibers for potential biomedical applications. J Mater Chem B 3(30):6194–6204

Kang X, Kirui A, Dickwella Widanage MC, Mentink-Vigier F, Cosgrove DJ, Wang T (2019) Lignin-polysaccharide interactions in plant secondary cell walls revealed by solid-state NMR. Nat Commun 10(1):347

Kaur R, Uppal S, Sharma P (2017) Antioxidant and antibacterial activities of sugarcane bagasse lignin and chemically modified lignins. Sugar Tech 19:675–680

Kim D, Jeong J, Ryu J-A, Choi SR, Lee JM, Bunch H (2020) In vitro evaluation of lignin-containing nanocellulose. Materials 13(15):3365

Kumar MNR (2000) A review of chitin and chitosan applications. React Funct Polym 46(1):1–27

Kumar R, Butreddy A, Kommineni N, Reddy PG, Bunekar N, Sarkar C, Dutt S, Mishra VK, Aadil KR, Mishra YK (2021) Lignin: drug/gene delivery and tissue engineering applications. Int J Nanomedicine 16:2419–2441

Lee E-S, Kim Y-O, Ha Y-M, Lim D, Hwang JY, Kim J, Park M, Cho JW, Jung YC (2018) Antimicrobial properties of lignin-decorated thin multi-walled carbon nanotubes in poly (vinyl alcohol) nanocomposites. Eur Polym J 105:79–84

Liao JJ, Abd Latif NH, Trache D, Brosse N, Hussin MH (2020) Current advancement on the isolation, characterization and application of lignin. Int J Biol Macromol 162:985–1024

Liu R, Dai L, Zou Z, Si C (2018) Drug-loaded poly (L-lactide)/lignin stereocomplex film for enhancing stability and sustained release of trans-resveratrol. Int J Biol Macromol 119:1129–1136

Liu J, Sun L, Xu W, Wang Q, Yu S, Sun J (2019) Current advances and future perspectives of 3D printing natural-derived biopolymers. Carbohydr Polym 207:297–316

Liu Y, Wang X, Wu Q, Pei W, Teo MJ, Chen ZS, Huang C (2022) Application of lignin and lignin-based composites in different tissue engineering fields. Int J Biol Macromol 222:994–1006

Lobato-Peralta DR, Duque-Brito E, Villafan-Vidales HI, Longoria A, Sebastian P, Cuentas-Gallegos AK, Arancibia-Bulnes CA, Okoye PU (2021) A review on trends in lignin extraction and valorization of lignocellulosic biomass for energy applications. J Clean Prod 293:126123

Long J, Qian K, Tan S, Liu J, Li J (2020) Macelignan protects against renal ischemia-reperfusion injury via inhibition of inflammation and apoptosis of renal epithelial cells. Cell Mol Biol 66(1):55–59

Lu FJ, Chu LH, Gau RJ (1998) Free radical-scavenging properties of lignin. Nutr Cancer 30:31–38

Luzi F, Tortorella I, Di Michele A, Dominici F, Argentati C, Morena F, Torre L, Puglia D, Martino S (2020) Novel nanocomposite PLA films with lignin/zinc oxide hybrids: design, characterization, interaction with mesenchymal stem cells. Nano 10(11):2176

Memic A, Abudula T (2021) Antioxidant, antibacterial, injectable lignin-gelatin composite cryogels for wound healing and tissue engineering. U.S. Patent US10881760B1

Nan N, Hu W, Wang J (2022) Lignin-based porous biomaterials for medical and pharmaceutical applications. Biomedicines 10(4):747

Ndaba B, Roopnarain A, Daramola MO, Adeleke R (2020) Influence of extraction methods on antimicrobial activities of lignin-based materials: a review. Sustain Chem Pharm 18:100342

Nevárez LAM, Casarrubias LB, Celzard A, Fierro V, Muñoz VT, Davila AC, Lubian JRT, Sánchez GG (2011) Biopolymer-based nanocomposites: effect of lignin acetylation in cellulose triacetate films. Sci Technol Adv Mater 12(4):045006

Parham S, Kharazi AZ, Bakhsheshi-Rad HR, Ghayour H, Ismail AF, Nur H, Berto F (2020) Electrospun nano-fibers for biomedical and tissue engineering applications: a comprehensive review. Materials 13(9):2153

Pérez-Rafael S, Ivanova K, Stefanov I, Puiggalí J, Del Valle LJ, Todorova K, Dimitrov P, Hinojosa-Caballero D, Tzanov T (2021) Nanoparticle-driven self-assembling injectable hydrogels provide a multi-factorial approach for chronic wound treatment. Acta Biomater 134:131–143

Qian Y, Zhong X, Li Y, Qiu X (2017) Fabrication of uniform lignin colloidal spheres for developing natural broad-spectrum sunscreens with high sun protection factor. Ind Crop Prod 101:54–60

Quraishi S, Martins M, Barros AA, Gurikov P, Raman S, Smirnova I, Duarte ARC, Reis RL (2015) Novel non-cytotoxic alginate–lignin hybrid aerogels as scaffolds for tissue engineering. J Supercrit Fluids 105:1–8

Rai S, Arun S, Kureel AK, Dutta P, Mehrotra G (2021) Preparation of dextran aldehyde and BSA conjugates from ligno-cellulosic biowaste for antioxidant and anti-cancer efficacy. Waste Biomass Valoriz 12:1327–1339

Ramiah P, Du Toit LC, Choonara YE, Kondiah PP, Pillay V (2020) Hydrogel-based bioinks for 3D bioprinting in tissue regeneration. Front Mater 7:76

Sadeghifar H, Venditti R, Jur J, Gorga RE, Pawlak JJ (2017) Cellulose-lignin biodegradable and flexible UV protection film. ACS Sustain Chem Eng 5(1):625–631

Salami MA, Kaveian F, Rafienia M, Saber-Samandari S, Khandan A, Naeimi M (2017) Electrospun polycaprolactone/lignin-based nanocomposite as a novel tissue scaffold for biomedical applications. J Med Signals Sens 7(4):228–238

Sato S, Norikura T, Mukai Y, Yamaoka S, Mikame K (2020) Lignin-derived low-molecular-weight oxidized lignophenol stimulates AMP-activated protein kinase and suppresses renal inflammation and interstitial fibrosis in high fat diet-fed mice. Chem Biol Interact 318:108977

Saudi A, Amini S, Amirpour N, Kazemi M, Kharazi AZ, Salehi H, Rafienia M (2019) Promoting neural cell proliferation and differentiation by incorporating lignin into electrospun poly (vinyl alcohol) and poly (glycerol sebacate) fibers. Mater Sci Eng C 104:110005

Shah S, Xu Q, Ullah M, Zahoor SS, Morales G, Sun J, Zhu D (2023) Lignin-based additive materials: A review of current status, challenges, and future perspectives. Addit Manuf 74:103711

Shu F, Jiang B, Yuan Y, Li M, Wu W, Jin Y, Xiao H (2021) Biological activities and emerging roles of lignin and lignin-based products— a review. Biomacromolecules 22(12):4905–4918

Shuai L, Amiri MT, Luterbacher JS (2016) The influence of interunit carbon–carbon linkages during lignin upgrading. Curr Opin Green Sustain Chem 2:59–63

Srisapoome P, Hamano K, Tsutsui I, Iiyama K (2018) Immunostimulation and yellow head virus (YHV) disease resistance induced by a lignin-based pulping by-product in black tiger shrimp (Penaeus monodon Linn.). Fish Shellfish Immunol 72:494–501

Terzioğlu P, Parın FN, Sıcak Y (2020) Lignin composites for biomedical applications: status, challenges and perspectives. In: Lignin: biosynthesis and transformation for industrial applications. Springer International Publishing, pp 253–273

Wahba SM, Darwish AS, Shehata IH, Abd Elhalem SS (2015) Sugarcane bagasse lignin, and silica gel and magneto-silica as drug vehicles for development of innocuous methotrexate drug against rheumatoid arthritis disease in albino rats. Mater Sci Eng C 48:599–610

Wang X, Han G, Shen Z, Sun R (2015a) Fabrication, property, and application of lignin-based nanocomposites. In: Eco-friendly polymer nanocomposites: chemistry and applications, vol 74. Springer India, pp 73–99

Wang Q, Mu H, Zhang L, Dong D, Zhang W, Duan J (2015b) Characterization of two water-soluble lignin metabolites with antiproliferative activities from Inonotus obliquus. Int J Biol Macromol 74:507–514

Wang D, Jang J, Kim K, Kim J, Park CB (2019) "Tree to bone": lignin/polycaprolactone nanofibers for hydroxyapatite biomineralization. Biomacromolecules 20(7):2684–2693

Wang H-M, Yuan T-Q, Song G-Y, Sun R-C (2021a) Advanced and versatile lignin-derived biodegradable composite film materials toward a sustainable world. Green Chem 23(11):3790–3817

Wang Y, Xiao X, Wang S, Li K, Jiang Y, Ma Y, Zhang T, Ran R (2021b) Exploration on UV-blocking performance of lignin from palm (Trachycarpus Fortunei) fiber. J Nat Fibers 18(1):71–79

Witzler M, Alzagameem A, Bergs M, El Khaldi-Hansen B, Klein SE, Hielscher D, Kamm B, Kreyenschmidt J, Tobiasch E, Schulze M (2018) Lignin-derived biomaterials for drug release and tissue engineering. Molecules 23(8):1885

Yang W, Fortunati E, Dominici F, Giovanale G, Mazzaglia A, Balestra GM, Kenny JM, Puglia D (2016) Effect of cellulose and lignin on disintegration, antimicrobial and antioxidant properties of PLA active films. Int J Biol Macromol 89:360–368

Yang X, Wang J, Guo H, Liu L, Xu W, Duan G (2020) Structural design toward functional materials by electrospinning: a review. E-Polymers 20(1):682–712

Yu O, Kim KH (2020) Lignin to materials: a focused review on recent novel lignin applications. Appl Sci 10(13):4626

Yuan X, Peng S, Lin W, Wang J, Zhang L (2019) Multistage pH-responsive mesoporous silica nanohybrids with charge reversal and intracellular release for efficient anticancer drug delivery. J Colloid Interface Sci 555:82–93

Zhang N (2020) Preparation of nanofibre material based on electrospinning technology and its application in rehabilitation of lower limb joint motion. Int J Nanotechnol 17(2–6):325–338

Zhao H, Li J, Wang P, Zeng S, Xie Y (2017) Lignin-carbohydrate complexes based spherical biocarriers: preparation, characterization, and biocompatibility. Int J Polym Sci 2017(1):4915185

Zhou Y, Han Y, Li G, Yang S, Xiong F, Chu F (2019) Preparation of targeted lignin–based hollow nanoparticles for the delivery of doxorubicin. Nano 9(2):188

10 Lignin Hybrid Materials and Blends for Biomedical Applications: A Life Cycle Analysis

Angela Daniela La Rosa

Abstract

Lignin is a biopolymer derived from lignocellulosic biomass that has garnered significant interest for its potential in biomedical applications, due to its unique properties such as high carbon content, thermal stability, biodegradability, and biocompatibility. Recent research has focused on developing lignin-based composites and hybrid materials for various medical uses, including tissue engineering scaffolds, wound dressings, and drug delivery systems. These materials offer several advantages, such as cost-effective processing and low energy requirements, making them attractive for sustainable biomedical applications. However, challenges remain in optimizing their properties and ensuring consistent performance in clinical settings. This chapter aims to provide with a short review on lignin hybrid materials and composites for biomedical applications, including advantages, challenges and future perspective.

Keywords

Scaffolds · Wound dressings · Drug delivery · Biocompatibility · Sustainability

10.1 Introduction

In recent years, significant research has focused on developing lignin-based hybrid materials and composites for various medical uses including tissue engineering scaffolds, wound dressings, and drug delivery systems. The incorporation of lignin

A. D. La Rosa (✉)
Department of Manufacturing and Civil Engineering, Norwegian University of Science and Technology (NTNU), Gjøvik, Norway
e-mail: angela.d.l.rosa@ntnu.no

M. N. Collins, M. Culebras (eds.), *Sustainable Biopolymers and Composites for Biomedical Applications*, Biomaterials, Bioengineering and Sustainability 5,
https://doi.org/10.1007/978-3-031-91972-5_10

into these materials enhances their mechanical properties, provides antioxidant benefits, and improves their overall biocompatibility (Sethulekshmi et al. 2023; Terzioğlu et al. 2020). The incorporation of lignin into biopolymers enhances their mechanical properties, providing the necessary support for cell attachment and proliferation. This is particularly important for applications in bone and cartilage tissue engineering (Witzler et al. 2018). Lignin has natural antioxidant properties, which can be beneficial in protecting cells from oxidative stress and damage (Liu et al. 2020); it is biocompatible and biodegradable, making it suitable for medical applications where these properties are crucial (Terzioğlu et al. 2020); it has emerged as a promising material for biomedical applications also due to its antimicrobial properties. Lignin's antimicrobial properties are primarily attributed to its complex polyphenolic structure, which includes phenolic hydroxyl and methoxy groups (Espinoza-Acosta et al. 2016). These groups are biologically active and can disrupt microbial cell walls, leading to the inhibition of bacterial and fungal growth (Sethulekshmi et al. 2023; Roy et al. 2023). Infact, the phenolic compounds in lignin can interfere with the cell membranes of microbes, causing cell lysis and death (Espinoza-Acosta et al. 2016). Lignin has shown effectiveness against a wide range of microorganisms, including bacteria, fungi, and viruses (Roy et al. 2023). When combined with other antimicrobial agents, lignin can enhance their effectiveness, making it a valuable component in composite materials (Alzagameem et al. 2019). Due to its antimicrobial properties, lignin is being explored for use in various applications such as wound dressings, coatings for medical devices, and packaging materials to prevent microbial contamination. Lignin is also cost-effective and sustainable. Infact, as a by-product of the paper and pulp industry, lignin is abundant and readily available, contributing to the sustainability of biomedical materials (Sethulekshmi et al. 2023; Terzioğlu et al. 2020).

Applications of lignin hybrid materials and composites are developing in several medical applications (Terzioğlu et al. 2020; Ma et al. 2021; O'brien 2011; Okur et al. 2019; Nan et al. 2022), e.g.: (i) tissue engineering: lignin-based composites are being explored for use in tissue engineering scaffolds. These scaffolds support cell growth and tissue regeneration (Terzioğlu et al. 2020); (ii) wound dressings: due to its antimicrobial properties, lignin can be used in wound dressing materials to prevent infections and promote healing (Terzioğlu et al. 2020); (iii) drug delivery: lignin's ability to form nanoparticles and its compatibility with various drugs make it a promising material for drug delivery systems. These systems can provide controlled and sustained release of medications (Ma et al. 2021); (iv) hydrogels and nanofibers: lignin can be used to create hydrogels and nanofibers, which are popular scaffold materials. Hydrogels provide a hydrated environment that mimics natural tissue, while nanofibers offer a high surface area for cell attachment and growth (Liang et al. 2022); (v) stem cell-based therapies: lignin-based scaffolds are being explored for use in stem cell-based therapies. These scaffolds can support the differentiation and proliferation of stem cells, aiding in the regeneration of damaged tissues. These applications highlight the versatility and potential of lignin-based materials in advancing medical technology and improving patient care.

10.2 Production of Lignin-Based Composites for Medical Applications

10.2.1 Type of Polymers

In the fabrication of lignin hybrid materials and composites for biomedical applications, various types of polymers are used to enhance their properties and functionality. Some commonly used polymers include:

- Polyethylene glycol (PEG), often used in drug delivery systems and tissue engineering for its biocompatibility and hydrophilicity;
- Poly(lactic acid) (PLA), a biodegradable polymer frequently used in medical implants and scaffolds (Domínguez-Robles et al. 2019);
- Polycaprolactone (PCL), a biodegradable polymer used in tissue engineering due to its slow degradation rate and good mechanical properties;
- Polyvinyl alcohol (PVA), used for its excellent film-forming, emulsifying, and adhesive properties;
- Chitosan, a natural polymer with antimicrobial properties, often used in wound dressings and tissue engineering.
- Gelatin, a natural polymer derived from collagen, used for its biocompatibility and biodegradability;
- Polyurethane (PU), known for its flexibility and durability, PU is used in various biomedical applications.

These polymers are combined with lignin to create composites that leverage the unique properties of both materials, such as enhanced mechanical strength, biodegradability, and biocompatibility. For example, in the case of lignin-PLA composites Lignin-PLA (poly-lactic acid) composites are gaining attention in biomedical applications due to their combined properties of biodegradability, biocompatibility, and mechanical strength. Lignin/PLA composites are used to manufacture scaffolds that support cell growth and tissue regeneration (Nan et al. 2022). The addition of lignin enhances the mechanical properties and provides antioxidant benefits, which can improve cell viability and proliferation. These composites are also explored for wound dressing applications. The antioxidant properties of lignin help in reducing oxidative stress at the wound site, promoting faster healing (Domínguez-Robles et al. 2019) https://www.mdpi.com/1999-4923/11/4/165. Additionally, the biocompatibility of PLA ensures that the dressing is safe for use on human skin (Domínguez-Robles et al. 2019). Lignin/PLA composites can be used to develop drug delivery systems that provide controlled release of therapeutic agents (see Fig. 10.1). The biodegradability of PLA allows for the gradual breakdown of the composite, releasing the drug over time. Lignin/PLA composites are suitable for 3D printing applications, particularly in creating customized medical devices and implants. The combination of lignin and PLA allows for the production of materials with specific mechanical and biological properties tailored to individual patient needs (Domínguez-Robles et al. 2019).

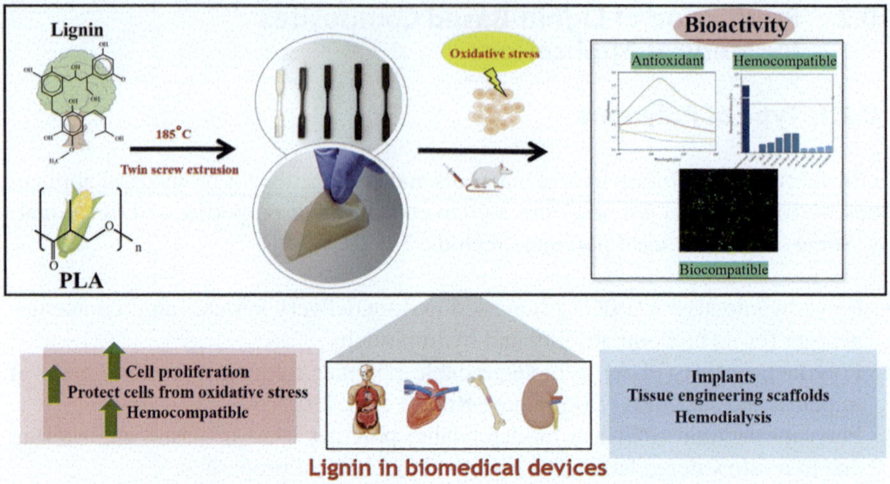

Fig. 10.1 Schematic representation of lignin/PLA composites and potential applications in biomedical industry. (With permission of Mearaj et al. (2023))

10.2.2 Lignin Extraction and Processing for Medical Use

Lignin extraction and processing for medical use involve several steps to ensure the material is suitable for biomedical applications (Spiridon 2020; Mondal et al. 2023). These methods and processes ensure that lignin is suitable for use in medical applications, leveraging its natural properties while enhancing its functionality through chemical modifications and advanced processing techniques. Some main extraction methods and processes are summarized in Fig. 10.2 and hereafter described:

Extraction Methods:

- Kraft Process. This is one of the most common methods, where lignin is extracted using sodium hydroxide and sodium sulfide. The resulting lignin, known as kraft lignin, is then purified (Spiridon 2020).
- Sulphite Process. In this method, lignin is extracted using sulfurous acid and its salts, producing lignosulfonates (Spiridon 2020).
- Organosolv Process. This involves using organic solvents to extract lignin, resulting in high-purity lignin suitable for medical applications (Spiridon 2020).
- Enzymatic Hydrolysis. This method uses enzymes to break down the plant biomass, releasing lignin in a more environmentally friendly manner (Spiridon 2020).

Processing Techniques:

- Purification. After extraction, lignin is purified to remove impurities and unwanted components. This step is crucial for medical applications to ensure biocompatibility (Mondal et al. 2023).

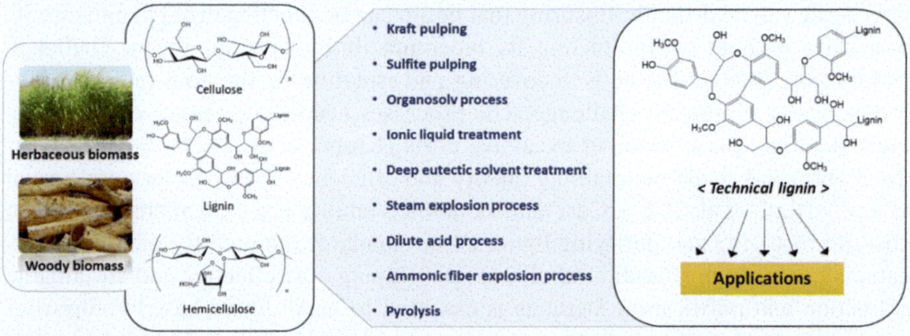

Fig. 10.2 Processes for the extraction of technical lignin. (Permission from Yu and Kim (2020))

- Functionalization: Lignin can be chemically modified to enhance its properties, such as increasing its solubility or adding functional groups that improve its antimicrobial activity (Wang et al. 2020).
- Nanoparticle Formation: Lignin can be processed into nanoparticles, which are useful in drug delivery systems due to their small size and high surface area (Wang et al. 2020).

After extraction and processing lignin can be combined with polymer by using different technology: Lignin is blended with other biocompatible polymers like cellulose, chitosan, or synthetic polymers to form composites (Kropat et al. 2021; Rath et al. 2024). Lignin can be processed into nanoparticles, which are then incorporated into composites to enhance their properties (Kropat et al. 2021). Advanced manufacturing techniques like 3D printing and electrospinning are used to create complex structures and scaffolds from lignin-based materials.

10.2.3 Challenges

To produce lignin-based composites for medical applications presents several challenges. One challenge is due to the heterogeneity of lignin. Lignin's complex and variable structure makes it difficult to achieve consistent quality and performance. This heterogeneity can affect the reproducibility of the final products (Kropat et al. 2021). Another issue is ensuring uniformity in lignin's chemical composition as it is crucial for medical applications, but this is challenging due to the natural variability in lignin sources (Kropat et al. 2021). Purity is another issue as lignin extracted from industrial processes often contains various organic and inorganic impurities. These impurities need to be removed to meet the stringent purity requirements for medical applications (Rath et al. 2024). Developing advanced purification techniques that are both efficient and cost-effective is essential to produce high-purity lignin (Rath et al. 2024). Chemical reactivity is another challenge in processing and functionalization. Achieving the desired chemical modifications consistently on a large scale can be difficult. Ensuring that lignin can be functionalized to enhance its properties without compromising its biocompatibility is a significant challenge (Rath et al. 2024). Efficiently recovering and isolating lignin from industrial by-products is a significant challenge. The processes need to be optimized to ensure high yield and purity without excessive costs (Kropat et al. 2021). Scalability of these processes while maintaining quality and efficiency is crucial for commercial viability (Rath et al. 2024). Cost and economic viability is a critical challenge. The cost of processing and purifying lignin to the standards required for medical applications can be high (Fazeli et al. 2024). Developing cost-effective and sustainable extraction and purification methods is essential to make lignin-based composites competitive with traditional materials (Fazeli et al. 2024). Finally, regulatory compliance, e.g.: meeting the stringent regulatory requirements for safety and efficacy in medical applications, can be complex and time-consuming. Addressing these challenges requires ongoing research and development to optimize extraction, purification, and processing methods, as well as collaboration between industry and regulatory bodies to ensure compliance and economic feasibility.

10.2.4 Successful Case Studies in Using Lignin-Based Materials for Medical Implants

There have been several successful case studies demonstrating the potential of lignin-based materials for medical implants. Here are a few notable examples:

10.3 Bone Regeneration Scaffolds

Researchers have developed lignin-based composite scaffolds for bone regeneration. These scaffolds combine lignin with other biocompatible materials like hydroxyapatite and chitosan. The resulting composites have shown excellent mechanical properties, biocompatibility, and the ability to support cell growth and differentiation, making them suitable for bone tissue engineering (Nan et al. 2022).

10.4 Antibacterial Coatings

Lignin has been used to create antibacterial coatings for medical implants. These coatings leverage lignin's natural antimicrobial properties to prevent infections associated with implants. Studies have shown that lignin-based coatings can effectively inhibit the growth of common pathogens such as staphylococcus aureus and escherichia coli (Radotić et al. 2023).

10.5 Drug-Eluting Implants

Lignin-based materials have been explored for use in drug-eluting implants. These implants can provide controlled and sustained release of therapeutic agents, improving the efficacy of treatments and reducing the need for frequent drug administration. Lignin's ability to form nanoparticles and its compatibility with various drugs make it an ideal candidate for such applications (Balk et al. 2023).

10.6 Cardiovascular Implants

In a recent study, lignin-based composites were used to develop cardiovascular implants, such as stents. These implants demonstrated good mechanical strength, flexibility, and biocompatibility. Additionally, the antioxidant properties of lignin helped in reducing oxidative stress, which is beneficial for cardiovascular health (Yu and Kim 2020).

These case studies highlight the versatility and potential of lignin-based materials in developing advanced medical implants that are biocompatible, sustainable, and effective (see Fig. 10.3).

10.7 Life Cycle Assessment (LCA) of Lignin Hybrid Materials and Composites

LCA involves evaluating the environmental impacts associated with their production, use, and disposal. Life cycle assessment enables calculation of product or service's potential environmental impacts at every stage of its life cycle, from the extraction of raw materials to the end of its useful life (ISO 14044 2006). To achieve this, the environmental effects must be allocated among the system's co-products. It is a complex analysis and comparative LCA is challenging due to lack of data and to the multi-output nature of lignin biorefineries, as several distinct products can be created, and various allocations functional unit and system boundaries are possible. Most of the LCA investigations available in literature do not include the end of life (EoL) but focus on a cradle-to-gate perspective (Lizundia et al. 2021). About the impact categories, assessment of the global warming potential (GWP) has received most of the attention, despite the fact that LCA permits the evaluation of additional effect categories such as eutrophication, land use, water use, or toxicity. The allocations related to economics, energy, mass, or allocation based on substituted impacts are particularly important among several possible allocations (Lizundia et al. 2021).

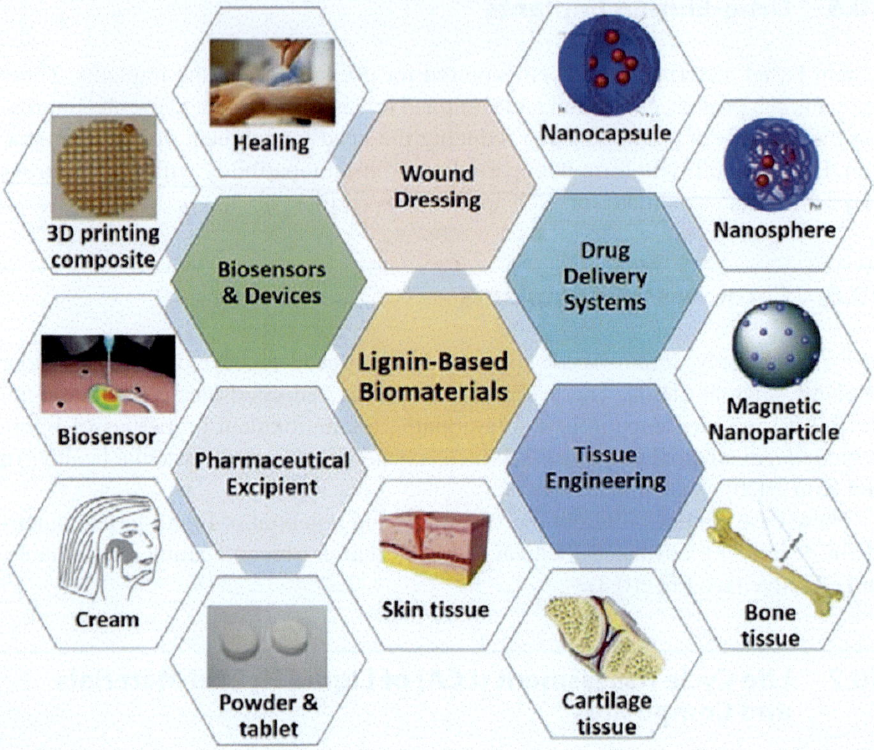

Fig. 10.3 Schematic illustration of the medical applications of lignin-based biomaterials. (Permission from Nan et al. (2022))

10.7.1 Comparative LCA Studies Between Lignin-Based and Synthetic Materials

Comparative LCA between lignin-based and synthetic materials have highlighted that lignin-based materials generally have a lower environmental impact compared to synthetic polymers. A study published by Lizundia et al. (2021) reviews that lignin-based nanocomposites have a significantly reduced carbon footprint and lower greenhouse gas emissions compared to their synthetic counterparts. The production of lignin-based materials often requires less energy. According to another review article (Shorey et al. 2024) the energy required for lignin extraction and processing is lower than that for producing synthetic polymers, contributing to overall energy savings. Being a by-product of the paper and pulp industry, lignin is produced by waste biomass, which helps in reducing the reliance on fossil fuels. This contrasts with synthetic materials that are typically derived from non-renewable petroleum sources (Bernier et al. 2013; Yang et al. 2024). Lignin-based materials are biodegradable, which reduces their environmental impact at the end of their life cycle while synthetic materials, often persist in the environment and contribute to pollution. Lignin-based materials generally exhibit lower toxicity levels compared to synthetic materials. This is crucial for biomedical applications where biocompatibility and safety are paramount. The LCA studies available in literature underscore the potential environmental benefits of lignin-based materials, making them a sustainable alternative to traditional synthetic polymer composites.

10.7.2 Optimization of the End-of-Life Disposal of Lignin Composites

Optimizing the end-of-life disposal of lignin composites for medical applications involves several strategies to ensure environmental sustainability and safety. Designing lignin composites to be fully biodegradable can significantly reduce their environmental impact. These materials can break down naturally in composting environments, returning nutrients to the soil (Ma et al. 2021). Establishing specialized composting facilities for medical waste can help manage the disposal of biodegradable lignin composites effectively. Recycling and reuse are other possible optimization ways. Developing processes to recover and recycle lignin from used medical devices can extend the lifecycle of the material (Yang et al. 2024). This involves separating lignin from other components and reprocessing it for new applications. Implementing closed-loop recycling systems within healthcare facilities can ensure that lignin-based materials are collected, processed, and reused efficiently (Yang et al. 2024; Ekielski and Mishra 2021). For lignin composites that cannot be composted or recycled, controlled incineration with energy recovery can be an effective disposal method. This process can convert waste into energy while minimizing environmental pollution. Ensuring that incineration facilities are equipped with advanced emission control technologies can reduce the release of harmful pollutants (Spiridon 2020). Innovative approaches to recycling lignin-based medical devices that focus on maximizing sustainability and minimizing environmental impact could be further developed. Some examples are listed below:

- Chemical Recycling
  - Depolymerization: this process breaks down lignin into its monomeric components, which can then be reused to create new lignin-based materials. Depolymerization can be achieved through chemical, thermal, or biological methods (Nan et al. 2022).
  - Solvent Extraction: using green solvents to extract and purify lignin from used medical devices allows for the recovery of high-purity lignin that can be reprocessed (Mondal et al. 2023).
- Mechanical Recycling
- Grinding and reprocessing: used lignin-based composites can be mechanically ground into fine particles and then reprocessed into new materials. This method is particularly useful for creating fillers or reinforcements in new composites (Mondal et al. 2023).

- Biological Recycling
- Microbial degradation: utilizing ligninolytic microorganisms to break down lignin into reusable components is an emerging approach. These microorganisms can convert lignin into valuable biochemicals that can be used in new medical applications (Rath et al. 2024).
- Advanced Material Recovery
  - Nanoparticle Recovery: for lignin-based nanoparticles used in medical devices, advanced separation techniques can recover these nanoparticles for reuse. This involves processes like centrifugation and filtration (Nan et al. 2022).
  - Composite Separation: techniques such as solvent-based separation can isolate lignin from other components in composite materials, allowing for the recovery and reuse of both lignin and the other materials (Spiridon 2020).

These innovative approaches highlight the potential for sustainable recycling of lignin-based medical devices, contributing to a more circular economy and reducing environmental impact.

10.8 Conclusions

Lignin hybrid materials and composites have shown significant promise in biomedical applications due to their unique properties and potential benefits. Here is a summary of Summarizing, the main advantages are biocompatibility and biodegradability, thermal stability, antioxidant and antimicrobial properties, cost-effectiveness and environmental sustainability. Among the challenges, the heterogeneity, because it can lead to variability in the properties of lignin-based materials and therefore not easy standardization. About future perspective, advanced functionalization (for more specific biomedical applications) and emphasis on sustainability, that will drive the exploration of lignin as a green alternative to synthetic polymers in biomedical applications. Overall, while there are challenges to overcome, the future of lignin hybrid materials and composites in the biomedical field looks promising, with ongoing research likely to unlock new potentials and applications.

Acknowledgement The author acknowledges the project 1-2-TRE-STEG: Steps towards circularity in wood-based. https://prosjektbanken.forskningsradet.no/project/FORISS/336488.

Conflict of Interest The author declares no potential conflict of interest.

References

Alzagameem A, Klein SE, Bergs M, Do XT, Korte I, Dohlen S, Hüwe C, Kreyenschmidt J, Kamm B, Larkins M et al (2019) Antimicrobial activity of lignin and lignin-derived cellulose and chitosan composites against selected pathogenic and spoilage microorganisms. Polymers 11:670

Balk M, Sofia P, Neffe AT, Tirelli N (2023) Lignin, the lignification process, and advanced, lignin-based materials. Int J Mol Sci 24(14)

Bernier E, Lavigne C, Robidoux PY (2013) Life cycle assessment of kraft lignin for polymer applications. Int J Life Cycle Assess 18:520–528

Domínguez-Robles J, Martin NK, Fong ML, Stewart SA, Irwin NJ, Rial-Hermida MI, Donnelly RF, Larrañeta E (2019) Antioxidant PLA composites containing lignin for 3D printing applications: a potential material for healthcare applications. Pharmaceutics 11(4):165

Ekielski A, Mishra PK (2021) Lignin for bioeconomy: the present and future role of technical lignin. Int J Mol Sci 22(1):63

Espinoza-Acosta JL, Torres-Chávez PI, Ramírez-Wong B, López-Saiz CM, Montaño-Leyva B (2016) Antioxidant, antimicrobial, and antimutagenic properties of technical lignins and their applications. BioRes 11(2):5452–5481

Fazeli M, Mukherjee S, Baniasadi H, Abidnejad R, Mujtaba M, Lipponen J, Jukka Seppälä J, Rojas OJ (2024) Lignin beyond the status quo: recent and emerging composite applications. Green Chem 26:593–630

ISO 14044:2006 Environmental management. Life cycle assessment. Requirements and guidelines

Kropat M, Liao M, Park H, Salem KS, Johnson S, Argyropoulos DS (2021) A perspective of lignin processing and utilization technologies for composites and plastics with emphasis on technical and market trends. Bioresources 16(1):2084–2115

Liang R, Yang X, Yew PYM et al (2022) PLA-lignin nanofibers as antioxidant biomaterials for cartilage regeneration and osteoarthritis treatment. J Nanobiotechnol 20:327

Liu R, Dai L, Xu C, Wang K, Zheng C, Si C (2020) Lignin-based micro- and nanomaterials and their composites in biomedical applications. Chem Sus Chem 13(17):4266–4283

Lizundia E, Sipponen MH, Greca LG, Balakshin M, Tardy BL, Rojas OJ, Puglia D (2021) Multifunctional lignin-based nanocomposites and nanohybrids. Green Chem 23:6698–6760

Ma C, Kim T-H, Liu K, Ma M-G, Choi S-E, Si C (2021) Multifunctional lignin-based composite materials for emerging applications. Front Bioeng Biotechnol 9:708976

Mearaj S, Ajaz AM, Kim MT, Choi JW (2023) Bioactive and hemocompatible PLA/lignin biocomposites: assessment of in vitro antioxidant activity for biomedical applications. ACS Appl Bio Mater 6(9):3648–3660

Mondal S, Jatrana A, Maan S et al (2023) Lignin modification and valorization in medicine, cosmetics, environmental remediation and agriculture: a review. Environ Chem Lett 21:2171–2197

Nan N, Hu W, Wang J (2022) Lignin-based porous biomaterials for medical and pharmaceutical applications. Biomedicines 10(4):747

O'brien FJ (2011) Biomaterials & scaffolds for tissue engineering. Mater Today 14(3):88–95

Okur NÜ, Hökenek N, Okur ME et al (2019) An alternative approach to wound healing field; new composite films from natural polymers for mupirocin dermal delivery. Saudi Pharm J 27(5):738–752

Radotić K, Spasojević D, Zmejkoski D (2023) Chapter 5. In: Joseph K, Wilson R, George G, Appukuttan S (eds) Lignin-based MaterialsHealth care and medical applications. The Royal Society of Chemistry, pp 85–105

Rath S, Pradhan D, Du H et al (2024) Transforming lignin into value-added products: perspectives on lignin chemistry, lignin-based biocomposites, and pathways for augmenting ligninolytic enzyme production. Adv Compos Hybrid Mater 7:27

Roy S, Priyadarshi R, Purohit SD, Rhim J (2023) Chapter 6. In: Joseph K, Wilson R, George G, Appukuttan S (eds) Lignin-based materials health care and medical applications. The Royal Society of Chemistry, pp 106–129

Sethulekshmi AS, Appukuttan S, George G, Wilson R, Joseph K (2023) Chapter 1. In: Joseph K, Wilson R, George G, Appukuttan S (eds) Lignin-based materials health care and medical applications. The Royal Society of Chemistry, pp 1–10

Shorey R, Salaghi A, Fatehi P, Mekonnen TH (2024) Valorization of lignin for advanced material applications: a review. RSC Sustain 2:804–831

Spiridon I (2020) Extraction of lignin and therapeutic applications of lignin-derived compounds. A review. Environ Chem Lett 18:771–785

Terzioğlu P, Parın FN, Sıcak Y (2020) Lignin composites for biomedical applications: status, challenges and perspectives. In: Sharma S, Kumar A (eds) Lignin, Springer Series on Polymer and Composite Materials. Springer, Cham

Wang Y-Y, Meng X, Pu Y, Ragauskas AJ (2020) Recent advances in the application of functionalized lignin in value-added polymeric materials. Polymers 12(10):2277

Witzler M, Alzagameem A, Bergs M, Khaldi-Hansen BE, Klein SE, Hielscher D, Kamm B, Kreyenschmidt J, Tobiasch E, Schulze M (2018) Lignin-derived biomaterials for drug release and tissue engineering. Molecules 23:1885

Yang Y, Guan Y, Li C et al (2024) Application and carbon footprint evaluation of lignin-based composite materials. Adv Compos Hybrid Mater 7:61

Yu O, Kim KH (2020) Lignin to materials: a focused review on recent novel lignin applications. Appl Sci 10(13):4626

Lignin Based Nanomaterials for Potential Biomedical Applications

11

Asmaa Dghoughi, Marya Raji, Mohammed-Ouadi Bensalah, Rachid Bouhfid, and Abouelkacem Qaiss

Abstract

The potential of lignin, a naturally occurring polymer obtained from plant biomass, in biological applications is examined in this chapter. Research into the extraction, modification, and application of lignin is being prompted by its underutilization despite its abundance. The chapter examines the difficulties presented by the intricate phenolic structure of lignin and highlights the effects of extraction techniques such as the Kraft, sulfite, alkaline and organosolv procedures on the characteristics of lignin. The creation of lignin-based nanomaterials, including nanoparticles, as well as chemical changes that improve lignin's functioning are also covered. The appealing uses of lignin nanoparticles in tissue engineering

A. Dghoughi (✉)
Laboratory of Mechanics and Materials (LMM), Faculty of Science, Mohammed V-University, Rabat, Morocco

Composites and Nanocomposites Center, Moroccan Foundation for Advanced Science, Innovation and Research, Rabat Design Center, Rue Mohamed El Jazouli, Madinat El Irfane, Rabat, Morocco

Mohammed VI Polytechnic University, Ben Guerir, Morocco
e-mail: a.dghoughi@mascir.ma

M. Raji · R. Bouhfid · A. Qaiss
Composites and Nanocomposites Center, Moroccan Foundation for Advanced Science, Innovation and Research, Rabat Design Center, Rue Mohamed El Jazouli, Madinat El Irfane, Rabat, Morocco

Mohammed VI Polytechnic University, Ben Guerir, Morocco

M.-O. Bensalah
Laboratory of Mechanics and Materials (LMM), Faculty of Science, Mohammed V-University, Rabat, Morocco

M. N. Collins, M. Culebras (eds.), *Sustainable Biopolymers and Composites for Biomedical Applications*, Biomaterials, Bioengineering and Sustainability 5,
https://doi.org/10.1007/978-3-031-91972-5_11

and drug and gene delivery are highlighted, as they enhance scaffold characteristics and drug stability. Overall, nanomaterials based on lignin present promising prospects in the biomedical domain; nonetheless, additional investigation is required to broaden their use in healthcare solutions.

Keywords

Lignin nanoparticles · Chemical modifications · Lignin-based nanomaterials biomedical applications

11.1 Introduction

Cellulose, hemicellulose, and lignin, the predominant natural polymers extracted from plants, continue to be the subject of intensive exploration within the scientific community, with a focus on the development of nanostructured materials (Barhoum et al. 2020). Substances and nanomaterials derived from starch, cellulose, hemicellulose, and natural fibers have recently attracted a lot of attention from scientists (Yu et al. 2021; Subbotina et al. 2022; Henschen et al. 2019; Daus and Heinze 2010; Ahmad et al. 2020; Sun 2017; Le Corre and Angellier-Coussy 2014). However, lignin has lately come under further investigation in an effort to ensure the most effective use of plant fiber reserves. First used in 1813 at the University of Geneva (Switzerland), the name "lignin" was initially coined by the Swiss botanist Augustin Pyramus de Candolle (1778–1841). The Latin word for wood, lignum, is the source of this term (horielmenc00cand). With its heterogeneous and amorphous structure, lignin is the second most widespread biopolymer after cellulose (Kai et al. 2016). It represents the predominant source of aromatic alcohols and simultaneously acts as a fundamental matrix for cell wall structuring within the plant (Norgren and Edlund 2014; Kim et al. 2015). Lignin is produced on a vast worldwide scale, with a market estimated to be valued at USD 954.5 million in 2019 and growing at an average of 2% per year by 2027 (Sugiarto et al. 2022). However, at present, only 2% of industrial lignin wastes are used for commercial purposes out of the total amount (Schoenherr et al. 2018). A significant amount of lignins is used as lignosulfonates, which are added to construction materials. The remaining lignins are mainly utilized for applications of low value, like adhesives, dispersants, and activated carbon, as low-grade fuel (Gosselink et al. 2004).

While the current use of industrial lignin wastes is still very restricted, innovative techniques are being investigated to separate, extract, and chemically convert these plentiful resources into a versatile array of bio-derived value-added materials (Duval and Lawoko 2014; Agrawal et al. 2014). Due to its complexity and the variety of linkages it contains, the removal of lignin during biomass fractionation is a challenging process. Fractionation methods fall into two groups: those that target the selective hydrolysis of polysaccharides, leaving lignin and other components as the solid residue, and those that solubilize lignin and separate the solid residue (Rodríguez (2020)). Following its removal from biomass, lignin can undergo a variety of chemical processes, including oxidation, depolymerization, functional group graft modification, and polymerization (Aro and Fatehi 2017; Eraghi et al. 2019;

Gao and Fatehi 2019). The breadth of these extraction and modification methods highlights the richness of lignin properties, which differ greatly based on its functional groups. These characteristics, which are absent from other natural polymers include strong antibacterial activity, good antioxidant capability, and excellent anti-UV properties (Witzler et al. 2018). Given the previously stated characteristics, lignin can be employed as a bioactive component in conjunction with commonly used biomaterials like cellulose (Sugiarto et al. 2022). Beyond its well-established function in materials science and environmental sustainability, lignin has emerged as a compelling candidate for biomedical applications. The biomedical field also attaches great importance to lignin for its intrinsic biocompatibility and structural variety, which is considering as promising assets for therapeutic interventions and regenerative medicine (Stanisz et al. 2022). Lignin proved its incredible role in biomedical fields, especially in drug/gene delivery, tissue engineering (Witzler et al. 2018; Kumar et al. 2021), 3D printing (Domínguez-Robles et al. 2019; Shavandi et al. 2020), and bioimaging (Myint et al. 2018). As part of lignin-based materials destined for biomedical uses, lignin has been reported as an immobilization matrix, crosslinking agent, nanofiller in many studies to create designed structures or to modify material properties (Stanisz et al. 2022; Cerrutti et al. 2015; Khadem et al. 2024).

Based on the promising developments in nanotechnology in biomedical engineering, nanolignin presents an appealing path to leverage its unique properties for enhanced therapeutic efficacy and a better comprehension of biological processes at the molecular level. The aim of this chapter is therefore to explore lignin-based nanomaterials and their potential for promising biomedical applications. Starting with an in-depth investigation of the properties and composition of lignin, as well as the techniques of extraction and chemical changes it undergoes, we offer an overview for comprehending its adaptability and potential. We then discuss the particular production of lignin-based nanomaterials, emphasizing their remarkable potential to address the expanding demands of tissue engineering, drug delivery, and targeted therapy in the biomedical industry. Finally, we discuss the preparation of lignin-based nanomaterials for various applications, underlining the potential of these nanomaterials for biomedical uses.

11.2 Structural organization of Lignin

One of the main elements of plant cell walls is lignin. Since it supports the polysaccharide structure of the cell wall, this robust, non-fibrous molecule is essential to a plant ability to grow stronger and more rigid. Lignin is an organic phenolic polymer possessing a high molecular weight, intricate chemistry, and intricate structure. Lignin is a natural phenolic polymer with a high molecular weight, complex composition, and structure. All vascular plants, with the interesting exception of tropical tree ferns (Dicksonia), have been demonstrated to have lignins using suitable color responses (Singh 2023). Mature plants have variable degrees of lignification in their stems, roots, bark, leaves, fruit shells, and seed hairs. Nonvascular algae, fungus, mushrooms, lichens, and liverworts lack lignins, and it is unclear if mosses have them (Lücking and Nelsen 2018). Although the specific structure of lignin has been thoroughly studied for several years, it remains unknown. It either reacts chemically with the carbohydrates or the high-molecular lignin creates a three-dimensional network within the wood (Chunbao and Ferdosian 2017). A model of the lignin structure is shown in Fig. 11.1, along with a list of frequent interunit connections and how commonly they occur in lignin from hardwood and softwood sources (Table 11.1).

Besides its inherent variability, the fundamental chemical structure of lignin consists of phenylpropane units connected by three aromatic alcohol precursors: p-coumaryl, coniferyl, and sinapyl alcohol. Depending on the lignin origin, the ratio

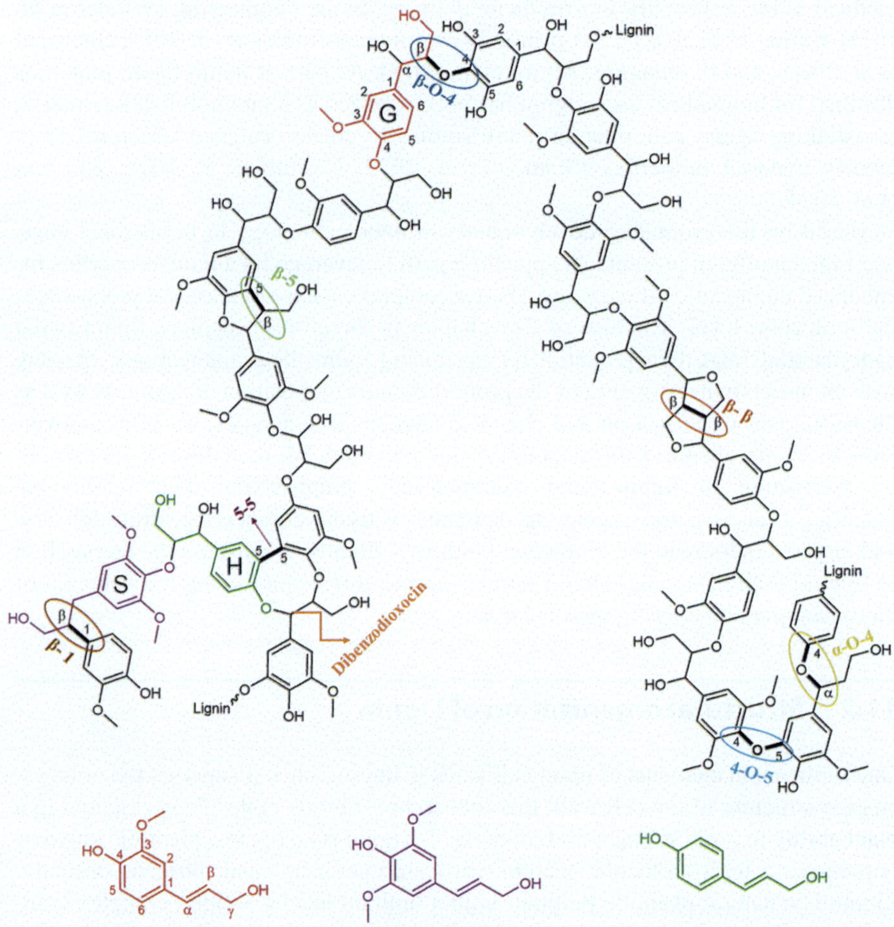

Conyferyl alcohol (G) | Sinapyl alcohol (S) | p-coumaryl alcohol (H)

Fig. 11.1 Model representation of the chemical structure of lignin. (Adapted from ref. Vanholme et al. (2010) under the CC-BY-3.0 license)

Table 11.1 Different linkages proportions in lignin molecules (Rodríguez (2020); Libretti et al. 2024)

Linkage type	Softwoods (%)	Hardwoods (%)
Ether linkages		
β-O-4	43–50	50–65
4-O-5	4	6–7
α-O-4	6–8	4–8
C-C linkages		
β-β	2–4	3–7
5-5	10–25	4–10
β-1	3–7	5–7
Dibenzodioxocin	0–2	5–7

of these ancestors might vary significantly (Feofilova and Mysyakina 2016). When integrated into the lignin macromolecule, the building blocks on which these monolignols are based comprise the p-hydroxyphenyl unit (H), the guaiacyl unit (G) and the syringyl unit (S) (Vanholme et al. 2010). These monomers are distributed differently in various plant species and tissues. While lignin from hardwood has almost equal quantities of G and S units but relatively tiny amounts of the H unit, lignin from softwood is primarily constituted of G units (up to 90%).

On the other hand, lignin from grasses is a roughly equimolar mixture of G, S, and H units (Faix 1991). According to Glasser, the type and proportion of linkages between benzene and propane units make up the majority of the lignin chemical structure (Glasser 2019). The fundamental bond types consist of α-O-4, β-O-4, 5–5, β–β, 4-O–5, and β-1.1. Norberg et al. (2013) reported that limited radicals to covalent connections in the 5-position on the syringyl unit lead hardwood lignin to have more β-O-4 links than softwood lignin (Norberg et al. 2013). Additionally, by forming β-5 and 5–5 connections in the free 5-position, the guaiacyl units in softwood lignins create a more branched and cross-linked structure than those in hardwood lignins (Norberg et al. 2013).

11.3 Separation and Extraction of Lignin

As the most complex phenolic natural biopolymer with a 3D network (Kubo and Kadla 2005), lignin is highly resistant to chemical and biological degradation (Ruiz-Dueñas and Martínez 2009). This inhibits biomass from being used to its full potential (Poveda-Giraldo et al. 2021). One of the critical processes in overcoming lignocellulose resistance is pretreatment (Liao et al. 2020). The various methods used for this purpose can be categorized into two groups based on how the lignin was fractionated: (i) methods that removed the lignin from the lignocellulosic biomass by separating the solid residue from the spent liquor, and (ii) methods that selectively hydrolyzed polysaccharides to leave behind lignin and a few products from the deconstruction of condensed carbohydrates as a solid residue (Rodríguez (2020)). However, there are advantages and disadvantages to each of these approaches. The extraction process also involves partial breaking of lignin bonds, which varies depending on the extraction technique used and alters the molecular weight, functional groups, and other characteristics of the separated lignins. Biomass pretreatment can be classified into several main groups, including chemical fractionation (using acidic or alkaline agents), solvent fractionation (e.g. ionic liquid, organosolv pretreatment, etc.), and mechanical fractionation (such as ball milling) (Perez-Cantu et al. 2013). Each of these methods has benefits as well as drawbacks. For instance, ionic liquids have taken the place of traditional solvents and solved a number of the disadvantages of conventional methods, such as equipment corrosion and high operating temperatures. Nevertheless, the cost of the raw ingredients needed for their synthesis and the additional steps and processes involved have restricted their industrial application (Liu et al. 2019a). It is imperative to comprehend these pretreatment techniques better in order to recognize lignin as a crucial building block for biofuel and renewable resources.

11.3.1 Kraft Process

The Kraft process, invented in 1879 and first used industrially in 1890, became the dominant method for pulping in the 1930s after the recovery boiler was introduced, allowing for chemical recovery and energy generation. Today, it produces around 130 million tons of pulp and 50–55 million metric tons of black liquor each year (Naseem et al. 2016; Bruijnincx et al. 2015), with about 75,000 tons of lignin extracted annually, primarily using the LignoBoost® process. Its widespread use is due to the high-quality pulp it produces, the ability to recover chemicals, and its energy efficiency (Rinaldi et al. 2016). In this approach, the β-aryl bonds existing between lignin-carbohydrate connections are cleaved by sodium hydroxide (NaOH) and sodium sulfide (NaS_2), acting as nucleophiles to produce chemically resistant cellulose (Lourençon et al. 2015). This process is carried out at elevated temperature (145–170 °C) and pressure, the pulp undergoes delignification and lignin depolymerization without hastening the solubilization or destruction of carbohydrates (Rodríguez (2020)). Following this step, the paste is washed, and the black liquor is filtered in order to concentrate it to 65% solids in direct-contact evaporators, by exposing the liquor to the exhaust gases from the recovery boiler. Subsequently, the black liquor is usually burned in the recovery boiler to provide energy and recuperate the chemicals needed to prepare white liquor (Huber et al. 2014). The extracted kraft lignin has an average molecular weight of 1000–3000 Da, but it can reach 15,000 Da. It is hydrophobic and typically soluble in alkali or organic solvents (Georgeta and Capraru 2013; Schutyser et al. 2018). Apart from the usual carboxyl, phenolic hydroxyl, and methoxy groups, kraft lignin also has a small quantity of sulfur groups (1–2 wt-%) on its structure (Doherty et al. 2011). Given these properties, precursors of kraft lignin can be directly applied as adhesives, emulsifiers, or dispersants. They can also be molecularly reduced to smaller entities for use in medicinal or cosmetic preparations, among many other applications (Vinardell et al. 2008; Gordobil et al. 2018). However, the kraft lignin is subjected to structural modifications through its extraction process, including the inclusion of thiol groups, ether bonds cleavage and the C-C bonds and phenolic hydroxyl groups increase.

These modifications produce a highly condensed lignin structure with low sulfur concentration and few -O-4 linkages, which makes the process of downstream valorization more difficult (Lange 2015). These disadvantages explain why lignin is used as a precursor for only around 2% of the total generated amount (Laurichesse and Avérous 2014). LignoBoost Technology has made kraft lignin commercially available by extracting lignin from pulp black liquor (Zakzeski et al. 2010). According to this process, lignin is first filtered via a chamber press filter before being precipitated through acidification with CO_2. Next, the filter cake is re-dispersed, acidified with H_2SO_4, filtered, and washed in a second chamber press filter utilizing displacement washing (Tomani (2010)). The key advantage of this process is that it is inexpensive, straightforward, and produces lignin with reduced ash and carbohydrate content impurities (Tomani (2010)).

11.3.2 Sulfite Process

The sulfite process, first invented in 1867 by B.C. Tilghman and marketed by Carl Ekman in 1874, emerged as the main pulp production process until the 1950s. Its declining popularity is attributable to the Kraft process, which responded to environmental concerns by allowing the use of a wider range of wood species, including softwoods, and offering better choices for chemical and energy recovery (Sixta et al. 2006). The first step in the pulping process is the reaction of lignin with a sulfite, which produces lignosulfonic acid when the lignin and free sulfurous acid react. Subsequently, the presence of counter ions such as calcium, sodium, ammonium, or magnesium promotes the production of water-soluble lignosulfonates, which are then fragmented (Vinardell et al. 2008; Zakzeski et al. 2010). In this approach, the reaction takes place at temperatures ranging from 120 to 180 °C, and the pH of the system can vary from 2 to 12 depending on the combination and dosage of the pulping chemicals (Laurichesse and Avérous 2014; Zakzeski et al. 2010). The introduction of polar sulfonic groups into the lignin structure generates hydrolysis and disintegration, while the cellulose retains solid (Galkin and Samec 2016; Azadi et al. 2013). As a result, the sulfur content of lignosulfonates can range from 4 to 8% by weight, and they also have greater average molecular weights (1000–50,000 Da) compared to kraft lignin, as sulfonate groups are incorporated into the lignin structure (Zakzeski et al. 2010; Galkin and Samec 2016; Azadi et al. 2013). Furthermore, the incorporation makes the catalytic transformation of lignosulfonates harder (Patil and Argyropoulos 2017). During this process, methoxyl groups are eliminated, ether linkages are broken, and new carbon-carbon bonds are created (Li et al. 2015a). In terms of potential applications, lignosulfonates show great promise as surfactants, flocculants, and dispersants in the concrete market (Aro and Fatehi 2017). By depolymerizing them, they can also be used as an advanced application to create vanillin for use in food applications (Rahimi et al. 2014). Nevertheless, the sulfite process has certain drawbacks, such as the creation of new C-C bonds that change the structure of lignin and the high amount of ash along with different impurities following isolation (Galkin and Samec 2016).

11.3.3 Alkaline Process

The most ancient method for producing lignin is alkaline pulping. Typically, the procedure is expanded to include non-woody biomass such as straw and bagasse (Rangan et al. 2021). With a worldwide production of 5% of the entire chemical pulp, the alkaline process is the third most significant pulping method. This approach involves the utilization of strong bases such as sodium hydroxide, calcium hydroxide, and hydrogen peroxide (Mondal et al. 2023). The lignin solubilization process has resemblance to the kraft approach, wherein the biomass undergoes digestion at temperatures ranging from 140 to 170 °C while an aqueous solution of sodium hydroxide containing 13–16% by weight is present (Laurichesse and Avérous 2014; Galkin and Samec 2016; Azadi et al. 2013). The key distinction of this method with the Kraft process is that it does not involve the employment of sodium sulfide as a reagent, which results in less effective lignin depolymerization since it lacks a potent nucleophile (G. Calvo-Flores et al. 2015). The extracted soda lignin from this process is difficult to isolate using filtration or centrifugation, owing to the high carboxylic acid content resulting from the aliphatic hydroxyl groups oxidation (Laurichesse and Avérous 2014). Additionally, due to the soda addition, soda lignin is quite free of contaminants but has low β-O-4 bonds and can exhibit a significant level of ash (Gillet et al. 2017). According to its carbon content, the mean molecular of alkaline lignin weight (MW) can vary from 1000 to 3000 Da (Galkin and Samec 2016; Azadi et al. 2013; Prinsen et al. 2013). To meet the massive and varied industrial demand for these kinds of compounds, the process of revalorization of this lignin is essential for the production of small aromatic building blocks. Among the various compounds thought to be possible for use in the food sector are cresols, catechols, resorcinols, quinones, vanillin, guaiacols, and numerous more that can be obtained by lignin catalytic reactions (Li et al. 2015a). This treatment method has the potential to become the primary method for creating lignin sulfur-free in the near future. Additionally, the reagents used are inexpensive and readily recovered. However, at the time, its large-scale adoption has been hampered by the lack of selectivity that leads to undesirable effects (Rodríguez (2020)).

11.3.4 Organosolv Process

One of the most potential substitutes for the existing traditional pulping techniques is the organosolv process, which treats biomass by using organic solvents as delignifying agents (Figueiredo et al. 2018). Research on this procedure commenced when Kleinert and Tayanthal identified, in 1931, that wood could be delignified with a combination of water and ethanol under increased temperature and pressure (Sixta et al. 2006). This approach has been used with a variety of solvents over the years, including alcohols like methanol; organic acids like acetic and formic acids, phenols, ketones, and ethylene glycol; and combined organic solvent-inorganic compounds (Alriols et al. 2009; Capolupo and Faraco 2016). Moreover, basic or acidic catalysts can be included to increase this process's effectiveness (Galkin and

Samec 2016). In order to delignify, organic solvent and water mixes are used, which dissolve some of the lignin and hemicellulose (Viell et al. 2013). Depending on the used solvent, the procedure is conducted at temperatures ranging from 100 to 250 °C and pressures up to 250 bar (Kiran and Balkan 1994). The lignin-carbohydrate and α-O-4 connections are primarily broken throughout this process, but when the lignin oligomers are separated from the lignocellulose matrix, β-O-4 may also be cleaved to some extent (Galkin and Samec 2016). Once the temperature, pH, and concentration of the organic solvent are all adjusted, the dissolved lignin and hemicelluloses can be recovered and separated by either evaporating the organic solvent or precipitating the lignin (Viell et al. 2013; Matsushita 2015). Since lignin produced using these methods has a low molecular weight (500–5000 Da) (Galkin and Samec 2016; Lora and Glasser 2002), no sulfur, and a low carbohydrate content, it is highly pure and can be used as a phenolic precursor or as a source of aromatic structures for glue, binders, and polymer substitutes (Zakzeski et al. 2010; Zhao et al. 2017). Considering the advantages of isolating cellulose, hemicellulose, and lignin, coupled with apprehensions regarding the environmental repercussions of conventional pulping, organosolv techniques are anticipated to garner increased attention for biomass fractionation in the future (Azadi et al. 2013). Despite the advantages it offers, this delignification method is rarely used routinely, as it severely corrodes equipment and produces pulp of inferior quality to that of soda and kraft pulping techniques (Laurichesse and Avérous 2014). Moreover, random condensation processes may take place instead of the depolymerization reactions in acidic environments. For instance, new C-C bonds may occur as a result of the synthesis of benzylic cations in acidic environments (Galkin and Samec 2016). In light of all of this, the natural structure of lignin is altered upon extraction. Additionally, depending on the plant source, kraft, organosolv, sulfate, and soda lignin possess different structures. Its structure, reactivity, and physical and chemical characteristics will therefore be crucial in determining its usage in new markets (Strassberger et al. 2014).

A summary of the discussed methods of lignin recovery as well as their characteristics and applications are summarized in Table 11.2.

11.4 Techniques of Lignin Modification

Lignin is a key ingredient for the development of innovative materials, either with or without chemical modification. While unmodified lignin can be incorporated directly to polymer matrices to improve properties like antioxidant and UV stability, its application is restricted to small amounts due to its thermal instability and mechanical limitations (Figueiredo et al. 2018). To exploit its full potential, different chemical modification techniques can be used. These involve depolymerization that yields smallest and usable fragments, the introduction of new reactive sites, modifications of the hydroxyl groups, and the formation of graft copolymers. Each strategy is dependent on the structural properties and particular reactivity of the functional groups of lignin, which ultimately affects the effectiveness and the

Table 11.2 Summary of the main extraction techniques of lignin, its properties and possible applications

Extraction technique	Symbol of lignin	Properties	Main applications
Kraft	KL	Hydrophobicity and solubility in alkali or organic solvents Diversity of functional groups in its structure including carboxyl, phenolic hydroxyl, and methoxy groups	Adhesives, emulsifiers, or dispersant Medicinal or cosmetic preparations
Sulfite (Lignosulfonate)	LS	Good solubility in alkaline conditions Sulfonic, carboxyl and phenolic hydroxyl groups are presented Good water solubility	Surfactants, flocculants, and dispersants in the concrete market Vanillin in the food industry
Alkaline	AL	High average molecular weight No sulfur content Inexpensive and readily recoverable reagents.	Cresols, catechols, resorcinols, quinones, vanillin, guaiacols in the food sector
Organosolv	OL	High purity with low molecular weight Sulfur-free Low carbohydrate content	Glue, binders, in polymer substitutions Phenolic precursor

suitability of the produced lignin-based materials for a range of applications (Laurichesse and Avérous 2014; Ragauskas et al. 2014).

The following section briefly investigates these various modification methods, each categorization can be divided into distinct submethods with its unique characteristics, benefits, and limitations.

11.4.1 Depolymerization of Lignin

Methods for lignin depolymerization seek to decompose lignin into low molecular weight molecules, such as vanillin, aromatic acids, aldehydes, and other useful chemicals (Amen-Chen et al.; Erdocia et al. 2012). These techniques aim to reveal the structure and composition of lignin, as well as to generate valuable components from waste lignin. In the last 60 years, a range of thermochemical conversion processes, such as pyrolysis, oxidation, hydrogenolysis, and gasification, have received considerable attention (Pandey and Kim 2011). These various depolymerization methods present distinct profiles in terms of their operational conditions, efficiency, and environmental implications, each catering to different aspects of lignin valorization.

Pyrolysis and gasification are thermal processes that break down lignin at high temperatures to make a range of products, notably bio-oils, gases and char (Figueiredo et al. 2018). Pyrolysis, carried out in the absence of oxygen, provides a wide range of products and enables high conversion rates, but it is limited by its high energy consumption and lack of selectivity (Pandey and Kim 2011; Huber et al. 2006; Tan et al. 2024). Gasification, while performed under regulated conditions of oxygen or steam, turns lignin into syngas, an essential building block for a number of chemicals and fuels. It is appropriate for integration into current energy systems because it generates cleaner-burning fuel, has higher energy conversion rates, and provides greater control and consistency (Samani et al. 2024).

On the other hand, more focused depolymerization pathways are provided by oxidation and hydrogenolysis. With the use of oxidizing agents like metal catalysts or peroxides, oxidation breaks down ether bonds to produce useful aromatic chemicals like vanillin with remarkable specificity (Laurichesse and Avérous 2014; Pandey and Kim 2011). This approach is outstanding for applications seeking precise aromatic product profiles but is constrained by the necessity for precise control to avoid over-oxidation and degradation of the intended end-products. Using hydrogen, hydrogenolysis breaks down lignin linkages at temperatures between 300 and 600 °C with a high degree of selectivity for particular monomers (Pandey and Kim 2011; Huber et al. 2006). Despite offering focused depolymerization with an emphasis on high-value products, hydrogenolysis is hindered by its dependence on expensive catalysts, the possibility of catalyst deactivation, and the need for high-pressure reactors, which render the process more complicated and raise operating costs (Shen et al. 2022). Ultimately, the intended product specificity, cost constraints, and environmental factors will influence the depolymerization technique selection.

11.4.2 Creation of New Active Sites on Lignin

Lignin comprises diverse functional groups including hydroxyl, methoxyl, carbonyl and carboxyl, positioning it as a versatile option for chemical modification. These modifications are designed to improve lignin solubility in organic solvents, decrease the brittleness of lignin-based polymers, and increase its chemical reactivity, thereby enabling improved processing and broader applications (Laurichesse and Avérous 2014). Hydroxyalkylation, amination, nitration, and sulfonation are common modifications that improve the reactivity of hydroxyl groups and provide new chemical active sites (Laurichesse and Avérous 2014). Through the process of hydroxyalkylation, lignin reacts with formaldehyde or other aldehydes to improve its adhesive qualities and significantly reduce its free formaldehyde concentration, which allows it for use in phenolic wood adhesives (Laurichesse and Avérous 2014; Saito et al. 2012). This technique uses non-toxic substitutes such glutaraldehyde to partially replace phenol in resin manufacturing, making the process more ecologically friendly (Lisý et al. 2022). Amination, on the other hand, incorporates amine functional groups to the lignin structure via reactions like the Mannich reaction, which can take place at different pH levels (Meister 2002; arend 1998; Du et al. 2014). This modification makes lignin more ionizable and positively charged properties, which renders it valuable for uses such as surfactants and asphalt emulsifiers (Du et al. 2014; Pan et al. 2013; Yuliestyan et al. 2018). Although amination enhances colloidal characteristics and improves the number of reactive sites, it frequently uses hazardous chemicals and extra procedures that can overcomplicate the process.

Usually, nitration takes place in non-aqueous solvents with agents such as nitric acid and acetic anhydride. The result is an amorphous powder that is yellow to brown, with a molecular weight between 600 and 2000 Da, and has a nitrogen concentration in the range of 6–7% (Laurichesse and Avérous 2014; Meister 2002; Zhang and Huang 2001). When utilized in polyurethane-nitro lignin (PU-NL) films, this modification improves lignin mechanical qualities, such as its stiffness, toughness, and tensile strength (Zhang and Huang 2001). Nevertheless, raising the NCO/OH molar ratio decreases film flexibility and recovery capacity because of the restricted movement of PU molecules induced by the strong cross-linking density (Zhang and Huang 2001). On the other hand, sulfomethylation uses methanol, alkali metal sulfite salts, and lignin to introduce methylene sulfonate groups into lignin in aqueous, neutral to basic conditions (Du et al. 2014; He and Fatehi 2015). By modifying the reaction conditions, the sulfonated lignin products can be produced to have improved dispersibility and be used as dye dispersants (Madzhidova et al. 1998). Furthermore, by adding sulfonate groups using sodium sulfite or sulfuric acid, sulfonation creates lignin with potent electrostatic repulsion characteristics, which are especially useful as dispersants in cement matrices (Du et al. 2014; Ouyang et al. 2009).

11.4.3 Chemical Modification of Active Functional Groups

Lignins comprise phenolic hydroxyl groups in addition to aliphatic hydroxyl groups situated at C-α and C-γ of their side chains. The most reactive functional components among them are phenolic hydroxyl groups, which have a major impact on the chemical reactivity of materials. When these hydroxyl groups are modified, lignin polyol derivatives are produced, which improves lignin solubility. These modifications increase the availability of highly reactive hydroxyl groups by converting a significant portion of phenolic hydroxyl groups to aliphatic hydroxyl units. Various functionalization techniques, including alkylation, esterification, etherification, phenolation, and urethanization, have been investigated in a number of research to introduce additional functional groups and increase the reactivity of lignin (Laurichesse and Avérous 2014).

Alkylation is the process that introduces alkyl groups to the lignin structure to make it more hydrophobic and compatible with non-polar matrices. This technique is particularly useful in increasing lignin dispersibility in hydrophobic polymers, making it excellent for composite applications. Nevertheless, alkylated lignin may be highly brittle, which could be undesirable in polymer blends (Li and Sarkanen 2002). Conversely, esterification creates ester groups through the reaction of hydroxyl groups in lignin with carboxylic acids or their byproducts. Through this process, the thermal stability and compatibility of lignin with other polymers are greatly increased, making it appropriate for use in coatings and thermoplastic composites. Compared to alkylation, esterification is comparatively simple and safer;

nonetheless, it might reduce the inherent antioxidant characteristics of lignin and frequently requires catalysts or high temperatures, which raises processing costs and decreases environmental friendliness (Kaur et al. 2017).

Etherification involves the reaction of lignin hydroxyl groups with alkyl halides or epoxides to produce ether linkages (Liu et al. 2019b). This approach is particularly useful for increasing lignin solubility in non-polar organic solvents and compatibility with a variety of polymer systems, including epoxy resins. Etherification often retains more of the original structure than alkylation, preserving its inherent characteristics while enhancing processability (Buono et al. 2016; Sameni et al. 2017). Nonetheless, one disadvantage of most lignin etherification procedures is that toxic solvents are employed, and hazardous wastes (halogenated species) are created, especially for homogeneous catalytic systems (Liu et al. 2019b). Another approach, phenolation, involves grafting phenol groups onto lignin to improve its reactivity with formaldehyde in resin compositions (Laurichesse and Avérous 2014; Effendi et al. 2008). This renders phenolated lignin an excellent precursor for phenolic resins used in adhesives, coatings, and foams. The resultant materials display better mechanical characteristics and thermal stability. However, the process often involves huge volumes of sulfuric acid, contributing to high costs and environmental challenges due to the requirement for complex recovery techniques (Eraghi et al. 2019). Urethanization involves the inclusion of urethane groups via isocyanate reactions, which considerably improves lignin compatibility with polyurethanes (Lee 2006). This is particularly useful in foam and elastomer applications. Although urethanization gives lignin-based materials flexibility and durability, its scalability for industrial applications is limited due to the use of hazardous and highly reactive isocyanates, require strict safety procedures and present environmental risks.

11.4.4 Production of Lignin Graft Copolymers

Lignin can be utilized to create lignin graft copolymers, which are star-like branching copolymers with a lignin core created by attaching polymer chains to the hydroxyl groups on the lignin structure (De Oliveira and Glasser 1994). Two main procedures have been carried out in order to develop the lignin graft copolymers: "grafting from" and "grafting to" strategies (Duval and Lawoko 2014).

There are noticeable trade-offs between the several processes used to produce lignin graft copolymers with regard to final material characteristics, efficiency, and process control. For applications requiring exact material characteristics, ring-opening polymerization (ROP) is excellent at producing well-defined copolymers with regulated molecular weights (Duval and Lawoko 2014; Cateto et al. 2009). However, it frequently requires strict reaction conditions and metal catalysts, which reduces its cost-effectiveness for large-scale production and increases the possibility of contamination. In contrast, radical polymerization is a more straightforward and adaptable method that enables the employment of a wide variety of monomers in mild environments (De Oliveira and Glasser 1994; Koshi Jima and Muraki 1968).

Its main drawback is its imprecise molecular weight control and homogeneity, which might result in inconsistent material characteristics.

Atom transfer radical polymerization (ATRP) gives improved control over polymerization, allowing the synthesis of copolymers with set chain lengths and tailored topologies (Laurichesse and Avérous 2014; Coessens et al.). This precision renders ATRP outstanding for advanced uses such as nanocomposites and biomedical materials. However, it entails extensive purification stages to remove metal residues and demands precise control over reaction conditions, which may restrict scalability and raise production costs. The "grafting to" process allows high control on the copolymer structure by connecting pre-synthesized polymers to lignin, which is advantageous for generating materials with specific features (Duval and Lawoko 2014). Nonetheless, it often results in inferior grafting density due to steric hindrance and can be time-consuming and expensive due to the requirement for pre-synthesized polymers and several reaction stages.

11.5 Lignin Based Nanomaterial Synthesis

Lignin is a key component in the synthesis of nanomaterials, owing to its abundance and unique chemical structure. It can be converted into multiple nanostructures, such as nanoparticles, nanotubes, nanofibers, nanocapsules and hydrogels. Lignin-based nanomaterials reveal improved mechanical and thermal performance, making them appropriate for various applications. The reactive functional groups found on the surface of lignin provide versatility since they make it simple to modify and interact with other materials in nanocomposites (Singh 2023). Methods such as anti-solvent precipitation, solvent exchange, polymerization and sonication are widely used for preparing lignin nanomaterials, enabling size, shape and distribution to be controlled (Zhao et al. 2016). The next section discusses some significant techniques for synthesizing lignin nanoparticles.

11.5.1 Solvent Exchange

The solvent shifting approach involves a solution of an organic compound in a water-miscible organic solvent, which is then mixed with an excess of water, leading to nanoparticle formation due to reduced solubility (Chauhan 2020). In the case of lignin, this process is carried out by dissolving lignin in an organic solvent such as Tetrahydrofuran (THF) or a THF/methanol mixture. After that, a dialysis membrane containing the lignin solution is immersed in deionized water for 24 hours. Lignin nanoparticles precipitate during this period when water gradually replaces the organic solvent, most likely via a nucleation-growth mechanism (Chauhan 2020; Lievonen et al. 2016). A wide array of applications exists for this technique, demonstrating a clear framework. However, the main drawback of this technique is the small solid content, which is about 1 weight percent (Beisl et al. 2017). Qian et al. (2014) synthesized colloidal lignin spheres measuring 110 nm for the first time using the self-assembly process, which involved dissolving acetylated lignin in THF and then gradually adding water (67%) to the mixture. As a result, hydrophobic interactions induced the lignin molecules to bind together (Qian et al. 2014). Among the parameters impacting the LNPs size, the pre-dialysis concentration of the lignin solution appears to have a key effect. Lievonen et al. (2016) investigated how particle size and PDI were affected by lignin concentrations ranging from 1 to 20 mg/mL. When the pre-dialysis lignin concentration was 1 mg/mL, the particle size and PDI decreased to a minimum of 200 nm and 0.15, respectively. Whereas when the starting concentration was 20 mg/mL, the particle size and PDI increased to 2000 nm and 0.56, respectively. This effect can be explained by the fact that more lignin is available to support the formation of nanoparticles at higher lignin concentrations. Higher size and PDI values are the outcome of the fast nucleation-growth process, which creates nanoparticles of different sizes. On the other hand, nucleus formation is less likely to occur at lower lignin concentrations, which lowers the average nanoparticle size and PDI values by decreasing the possibility of bigger particle creation (Lievonen et al. 2016). Another important parameter for controlling LNPs size and uniformity is the order of solvent addition. This parameter was studied by Zhang et al. (2022) in their research, where they explored the effectiveness of LNPs in UV protection for PVA composite films. They employed two techniques: the conventional anti-solvent method and the trans anti-solvent method. The conventional procedure, as shown in Fig. 11.2, entails introducing deionized water to a lignin solution gradually. This causes phase separation and the development of bigger, irregular nanoparticles. On the other hand, the trans anti-solvent approach produces smaller, more homogeneous LNPs by introducing deionized water dropwise into the lignin solution, which promotes supersaturation. When incorporated into PVA films, these well-stabilized nanoparticles which are driven by π-π interactions showed improved UV-blocking efficiency (Zhang et al. 2022).

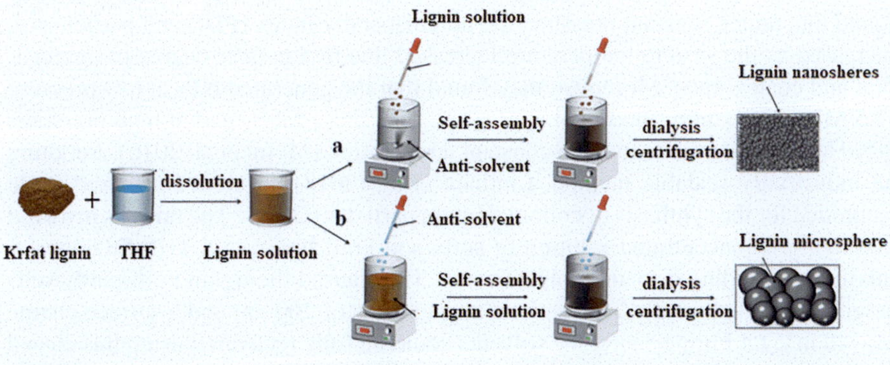

Fig. 11.2 The synthetic pathway adopted to produce lignin micro/nanospheres: (**a**) trans anti-solvent process for lignin nanospheres; (**b**) conventional anti-solvent process for lignin microspheres (Zhang et al. 2022)

11.5.2 Anti-solvent Precipitation

The capacity of anti-solvent precipitation techniques for producing microparticles and microparticulate components led to their investigation. This technique involves agitating an aqueous solution while adding an organic solution containing the desired polymer. Removal of the organic solvent by extraction or evaporation leads to polymer precipitation and the production of solid microparticles. Among the often-utilized anti-solvents are methanol, ethanol, and acetone (Zasadowski et al. 2014). Temperature at solvent evaporation and the existence of emulsifiers are two critical factors influencing nanoparticle formation and thus its size. Researchers have proposed that with the use of higher temperatures, smaller nanoparticles are formed throughout the precipitation process. Maintaining the temperature at least 20 °C below the organic solvent boiling point will yield the best nanoparticle properties (Mondal et al. 2023). Besides the aforementioned factors, further parameters such as pressure, rate of the solution injection, starting concentration of lignin solution, can be adjusted to control the size and shape of the obtained NPs (Myint et al. 2016). For instance, the impact of water drop speed on lignin nanosphere size was investigated by Xiong et al. (2017). Once water was added to an enzymatic hydrolysis lignin solution in THF at a starting concentration of 0.5 mg/ml at dropping rates of 2 to 8 mL/min, the size of the nanospheres reduced from around 315 nm to 190 nm, respectively (Xiong et al. 2017). Using ethanol, methanol, and acetone, Al-Rudainy et al. (2018) investigated the antisolvent precipitation method and evaluated the effects of temperature, pH, and solute concentration. Methanol produced the lowest yield, whilst acetone produced the greatest. While temperatures over 25 °C and higher pH values (up to 11.8) greatly enhanced precipitation, increased solute dilution resulted in lower yields. According to the study, the procedure was optimized by heating samples and anti-solvents and modifying pH with sodium hydroxide; the highest yield was recorded at pH 11.8 (Wallberg et al. 2018). In another study which was conducted by Myint et al. (2016), compressed liquid CO_2 was used as an anti-solvent and DMF was used to dissolve the kraft lignin to examine the effects of temperature and pressure on the size and shape of the NPs. They found that under constant pressure, the polydispersity index (PDI) and particle size increased as the system temperature increased due to a greater degree of aggregation and coalescence. Moreover, they found that the generated NPs at low pressure (7.5 MPa) were more fused and aggregated than those fabricated at high pressures (15.0 MPa) while maintaining a constant temperature (Myint et al. 2016). Adopting an industrially scalable method, Lintinen et al. (2018) developed a closed cycle technique for the synthesis of colloidal lignin particles (CLPs). The process involved dissolving a concentrated solution of softwood kraft lignin in a THF/EtOH/water mixture and adding it to anti-solvent water. This caused the lignin to instantly self-assemble into spherical CLPs with an average size of 200 nm and a surface charge of −40 mV.7.4 Furthermore, the solvents could be fully recovered using this closed cycle system with minimal energy usage (Lintinen et al. 2018).

11.5.3 Self-Assembly Method

Self-assembly is a process in which pre-existing components autonomously arrange into a structured or ordered system due to precise intermolecular interactions, including electrostatic, hydrophobic, hydrogen bonding, and Van der Waals forces without external direction (Chauhan 2020; Zhang et al. 2022). This technique is commonly used for nanoparticle synthesis, as it depends on noncovalent interactions to establish an organized configuration of particles. Qian et al. (2017) developed a straightforward and effective self-assembly technique to produce large, medium, and small lignin-based colloidal spheres utilizing enzymatic hydrolysis lignin (EHL) and organosolv lignin (OL) as raw ingredients. Using EHL as a case study, substantial colloidal spheres were synthesized by incrementally introducing NaCl aqueous solutions into the 10 g/L EHL acetone/water (8:1, vol/vol) solution. Midsize colloidal spheres were produced similarly, however NaCl aqueous solutions had to be substituted with water. The concentration of the EHL acetone/water (8:1, vol/vol) solution would be reduced to 0.1 g/L if small spheres were needed. EHL solutions were then added to water to create nanoscale particles. Lignin-based colloidal spheres of various diameters might be effectively produced by simply modifying a few parameters. Another study by Li et al. (2016) suggested a simple and useful technique for creating complex spherical micelles based on lignin in green solvents with pH-responsive characteristics. Following quaternization, the alkali lignin (AL) was allowed to self-assemble to create complex lignin-based micelles using sodium dodecyl benzene sulfonate (SDBS) in an ethanol/water blend as the water content increased, from 0 to over 86% (Li et al. 2017). Liu et al. (2019c) synthesized LNPs utilizing the Sequential Organosolv Fragmentation Approach (SOFA) with ethanol and several phases of catalysts to selectively dissolve lignin from corn stover. This approach was used to create uniform lignin streams and adjust their chemical characteristics and reactivity, enabling the production of consistent grade LNPs by self-assembly. The optimal particle diameter remained consistent across the stages: stage 1 (50% ethanol +1% sulfuric acid), stage 3 (50% ethanol), and stage 2 (50% ethanol +1% formic acid). As a result, the SOFA process with ethanol and sulfuric acid yielded the lowest particle diameter, around 130 nm (Liu et al. 2019c). In a recent research, carried out by Tanganini et al. (2023), authors examined the use of elephant grass lignin to produce lignin nanoparticles. The lignin extraction technique featured a sequential acid-alkaline pretreatment process, which produced very pure lignin, then LNPs self-assembly by dissolving lignin in acetone and using water as an antisolvent. As can be seen from Fig. 11.3, the method produced spherical nanoparticles with a smooth surface and an average diameter of about 80 nm. The self-assembly mechanism is governed by the amphiphilic character of lignin, with hydrophobic fragments forming the inner core of nanoparticles and hydrophilic functional groups exposing the surface, thereby improving their colloidal stability (Tanganini et al. 2023).

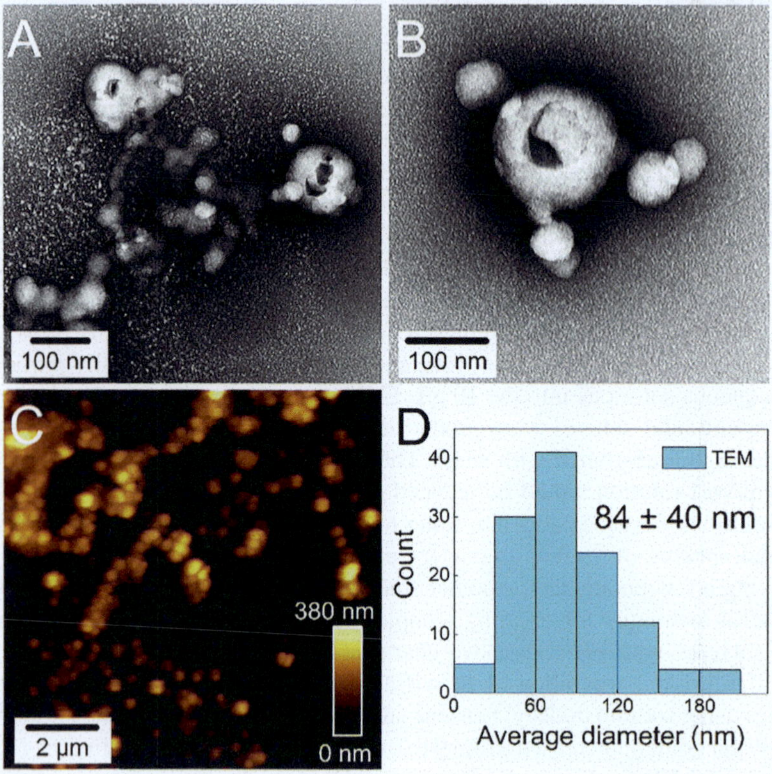

Fig. 11.3 (**a**, **b**) TEM images of SA-LNPs. (**c**) AFM topography images of SA-LNPs. (**d**) Histogram of the average diameter size distribution of lignin nanoparticles obtained from TEM image measurements using ImageJ software, reused from ref (Tanganini et al. 2023) under the CC-BY-3.0 license

11.5.4 Acid Precipitation Method

This is one of the most widely known and commonly utilized procedures, resulting in irregular network structure forms and unstable sedimentation caused by the protonation of lignin's charged groups, which has an impact on LNP stability. The most often utilized acids include HCl, HNO_3, and H_2SO_4 (Parvathy et al. 2021). Acid precipitation occurs when the pH of lignin solution is changed to almost 2, resulting in the precipitation of lignin nanoparticles. Frangville et al. (2012) discovered an innovative acid preparation process for producing lignin nanoparticles. This study proposed two alternate approaches. The first approach produced lignin nanoparticles in the form of precipitates by adding hydrochloric acid to the ethylene glycol solution of lignin, followed by cross-linking and water dialysis, which remained stable over a wide pH range. In the second technique, the lignin nanoparticles were generated by quickly introducing HNO_3 solutions into the high pH aqueous lignin solutions, which was stable only at low pH (Frangville et al. 2012). Pang et al.

(2017) produced lignin nanoparticles using an alkaline lignin solution by changing the pH to 11 with sodium hydroxide solution while stirring constantly. After agitating the resultant solution for a full night to dissolve the lignin particles, sodium dodecyl sulfate was added while stirring, and LNPs were produced by using HCL to bring the pH of the solution to 2.5 while stirring continuously. The solution was then dialyzed for five days in ultra-pure water. The findings showed that the nanoparticles size reduced and stayed in the 50–250 nm range when the sodium dodecyl sulfate concentration increased (Pang et al. 2017). In their study, Obrzut et al. (2024) investigated the effects of pH and salt type on the formation and characteristics of lignin nanoparticles through a biorefinery procedure integrated with microbial electrolysis. The authors employed various salts, such as phosphate, carbonate, nitrate, and chloride, to adjust the size and shape of LNPs, while systematically altering the pH. Their findings indicated that various salts led to the development of unique nanoparticle shapes: spherical LNPs were generated with phosphate salts, rod-like structures were formed with nitrate and chloride, and flower-like morphologies with carbonate salts (Fig. 11.4). SEM analyses demonstrated that the flower-like LNPs, produced at basic pH in carbonate solutions, displayed the highest surface

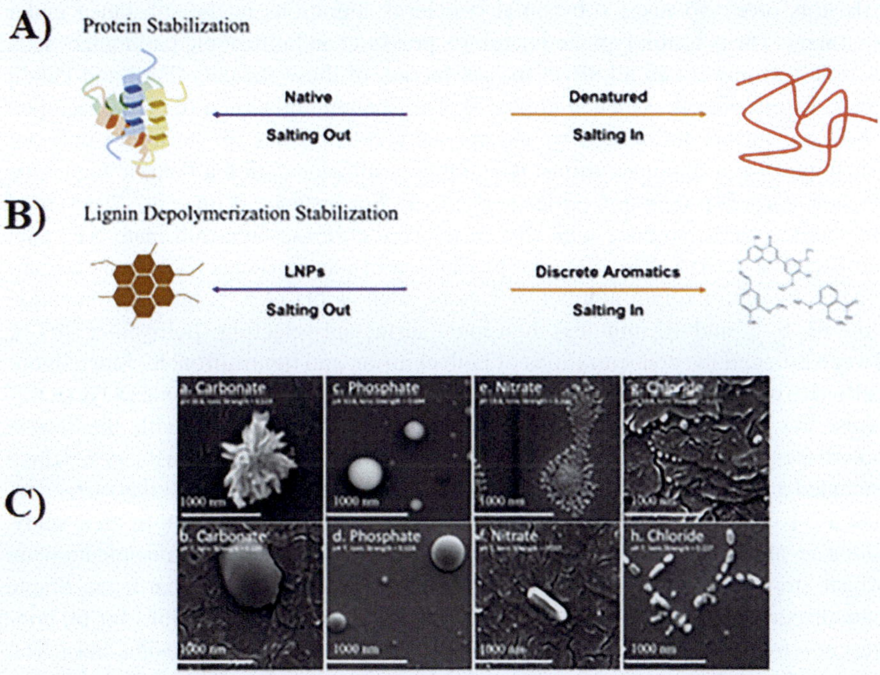

Fig. 11.4 (**a**) The Hofmeister series effect on protein stabilization. (**b**) The hypothesized stability of depolymerized lignin with respect to ion type is illustrated. (**c**) SEM images of select LNPs, all taken at t = 7 d. (**a**) carbonate, basic, I = 0.529; (**b**) carbonate, neutral, I = 0.185; (**c**) phosphate, basic, I = 0.694; (**d**) phosphate, neutral, I = 0.526; (**e**) nitrate, basic, I = 0.227; (**f**) nitrate, neutral, I = 0.227; (**g**) chloride, basic, I = 0.227; (**h**) chloride, neutral, I = 0.227 (Reproduced from ref. Obrzut et al. (2024) under the CC-BY-3.0 license)

area-to-volume ratio, leading to enhanced antioxidant activity similar to the commercial standard antioxidant, Trolox. The researchers also examined the influence of pH and the Hofmeister effect on the stability of LNPs through the use of previously mentioned salts. They addressed how these factors affect the stability of LNP at different pH values. They discovered that the LNPs stability was improved, particularly at higher pH values in solutions that contained kosmotropic salts like phosphate. On the other hand, especially at lower pH values, chaotropic salts such as chloride were less successful in stabilizing the nanoparticles. Overall, their findings reveal that the pH level and salt type have a significant impact on regulating the colloidal stability of LNPs, which is important for applications including cosmetics and pharmaceuticals where long-term stability is crucial (Obrzut et al. 2024).

11.5.5 Ultrasonication Method

Ultrasonication is a process based on the cavitation phenomenon, in which millions of vapor bubbles develop in a liquid and then burst or implode, producing high pressure and temperatures quickly (Mondal et al. 2023). In addition to producing radicals, this process causes substantial structural alterations in the substance under treatment. The solution type, temperature, pressure, and ultrasonic parameters such as time and power can all affect the production of these radicals (Patil and Pandit 2007; Kuijpers et al.; Gilca et al. 2015). The content and structure of the resultant LNPs are further influenced by the special characteristics of the lignin polymer when applied to lignin solutions, which makes ultrasonication a flexible technique for nanoparticle production (Gilca et al. 2015). For instance, Kim et al. (2013) used ultrasonication to produce ionically crosslinked chitosan–lignosulfonate NPs with antibacterial activity. The effective production of nanoparticles (NPs) was accomplished by optimizing a number of factors, such as pH (4.5, 5, and 6), sonication time (2, 5, 8, and 10 minutes), non-ionic surfactant selection (poloxamer 407 or Tween 80), and the concentrations of both chitosan and lignosulfonate. Since lignosulfonate contains sulfonate groups (SO_3-), which function as anionic polyelectrolytes, the chitosan NPs were more stable. The smallest NPs with the lowest polydispersity index (PDI) were produced under the best circumstances, which included a pH of 5, 8 minutes of sonication, 1% (v/v) poloxamer as the surfactant, and a 2:1 mass ratio of chitosan to lignosulfonate (Kim et al. 2013). In their study, Gilca et al. (2015) investigated the sonochemical process of ultrasonication on wheat straw and Sarkanda grass lignins to produce lignin nanoparticles. Stable nanodispersions were produced by sonicating aqueous lignin solutions for 60 minutes at a frequency of 20 kHz and a power of 600 W using an ultrasonic horn. The average diameter decreased from the micron to the nanometer scale (0.01–0.05 μm), indicating a considerable drop in particle size. Further confirmation of the development of distinct lignin nanoparticles smaller than 100 nm was provided by TEM investigation. Furthermore, a decrease of the PDI and molecular weight was noticed, indicating that the sonication method caused lignin depolymerization, especially for Sarkanda grass lignin (Gilca et al. 2015). In a related study, Gonzalez et al. (2017)

used ultrasonication to synthesize lignin nanoparticles from softwood kraft lignin. In their research, they prepared a 0.1% (wt.) lignin suspension in water and ultrasonically sonicated it at a frequency of 20 kHz with a 130 W power source and a 95% oscillation amplitude. Using an ultrasonic tip, the sonication procedure was conducted for 2, 4, and 6 hours at different intervals. Following each treatment, they noticed that the resulting LNPs had irregular morphologies with a noticeable decrease in particle size. Indeed, following a 6-hour treatment period, they produced lignin nanoparticles ranging from 10 to 50 nm, beginning with lignin agglomerates that had dimensions between 1 and 3 μm (Garcia Gonzalez et al. 2017).

11.5.6 Interfacial Crosslinking

The interfacial crosslinking process involves mixing an aqueous and an oily phase, either by using or not using surfactants or crosslinking agents, to form precursor microemulsions that produce particles after the dispersed materials have been crosslinked (Nypelö et al. 2015; Tortora et al. 2014). Using this process, Li et al. (2015b) fabricated porous lignosulfonate spheres from the cross-linking reaction of lignosulfonate and sodium alginate using epichlorohydrin as a cross-linking agent followed by dropwise adding into CaCl2 solutions for gelation and solidification. The produced lignosulfonate spheres demonstrated a clear porous structure with significant porosity and a big pore volume (Li et al. 2015b). Chen et al. (2016) also employed lignosulfonate to produce oil-in-water microemulsions and pH-sensitive nanocapsules for encapsulating hydrophobic compounds. Lignosulfonate was first modified by grafting allyl groups via etherification. Once this step had been completed, a microemulsion was prepared using ultrasound. In this formulation, the modified lignosulfonate and the surfactant sodium dodecyl sulfate were dissolved in the aqueous phase. The oil phase consisted of butyl acetate, accompanied by a co-stabilizer (hexadecane), an initiator and a cross-linking agent. At the water-oil interface, lignosulfonate and the cross-linker were in contact and underwent a thiol-ene crosslinking reaction induced by free radicals (Chen et al. 2016). In their research, Wang et al. (2024) investigated the use of interfacial crosslinking with a deep eutectic solvent (DES) to manufacture lignin microcapsules as an environmentally friendly substitute for traditional organic solvents. After dissolving lignin in a choline chloride-lactic acid-based DES, the authors emulsified the mixture with soybean oil that contained epichlorohydrin or poly(ethylene glycol) diglycidyl ether (PEGDE) as crosslinking agents. In order to produce microcapsules, the technique required vigorous mixing to form emulsions and then heating to promote crosslinking at the interface between oil and water. According to their findings, epichlorohydrin enabled the production of smaller, more uniform microcapsules, around 2 μm in size, whereas PEGDE generated larger microcapsules with a wider size dispersion (Wang et al. 2024).

11.6 Applications of Lignin Nanoparticles

The production of lignin-based nanomaterials has significant advantages, such as improved characteristics of polymer blends and increased antioxidant activity attributable to high surface area-to-volume ratios (Nair et al. 2014; Yearla and Padmasree 2016; Lu et al. 2012). Furthermore, the availability of functional groups on the lignin structure that could be easily chemically transformed expands the potential of LNPs for a wide range of biomedical applications (Figueiredo et al. 2018).Their prospective uses encompass drug delivery systems, tissue engineering, and wound healing, providing revolutionary solutions in healthcare (see Fig. 11.5). The following section will explore these applications in further detail, analyzing their mechanisms and potential effects.

11.6.1 Drug and Gene Delivery

Drug delivery systems are sophisticated technologies aimed at improving the therapeutic effectiveness of pharmaceutical agents or natural chemicals at specific places, such as tumors, while reducing potential hazardous side effects (Alqahtani et al. 2019). The primary advantages of these nanostructures encompass safeguarding the drugs from quick disintegration upon systemic administration and employing specialized ligands to target the drug to cancer cells, therefore improving its absorption

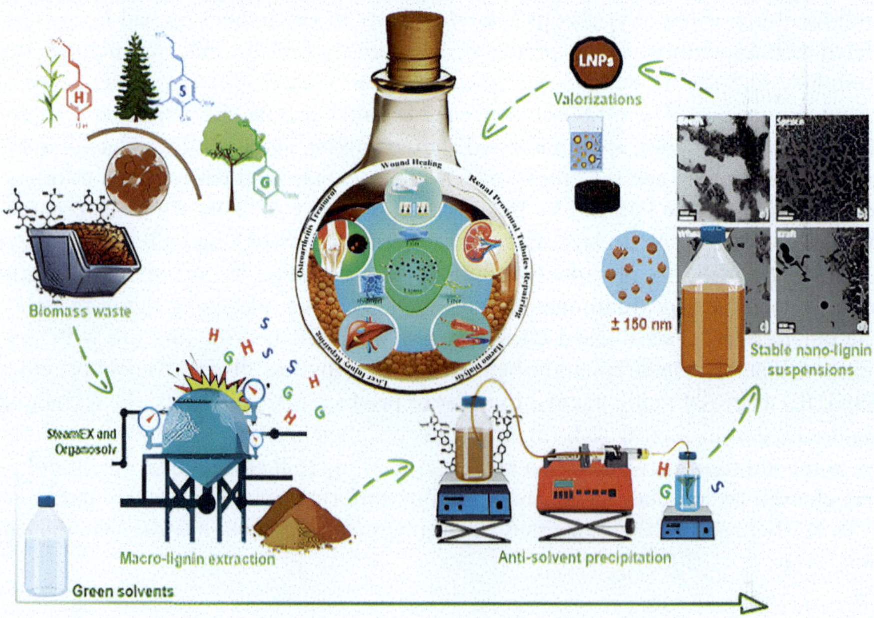

Fig. 11.5 Overview of lignin production and applications in different medical applications fields

by tumors (Khadem et al. 2024). Engineered nanoparticles demonstrate significant utility in the field of biomedicine, attributed to their enhanced surface to mass ratio relative to other particles. This distinctive characteristic allows nanoparticles to possess improved ability to bind, adsorb, and transport valuable compounds, including drugs, genes, and proteins (De Jong and Borm 2008). Among the natural and biodegradable carriers of drugs available, lignin nanoparticles seem to be the most promising green instrument for drug delivery because of the low-cost raw material, easy and controllable transformation into uniform NPs (Tian et al. 2017). Drugs can be encapsulated or dispersed using lignin in particle systems such as nanoparticles, nanocapsules, nanospheres, nanoemulsions, and micelles (Glasser et al. 1993; Dehne et al. 2017). For instance, Alqahtani et al. (2019) demonstrated the feasibility of using cross-linked organosolv lignin nanoparticles for drug delivery. In their investigation, the authors succeeded in encapsulating curcumin, a lipophilic drug model, in lignin nanoparticles (LNPs) averaging 104 nm in size, with a 92% encapsulation efficiency. The LNPs exhibited a desirable gradual release in intestinal conditions and great stability in simulated stomach environments, according to in vitro release studies. The encapsulated curcumin also showed stability during storage conditions. Furthermore, compared to free curcumin, curcumin-loaded LNPs significantly improved intestinal penetration and cellular uptake while showing minimal damage to Caco-2 cells, according to bioavailability and absorption assays. Notably, when LNPs were incubated on a Caco-2 cell monolayer, their apparent permeability increased fivefold, whereas when curcumin was formulated with LNPs, its bioavailability increased tenfold over the unformulated form. Their work showed the potential of LNPs as a non-toxic enhancement for the absorption of lipophilic oral drugs (Alqahtani et al. 2019). Another promising nanodrug carrier has been developed by Chai et al. (2021) using a straightforward microfluidic method for anticancer drugs. Lignin/chitosan nanoparticles were prepared using a solvent-shifting process, which resulted in an average particle size of about 180 nm. The electrostatic co-assembly of lignin and chitosan is achieved by interaction between carboxyl groups in lignin and amino groups in chitosan. The lignin/chitosan nanoparticles (Lig/ChiNPs) comprised two hydrophobic anticancer drugs, curcumin (CCM) and docetaxel (DTX). To examine the efficiency of the nanoparticles, in vitro drug release experiments were done using dialysis, as well as cytotoxicity assessments on HeLa cells using the CCK-8 assay. Both DTX@Lig/ChiNPs and CCM@Lig/ChiNPs demonstrated strong cytotoxic effects on HeLa cells, with drug release occurring in an acidic environment that mimicked the tumor microenvironment (Chai et al. 2021). To comprehend the impact of lignin nanoparticles on cancer drug delivery when combined with metal nanocarriers, Figueiredo et al. (2017) have developed three distinct types of lignin nanoparticles including LNPs, iron (III)-complexed lignin nanoparticles (Fe-LNPs), and Fe_3O infused lignin nanoparticles (Fe_3O_4- LNPs). The nanocarriers were loaded with varying quantities of the poorly water-soluble drugs sorafenib and benzazulene, which demonstrated an improved release profile and an antiproliferative activity against several cell lines. Consequently, it might be claimed that the superparamagnetic behavior of Fe_3O_4, combined with LNPs, has great potential for drug delivery in cancer treatment

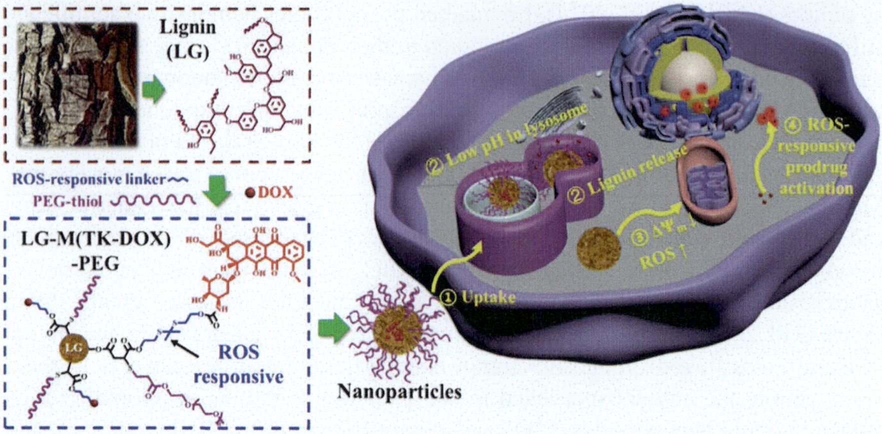

Fig. 11.6 Schematic Illustration for the Construction of LG-M(TK-DOX)-PEG Nanoparticles and the Mechanism of Oxidative Stress Amplification in Cancer Cells for ROS-Responsive DOX Drug Release (Reproduced with permission from ref. Zhou et al. (2024)

(Figueiredo et al. 2017). In a recent study, Zhou et al. (2024) developed lignin-based nanoparticles to improve tumor treatment by enhancing reactive oxygen species (ROS)-responsive drug release and amplifying oxidative stress. In order to produce the LNPs, an LG-M(TK)-PEG copolymer was produced by combining polyethylene glycol (PEG), thioketal (TK) linkages, and maleic anhydride-modified lignin (LG-M). The ROS-cleavable TK bond was attached to the anticancer drug DOX (doxorubicin) to create a ROS-activatable prodrug (LG-M(TK-DOX)-PEG). (Fig. 11.6). Nanoparticles with an average size of 125.7 nm were created by solvent-antisolvent precipitation. The researchers discovered that cancer cells absorb the LNPs more efficiently, resulting in selective ROS formation and drug release in tumor settings, as evidenced by the high ROS levels in breast cancer 4 T1 cells. Additionally, DOX-loaded nanoparticles demonstrated a regulated release under high ROS conditions, leading to considerable tumor inhibition with less systemic toxicity than free DOX treatment (Zhou et al. 2024).

11.6.2 Tissue Engineering

Tissue engineering has been recognized as a promising approach in the regenerative medicine domain for repairing, replacing, and improving the function of a given tissue or organ, employing biodegradable and biocompatible polymers (Khadem et al. 2024; Jagur-Grodzinski 2006). The field relies extensively on the utilization of scaffolds as biomaterials to simulate the extracellular matrix (ECM). Proper scaffold characteristics are necessary while establishing or determining the convenience of a scaffold for tissue engineering (O'Brien 2011). Alongside the physical and biological considerations, biocompatibility, precise mechanical characteristics,

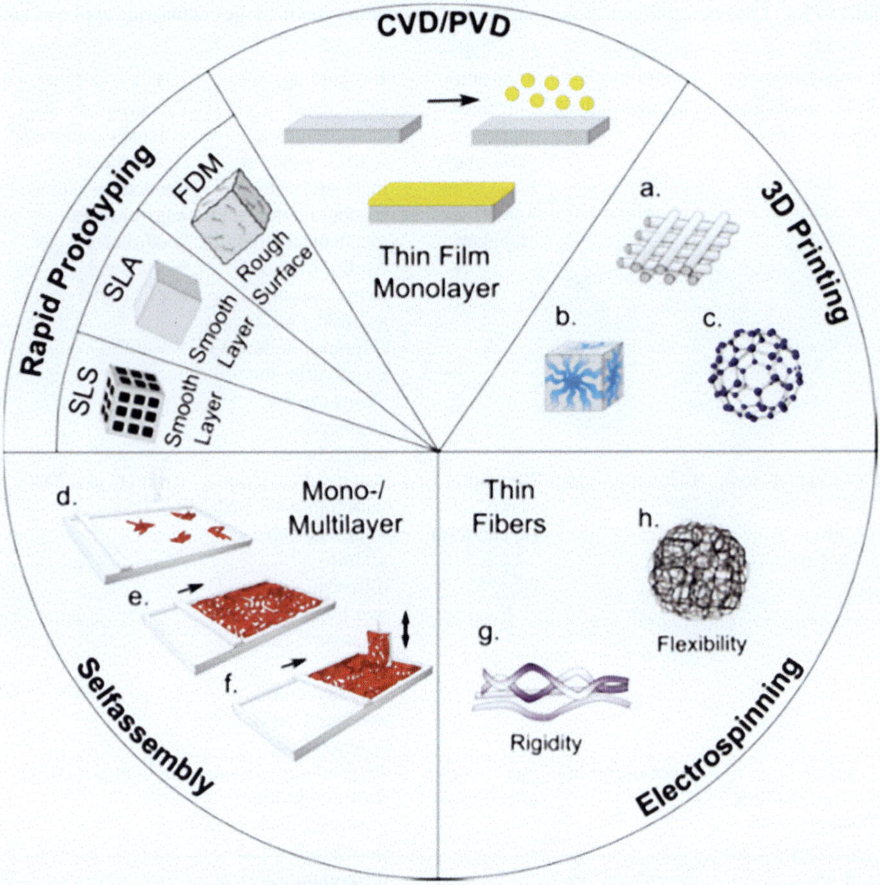

Fig. 11.7 Fabrication methods used for the development of nanostructured scaffolds for tissue engineering applications: 3D printing, electrospinning, rapid prototyping and self-assembly techniques such as Langmuir-Blodgett (Witzler et al. 2018)

porosity, surface structure, and topography are the essential parameters influencing the regeneration process (Nazeer et al. 2019). Figure 11.7 depicts the techniques utilized to create various scaffold materials for tissue engineering. These techniques include rapid prototyping (RP) methods such as selective laser sintering (SLS), selective laser ablation (SLA), chemical and physical vapor deposition (CVD, PVD), fused deposition modeling (FDM), 3D printing methods resulting in tailor-made layered, cubic and spherical structures (Witzler et al. 2018).

Multiple research has been undertaken on the potential use of lignin in various types of materials and processing processes for tissue engineering applications due to its non-toxic, ultraviolet protecting, antioxidant, and antibacterial properties (Sugiarto et al. 2022). Table 11.3 summarizes the different studies investigating lignin-based nanofibers and nanocomposites for tissue engineering applications. In

Table 11.3 Overview of lignin-Based nanofibers/nanocomposites in tissue engineering applications

Composition	Processing methodology	Potential application	Key findings	Ref
Polycaprolactone (PCL), Lignin	Electrospinning	Soft tissue scaffolds, particularly for skin and bone tissue engineering	PCL/lignin nanocomposite scaffolds showed increased porosity, biodegradation, and mechanical strength. Addition of 10% lignin optimized the scaffold's biological response, indicating its potential for various tissue engineering applications.	Electrospun polycaprolactone/lignin-based nanocomposite as a novel tissue scaffold for biomedical applications (2017)
Polycaprolactone (PCL) with Lignin Nanoparticles	Electrospinning	Peripheral nerve regeneration	Aligned PCL fibers with lignin showed improved cell viability, differentiation, and neurite length extension. In vivo studies demonstrated enhanced nerve regeneration.	Amini et al. (2020)
Poly(vinyl alcohol) (PVA), Poly(glycerol sebacate) (PGS), Lignin	Electrospinning	Nerve tissue engineering	Aligned electrospun fibers with lignin improved nerve cell proliferation and differentiation. 5% lignin in PVA-PGS showed enhanced cell growth and differentiation, indicating potential for neural tissue scaffolding.	Saudi et al. (2019)
Polyacrylamide (PAM), Lignin nanoparticles (LNP)	Free radical polymerization	Tissue regeneration, artificial muscles	PAM/LNP hydrogel displayed high compressive and tensile strength, enhanced by lignin nanoparticles acting as cross-linking junctions. The hydrogel's excellent mechanical properties make it suitable for biomedical applications.	Chen et al. (2019)

(continued)

Table 11.3 (continued)

Composition	Processing methodology	Potential application	Key findings	Ref
Poly(ε-caprolactone)-lignin nanofiber membranes	Electrospinning	PCL-lignin nanofibers exhibited high antioxidant activity, low cytotoxicity, and reduced oxidative stress, making them suitable for OA therapy.	Promote the proliferation and interaction of human dermal fibroblasts which is promising for tissue engineering.	Liang et al. (2020)
Lignin/Silica Nanohybrids)	Chemical Precipitation and Hydrothermal	Bone tissue engineering	Lignin/silica nanohybrids from rice husk showed excellent cytocompatibility and enhanced osteogenic differentiation in human mesenchymal stem cells.	Athinarayanan et al. (2023)

this context, electrospinning is recognized as a viable, inexpensive method for fabricating polymeric scaffolds that replicate the extracellular matrix, rendering it suitable for soft tissue engineering. A significant example is the development of nanocomposites from polycaprolactone (PCL) and lignin, in which different amounts of lignin (0, 5, 10, and 15% by weight) were introduced into PCL scaffolds. According to research on the shape, mechanical properties, swelling behavior, and bioactivity of the scaffold, the 10 wt.% nanocomposite had the optimal characteristics, such as suitable porosity, improved biodegradation, decreased fiber diameter, and increased tensile strength. Furthermore, the incorporation of lignin accelerated the degradation rate of PCL scaffold by 10%, demonstrating its potential to degrade more quickly in biological settings (Salami et al. 2017). In a similar trend, Amini et al. (2020) deployed the bioactivity of lignin nanoparticles in aligned PCL fibers to promote peripheral nerve regeneration. Smooth, homogeneous fibers with improved wettability, higher water uptake, and rapid breakdown were the result of the lignin addition. Stronger mechanical characteristics were indicated by mechanical testing, which demonstrated that the Young's modulus improved with increasing lignin content. On the other hand, the biological assessments demonstrated that incorporating lignin into PC12 and human adipose-derived stem cells (hADSCs) enhanced their cell survival, adhesion, and neural development. Significant enhancements in neurite outgrowth and the expression of neuronal markers including MAP2 and β-Tubulin III were observed at higher lignin amounts, particularly 15% (Amini et al. 2020). A study performed by Saudi et al. (2019) investigated the incorporation of lignin at different concentrations (0, 1, 3, and 5% wt) into electrospun poly(vinyl alcohol) (PVA) and poly(glycerol sebacate) (PGS) fibers to improve nerve tissue scaffolds. The results revealed that the produced fibers displayed smooth and homogeneous surfaces with a decreasing diameter profile from 530 nm to 370 nm. The incorporation of lignin also enhanced the hydrophilicity and degrading behavior of the fibers, as well as their mechanical characteristics, increasing their modulus of elasticity from 0.1 to 0.4 MPa. In vitro assays on PC12 cells revealed that lignin improved both cell proliferation and adhesion, while immunocytochemistry and gene expression analysis demonstrated its favorable impact on neuronal differentiation. Notably, fibers containing 5% lignin (VGL5) showed the best results, stimulating cell differentiation and growth (Saudi et al. 2019). In another study, Chen et al. (2019) have successfully created a polyacrylamide/lignin nanoparticle (PAM/LNP) nanocomposite hydrogel using a simple in-situ free radical polymerization procedure. Compared to pure PAM hydrogels, the mechanical characteristics were much improved in the case of hydrogels filled with LNPs as cross-linking junctions. This resulted in remarkable compressive and tensile strengths, as well as fracture strengths. The remarkable properties of the PAM/LNP hydrogel are due to the combined effects of its structure and the reversible energy absorption supplied by the strong hydrogen bonds between the polymer chains. This efficient hydrogel material, characterized by superior mechanical properties, straightforward synthesis, and non-cytotoxicity, exhibits considerable potential for various biomedical uses, including tissue engineering, regenerative medicine, artificial muscles, and durable underwater antifouling materials (Chen et al. 2019). Liang et al. (2020) investigated another unique use of lignin-based nanomaterials to treat osteoarthritis (OA). Treatments for osteoarthritis are often of limited effectiveness, as antioxidants are rapidly eliminated and have low bioavailability. Poly(ε-caprolactone)-grafted lignin (PCL-g-lignin) nanofibers, which combine the mechanical strength of PCL with the antioxidant qualities of lignin, were therefore suggested by the authors as an alternative option. Experiments conducted both in vitro and in vivo showed that PCL-lignin nanofibers efficiently minimize oxidative stress, boost cell viability, and inhibit inflammation and cartilage deterioration. These nanofibers promote the synthesis of antioxidant enzymes by activating the Keap1-Nrf2 pathway, offering long-term therapeutic advantages without the need for regular administration which is necessary for traditional treatments (Liang et al. 2020). In a recent study, lignin/silica nanohybrids (LiSNHs) were successfully produced from rice husk (RH) using a simple approach, establishing RH as an environmentally benign bioprecursor for emerging biomaterials. The RH-derived LiSNHs have silica nanostructures (5–35 nm) attached onto lignin spheres (~200 nm) with exceptional thermal stability. Cell viability studies and microscopic analysis confirmed the nanohybrids cytocompatibility, with no deleterious effects on human mesenchymal stem cells (hMSCs). LiSNHs have also been shown to stimulate osteogenic differentiation in hMSCs. These findings emphasize the potential of RH-derived LiSNHs as an appealing material for bone tissue creation, providing both biomedical functionality and sustainability (Athinarayanan et al. 2023).

11.6.3 Wound Healing

Wound healing is an intricate physiological procedure that aims to restore skin barrier function (Sezer et al. 2011; Portela et al. 2019). The regeneration of dermal and epidermal tissues is the foundation of the healing process (Üstündağ Okur et al. 2019). Appropriate wound dressing materials are the primary healthcare prerequisites for appropriate wound healing. Conventional dressings, including gauze, bandages, gauze-woven cotton and absorbent cotton composites, do not provide an adequate healing environment. Maintaining a moist environment, preventing bacterial contamination, allowing gas exchange, absorbing excess exudate, and minimizing discomfort are all characteristics of the optimal wound dressing (Mutlu et al. 2018). Additionally, it should be hygienic, nontoxic, nonallergic, nonadherent, and comfortable (Mutlu et al. 2018). Thus, a great deal of research has been conducted to develop more effective goods that effectively heal wounds. In this context, lignin-based skin wound healing solutions have drawn great attention from the market owing to their unique characteristics, which include superior tissue adhesion, biocompatibility, hemocompatibility, and antimicrobial properties (Nan et al. 2022; Xu et al. 2021; Liu et al. 2022). Alqahtani et al. (2020) synthesized curcumin-loaded LNPs and investigated their wound healing potential. During wound healing, authors discovered that the LNPs had no harmful effects and were compatible with skin keratinocytes. Significant antibacterial activity was also shown by the curcumin-loaded LNPs against gram-positive bacterial pathogens, particularly S. aureus, which is frequently found in wounds. In addition, a scratch experiment revealed that curcumin-loaded LNP therapy stimulated fibroblast cell migration.

In order to develop a self-healing hydrogel dressing with strong mechanical properties, antibacterial capacity, and antioxidant abilities (Alqahtani et al. 2020). Zhang et al. (2020) employed supramolecular interactions between lignin and poly(ionic liquid) compounds. According to the results, the characteristics of hydrogel dressing including its tensile strength, breaking elongation, and elastic modulus were all improved by the 3D structure of lignin. The antibacterial tests showed that the hydrogel dressings might offer consistent, long-term antibacterial properties and be used repeatedly. Furthermore, the wound healing model demonstrated how to efficiently accelerate wound healing by creating lignin-based composite hydrogels (Zhang et al. 2020). A further study confirmed that hydrogels comprising LNPs were harmless for skin tissue and biocompatible. Silver-lignin nanoparticles (Ag-Lignin NPs) were used in this study to create a plant-inspired adhesive hydrogel that activated a dynamic redox catechol chemistry system. The hydrogel was created using a straightforward in-situ polymerization process that requires no UV or thermal treatment, making it biocompatible and appropriate for use in biomedical uses. Catechol groups were continually produced by Ag-Lignin NPs, resulting in consistent and long-lasting adhesiveness. Furthermore, the antibacterial characteristics of Ag-Lignin NPs provided the hydrogel outstanding antibacterial capacity while simultaneously increasing cell affinity (Gan et al. 2019). In another investigation (Du et al. 2022), a droplet nanoprecipitation process was used to create lignin nanoparticles (LNPs) for possible wound healing purposes. The method succeeds in

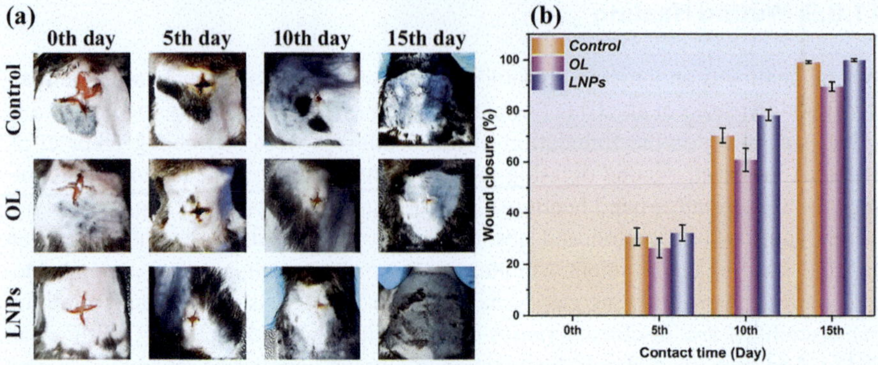

Fig. 11.8 (**a**) Photographs of wounds with control, OL and LNPs on the 0th, fifth, tenth and 15th day, and (**b**) the wound recovery rate calculated from the wound recovery area treated with control, OL and LNP. (Reproduced with permission from Du et al. (2022))

producing consistent LNPs with adjustable sizes, between 50 and 350 nm without altering the lignin chemical structure. The produced LNPs were extremely biocompatible for use in biomedical applications due to their significant bactericidal activity, great water stability, and antioxidant abilities. In vivo experiments on mice revealed that LNPs promoted wound healing, with quicker closure rates and progressed granulation tissue production as compared to untreated and OL-treated groups (Fig. 11.8) (Du et al. 2022).

11.7 Conclusion

The reuse of materials previously classified as manufacturing waste to make new materials offers a significant economic opportunity in an industry with a growing awareness of environmental sustainability. Bioengineering and nanotechnology are being explored to create promising vehicles for many applications in order to accomplish this purpose. Because of its essential characteristics, which include antioxidant, antibacterial, and stabilizing qualities, lignin has demonstrated significant potential as a component of novel green materials, making this biopolymer promising for end-use applications. In the chemical and pharmaceutical industries, lignin valorization offers a significant chance to produce high-value products from renewable resources. Lignin can be used as a carbon source and ingredient in polymer blends as a substitute for fossil fuels. However, its wider use is hampered by its high polydispersity and changing chemical structure. Compatibility with non-polar matrices can be improved by chemical modifications. Lignin-based nanoscale materials offer improved property control, which in turn enables biomedical applications, but research into their application in drug delivery and cytotoxicity testing is still limited. Ultimately, advances in lignin modification imply that its valorization and nanoscale applications will emerge as important study fields in the near future.

References

Agrawal A, Kaushik N, Biswas S (2014) Derivatives and applications of lignin–an insight. SciTech J 1(7):30–36

Ahmad M, Gani A, Hassan I, Huang Q, Shabbir H (2020) Production and characterization of starch nanoparticles by mild alkali hydrolysis and ultra-sonication process. Sci Rep 10:3533. https://doi.org/10.1038/s41598-020-60380-0

Alqahtani MS, Alqahtani A, Al-Thabit A, Roni M, Syed R (2019) Novel lignin nanoparticles for oral drug delivery. J Mater Chem B 7:4461–4473. https://doi.org/10.1039/c9tb00594c

Alqahtani MS, Alqahtani A, Kazi M, Ahmad MZ, Alahmari A, Alsenaidy MA, Syed R (2020) Wound-healing potential of curcumin loaded lignin nanoparticles. J Drug Deliv Sci Technol 60:102020. https://doi.org/10.1016/j.jddst.2020.102020

Alriols MG, Tejado A, Blanco M, Mondragon I, Labidi J (2009) Agricultural palm oil tree residues as raw material for cellulose, lignin and hemicelluloses production by ethylene glycol pulping process. Chem Eng J 148:106–114. https://doi.org/10.1016/j.cej.2008.08.008

Amen-Chen C, Pakdel H, Roy C Production of monomeric phenols by thermochemical conversion of biomass: a review

Amini S, Saudi A, Amirpour N, Jahromi M, Najafabadi SS, Kazemi M, Rafienia M, Salehi H (2020) Application of electrospun polycaprolactone fibers embedding lignin nanoparticle for peripheral nerve regeneration: in vitro and in vivo study. Int J Biol Macromol 159:154–173. https://doi.org/10.1016/j.ijbiomac.2020.05.073

arend 1998

Aro T, Fatehi P (2017) Production and application of lignosulfonates and sulfonated lignin. ChemSusChem 10:1861–1877

Athinarayanan J, Periasamy VS, Alshatwi AA (2023) Assessment of osteogenic differentiation potential of cytocompatible rice husk-derived lignin/silica nanohybrids for bone tissue engineering. SILICON 15:7235–7245. https://doi.org/10.1007/s12633-023-02573-6

Azadi P, Inderwildi OR, Farnood R, King DA (2013) Liquid fuels, hydrogen and chemicals from lignin: a critical review. Renew Sust Energ Rev 21:506–523

Barhoum A, Jeevanandam J, Rastogi A, Samyn P, Boluk Y, Dufresne A, Danquah MK, Bechelany M (2020) Plant celluloses, hemicelluloses, lignins, and volatile oils for the synthesis of nanoparticles and nanostructured materials. Nanoscale 12:22845–22890

Beisl S, Miltner A, Friedl A (2017) Lignin from micro- to nanosize: production methods. Int J Mol Sci 18

Bruijnincx PCA, Rinaldi R, Weckhuysen BM (2015) Unlocking the potential of a sleeping giant: lignins as sustainable raw materials for renewable fuels, chemicals and materials. Green Chem 17:4860–4861

Buono P, Duval A, Verge P, Averous L, Habibi Y (2016) New insights on the chemical modification of lignin: acetylation versus silylation. ACS Sustain Chem Eng 4:5212–5222. https://doi.org/10.1021/acssuschemeng.6b00903

Capolupo L, Faraco V (2016) Green methods of lignocellulose pretreatment for biorefinery development. Appl Microbiol Biotechnol 100:9451–9467

Cateto CA, Barreiro MF, Rodrigues AE, Belgacem MN (2009) Optimization study of lignin oxypropylation in view of the preparation of polyurethane rigid foams. Ind Eng Chem Res 48:2583–2589. https://doi.org/10.1021/ie801251r

Cerrutti BM, Moraes ML, Pulcinelli SH, Santilli CV (2015) Lignin as immobilization matrix for HIV p17 peptide used in immunosensing. Biosens Bioelectron 71:420–426. https://doi.org/10.1016/j.bios.2015.04.054

Chai Y, Wang Y, Li B, Qi W, Su R, He Z (2021) Microfluidic synthesis of lignin/chitosan nanoparticles for the pH-responsive delivery of anticancer drugs. Langmuir 37:7219–7226. https://doi.org/10.1021/acs.langmuir.1c00778

Chauhan PS (2020) Lignin nanoparticles: eco-friendly and versatile tool for new era. Bioresour Technol Rep 9:100374

Chen N, Dempere LA, Tong Z (2016) Synthesis of pH-responsive lignin-based Nanocapsules for controlled release of hydrophobic molecules. ACS Sustain Chem Eng 4:5204–5211. https://doi.org/10.1021/acssuschemeng.6b01209

Chen Y, Zheng K, Niu L, Zhang Y, Liu Y, Wang C, Chu F (2019) Highly mechanical properties nanocomposite hydrogels with biorenewable lignin nanoparticles. Int J Biol Macromol 128:414–420. https://doi.org/10.1016/j.ijbiomac.2019.01.099

Chunbao X, Ferdosian F (2017) Structure and properties of lignin. In: Conversion of lignin into bio-based chemicals and materials. Springer, Berlin Heidelberg, Berlin, Heidelberg, pp 1–12

Coessens V, Pintauer T, Matyjaszewski K Functional polymers by atom transfer radical polymerization

Daus S, Heinze T (2010) Xylan-based nanoparticles: prodrugs for ibuprofen release. Macromol Biosci 10:211–220. https://doi.org/10.1002/mabi.200900201

De Candolle M (1813) Theorie elementaire de la botanique ou exposition des principes de la classification naturelle et de l'Art de decrire et d'etudier les vegetaux. Paris: Detervill

De Jong WH, Borm PJ (2008) Drug delivery and nanoparticles: applications and hazards

De Oliveira W, Glasser WG (1994) Multiphase materials with lignin. 11. Starlike copolymers with caprolactone

Dehne L, Vila C, Saake B, Schwarz KU (2017) Esterification of Kraft lignin as a method to improve structural and mechanical properties of lignin-polyethylene blends. J Appl Polym Sci 134. https://doi.org/10.1002/app.44582

Doherty WOS, Mousavioun P, Fellows CM (2011) Value-adding to cellulosic ethanol: lignin polymers. Ind Crop Prod 33:259–276

Domínguez-Robles J, Martin NK, Fong ML, Stewart SA, Irwin NJ, Rial-Hermida MI, Donnelly RF, Larrañeta E (2019) Antioxidant pla composites containing lignin for 3D printing applications: a potential material for healthcare applications. Pharmaceutics 11. https://doi.org/10.3390/pharmaceutics11040165

Du X, Li J, Lindström ME (2014) Modification of industrial softwood kraft lignin using Mannich reaction with and without phenolation pretreatment. Ind Crop Prod 52:729–735. https://doi.org/10.1016/j.indcrop.2013.11.035

Du B, Li W, Bai Y, Pan Z, Wang Q, Wang X, Ding H, Lv G, Zhou J (2022) Fabrication of uniform lignin nanoparticles with tunable size for potential wound healing application. Int J Biol Macromol 214:170–180. https://doi.org/10.1016/j.ijbiomac.2022.06.066

Duval A, Lawoko M (2014) A review on lignin-based polymeric, micro- and nano-structured materials. React Funct Polym 85:78–96. https://doi.org/10.1016/j.reactfunctpolym.2014.09.017

Effendi A, Gerhauser H, Bridgwater AV (2008) Production of renewable phenolic resins by thermochemical conversion of biomass: a review. Renew Sust Energ Rev 12:2092–2116

Eraghi Kazzaz A, Hosseinpour Feizi Z, Fatehi P (2019) Grafting strategies for hydroxy groups of lignin for producing materials. Green Chem 21:5714–5752

Erdocia X, Toledano A, Corcuera MÁ, Labidi J (2012) Organosolv black liquor hydrolysis to obtain low molecular weight phenolic compounds. In: Chemical Engineering Transactions. Italian Association of Chemical Engineering - AIDIC, pp. 535–540

Faix O (1991) Supplement classification of lignins from different botanical origins by FT-IR spectroscopy

Feofilova EP, Mysyakina IS (2016) Lignin: chemical structure, biodegradation, and practical application (a review). Appl Biochem Microbiol 52:573–581

Figueiredo P, Lintinen K, Kiriazis A, Hynninen V, Liu Z, Bauleth-Ramos T, Rahikkala A, Correia A, Kohout T, Sarmento B, Yli-Kauhaluoma J, Hirvonen J, Ikkala O, Kostiainen MA, Santos HA (2017) In vitro evaluation of biodegradable lignin-based nanoparticles for drug delivery and enhanced antiproliferation effect in cancer cells. Biomaterials 121:97–108. https://doi.org/10.1016/j.biomaterials.2016.12.034

Figueiredo P, Lintinen K, Hirvonen JT, Kostiainen MA, Santos HA (2018) Properties and chemical modifications of lignin: towards lignin-based nanomaterials for biomedical applications. Prog Mater Sci 93:233–269

Frangville C, Rutkevičius M, Richter AP, Velev OD, Stoyanov SD, Paunov VN (2012) Fabrication of environmentally biodegradable lignin nanoparticles. ChemPhysChem 13:4235–4243. https://doi.org/10.1002/cphc.201200537

G. Calvo-Flores F, Dobado J, Isac-García J, Martin-Martinez F (2015) Lignin and lignans as renewable raw materials: chemistry, technology and applications

Galkin MV, Samec JSM (2016) Lignin valorization through catalytic lignocellulose fractionation: a fundamental platform for the future biorefinery. ChemSusChem 9:1544–1558

Gan D, Xing W, Jiang L, Fang J, Zhao C, Ren F, Fang L, Wang K, Lu X (2019) Plant-inspired adhesive and tough hydrogel based on Ag-Lignin nanoparticles-triggered dynamic redox catechol chemistry. Nat Commun 10:1487. https://doi.org/10.1038/s41467-019-09351-2

Gao W, Fatehi P (2019) Lignin for polymer and nanoparticle production: current status and challenges. Can J Chem Eng 97:2827–2842. https://doi.org/10.1002/cjce.23620

Garcia Gonzalez MN, Levi M, Turri S, Griffini G (2017) Lignin nanoparticles by ultrasonication and their incorporation in waterborne polymer nanocomposites. J Appl Polym Sci 134. https://doi.org/10.1002/app.45318

Cazacu Georgeta and Capraru M and PVI (2013) Advances concerning lignin utilization in new materials. In: Thomas Sabu and Visakh PM and MAjiP (ed) Advances in natural polymers: Composites and nanocomposites. Springer Berlin Heidelberg, Berlin, Heidelberg, pp. 255–312

Gilca IA, Popa VI, Crestini C (2015) Obtaining lignin nanoparticles by sonication. Ultrason Sonochem 23:369–375. https://doi.org/10.1016/j.ultsonch.2014.08.021

Gillet S, Aguedo M, Petitjean L, Morais ARC, Da Costa Lopes AM, Łukasik RM, Anastas PT (2017) Lignin transformations for high value applications: towards targeted modifications using green chemistry. Green Chem 19:4200–4233

Glasser WG (2019) About making lignin great again—some lessons from the past. Front Chem 7

Glasser WG, Davé V, Frazier CE (1993) Molecular weight distribution of (semi-) commercial lignin derivatives. J Wood Chem Technol 13:545–559. https://doi.org/10.1080/02773819308020533

Gordobil O, Herrera R, Yahyaoui M, Ilk S, Kaya M, Labidi J (2018) Potential use of Kraft and organosolv lignins as a natural additive for healthcare products. RSC Adv 8:24525–24533. https://doi.org/10.1039/c8ra02255k

Gosselink RJA, De Jong E, Guran B, Abächerli A (2004) Co-ordination network for lignin - standardisation, production and applications adapted to market requirements (EUROLIGNIN). In: Industrial crops and products. pp. 121–129

He W, Fatehi P (2015) Preparation of sulfomethylated softwood kraft lignin as a dispersant for cement admixture. RSC Adv 5:47031–47039. https://doi.org/10.1039/c5ra04526f

Henschen J, Li D, Ek M (2019) Preparation of cellulose nanomaterials via cellulose oxalates. Carbohydr Polym 213:208–216. https://doi.org/10.1016/j.carbpol.2019.02.056

Huber GW, Iborra S, Corma A (2006) Synthesis of transportation fuels from biomass: chemistry, catalysts, and engineering. Chem Rev 106:4044–4098

Huber P, Burnet A, Petit-Conil M (2014) Scale deposits in Kraft pulp bleach plants with reduced water consumption: a review. J Environ Manag 141:36–50

Jagur-Grodzinski J (2006) Polymers for tissue engineering, medical devices, and regenerative medicine. Concise general review of recent studies. Polym Adv Technol 17:395–418

Kai D, Ren W, Tian L, Chee PL, Liu Y, Ramakrishna S, Loh XJ (2016) Engineering poly(lactide)-lignin nanofibers with antioxidant activity for biomedical application. ACS Sustain Chem Eng 4:5268–5276. https://doi.org/10.1021/acssuschemeng.6b00478

Kaur R, Uppal SK, Sharma P (2017) Antioxidant and antibacterial activities of sugarcane bagasse lignin and chemically modified lignins. Sugar Tech 19:675–680. https://doi.org/10.1007/s12355-017-0513-y

Khadem E, Ghafarzadeh M, Kharaziha M, Sun F, Zhang X (2024) Lignin derivatives-based hydrogels for biomedical applications. Int J Biol Macromol 261:129877

Kim S, Fernandes MM, Matamá T, Loureiro A, Gomes AC, Cavaco-Paulo A (2013) Chitosan-lignosulfonates sono-chemically prepared nanoparticles: characterisation and potential applications. Colloids Surf B Biointerfaces 103:1–8. https://doi.org/10.1016/j.colsurfb.2012.10.033

Kim YS, Youe WJ, Kim SJ, Lee OK, Lee SS (2015) Preparation of a thermoplastic lignin-based biomaterial through atom transfer radical polymerization. J Wood Chem Technol 35:251–259. https://doi.org/10.1080/02773813.2014.937006

Kiran E, Balkan H (1994) High-pressure extraction and delignification of red spruce with binary and ternary mixtures of acetic acid, water, and supercritical carbon dioxide+

Koshi Jima T, Muraki E (1968) Radical grafting on lignin. Hydrochloric acid lignin part I. Radiation-induced grafting of styrene onto hydrochloric acid lignin

Kubo S, Kadla JF (2005) Hydrogen bonding in lignin: a fourier transform infrared model compound study. Biomacromolecules 6:2815–2821. https://doi.org/10.1021/bm050288q

Kuijpers MWA, Kemmere MF, Keurentjes JTF Calorimetric study of the energy efficiency for ultrasound-induced radical formation

Kumar R, Butreddy A, Kommineni N, Guruprasad Reddy P, Bunekar N, Sarkar C, Dutt S, Mishra VK, Aadil KR, Mishra YK, Oupicky D, Kaushik A (2021) Lignin: drug/gene delivery and tissue engineering applications. Int J Nanomedicine 16:2419–2441

Lange J (2015) Nachwachsende Rohstoffe: das Problem der Katalysatordesaktivierung und Wege zu seiner Lösung. Angew Chem 127:13382–13394. https://doi.org/10.1002/ange.201503595

Laurichesse S, Avérous L (2014) Chemical modification of lignins: towards biobased polymers. Prog Polym Sci 39:1266–1290

Le Corre D, Angellier-Coussy H (2014) Preparation and application of starch nanoparticles for nanocomposites: a review. React Funct Polym 85:97–120

Lee NC (2006) Practical guide to blow moulding. Rapra Technology Ltd.

Li Y, Sarkanen S (2002) Alkylated kraft lignin-based thermoplastic blends with aliphatic polyesters. Macromolecules 35:9707–9715. https://doi.org/10.1021/ma021124u

Li C, Zhao X, Wang A, Huber GW, Zhang T (2015a) Catalytic transformation of lignin for the production of chemicals and fuels. Chem Rev 115:11559–11624

Li Z, Ge Y, Wan L (2015b) Fabrication of a green porous lignin-based sphere for the removal of lead ions from aqueous media. J Hazard Mater 285:77–83. https://doi.org/10.1016/j.jhazmat.2014.11.033

Li Y, Wu M, Wang B, Wu Y, Ma M, Zhang X (2016) Synthesis of magnetic lignin-based hollow microspheres: a highly adsorptive and reusable adsorbent derived from renewable resources. ACS Sustain Chem Eng 4:5523–5532. https://doi.org/10.1021/acssuschemeng.6b01244

Li Y, Qiu X, Qian Y, Xiong W, Yang D (2017) pH-responsive lignin-based complex micelles: preparation, characterization and application in oral drug delivery. Chem Eng J 327:1176–1183. https://doi.org/10.1016/j.cej.2017.07.022

Liang R, Zhao J, Li B, Cai P, Loh XJ, Xu C, Chen P, Kai D, Zheng L (2020) Implantable and degradable antioxidant poly(ε-caprolactone)-lignin nanofiber membrane for effective osteoarthritis treatment. Biomaterials 230:119601. https://doi.org/10.1016/j.biomaterials.2019.119601

Liao JJ, Latif NHA, Trache D, Brosse N, Hussin MH (2020) Current advancement on the isolation, characterization and application of lignin. Int J Biol Macromol 162:985–1024

Libretti C, Santos Correa L, Meier MAR (2024) From waste to resource: advancements in sustainable lignin modification. Green Chem 26:4358–4386

Lievonen M, Valle-Delgado JJ, Mattinen ML, Hult EL, Lintinen K, Kostiainen MA, Paananen A, Szilvay GR, Setälä H, Österberg M (2016) A simple process for lignin nanoparticle preparation. Green Chem 18:1416–1422. https://doi.org/10.1039/c5gc01436k

Lintinen K, Xiao Y, Bangalore Ashok R, Leskinen T, Sakarinen E, Sipponen M, Muhammad F, Oinas P, Österberg M, Kostiainen M (2018) Closed cycle production of concentrated and dry redispersible colloidal lignin particles with a three solvent polarity exchange method. Green Chem 20:843–850. https://doi.org/10.1039/c7gc03465b

Lisý A, Ház A, Nadányi R, Jablonský M, Šurina I (2022) About Hydrophobicity of lignin: A review of selected chemical methods for lignin valorisation in biopolymer production. Energies (Basel) 15

Liu Y, Zheng J, Xiao J, He X, Zhang K, Yuan S, Peng Z, Chen Z, Lin X (2019a) Enhanced enzymatic hydrolysis and lignin extraction of wheat straw by triethylbenzyl ammonium chloride/

lactic acid-based deep eutectic solvent pretreatment. ACS Omega 4:19829–19839. https://doi.org/10.1021/acsomega.9b02709

Liu LY, Hua Q, Renneckar S (2019b) A simple route to synthesize esterified lignin derivatives. Green Chem 21:3682–3692. https://doi.org/10.1039/c9gc00844f

Liu ZH, Hao N, Shinde S, Pu Y, Kang X, Ragauskas AJ, Yuan JS (2019c) Defining lignin nanoparticle properties through tailored lignin reactivity by sequential organosolv fragmentation approach (SOFA). Green Chem 21:245–260. https://doi.org/10.1039/c8gc03290d

Liu Y, Wang X, Wu Q, Pei W, Teo MJ, Chen ZS, Huang C (2022) Application of lignin and lignin-based composites in different tissue engineering fields. Int J Biol Macromol 222:994–1006

Lora JH, Glasser WG (2002) Recent industrial applications of lignin: a sustainable alternative to nonrenewable materials

Lourençon TV, Hansel FA, Da Silva TA, Ramos LP, De Muniz GIB, Magalhães WLE (2015) Hardwood and softwood kraft lignins fractionation by simple sequential acid precipitation. Sep Purif Technol 154:82–88. https://doi.org/10.1016/j.seppur.2015.09.015

Lu Q, Zhu M, Zu Y, Liu W, Yang L, Zhang Y, Zhao X, Zhang X, Zhang X, Li W (2012) Comparative antioxidant activity of nanoscale lignin prepared by a supercritical antisolvent (SAS) process with non-nanoscale lignin. Food Chem 135:63–67. https://doi.org/10.1016/j.foodchem.2012.04.070

Lücking R, Nelsen MP (2018) Ediacarans, Protolichens, and lichen-derived Penicillium: a critical reassessment of the evolution of Lichenization in fungi. In: Transformative Paleobotany: papers to commemorate the life and legacy of Thomas N. Taylor. Elsevier, pp 551–590

Madzhidova VE, Dalimova GN, Abduazimov KA (1998) Sulfomethylation of lignins

Matsushita Y (2015) Conversion of technical lignins to functional materials with retained polymeric properties. J Wood Sci 61:230–250. https://doi.org/10.1007/s10086-015-1470-2

Meister JJ (2002) Modification of lignin. J Macromol Sci 42:235–289. https://doi.org/10.1081/MC-120004764

Mondal S, Jatrana A, Maan S, Sharma P (2023) Lignin modification and valorization in medicine, cosmetics, environmental remediation and agriculture: a review. Environ Chem Lett 21:2171–2197

Mutlu G, Calamak S, Ulubayram K, Guven E (2018) Curcumin-loaded electrospun PHBV nanofibers as potential wound-dressing material. J Drug Deliv Sci Technol 43:185–193. https://doi.org/10.1016/j.jddst.2017.09.017

Myint AA, Lee HW, Seo B, Son WS, Yoon J, Yoon TJ, Park HJ, Yu J, Yoon J, Lee YW (2016) One pot synthesis of environmentally friendly lignin nanoparticles with compressed liquid carbon dioxide as an antisolvent. Green Chem 18:2129–2146. https://doi.org/10.1039/c5gc02398j

Myint AA, Rhim WK, Nam JM, Kim J, Lee YW (2018) Water-soluble, lignin-derived carbon dots with high fluorescent emissions and their applications in bioimaging. J Ind Eng Chem 66:387–395. https://doi.org/10.1016/j.jiec.2018.06.005

Nair SS, Sharma S, Pu Y, Sun Q, Pan S, Zhu JY, Deng Y, Ragauskas AJ (2014) High shear homogenization of lignin to nanolignin and thermal stability of nanolignin-polyvinyl alcohol blends. ChemSusChem 7:3513–3520. https://doi.org/10.1002/cssc.201402314

Nan N, Hu W, Wang J (2022) Lignin-based porous biomaterials for medical and pharmaceutical applications. Biomedicines 10

Naseem A, Tabasum S, Zia KM, Zuber M, Ali M, Noreen A (2016) Lignin-derivatives based polymers, blends and composites: a review. Int J Biol Macromol 93:296–313. https://doi.org/10.1016/j.ijbiomac.2016.08.030

Nazeer MA, Yilgor E, Yilgor I (2019) Electrospun polycaprolactone/silk fibroin nanofibrous bioactive scaffolds for tissue engineering applications. Polymer (Guildf) 168:86–94. https://doi.org/10.1016/j.polymer.2019.02.023

Norberg I, Nordström Y, Drougge R, Gellerstedt G, Sjöholm E (2013) A new method for stabilizing softwood kraft lignin fibers for carbon fiber production. J Appl Polym Sci 128:3824–3830. https://doi.org/10.1002/app.38588

Norgren M, Edlund H (2014) Lignin: recent advances and emerging applications. Curr Opin Colloid Interface Sci 19:409–416

Nypelö TE, Carrillo CA, Rojas OJ (2015) Lignin supracolloids synthesized from (W/O) microemulsions: use in the interfacial stabilization of Pickering systems and organic carriers for silver metal. Soft Matter 11:2046–2054. https://doi.org/10.1039/c4sm02851a

O'Brien FJ (2011) Biomaterials & scaffolds for tissue engineering. Mater Today 14:88–95

Obrzut N, Hickmott R, Gray K (2024) Tailoring lignin nanoparticle properties: the effects of pH and salt on shape and antioxidant capacity. RSC Sustain 2:988–994. https://doi.org/10.1039/d3su00380a

Ouyang X, Ke L, Qiu X, Guo Y, Pang Y (2009) Sulfonation of alkali lignin and its potential use in dispersant for cement. J Dispers Sci Technol 30:1–6. https://doi.org/10.1080/01932690802473560

Pan H, Sun G, Zhao T (2013) Synthesis and characterization of aminated lignin. Int J Biol Macromol 59:221–226. https://doi.org/10.1016/j.ijbiomac.2013.04.049

Pandey MP, Kim CS (2011) Lignin depolymerization and conversion: a review of thermochemical methods. Chem Eng Technol 34:29–41

Pang Y, Wang S, Qiu X, Luo Y, Lou H, Huang J (2017) Preparation of lignin/sodium dodecyl sulfate composite nanoparticles and their application in pickering emulsion template-based microencapsulation. J Agric Food Chem 65:11011–11019. https://doi.org/10.1021/acs.jafc.7b03784

Parvathy G, Sethulekshmi AS, Jayan JS, Raman A, Saritha A (2021) Lignin based nano-composites: synthesis and applications. Process Saf Environ Prot 145:395–410

Patil SV, Argyropoulos DS (2017) Stable organic radicals in lignin: a review. ChemSusChem 10:3284–3303

Patil MN, Pandit AB (2007) Cavitation - a novel technique for making stable nano-suspensions. Ultrason Sonochem 14:519–530. https://doi.org/10.1016/j.ultsonch.2006.10.007

Perez-Cantu L, Schreiber A, Schütt F, Saake B, Kirsch C, Smirnova I (2013) Comparison of pretreatment methods for rye straw in the second generation biorefinery: effect on cellulose, hemicellulose and lignin recovery. Bioresour Technol 142:428–435. https://doi.org/10.1016/j.biortech.2013.05.054

Portela R, Leal CR, Almeida PL, Sobral RG (2019) Bacterial cellulose: a versatile biopolymer for wound dressing applications. Microb Biotechnol 12:586–610

Poveda-Giraldo JA, Solarte-Toro JC, Cardona Alzate CA (2021) The potential use of lignin as a platform product in biorefineries: a review. Renew Sust Energ Rev 138:110688

Prinsen P, Rencoret J, Gutiérrez A, Liitiä T, Tamminen T, Colodette JL, Berbis MÁ, Jiménez-Barbero J, Martínez ÁT, Del Río JC (2013) Modification of the lignin structure during alkaline delignification of eucalyptus wood by kraft, soda-AQ, and soda-O2 cooking. Ind Eng Chem Res 52:15702–15712. https://doi.org/10.1021/ie401364d

Qian Y, Deng Y, Qiu X, Li H, Yang D (2014) Formation of uniform colloidal spheres from lignin, a renewable resource recovered from pulping spent liquor. Green Chem 16:2156–2163. https://doi.org/10.1039/c3gc42131g

Qian Y, Zhong X, Li Y, Qiu X (2017) Fabrication of uniform lignin colloidal spheres for developing natural broad-spectrum sunscreens with high sun protection factor. Ind Crop Prod 101:54–60. https://doi.org/10.1016/j.indcrop.2017.03.001

Ragauskas AJ, Beckham GT, Biddy MJ, Chandra R, Chen F, Davis MF, Davison BH, Dixon RA, Gilna P, Keller M, Langan P, Naskar AK, Saddler JN, Tschaplinski TJ, Tuskan GA, Wyman CE (2014) Lignin valorization: improving lignin processing in the biorefinery. Science 1979:344

Rahimi A, Ulbrich A, Coon JJ, Stahl SS (2014) Formic-acid-induced depolymerization of oxidized lignin to aromatics. Nature 515:249–252. https://doi.org/10.1038/nature13867

Rangan A, Manjula MV, Satyanarayana KG, Menon R (2021) Lignin nanoparticles and their biodegradable composites. In: Sabu T, Balakrishnan P (eds) Green composites. Springer Singapore, Singapore, pp 295–327

Rinaldi R, Jastrzebski R, Clough MT, Ralph J, Kennema M, Bruijnincx PCA, Weckhuysen BM (2016) Wege zur Verwertung von Lignin: Fortschritte in der Biotechnik, der Bioraffination und der Katalyse. Angew Chem 128:8296–8354. https://doi.org/10.1002/ange.201510351

Rodríguez JF (2020) Lignin as a source of phenolic compounds: from lignin extraction to its transformation by different route

Ruiz-Dueñas FJ, Martínez ÁT (2009) Microbial degradation of lignin: how a bulky recalcitrant polymer is efficiently recycled in nature and how we can take advantage of this. Microb Biotechnol 2:164–177

Saito T, Brown RH, Hunt MA, Pickel DL, Pickel JM, Messman JM, Baker FS, Keller M, Naskar AK (2012) Turning renewable resources into value-added polymer: development of lignin-based thermoplastic. Green Chem 14:3295–3303. https://doi.org/10.1039/c2gc35933b

Salami M, Kaveian F, Rafienia M, et al (2017) Electrospun Polycaprolactone/lignin-based Nanocomposite as a Novel Tissue Scaffold for Biomedical Applications. J Med Signals Sens

Samani N, Khalil R, Seljeskog M, Bakken J, Thapa RK, Eikeland MS (2024) Experimental and simulation studies of oxygen-blown, steam-injected, entrained flow gasification of lignin. Fuel 362:130713. https://doi.org/10.1016/j.fuel.2023.130713

Sameni J, Krigstin S, Sain M (2017) Acetylation & lignin solubility

Saudi A, Amini S, Amirpour N, Kazemi M, Zargar Kharazi A, Salehi H, Rafienia M (2019) Promoting neural cell proliferation and differentiation by incorporating lignin into electrospun poly(vinyl alcohol) and poly(glycerol sebacate) fibers. Mater Sci Eng C 104:110005. https://doi.org/10.1016/j.msec.2019.110005

Schoenherr S, Ebrahimi M, Czermak P (2018) Lignin degradation processes and the purification of valuable products. In: Lignin - Trends and applications. InTech

Schutyser W, Renders T, Van Den Bosch S, Koelewijn SF, Beckham GT, Sels BF (2018) Chemicals from lignin: an interplay of lignocellulose fractionation, depolymerisation, and upgrading. Chem Soc Rev 47:852–908

Sezer AD, Cevher E (2011) Biopolymers as Wound Healing Materials: Challenges and New Strategies. In: Pignatello R (ed) Biomaterials. IntechOpen, Rijeka

Shavandi A, Hosseini S, Okoro OV, Nie L, Eghbali Babadi F, Melchels F (2020) 3D bioprinting of lignocellulosic biomaterials. Adv Healthc Mater 9:e2001472

Shen X, Zhang C, Han B, Wang F (2022) Catalytic self-transfer hydrogenolysis of lignin with endogenous hydrogen: road to the carbon-neutral future. Chem Soc Rev 51:1608–1628. https://doi.org/10.1039/D1CS00908G

Singh SP (2023) Lignin and their role in nanomaterials synthesis and applications. In: Secondary metabolites based green synthesis of nanomaterials and their applications. Springer Nature Singapore, pp 119–139

Sixta H, Potthast A, Krotschek AW (2006) Chemical Pulping Processe. In: Handbook of Pulp. John Wiley & Sons, Ltd, pp 109–229

Stanisz M, Klapiszewski CMN, Jesionowski T (2022) Recent progress in biomedical and biotechnological applications of lignin-based spherical nano- and microstructures: a comprehensive review. Mater Today Chem 26:101198

Strassberger Z, Tanase S, Rothenberg G (2014) The pros and cons of lignin valorisation in an integrated biorefinery. RSC Adv 4:25310–25318. https://doi.org/10.1039/c4ra04747h

Subbotina E, Ram F, Dvinskikh SV, Berglund LA, Olsén P (2022) Aqueous synthesis of highly functional, hydrophobic, and chemically recyclable cellulose nanomaterials through oxime ligation. Nat Commun 13:6924. https://doi.org/10.1038/s41467-022-34697-5

Sugiarto S, Leow Y, Tan CL, Wang G, Kai D (2022) How far is lignin from being a biomedical material? Bioact Mater 8:71–94

Sun Q (2017) Starch nanoparticles. In: Starch in food: structure, function and applications. Elsevier, pp 691–745

Tan Z, Li Y, Chen F, Liu J, Zhong J, Guo L, Zhang R, Chen R (2024) Challenges and perspectives of the conversion of lignin waste to high-value chemicals by pyrolysis. PRO 12

Tanganini IC, Camargos CHM, Jackson JC, Rezende CA, Ceccato-Antonini SR, Faria AF (2023) Self-assembled lignin nanoparticles produced from elephant grass leaves enable selective inactivation of Gram-positive microorganisms. RSC Sustain 2:459–474. https://doi.org/10.1039/d3su00400g

Tian D, Hu J, Chandra RP, Saddler JN, Lu C (2017) Valorizing recalcitrant cellulolytic enzyme lignin via lignin nanoparticles fabrication in an integrated biorefinery. ACS Sustain Chem Eng 5:2702–2710. https://doi.org/10.1021/acssuschemeng.6b03043

Tomani P (2010) The lignoboost process. Cellulose Chemistry and Technology 44:53–58
Tortora M, Cavalieri F, Mosesso P, Ciaffardini F, Melone F, Crestini C (2014) Ultrasound driven assembly of lignin into microcapsules for storage and delivery of hydrophobic molecules. Biomacromolecules 15:1634–1643. https://doi.org/10.1021/bm500015j
Üstündağ Okur N, Hökenek N, Okur ME, Ayla Ş, Yoltaş A, Siafaka PI, Cevher E (2019) An alternative approach to wound healing field; new composite films from natural polymers for mupirocin dermal delivery. Saudi Pharma J 27:738–752. https://doi.org/10.1016/j.jsps.2019.04.010
Vanholme R, Demedts B, Morreel K, Ralph J, Boerjan W (2010) Lignin biosynthesis and structure. Plant Physiol 153:895–905. https://doi.org/10.1104/pp.110.155119
Viell J, Harwardt A, Seiler J, Marquardt W (2013) Is biomass fractionation by Organosolv-like processes economically viable? A conceptual design study. Bioresour Technol 150:89–97. https://doi.org/10.1016/j.biortech.2013.09.078
Vinardell MP, Ugartondo V, Mitjans M (2008) Potential applications of antioxidant lignins from different sources. Ind Crop Prod 27:220–223. https://doi.org/10.1016/j.indcrop.2007.07.011
Wallberg O, Al-Rudainy B, Galbe M, Schagerlöf H (2018) Antisolvent precipitation of hemicelluloses, lignosulfonates and their complexes from ultrafiltrated spent sulfite liquor (SSL). Holzforschung 72:839–850. https://doi.org/10.1515/hf-2017-0218
Wang Y, Xu B, Ge S, Yan L (2024) Preparation of lignin microcapsules via interfacial crosslinking using deep eutectic solution to dissolve lignin. Sustain Chem Environ 6:100120. https://doi.org/10.1016/j.scenv.2024.100120
Witzler M, Alzagameem A, Bergs M, El K-HB, Klein SE, Hielscher D, Kamm B, Kreyenschmidt J, Tobiasch E, Schulze M (2018) Lignin-derived biomaterials for drug release and tissue engineering. Molecules 23
Xiong F, Han Y, Wang S, Li G, Qin T, Chen Y, Chu F (2017) Preparation and formation mechanism of size-controlled lignin nanospheres by self-assembly. Ind Crop Prod 100:146–152. https://doi.org/10.1016/j.indcrop.2017.02.025
Xu J, Xu JJ, Lin Q, Jiang L, Zhang D, Li Z, Ma B, Zhang C, Li L, Kai D, Yu HD, Loh XJ (2021) Lignin-incorporated nanogel serving as an antioxidant biomaterial for wound healing. ACS Appl Biol Mater 4:3–13
Yearla SR, Padmasree K (2016) Preparation and characterisation of lignin nanoparticles: evaluation of their potential as antioxidants and UV protectants. J Exp Nanosci 11:289–302. https://doi.org/10.1080/17458080.2015.1055842
Yu S, Sun J, Shi Y, Wang Q, Wu J, Liu J (2021) Nanocellulose from various biomass wastes: its preparation and potential usages towards the high value-added products. Environ Sci Ecotechnol 5:100077
Yuliestyan A, Gabet T, Marsac P, et al (2018) Sustainable asphalt mixes manufactured with reclaimed asphalt and modified-lignin-stabilized bitumen emulsions. Constr Build Mater 173:662–671. https://doi.org/10.1016/J.CONBUILDMAT.2018.04.044
Zakzeski J, Bruijnincx PCA, Jongerius AL, Weckhuysen BM (2010) The catalytic valorization of lignin for the production of renewable chemicals. Chem Rev 110:3552–3599. https://doi.org/10.1021/cr900354u
Zasadowski D, Yang J, Edlund H, Norgren M (2014) Antisolvent precipitation of water-soluble hemicelluloses from TMP process water. Carbohydr Polym 113:411–419. https://doi.org/10.1016/j.carbpol.2014.07.033
Zhang L, Huang J (2001) Effects of nitrolignin on mechanical properties of polyurethane-Nitrolignin films
Zhang Y, Yuan B, Zhang Y, Cao Q, Yang C, Li Y, Zhou J (2020) Biomimetic lignin/poly(ionic liquids) composite hydrogel dressing with excellent mechanical strength, self-healing properties, and reusability. Chem Eng J 400:125984. https://doi.org/10.1016/j.cej.2020.125984
Zhang J, Tian Z, Ji X, Zhang F (2022) Fabrication mechanisms of lignin nanoparticles and their ultraviolet protection ability in PVA composite film. Polymers (Basel) 14. https://doi.org/10.3390/polym14194196
Zhao W, Simmons B, Singh S, Ragauskas A, Cheng G (2016) From lignin association to nano–/micro-particle preparation: extracting higher value of lignin. Green Chem 18:5693–5700

Zhao X, Li S, Wu R, Liu D (2017) Organosolv fractionating pre-treatment of lignocellulosic biomass for efficient enzymatic saccharification: chemistry, kinetics, and substrate structures. Biofuels Bioprod Biorefin 11:567–590

Zhou Z, Wang J, Xu X, Wang Z, Mao L, Zhang S, Zhang H, Li Y, Yu Q, Jiang N, Zhang G, Gan Z, Ning Z (2024) Lignin-based nanoparticles for combination of tumor oxidative stress amplification and reactive oxygen species responsive drug release. Bioconjug Chem 35:1207–1217. https://doi.org/10.1021/acs.bioconjchem.4c00261

Lignin as a Drug Encapsulant 12

Kushal Chakraborty, Jeong Man An, Dong Yun Lee,
and Yong-kyu Lee

Abstract

Lignin, an abundant natural biopolymer derived from lignocellulosic biomass, has gained increasing attention for its potential in biomedical applications, particularly as a sustainable drug encapsulant. Its unique structural characteristics including diverse functional groups, high carbon content, and inherent biodegradability enable lignin to serve as a promising platform for the controlled delivery of therapeutic agents. This chapter delves into the structural complexity

K. Chakraborty
Department of IT and Energy Convergence (BK21 FOUR), Korea National University of Transportation, Chungju, Republic of Korea

J. M. An
Department of Bioengineering, College of Engineering, Hanyang University, Seoul, Republic of Korea

D. Y. Lee (✉)
Department of Bioengineering, College of Engineering, and BK FOUR Biopharmaceutical Innovation Leader for Education and Research Group, Hanyang University, Seoul, Republic of Korea

Institute of Nano Science and Technology (INST), Hanyang University, Seoul, Republic of Korea

Institute for Bioengineering and Biopharmaceutical Research (IBBR), Hanyang University, Seoul, Republic of Korea
e-mail: dongyunlee@hanyang.ac.kr

Y.-k. Lee (✉)
Department of Green Bio Engineering, Graduate School, Korea National University of Transportation, Chungju, Republic of Korea

4D Convergence Technology Institute, Korea National University of Transportation, Jeungpyeong, Republic of Korea
e-mail: leeyk@ut.ac.kr

M. N. Collins, M. Culebras (eds.), *Sustainable Biopolymers and Composites for Biomedical Applications*, Biomaterials, Bioengineering and Sustainability 5,
https://doi.org/10.1007/978-3-031-91972-5_12

of lignin, its various sources, functional groups, and interunit linkages that influence its behavior in drug encapsulation. A range of lignin-based materials, including nanoparticles, hydrogels, films, and scaffolds, are discussed in relation to their capacity to entrap, encapsulate, and adsorb active pharmaceutical ingredients. Various fabrication methods such as nanoprecipitation, emulsification, and chemical conjugation are presented, highlighting lignin's adaptability for targeted, stimuli-responsive, and sustained drug release. The chapter also reviews recent advances in lignin-based drug delivery for cancer therapy, wound healing, and imaging, while addressing toxicological concerns and regulatory challenges. Overall, lignin emerges as a versatile, eco-friendly, and biocompatible candidate for next-generation drug delivery systems.

Keywords

Sustainable materials · Lignin · Nanocarriers · Drug delivery · Encapsulation · Controlled release

12.1 Introduction

Lignocellulosic biomass, with its abundant availability, serves as a substantial reservoir for the environmentally conscious generation of renewable fuels, chemicals, and materials that cater to the needs of humanity. Biomass, particularly wood, has been employed for countless centuries as a fundamental component in the realm of construction and building, serving a multitude of purposes and functioning as a vital source of thermal energy. The preponderance of mass in plants is concentrated within the cellular walls, which consist predominantly of the polysaccharide cellulose, hemicellulose, and pectin, in conjunction with the alkyl-aromatic heteropolymer known as lignin (Mosier 2005; Kumar et al. 2008; Cai et al. 2017; Zhang et al. 2011; Wu et al. 2018; Gopinath et al. 2022; Thakur et al. 1997).

Being the second-most abundant natural polymer in the kingdom Plantae (second only to cellulose), lignin, frequently associates with cellulose and hemicellulose, thereby constituting the primary structural framework of plants (Vasile and Baican 2023). Regrettably, the intricate composition of lignin renders it arduous to comprehend and employ. Lignin, nonetheless, is widely considered to be an exceptional biomass chemical raw material and garners significant attention within the realm of materials (Yoo et al. 2020). The aforementioned characteristics, namely its diverse functional group, capacity for renewal, ability to degrade, lack of toxicity, and affordability (owing to the possibility of lignin being generated as a by-product in the paper industry), contribute to the rationale behind this assertion. In recent years, there has been a significant increase in the interest of researchers towards lignin. The researchers are currently engaged in comprehending the established characteristics and investigating the novel physicochemical phenomena exhibited by lignin. Furthermore, they are endeavouring to utilise this knowledge in a wide array of applications spanning across various disciplines such as materials science, drug delivery, tissue engineering, food science, etc. From this point forward, the amount of research, specifically in the biomedical application of lignin, is rapidly increasing (Dizhbite 2004; Domínguez-Robles et al. 2019; Iravani 2020; Nan et al. 2022; Witzler et al. 2018; Kai et al. 2015; Quraishi et al. 2015; Tao et al. 2020).

The scientific community utilises a range of naturally occurring and chemically synthesised lignins for research purposes. These include Kraft or softwood lignin, lignin alkali or soda lignin, hardwood lignin, lignosulphonates, and Organosolv lignin (Gellerstedt 2015; Lapierre et al. 1995; Mousavioun and Doherty 2010; Gonçalves et al. 2021; Xu et al. 2006). Within the domain of softwood lignin, it is observed that the guaiacyl structure holds a position of dominance. Conversely, in the context of hardwood lignin, it is noteworthy that both the S (syringy) and G (guaiacyl) structures exhibit a state of dominance. The production of lignin on a global scale is primarily dominated by softwood lignin, accounting for approximately 85% of the total lignin production (Doherty et al. 2011; Chakar and Ragauskas 2004; Crestini et al. 2017; Sakakibara 1980). The pulping process employed for the production of wood pulp, utilising sodium hydroxide as the cooking agent, is commonly referred to as the soda pulping process. In this particular method, the primary by-product obtained is known as soda lignin. The aforementioned statement primarily pertains to the acquisition of the desired outcome through the utilisation of a cooking method that is devoid of any traces of sulphur (Joffres et al. 2014; Nagieb and Shukry 1984). Lignosulphonates, which are classified as water-soluble anionic polyelectrolytes, are characterised by the presence of numerous charged groups. The lignin in question is derived from a sulphate cooking process, wherein wood is subjected to delignification through the action of HSO_3^- and SO_3^- ions. These lignins typically exhibit high molecular weights (Aro and Fatehi 2017; Ruwoldt 2020). Organosolv lignins are typically generated via a pulping procedure wherein a variety of organic solvents, such as formic acid, ethanol, and acetic acid, are employed (de la Torre et al. 2013; El Hage et al. 2009).

12.2 Lignin: A Structural Perspective

The three-dimensional structure of lignin is formed through the chemical bonding of various alkyl and aryl groups, specifically alkyl-alkyl, alkyl-aryl, and aryl-aryl linkages. Extensive research conducted by Freudenberg and colleagues from 1940 to 1970 has shed light on the precursors of lignin synthesis in nature. These precursors consist of p-coumaryl alcohol (4-hydroxyphenylpropane), coniferyl alcohol (3-methoxy-4-hydroxyphenylpropane), and sinapyl alcohol (3,5-dimethoxy-4-hydr oxyphenylpropane) (Terashima 2001). The composition of natural lignin is not merely a straightforward concatenation of monomers; rather, it arises from the non-uniform coupling or addition of precursor alcohols. There exist notable disparities in the lignin content across various tissues or cell walls. Several ecological factors, including but not limited to plant growth, illumination, climate, and nutrition have been found to exert an influence on the chemical composition of lignin (Nimz 1974; Chen 2014; Welker et al. 2015; Hatfield and Vermerris 2001).

The elucidation of the chemical structure of lignin remains one of the most formidable challenges that persists within the discipline of natural polymers. The molecules of lignin and its degradation products exhibit numerous asymmetric centres; however, they do not possess optical activity. Consequently, lignin is not structured in a manner akin to cellulose or protein, which are characterised by a singular key-type linkage. There exist numerous carbon-carbon bonds among the structural entities, nevertheless, the overall molecular structure remains indiscernible through the conventional decomposition technique. The examination of the structural characteristics of residual lignins holds significant importance in the realm of pulp delignification and bleaching investigations. The elucidation of the chemical structure of residual lignin provides valuable insights into the reactivity of the lignin during the subsequent bleaching stages. Furthermore, it is worth noting that the chemical treatments employed in various experiments can be effectively evaluated by examining the alterations in the residual lignin structure (Lu et al. 2020).

The extraction of lignin from plant tissue remains a significant challenge in the field of lignin chemistry (Radotić and Mićić 2016). Conventional acidolysis and enzymatic hydrolysis are used to extract lignin from the pulp matrix (Fu et al. 2010). Although several other methods are in play but when quantitative measurements are in question, these are unemployable. Additionally, it is worth mentioning that the plant exhibits a sophisticated regulatory mechanism. As a result, the composition of lignin in certain wood specimens predominantly consists of guaiacum lignin, while others primarily contain syringa lignin. It is also important to acknowledge that the formation of wood quality stress is influenced by various factors, including the diverse plant growth environments (Tribot et al. 2019). Henceforth, it can be stated that lignin belongs to the category of intricate molecular structures consisting of polymers that defy description through a mere structural formula. The characteristics of lignin can solely be elucidated by considering the constituent elements, functional groups, and the amalgamation of each individual unit (Spiridon 2020; Ye et al. 2012; Watkins et al. 2015; Adler 1957).

12.2.1 Components of Lignin

The primary components of natural lignin are carbon, hydrogen, and oxygen, with a significantly higher carbon content compared to carbohydrates. The carbon percentage of softwood lignin is approximately 60% to 65%, whereas the carbon content of hardwood lignin is around 56% to 60% (Nimz 1974). Hardwood lignin has a comparatively high methoxy concentration, resulting in a higher oxygen content compared to softwood. Wood lignin is typically regarded as lacking nitrogen elements (Harris et al. 1938). However, it is worth noting that the lignin found in grasses does contain a small quantity of nitrogen. The element contents of various lignin samples exhibit slight variations depending on the specific raw material and the methods employed for separation (Toledano et al. 2010).

The elemental analysis results of lignin are typically presented in relation to the element composition of the average C9 unit. Specifically, this refers to the benzene propane (C6-C3) unit, which is employed to eliminate methoxy, along with the hydrogen, oxygen atoms, and methyl oxygen bases associated with each C9 unit (Nimz 1974; Adler 1957).

Lignin has the capability to incorporate new elements through specific chemical reactions. For instance, sulphur elements can be introduced to the lignin through the processes of kraft pulping and sulphite pulping. For instance, in the lignosulfonate case, the presence of -SO_3H group actively influence the sulphur percentage in the molecular building block compared to the organic solvent lignin whereas the sulphur percentage in sulphate lignin solely depends on the presence of hydrosulphonyl group (Gellerstedt and Lindfors 1984; Magina et al. 2015).

12.2.2 Functional Groups

The presence of functional groups such as phenolic hydroxyl groups, alcohol hydroxyl groups, etc. are significant structural features of lignin. The spectral properties, diffusion characteristics and chemical response of lignin are directly determined by it. Therefor both quantitative and qualitative measurement of these parts play a crucial role while investigating the structural aspects of lignin.

12.2.2.1 Hydroxyl Groups

Hydroxyl groups, encompassing both aliphatic hydroxyl groups and phenolic hydroxyl groups, are functional groups that exhibit a higher concentration of lignin. These groups are of utmost significance in the process of modifying lignin to create functional materials. The preparation method employed for lignin extraction exhibits notable variations, leading to distinct hydroxyl content in the resulting lignin samples. It is imperative to eliminate any remaining carbohydrates in the process of preparing lignin, as their presence can have an impact on the accurate determination of the aliphatic hydroxyl group (Lee et al. 2021; Li et al. 2018; Serrano et al. 2018).

Mostly employed methods for quantitative determination of hydroxyl groups are, (i) methoxyl group determination of diazomethane-methylated lignin, (ii) methanol determination after periodate oxidation, (iii) ^{1}H-NMR of acylated lignin, (iv) potentiometric or conductometric titration, (v) ionisation differential spectroscopy, and (vi) Folin–Ciocalteu Reagent method (Månsson 1983; Pérez et al. 2023).

For unaltered kraft and milled wood lignins, these procedures often yield findings that are quite consistent in general. Within modified lignins, the analysis is disrupted by the presence of undetermined amounts of diverse functional groups, such as esters, catechol groups, and so forth.

The initial approach necessitates a quantitative assessment of methylation. Regarding the phenolic hydroxyls, it is worth noting that their determination can pose certain challenges (Brauns 1939). In the second method, known as periodate oxidation, the determination is limited to phenol groups that are adjacent to a methoxyl group (Gosselink et al. 2011). Consequently, phenol units that do not contain a methoxyl group, such as catechols, are not taken into consideration. In method three, the spectra exhibit a characteristic of broad overlapping signals. The acquisition of data in this context introduces a certain level of uncertainty to the process of integration (Lundquist and Stern 1989). The uncertainty of method four arises from the broad range of ionisation constants exhibited by the phenolic hydroxyls, as well as the presence of an indeterminate quantity of diverse carboxylic groups. The fifth method is not absolute and requires calibration using suitable model substances, which can pose challenges, particularly when dealing with modified lignins (Timell 1960; Richel et al. 2012). Method six or Folin-Ciocalteu reagent method is a well-established quantitative approach which utilises phenol as a reducing agent to restore the complex under alkaline conditions. This restoration process leads to the formation of blue reaction products, which can be conveniently detected at a wavelength of 765 nm. The aforementioned method has been successfully employed in the analysis and quantification of phenolic hydroxyl groups present in lignin and its various derivatives (Ainsworth and Gillespie 2007).

12.2.2.2 Carbonyl Groups

Lignin also exhibits a significant abundance of carbonyl groups including ketone, carboxyl and aldehyde groups. The presence of these carbonyl groups is not inherent in the mother structure of lignin; rather, it is formed through a process of degradation and refashion of lignin's polymeric network (Adler 1957; Fumoto et al. 2022). The carbonyl group in the original lignin is composed of both conjugated and nonconjugated carbonyls. The carbonyl moiety that is attached to the α-carbon atom can be identified as the conjugated carbonyl in the form of a ketone ($C_\alpha = O$). On the other hand, the carbonyl group located on the γ-carbon atom is observed to exist as a conjugated aldehyde ($C_\gamma HO$). For the account of non-conjugated carbonyl, it is designated as $C_\beta = O$.

The aromatic ring-conjugated carbonyl group is a reactive moiety found in the structure of lignin. The quantity of this group present in lignin has a significant impact on the rate of degradation reactions of lignin (Adler and Marton 1961). Furthermore, it is responsible for the occurrence of yellowing in pulp products subsequent to heating or exposure to UV irradiation during the pulping process. The various categories of cyclic conjugated carbonyl compounds can be quantitatively detected through the utilisation of reductive differential spectrometry (Chen 1992). Another popular method for successful quantification of aromatic carbonyl groups involves the chemical reaction with hydroxylamine hydrochloride followed by the titration. Although this method encounters with incomplete reduction of the carbonyl groups, to mitigate this problem, a new approach was developed, where sodium borohydride was used for complete reduction of the carbonyl groups followed by infrared spectroscopic determination of all conjugated carbonyl groups (Marton et al. 1961). However, it is important to note that the accuracy of this spectral method is contingent upon the lignin model and can be influenced by the specific source of lignin.

12.2.3 Closer Look into Interunit Linkage in Lignin

The complex macromolecular substance, lignin, goes through a series of interconnected bond breaking and making to for a three-dimensional array. The composition and arrangement of chemical connection between benzene-propane units decide the final fate of the structure. In order to ascertain interunit linkages, the process typically involves the degradation of lignin into low molecular weight constituents such as monomers, dimers, and oligomers (Chakar and Ragauskas 2004). Subsequently, the resulting products are subjected to analysis through the utilisation of Gas Chromatography-Mass Spectrometry (GC-MS), Liquid Chromatography-Mass Spectrometry (LC-MS), and Nuclear Magnetic Resonance (NMR) techniques (Mullen and Boateng 2010; Syrjänen et al. 2000; Chen and Robert 1988). Through the utilisation of various methodologies and the application of computational modelling, researchers have successfully derived estimations pertaining to the nature and proportional prevalence of interunit linkages. Within the realm of interunit linkages, the primary structures consist of the β-O-4, β-β, β-5, and 5–5′ units. Notably, the recently uncovered units include dibenzodioxocin, spirodienone, and benzodioxane. Other linkages, such as β-1, 4-O-5 diphenyl and α-O-4, are considered to be relatively uncommon in nature (Lapierre 2015; Figueiredo et al. 2018). The relative abundance of each linkage is contingent upon the specific species of biomass, the type of lignin present, and the method employed for isolation.

12.2.3.1 Aryl Ether or β-O-4

The prevalent β-O-4 structure observed in lignin is known as aryl propyl alcohol-β-aryl ether, which is readily formed during the acid and alcohol hydrolysis reaction. Adler and colleagues postulated that the guaiacylglycerol-β-aryl ether present in lignin undergoes degradation via acidolysis, resulting in the formation of Hilbert ketones. This process leads to the production of a solid product that is both insoluble in water and ether. They effectively demonstrated the existence of a 0.31 aryl glycerol unit (per OCH_3) that possesses an aryl ether linkage in the β position of the side chain. This was accomplished through the implementation of acidolysis with hydrochloric acid on Björkman lignin (Adler et al. 1957). Previously C. Lapierre and colleagues demonstrated a solvolysis method in dioxane-ethanethiol sovent with boron trifluoride etherate, named thioacidolysis for estimation of uncondensed alkyl aryl ether structures in lignin by specifically cleaving the β-O-4 structure. Although it was widely celebrated method, the solvent extraction was a critical turn which accentuate the calibre of experimentalist (Rolando et al. 1992). Utilising spectroscopic analyses, the estimation of the β-O-4 linkage can be achieved through the use of ^{1}H NMR on acetylated lignin samples and the quantitative ^{13}C NMR on non-derivatized lignin samples. In more recent studies, a demonstration has been conducted to showcase the capabilities of the advanced two-dimensional Nuclear Magnetic Resonance (NMR) technique or HSQC. This technique has been shown to have the ability to accurately measure the relative quantities of β-O-4 units present in the entirety of the cell wall (Marita et al. 1999).

12.2.3.2 Phenylcoumaran or β-5

The β-5 bond, pertains to the specific chemical bond that arises from the interaction between the β-carbon atom of phenyl propane and the fifth carbon atom of the benzene ring within a distinct structural unit. The structure of phenyl coumarin is often employed to represent this. To analytically evaluate this, the pyrolysis of spurce milled wood lignin can be employed (Kuroda and Nakagawa-izumi 2006). The relative stereochemistry of the β-5 linking motif has been determined to be predominantly trans, with the presence of cis configuration being observed in minimal quantities, if at all. A comprehensive computational investigation was undertaken employing model substrates in order to elucidate the underlying factors responsible for the observed stereochemistry. It has been determined that the ring-closing reaction, subsequent to the radical dimerization process, results in the creation of the β-5 bond. The process of ring closure is believed to be influenced by thermodynamic factors, which tend to promote the formation of the more stable trans relationship between the substituents, if the process takes place at all (Orlandi et al. 2001).

12.2.3.3 Resinol or β-β

The β-β linking motif, which is observed during lignification in planta, exhibits an unusual characteristic. Unlike chain elongation reactions, this motif can only be formed through monolignol dimerization reactions. The pinoresinol structure was initially identified within the enzymatic dehydrogenation polymer (DHP) derived from coniferyl alcohol. Additionally, various other resinol units, including syringaresinol, dimethoxylariciresinol, and lariciresinol, have been successfully isolated from percolation hydrolysate and hydrogenation products obtained from hardwood sources (Katahira et al. 2018). The β-β linking motif has been observed to constitute approximately 3–12% of the total linking motifs present in lignin. Various methodologies have been employed in the synthesis of the fundamental building block of the β-β linking motif, as these compounds have garnered attention due to their potential biological attributes, such as antitumor, antiviral, immunosuppressant, and anti-inflammatory effects (Lahive et al. 2020).

12.2.3.4 Biphenyl or 5-5′

The confirmation of the biphenyl structure was achieved through the isolation of dehydrodivanillin from the oxidation products of nitrobenzene. John C. Pew's findings have demonstrated that the structural linkage between the fifth carbon atoms of the two phenyl propane cells was not a result of a chemical reaction, but rather it was found to naturally exist within the wood lignin (Pew 1955).

12.2.3.5 Pine Resin Phenol or β-β′

The β-β′ bond, also known as the beta-beta prime bond, is a prominent feature in the chemical structure of lignin-phenolic compounds, such as pine resin phenol. The pine resin phenol was derived through the process of dehydrogenation polymerization of coniferyl alcohol. Subsequently, the structure of said phenol was identified during the decomposition of spruce lignin using methanol under ambient conditions. The content of this particular structure is found to be significantly lower in softwood lignin, whereas it tends to be relatively higher in hardwood lignin (Nimz et al. 1984).

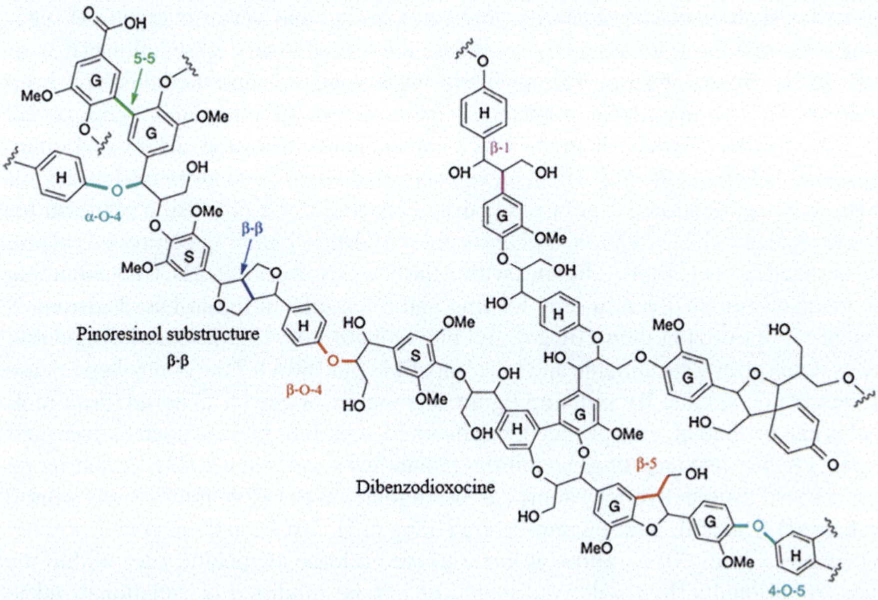

Fig. 12.1 Different types of interunit linkage present in a lignin motif. (Reproduced with permission (Figueiredo et al. 2018), copyright Elsevier)

12.2.3.6 Other Linkages

In addition to aforementioned bonds, α-O-4, 4-O-5 bonds also happen to exist in lignin structure (Evstigneyev et al. 2017). The formation of the 4-O-5 linking motif does not occur in the early stages of the lignification process. Instead, it is formed through the coupling of lignin oligomers or dimers. It makes up about 2% of the linking motifs in lignin, serving as a minor motif (Yue et al. 2016).

After the chemical pulping process is finished on plant materials, a little amount of lignin, known as residual lignin, remains in the resulting pulp. The chemical bond present in residual lignin displays unique properties in comparison to those observed in wood. The main reason for this difference is the increased occurrence of a polycondensation structure in lignin. After comparing traditional conventional kraft cooking (CK) with extended modified continuous cooking (EMCC), it was found that the residual lignin structure of the pulp was impacted. More precisely, the analysis revealed that the amount of β-O-4 in the residual lignin from the pulp produced by EMCC was lower, whereas the concentration of condensation-type structures was higher (Froass et al. 1998; McCarthy and Islam 1999). The main lignin linkages are summarized in Fig. 12.1.

12.3 Lignin Based Materials and Methods for Active Substance Loading

Lignin, a complex aromatic polymer abundant in plant cell walls, has emerged as a promising material for the development of drug delivery vehicles due to its renewable nature, biocompatibility, and tunable properties. Lignin possesses unique properties such as biodegradability, low cytotoxicity, and versatile chemical functionalities, making it an attractive candidate for drug delivery applications (Kumar et al. 2021). In recent years, various lignin-based materials and methods have been explored for loading active substances, including small molecules (Zhou et al. 2019a), proteins (Figueiredo et al. 2017), nucleic acids (Ten et al. 2014), and imaging agents (Zhang et al. 2023) to achieve controlled release and targeted delivery for therapeutic applications. Lignin-based drug carriers offer a promising platform for the entrapment, encapsulation, and absorption of drugs, enabling controlled release and targeted delivery to specific sites within the body (Nan et al. 2022). Understanding the mechanisms involved in drug loading and release from lignin-based carriers is crucial for optimizing their efficacy and biocompatibility. Lignin-based drug delivery systems offer a sustainable and biocompatible platform for the controlled release of therapeutic agents. By utilizing lignin as a matrix or carrier material, drug molecules can be loaded, encapsulated, or adsorbed, enabling precise control over their release kinetics and targeting capabilities (Chaudhary and Sinha 2023). Furthermore, lignin-based drug delivery systems can be engineered to respond to various stimuli such as pH (Lu et al. 2023), temperature (Jiang et al. 2018), and enzymatic activity (Yiamsawas et al. 2017), allowing for triggered release at specific sites within the body. Additionally, lignin-derived materials can be modified or functionalized to enhance their biocompatibility, stability, and pharmacokinetic profiles, paving the way for the development of novel therapeutics for a wide range of medical conditions (Riley and Vermerris 2022).

Lignin-based materials encompass a diverse range of formulations, including lignin nanoparticles (Tang et al. 2020), micro/nanogels (Xu et al. 2021), hydrogels (Meng et al. 2019), films (Zadeh et al. 2018), and scaffolds (Silva-Barroso et al. 2023), each offering distinct advantages for active substance loading and delivery. Lignin nanoparticles, typically prepared through methods such as nanoprecipitation, emulsion templating, or self-assembly, provide a high surface area-to-volume ratio and colloidal stability, making them ideal carriers for hydrophobic drugs and imaging agents (Schneider et al. 2021). Lignin micro/nanogels, formed via crosslinking or self-assembly of lignin molecules, offer tunable porosity, swelling behavior, and responsiveness to environmental stimuli, enabling the encapsulation and release of both hydrophilic and hydrophobic drugs (Rico-García et al. 2020). Lignin-based hydrogels, fabricated through the crosslinking of lignin with other polymers or crosslinkers, exhibit high water retention capacity and mechanical strength, making them suitable for sustained release and tissue engineering applications (Culebras et al. 2021).

Several methods have been employed for loading active substances into lignin-based drug delivery vehicles, including physical adsorption, chemical conjugation, co-precipitation, and emulsification (Morales et al. 2022; Gao et al. 2022; Zhou et al. 2019b). Physical adsorption involves the non-covalent attachment of drugs onto the surface or within the pores of lignin-based carriers, driven by interactions such as hydrogen bonding, hydrophobic interactions, and π-π stacking (Shi et al. 2013; McMichael et al. 2024). Chemical conjugation entails the covalent linkage of drugs to lignin molecules via reactive functional groups, enabling precise control over drug loading and release kinetics. Co-precipitation involves the simultaneous precipitation of lignin and drugs from solution, leading to the formation of composite nanoparticles or complexes with enhanced stability and encapsulation efficiency (Sharma et al. 2023). Emulsification techniques, such as solvent evaporation or solvent diffusion, enable the encapsulation of hydrophobic drugs within lignin-based nanoparticles or microspheres, providing protection against degradation and improving bioavailability (Moreno and Sipponen 2020).

Lignin-based drug delivery vehicles loaded with active substances hold immense potential for various biomedical applications, including cancer therapy (Garg et al. 2022), regenerative medicine (Witzler et al. 2018), infectious disease treatment (Morena and Tzanov 2022), and diagnostic imaging (Ali and Mehanna 2022). By tailoring the physicochemical properties of lignin-based materials and optimizing the loading and release parameters, researchers can achieve precise control over drug delivery kinetics, site-specific targeting, and therapeutic efficacy. Future research directions may focus on enhancing the biodegradability, biocompatibility, and stimuli-responsiveness of lignin-based drug delivery vehicles, as well as exploring novel strategies for multi-modal imaging, combination therapy, and personalized medicine (Karagoz et al. 2023; Stanisz et al. 2022).

12.4 Entrapment Encapsulation and Absorption

Entrapment involves the physical entrapment of drugs within the porous structure of lignin-based carriers. Lignin, with its highly porous and heterogeneous structure, provides ample space for drug molecules to be trapped within its matrix through various mechanisms such as adsorption, absorption, and physical entanglement (Nan et al. 2022). The entrapment process is influenced by factors such as the surface area, pore size distribution, and surface chemistry of lignin, as well as the physicochemical properties of the drug molecules (Abdullah et al. 2023).

During entrapment, drug molecules diffuse into the pores of lignin-based carriers driven by concentration gradients. Once inside the pores, the drugs may interact with lignin through non-covalent interactions such as hydrogen bonding, hydrophobic interactions, and π-π stacking, leading to their retention within the carrier matrix (Kumar et al. 2021; Verdini et al. 2022; Wijaya et al. 2021). The entrapment of drugs in lignin-based carriers offers protection against premature degradation and enhances their stability during storage and transportation.

Encapsulation involves the formation of a protective shell or coating around drug molecules, confining them within discrete particles or vesicles. In lignin-based drug delivery systems, encapsulation can be achieved through various techniques such as nanoprecipitation, emulsification, and coacervation. Lignin, owing to its amphiphilic nature and self-assembly properties, can spontaneously form nanostructures such as micelles, vesicles, and nanoparticles in aqueous solutions, facilitating the encapsulation of hydrophobic and hydrophilic drugs alike (Alqahtani et al. 2019; Lee et al. 2022). During encapsulation, drug molecules are solubilized or dispersed within the core of lignin-based nanoparticles or vesicles, which are then stabilized by the surrounding lignin matrix or surface-functionalized ligands. The encapsulation process not only improves the solubility and bioavailability of poorly water-soluble drugs but also enables sustained release and targeted delivery to specific tissues or cells. Additionally, the encapsulation of drugs within lignin-based carriers can minimize systemic toxicity and off-target effects, enhancing their therapeutic efficacy and safety profile.

Absorption involves the adhesion or attachment of drug molecules onto the surface of lignin-based carriers through interactions such as electrostatic attraction (Witzler et al. 2018; Zongo and Lange 2023), Van der Waals forces (Mishra and Ekielski 2019), and chemical bonding (Zheng et al. 2024). Lignin, with its rich abundance of functional groups including hydroxyl, carboxyl, and phenolic moieties, offers numerous sites for the adsorption of drugs via hydrogen bonding, ion exchange, and covalent conjugation.

During absorption, drug molecules adsorb onto the surface of lignin-based carriers, forming a monolayer or multilayer coating depending on the concentration and affinity of the drugs. The adsorbed drugs can be released from the carrier surface through desorption processes triggered by changes in environmental conditions such as pH, temperature, and ionic strength (Rico-García et al. 2020). The absorption of drugs onto lignin-based carriers can enhance their stability, prolong their circulation time in the bloodstream, and facilitate their uptake by target cells or tissues through receptor-mediated endocytosis or passive diffusion (Pathania et al. 2023; Dai et al. 2021).

The entrapment, encapsulation, and absorption of drugs in lignin-based drug carriers represent versatile strategies for achieving controlled release, targeted delivery, and enhanced therapeutic outcomes. By harnessing the unique properties of lignin, researchers continue to explore novel formulations and delivery platforms to address unmet needs in drug delivery and improve patient care. Lignin-based materials and methods offer versatile platforms for loading active substances in drug delivery vehicles, with the potential to revolutionize the field of biomedicine (Domínguez-Robles et al. 2020). By leveraging the unique properties of lignin and advancing innovative fabrication techniques, researchers can unlock new opportunities for developing next-generation therapeutics with improved safety, and efficacy (Tian et al. 2022). Additionally, the biocompatibility, biodegradability, and tunable properties of lignin make it an attractive candidate for the development of sustainable drug delivery systems, aligning with the growing demand for eco-friendly and bio-based materials in healthcare (Hachimi Alaoui et al. 2023). Furthermore, the ability of lignin-based carriers to respond to external stimuli and target specific tissues or cells holds promise for personalized medicine applications, enabling tailored treatment strategies and improved patient outcomes (Elumalai et al. 2024).

Lubna et al. developed Hyaluronic acid (HA) coated irinotecan loaded lignin nanoparticles (HDLNPs) using ionic interaction (Siddiqui et al. 2023). Nanoparticles optimized for enhanced chemotherapeutic targeting to cancer cells with over-expressed CD44 receptors were characterized. Hemocompatibility of HDLNPs was supported by interaction studies with blood components, demonstrating sustained plasma residence. Studies on HT-29 cells revealed significantly improved chemotherapeutic efficacy of HDLNPs, with retention of antioxidant activity of lignin observed in vitro. In vivo biodistribution studies in tumor-bearing mice confirmed enhanced drug localization at the tumor site over an extended period. Furthermore, ligand-assisted targeting chemotherapy showed efficacy in tumor regression, as indicated by histopathological studies. Encapsulation of irinotecan in HA-coated lignin nanoparticles suggested potential mitigation of myelosuppression, liver steatosis, and kidney failure associated with conventional therapy. HDLNPs demonstrated stability over 12 months.

Yeyan et al. developed LPC-MWCNT (Lignin/Poly(vinyl alcohol)-Multiwalled carbon nanotubes) hydrogel wound dressings utilizing lignin sourced from various low-cost, environmentally friendly materials, emphasizing its favorable biocompatibility (Chao et al. 2023). The mechanical properties and antioxidant activity of the hydrogels were found to be correlated with lignin content, exhibiting significant enhancement compared to PVA hydrogels. Lignin imparted antioxidant properties to the hydrogels, contributing to wound healing promotion and aligning with clean energy development. Additionally, carbon nanotubes conferred broad-spectrum photothermal antibacterial activity to the hydrogels. In vitro antibacterial assays demonstrated excellent bactericidal efficacy against E. coli and S. aureus. In a full-thickness skin defect wound model in mice, the hydrogel exhibited accelerated wound healing effects. Tissue staining experiments further validated the hydrogel's advantages in skin wound repair. The proposed hydrogel dressings exhibit potent antibacterial properties and robust wound healing capabilities, with potential for cost-effective large-scale production, facilitating clinical translation as next-generation biomass wound dressings.

Xiaojun et al. synthesized nitrogen and lanthanum co-doped multifunctional lignin-based carbon quantum dots ((N, La)-CQDs) via a straightforward one-step hydrothermal approach using enzymatic hydrolysis lignin as the substrate (Zhang et al. 2023). The resulting (N, La)-CQDs demonstrated the capability to detect specific ions in water samples, live cells, and zebrafish. These (N, La)-CQDs were employed as probes for the detection of Fe^{3+}, Sn^{2+}, and ClO^-, with detection limits of 0.99 μM, 1.1 μM, and 1.1 μM, respectively, and linear fit R2 values of 0.9997, 0.9943, and 0.9941, respectively. Assessment using 4 T1 cells as a model for cytotoxicity and cell imaging revealed that (N, La)-CQDs were non-toxic and emitted bright blue fluorescence within the cells. Furthermore, (N, La)-CQDs were successfully applied for zebrafish embryo imaging, displaying blue fluorescence within the zebrafish. The fluorescence intensity of zebrafish containing (N, La)-CQDs progressively decreased with increasing concentrations of Sn2+ solution. In conclusion, the non-cytotoxic (N, La)-CQDs exhibit promising potential as a material for selective ion detection in living organisms and aqueous environments, suggesting their suitability for applications in cell imaging and ion detection within the medical field.

12.5 Toxicological Parameters

Whilst engineered nanomaterials consist of materials that have been widely recognised for many decades, the assessment of their properties presents a unique and complex regulatory obstacle. The European Commission (EC) and the Food and Drug Administration (FDA) are currently engaged in a concerted endeavour aimed at achieving greater harmonisation in testing and assessment criteria (Rauscher et al. 2017; Sipponen et al. 2019). Historically, the classification of nanomaterials was primarily determined by their physical dimensions. However, contemporary regulatory measures and guidelines implemented by revered organisations such as the FDA and the EC have moved away from rigid size criteria. Consequently, the scope of the nanomaterial family has been expanded to include agglomerates of microsized particles.

Recent scholarly investigations have been dedicated to the pursuit of establishing a uniform approach to the toxicological evaluation of nanomaterials. Furthermore, it has been suggested that a number of preliminary measures should be taken in order to enhance the analysis of the ecological toxicity of nanomaterials. This observation is particularly significant due to the fact that nanomaterials are increasingly permeating various domains of contemporary existence, encompassing biomedical materials, agricultural commodities, home and personal care products, and numerous others. Furthermore, it is worth noting that engineered nanomaterials, even those comprised of otherwise harmless natural substances, exhibit a range of short- and long-term effects that have not yet been comprehensively elucidated.

Since the inception of debates surrounding the potential dangers associated with nanomaterials, the concept of Risk Assessment (RA) for chemicals has emerged as the most pertinent methodology for comprehending and pragmatically estimating said hazards (Hristozov et al. 2012). Being a naturally occurring substance, it can be stated that the fundamental ecotoxicity of lignin does not give rise to a substantial cause for concern. Nevertheless, it is important to acknowledge that, potential issues may arise as a result of chemical modifications that occur during the fabrication process. The utilisation of materials wherein the nanostructure emerges exclusively from macromolecular interactions of lignin presents inherently fewer challenges when contrasted with those incorporating chemically modified lignins. As an exemplification, the procedure of cross-linking lignin possesses the potentiality to markedly diminish its biodegradability. The phenomenon in question arises as a consequence of the hindrance of the phenolic hydroxyl (OH) groups, which function as the principal sites for enzymatic breakdown of lignins in their indigenous surroundings (Barclay et al. 1997; Gärtner et al. 1999; Ragnar et al. 2000). One persistent issue remains, regardless of whether or not lignin has been modified: A micro- or nanoparticle, in its fundamental nature, encapsulates a heightened concentration that is restricted within a condensed structure within the encompassing milieu. It is of utmost importance to acknowledge that the aforementioned concentration is not inherently natural. This specific piece of information possesses the inherent capacity to give rise to an "unanticipated" ecological toxicity, which becomes evident through an increased occurrence of Fenton-like oxidation by-products (Mai et al. 2000). It is abundantly clear that additional inquiry is imperative to shed light on the safety and environmental implications of utilising lignin-based nanomaterials in a wide range of emerging applications.

12.6 Conclusion

The rising demand for green biomaterials can be attributed to their cost-effectiveness in production and their environmentally friendly characteristics, such as biocompatibility and biodegradability. In order to achieve this heightened level of utilisation, the fields of bioengineering and nanotechnology are currently being advanced with the aim of creating highly promising means of transportation for various purposes. As lignin exhibits remarkable potential as a constituent of novel environmentally friendly materials, owing to its pivotal attributes, including its antioxidant, antimicrobial, and stabilising properties, which render this biopolymer highly promising for various practical applications (Alqahtani et al. 2019). The utilisation of lignin in the field of drug delivery systems has predominantly focused on harnessing its reflexive functionality. This includes its ability to adsorb and trap active substances, scavenge UV radiation, and facilitate pH-triggered release mechanisms (Li et al. 2017). At this juncture, we find ourselves on the cusp of a significant turning point, wherein our endeavours shall be directed towards the complex development of functional materials that are derived from lignin and possess inherent activity. The field of biomedical engineering, particularly in relation to lignin, is expected to draw insights and inspiration from the advancements made in the realm of other polymers and colloidal materials-based drug delivery systems. Furthermore, there exists a profound venture to expand the repertoire of distinct, precisely defined nanoscale constituents. It is within our vision that the establishment of a standardised approach to the manufacturing process of spherical lignin nanoparticles, lignin nanofibres, and lignin capsules (Iravani and Varma 2020; Fang et al. 2017; Sinha et al. 2022), will result in the attainment of uniform material characteristics and consequently facilitate the advancement of novel drug carriers in the future. In order to enhance the evaluation of different carrier materials derived from lignin, we strongly encourage researchers to employ clear and precise reporting of the values pertaining to encapsulation efficiency and loading capacity, in addition to other pertinent findings.

Several of the reports primarily centre their attention on the exploration of potential applications for lignin, yet they do not delve extensively into harnessing its distinctive properties. The future entails a more proactive utilisation of the distinctive chemical properties of lignins, such as their pH-responsive solubility and customisable thermal characteristics, in order to enhance their value in the drug chemistry. The importance of specific functionality cannot be overstated in numerous applications within the field of biomedicine, biosensors, and other high value-added domains. The next generation systems will consist of materials that contain multiple active substances, exhibiting potential for controlled sequential release or synergistic simultaneous action of entrapped or encapsulated substances. Typically, controlled release materials consist of a substrate that is sensitive to enzymes, which is connected to another component that induces alterations in the overall conformation at a macroscopic level.

It is of utmost importance to acknowledge that the existing corpus of scholarly investigations concerning the utilisation of lignin in the fabrication of nanoscale materials for the purpose of drug and gene delivery, along with other biomedical applications, remains rather limited in its extent. Furthermore, the examination of lignin nanoparticles using in vitro and in vivo analyses is significantly constrained, with only a small number of studies existing on the assessment of cytotoxicity. Furthermore, the progress made in the field of lignin-based hydrogels presents a significant opportunity for the replacement of conventional synthetic materials across a range of biomedical and industrial applications, in conjunction with the development of nanomaterials. Given the notable progress achieved in the realm of modification chemistry, one can reasonably predict that the domain of lignin valorisation, particularly in relation to its expanding capabilities at the nanoscale, will undoubtedly emerge as a prominent and noteworthy area of academic study in the coming years.

References

Abdullah T, İlyasoğlu G, Memić A (2023) Designing lignin-based biomaterials as carriers of bioactive molecules. Pharmaceutics 15:1114

Adler E (1957) Structural elements of lignin. Ind Eng Chem 49:1377–1383

Adler E, Marton J (1961) Carbonyl groups in lignin. Acta Chem Scand 15:9–369

Adler E, Pepper JM, Eriksoo E (1957) Action of mineral acid on lignin and model substances of Guaiacylglycerol-β-aryl ether type. Ind Eng Chem 49:1391–1392

Ainsworth EA, Gillespie KM (2007) Estimation of total phenolic content and other oxidation substrates in plant tissues using Folin–Ciocalteu reagent. Nat Protoc 2:875–877

Ali DA, Mehanna MM (2022) Role of lignin-based nanoparticles in anticancer drug delivery and bioimaging: an up-to-date review. Int J Biol Macromol 221:934–953

Alqahtani MS, Alqahtani A, Al-Thabit A, Roni M, Syed R (2019) Novel lignin nanoparticles for oral drug delivery. J Mater Chem B 7:4461–4473

Aro T, Fatehi P (2017) Production and application of Lignosulfonates and sulfonated lignin. ChemSusChem 10:1861–1877

Barclay LRC, Xi F, Norris JQ (1997) Antioxidant properties of phenolic lignin model compounds. J Wood Chem Technol 17:73–90

Brauns FE (1939) Native lignin 1 I. Its isolation and methylation. J Am Chem Soc 61:2120–2127

Cai J et al (2017) Review of physicochemical properties and analytical characterization of lignocellulosic biomass. Renew Sust Energ Rev 76:309–322

Chakar FS, Ragauskas AJ (2004) Review of current and future softwood Kraft lignin process chemistry. Ind Crop Prod 20:131–141

Chao Y et al (2023) Architecting lignin/poly(vinyl alcohol) hydrogel with carbon nanotubes for Photothermal antibacterial therapy. ACS Appl Bio Mater 6:1525–1535

Chaudhary M, Sinha VR (2023) Lignin-based carriers for drug delivery applications: from an industrial waste to a pharmaceutical aid. Eur Polym J 195:112206

Chen C-L (1992) Determination of Carbonyl Groups. In: Lin SY, Dence CW (eds) Methods in Lignin chemistry. Springer, Berlin, Heidelberg, pp 446–457. https://doi.org/10.1007/978-3-642-74065-7_30

Chen H (2014) Chemical composition and structure of natural lignocellulose. In: Biotechnology of lignocellulose. Springer Netherlands, pp 25–71. https://doi.org/10.1007/978-94-007-6898-7_2

Chen C-L, Robert D (1988) Characterization of lignin by 1H and 13C NMR spectroscopy. Methods Enzymol 161:137–174. https://doi.org/10.1016/0076-6879(88)61017-2
Crestini C, Lange H, Sette M, Argyropoulos DS (2017) On the structure of softwood Kraft lignin. Green Chem 19:4104–4121
Culebras M, Barrett A, Pishnamazi M, Walker GM, Collins MN (2021) Wood-derived hydrogels as a platform for drug-release systems. ACS Sustain Chem Eng 9:2515–2522
Dai L, Liu R, Si C-L (2021) Lignin-based materials for drug and gene delivery. In: Lignin-based materials for biomedical applications. Elsevier, pp 327–370. https://doi.org/10.1016/B978-0-12-820303-3.00006-0
de la Torre MJ, Moral A, Hernández MD, Cabeza E, Tijero A (2013) Organosolv lignin for biofuel. Ind Crop Prod 45:58–63
Dizhbite T (2004) Characterization of the radical scavenging activity of lignins? Natural antioxidants. Bioresour Technol 95:309–317
Doherty WOS, Mousavioun P, Fellows CM (2011) Value-adding to cellulosic ethanol: lignin polymers. Ind Crop Prod 33:259–276
Domínguez-Robles J et al (2019) Lignin and cellulose blends as pharmaceutical excipient for tablet manufacturing via direct compression. Biomol Ther 9:423
Domínguez-Robles J et al (2020) Lignin for pharmaceutical and biomedical applications—could this become a reality? Sustain Chem Pharm 18:100320
El Hage R et al (2009) Characterization of milled wood lignin and ethanol organosolv lignin from miscanthus. Polym Degrad Stab 94:1632–1638
Elumalai K, Srinivasan S, Shanmugam A (2024) Review of the efficacy of nanoparticle-based drug delivery systems for cancer treatment. Biomed Tech 5:109–122
Evstigneyev EI, Kalugina AV, Ivanov AY, Vasilyev AV (2017) Contents of α-O-4 and β-O-4 bonds in native lignin and isolated lignin preparations. J Wood Chem Technol 37:294–306
Fang W, Yang S, Wang X-L, Yuan T-Q, Sun R-C (2017) Manufacture and application of lignin-based carbon fibers (LCFs) and lignin-based carbon nanofibers (LCNFs). Green Chem 19:1794–1827
Figueiredo P et al (2017) In vitro evaluation of biodegradable lignin-based nanoparticles for drug delivery and enhanced antiproliferation effect in cancer cells. Biomaterials 121:97–108
Figueiredo P, Lintinen K, Hirvonen JT, Kostiainen MA, Santos HA (2018) Properties and chemical modifications of lignin: towards lignin-based nanomaterials for biomedical applications. Prog Mater Sci 93:233–269
Froass PM, Ragauskas AJ, Jiang JE (1998) NMR studies part 3: analysis of Lignins from modern Kraft pulping technologies. Holzforschung 52:385–390
Fu D, Mazza G, Tamaki Y (2010) Lignin extraction from straw by ionic liquids and enzymatic hydrolysis of the cellulosic residues. J Agric Food Chem 58:2915–2922
Fumoto E et al (2022) Determination of carbonyl functional groups in lignin-derived fraction using infrared spectroscopy. Fuel 318:123530
Gao K et al (2022) Lignin nanoparticles as highly efficient, recyclable emulsifiers for enhanced oil recovery. ACS Sustain Chem Eng 10:9334–9344
Garg J et al (2022) Applications of lignin nanoparticles for cancer drug delivery: an update. Mater Lett 311:131573
Gärtner A, Gellerstedt G, Tamminen T (1999) Determination of phenolic hydroxyl groups in residual lignin using a modified UV-method. Nord Pulp Pap Res J 14:163–170
Gellerstedt G (2015) Softwood Kraft lignin: raw material for the future. Ind Crop Prod 77:845–854
Gellerstedt G, Lindfors E-L (1984) Structural changes in lignin during Kraft pulping. Holzforschung 38:151–158
Gonçalves S et al (2021) Lignosulphonates as an alternative to non-renewable binders in wood-based materials. Polymers (Basel) 13:4196
Gopinath V et al (2022) Multifunctional applications of natural polysaccharide starch and cellulose: an update on recent advances. Biomed Pharmacother 146:112492
Gosselink RJA et al (2011) Effect of periodate on lignin for wood adhesive application. Holzforschung 65:155–162

Hachimi Alaoui C, Réthoré G, Weiss P, Fatimi A (2023) Sustainable biomass lignin-based hydrogels: a review on properties, formulation, and biomedical applications. Int J Mol Sci 24:13493

Harris EE, D'Ianni J, Adkins H (1938) Reaction of hardwood lignin with hydrogen. J Am Chem Soc 60:1467–1470

Hatfield R, Vermerris W (2001) Lignin formation in plants. The dilemma of linkage specificity. Plant Physiol 126:1351–1357

Hristozov DR, Gottardo S, Critto A, Marcomini A (2012) Risk assessment of engineered nanomaterials: a review of available data and approaches from a regulatory perspective. Nanotoxicology 6:880–898

Iravani S (2020) Biomedical applications of lignin-based nanoparticles. In: *Nanoparticles and their biomedical applications*. Springer Singapore, pp 217–224. https://doi.org/10.1007/978-981-15-0391-7_8

Iravani S, Varma RS (2020) Greener synthesis of lignin nanoparticles and their applications. Green Chem 22:612–636

Jiang P et al (2018) Preparation and characterization of thermo-sensitive gel with phenolated alkali lignin. Sci Rep 8:14450

Joffres B et al (2014) Catalytic hydroconversion of a wheat straw soda lignin: characterization of the products and the lignin residue. Appl Catal B Environ 145:167–176

Kai D, Jiang S, Low ZW, Loh XJ (2015) Engineering highly stretchable lignin-based electrospun nanofibers for potential biomedical applications. J Mater Chem B 3:6194–6204

Karagoz P et al (2023) Pharmaceutical applications of lignin-derived chemicals and lignin-based materials: linking lignin source and processing with clinical indication. Biomass Convers Biorefinery 14:26553–26574. https://doi.org/10.1007/s13399-023-03745-5

Katahira R, Elder TJ, Beckham GT (2018) Chapter 1. A Brief introduction to lignin structure. In: Lignin valorization: emerging approaches, pp 1–20. https://doi.org/10.1039/9781788010351-00001

Kumar R, Singh S, Singh OV (2008) Bioconversion of lignocellulosic biomass: biochemical and molecular perspectives. J Ind Microbiol Biotechnol 35:377–391

Kumar R et al (2021) Lignin: drug/gene delivery and tissue engineering applications. Int J Nanomedicine 16:2419–2441

Kuroda K, Nakagawa-izumi A (2006) Analytical pyrolysis of lignin: products stemming from β-5 substructures. Org Geochem 37:665–673

Lahive CW, Kamer PCJ, Lancefield CS, Deuss PJ (2020) An introduction to model compounds of lignin linking motifs; synthesis and selection considerations for reactivity studies. ChemSusChem 13:4238–4265

Lapierre C (2015) Application of new methods for the investigation of Lignin structure. In: Applied statistics in agricultural, biological, and environmental sciences, pp 133–166. https://doi.org/10.2134/1993.foragecellwall.c6

Lapierre C, Pollet B, Rolando C (1995) New insights into the molecular architecture of hardwood lignins by chemical degradative methods. Res Chem Intermed 21:397–412

Lee JH, Kim TM, Choi I-G, Choi JW (2021) Phenolic hydroxyl groups in the lignin polymer affect the Formation of lignin nanoparticles. Nano 11:1790

Lee JH, Im JS, Jin X, Kim TM, Choi JW (2022) In vitro and in vivo evaluation of drug-encapsulated lignin nanoparticles for release control. ACS Sustain Chem Eng 10:5792–5802

Li Y, Qiu X, Qian Y, Xiong W, Yang D (2017) pH-responsive lignin-based complex micelles: preparation, characterization and application in oral drug delivery. Chem Eng J 327:1176–1183

Li Q et al (2018) Tuning hydroxyl groups for quality carbon fiber of lignin. Carbon N Y 139:500–511

Lu Y-C, Lu Y, Fan X (2020) Structure and characteristics of Lignin. In: Lignin, pp 17–75. https://doi.org/10.1007/978-3-030-40663-9_2

Lu F et al (2023) Preparation of pH-sensitive lignin nanoparticles and its application in hydrophobic drug delivery. Ind Crop Prod 202:117012

Lundquist K, Stern K (1989) Analysis of lignins by 1H NMR spectroscopy. Nord Pulp Pap Res J 4:210–213

Magina S, Marques AP, Evtuguin DV (2015) Study on the residual lignin in Eucalyptus globulus sulphite pulp. Holzforschung 69:513–522

Mai C, Majcherczyk A, Hüttermann A (2000) Chemo-enzymatic synthesis and characterization of graft copolymers from lignin and acrylic compounds. Enzym Microb Technol 27:167–175

Månsson P (1983) Quantitative determination of phenolic and Total hydroxyl groups in Lignins. Holzforschung 37:143–146

Marita JM, Ralph J, Hatfield RD, Chapple C (1999) NMR characterization of lignins in Arabidopsis altered in the activity of ferulate 5-hydroxylase. Proc Natl Acad Sci 96:12328–12332

Marton J et al (1961) Carbonyl groups in lignin. IV. Infrared absorption studies and examination of the volumetric borohydride method. Acta Chem Scand 15:384–392

McCarthy JL, Islam A (1999) Lignin chemistry, technology, and utilization: a brief history. In: Lignin: historical, biological, and materials perspectives. ACS Publications, Washington, DC, pp 2–99. https://doi.org/10.1021/bk-2000-0742.ch001

McMichael PS, Hoque M, dos Santos FB, French V, Foster EJ (2024) Binary mixture of subcritical water and acetone: a hybrid solvent system towards the production of lignin nanoparticles. React Chem Eng 9:226–234

Meng Y, Lu J, Cheng Y, Li Q, Wang H (2019) Lignin-based hydrogels: a review of preparation, properties, and application. Int J Biol Macromol 135:1006–1019

Mishra PK, Ekielski A (2019) The self-assembly of lignin and its application in nanoparticle synthesis: a short review. Nano 9:243

Morales A, Labidi J, Gullón P (2022) Influence of lignin modifications on physically crosslinked lignin hydrogels for drug delivery applications. Sustain Mater Technol 33:e00474

Morena AG, Tzanov T (2022) Antibacterial lignin-based nanoparticles and their use in composite materials. Nanoscale Adv 4:4447–4469

Moreno A, Sipponen MH (2020) Lignin-based smart materials: a roadmap to processing and synthesis for current and future applications. Mater Horizons 7:2237–2257

Mosier N (2005) Features of promising technologies for pretreatment of lignocellulosic biomass. Bioresour Technol 96:673–686

Mousavioun P, Doherty WOS (2010) Chemical and thermal properties of fractionated bagasse soda lignin. Ind Crop Prod 31:52–58

Mullen CA, Boateng AA (2010) Catalytic pyrolysis-GC/MS of lignin from several sources. Fuel Process Technol 91:1446–1458

Nagieb ZA, Shukry N (1984) Investigation of lignins from soda and sulphate cooking of rice straw and corn stalks. Die Angew Makromol Chemie 127:67–87

Nan N, Hu W, Wang J (2022) Lignin-based porous biomaterials for medical and pharmaceutical applications. Biomedicines 10:747

Nimz H (1974) Beech lignin—proposal of a constitutional scheme. Angew Chemie Int Ed English 13:313–321

Nimz HH, Tschirner U, Stähle M, Lehmann R, Schlosser M (1984) Carbon-13 NMR spectra of Lignins, 10. 1 comparison of structural units in spruce and beech lignin. J Wood Chem Technol 4:265–284

Orlandi M, Rindone B, Molteni G, Rummakko P, Brunow G (2001) Asymmetric biomimetic oxidations of phenols: the mechanism of the diastereo- and enantioselective synthesis of dehydrodiconiferyl ferulate (DDF) and dehydrodiconiferyl alcohol (DDA). Tetrahedron 57:371–378

Pathania K et al (2023) Green synthesis of lignin-based nanoparticles as a bio-carrier for targeted delivery in cancer therapy. Int J Biol Macromol 229:684–695

Pérez M, Dominguez-López I, Lamuela-Raventós RM (2023) The chemistry behind the folin–ciocalteu method for the estimation of (poly)phenol content in food: total phenolic intake in a mediterranean dietary pattern. J Agric Food Chem 71:17543–17553

Pew JC (1955) Nitrobenzene oxidation of lignin model compounds, spruce wood and spruce "native lignin". J Am Chem Soc 77:2831–2833

Quraishi S et al (2015) Novel non-cytotoxic alginate–lignin hybrid aerogels as scaffolds for tissue engineering. J Supercrit Fluids 105:1–8

Radotić K, Mićić M (2016) Methods for extraction and purification of lignin and cellulose from plant tissues. In: Micic M (ed) Sample preparation techniques for soil, plant, and animal samples. Humana Press, New York, pp 365–376. https://doi.org/10.1007/978-1-4939-3185-9_26

Ragnar M, Lindgren CT, Nilvebrant N-O (2000) pK a -values of Guaiacyl and Syringyl phenols related to lignin. J Wood Chem Technol 20:277–305

Rauscher H, Rasmussen K, Sokull-Klüttgen B (2017) Regulatory aspects of nanomaterials in the EU. Chemie Ing Tech 89:224–231

Richel A, Vanderghem C, Simon M, Wathelet B, Paquot M (2012) Evaluation of matrix-assisted laser desorption/ionization mass spectrometry for second-generation lignin analysis. Anal Chem Insights 7:ACI.S10799

Rico-García D et al (2020) Lignin-based hydrogels: synthesis and applications. Polymers (Basel) 12:81

Riley MK, Vermerris W (2022) Delivery of DNA into human cells by functionalized lignin nanoparticles. Materials (Basel) 15:303

Rolando C, Monties B, Lapierre C (1992) Thioacidolysis. In: Lin SY, Dence CW (eds) Methods in Lignin chemistry. Springer, Berlin, Heidelberg, pp 334–349. https://doi.org/10.1007/978-3-642-74065-7_23

Ruwoldt J (2020) A critical review of the physicochemical properties of Lignosulfonates: chemical structure and behavior in aqueous solution, at surfaces and interfaces. Surfaces 3:622–648

Sakakibara A (1980) A structural model of softwood lignin. Wood Sci Technol 14:89–100

Schneider WDH, Dillon AJP, Camassola M (2021) Lignin nanoparticles enter the scene: a promising versatile green tool for multiple applications. Biotechnol Adv 47:107685

Serrano L et al (2018) Fast, easy, and economical quantification of lignin phenolic hydroxyl groups: comparison with classical techniques. Energy Fuel 32:5969–5977

Sharma S et al (2023) Lignin nanoparticles as a novel carrier for efficacious delivery of toll like receptor 7/8 agonist: physicochemical and in-vitro evaluation. J Indian Chem Soc 100:101008

Shi Y et al (2013) Π–Π stacking increases the stability and loading capacity of thermosensitive polymeric micelles for chemotherapeutic drugs. Biomacromolecules 14:1826–1837

Siddiqui L et al (2023) CD44 mediated colon cancer targeting mutlifaceted lignin nanoparticles: synthesis, in vitro characterization and in vivo efficacy studies. Int J Pharm 643:123270

Silva-Barroso AS, Cabral CSD, Ferreira P, Moreira AF, Correia IJ (2023) Lignin-enriched tricalcium phosphate/sodium alginate 3D scaffolds for application in bone tissue regeneration. Int J Biol Macromol 239:124258

Sinha A, Lim DZH, Wei J (2022) A lignin-based capsule system with tunable properties tailored for robust self-healing concrete. Cem Concr Compos 132:104643

Sipponen MH, Lange H, Crestini C, Henn A, Österberg M (2019) Lignin for Nano- and Microscaled carrier systems: applications, trends, and challenges. ChemSusChem 12:2039–2054

Spiridon I (2020) Extraction of lignin and therapeutic applications of lignin-derived compounds. A review. Environ Chem Lett 18:771–785

Stanisz M, Klapiszewski Ł, Collins MN, Jesionowski T (2022) Recent progress in biomedical and biotechnological applications of lignin-based spherical nano- and microstructures: a comprehensive review. Mater Today Chem 26:101198

Syrjänen K, Sipilä J, Björk H, Brunow G (2000) The identification of Dilignols from dehydrogenation mixtures of Coniferyl alcohol and Apocynol [4-(1-hydroxyethyl)-2-methoxyphenol] by LC-ES-MS/MS. J Agric Food Chem 48:5211–5215

Tang Q et al (2020) Lignin-based nanoparticles: a review on their preparations and applications. Polymers (Basel). 12:2471

Tao J et al (2020) Lignin—an underutilized, renewable and valuable material for food industry. Crit Rev Food Sci Nutr 60:2011–2033

Ten E et al (2014) Lignin nanotubes as vehicles for gene delivery into human cells. Biomacromolecules 15:327–338

Terashima N (2001) Possible approaches for studying three dimensional structure of Lignin. Prog Biotechnol 18:257–262. https://doi.org/10.1016/S0921-0423(01)80080-0

Thakur BR, Singh RK, Handa AK, Rao MA (1997) Chemistry and uses of pectin — a review. Crit Rev Food Sci Nutr 37:47–73

Tian H et al (2022) Enhancing the therapeutic efficacy of nanoparticles for cancer treatment using versatile targeted strategies. J Hematol Oncol 15:132

Timell TE (1960) Isolation and properties of an O-Acetyl-4-O-methylglucurono-xyloglycan from the wood of white birch (Betula papyrifera) 1. J Am Chem Soc 82:5211–5215
Toledano A, García A, Mondragon I, Labidi J (2010) Lignin separation and fractionation by ultrafiltration. Sep Purif Technol 71:38–43
Tribot A et al (2019) Wood-lignin: supply, extraction processes and use as bio-based material. Eur Polym J 112:228–240
Vasile C, Baican M (2023) Lignins as promising renewable biopolymers and bioactive compounds for high-performance materials. Polymers (Basel). 15:3177
Verdini F et al (2022) Lignin as a natural carrier for the efficient delivery of bioactive compounds: from waste to health. Molecules 27:3598
Watkins D, Nuruddin M, Hosur M, Tcherbi-Narteh A, Jeelani S (2015) Extraction and characterization of lignin from different biomass resources. J Mater Res Technol 4:26–32
Welker C et al (2015) Engineering plant biomass lignin content and composition for biofuels and bioproducts. Energies 8:7654–7676
Wijaya CJ, Ismadji S, Gunawan S (2021) A review of Lignocellulosic-derived nanoparticles for drug delivery applications: lignin nanoparticles, Xylan nanoparticles, and cellulose nanocrystals. Molecules 26:676
Witzler M et al (2018) Lignin-derived biomaterials for drug release and tissue engineering. Molecules 23:1885
Wu X et al (2018) Solar energy-driven lignin-first approach to full utilization of lignocellulosic biomass under mild conditions. Nat Catal 1:772–780
Xu F, Sun J-X, Sun R, Fowler P, Baird MS (2006) Comparative study of organosolv lignins from wheat straw. Ind Crop Prod 23:180–193
Xu J et al (2021) Lignin-incorporated Nanogel serving as an antioxidant biomaterial for wound healing. ACS Appl Bio Mater 4:3–13
Ye Y, Zhang Y, Fan J, Chang J (2012) Novel method for production of Phenolics by combining lignin extraction with lignin Depolymerization in aqueous ethanol. Ind Eng Chem Res 51:103–110
Yiamsawas D, Beckers SJ, Lu H, Landfester K, Wurm FR (2017) Morphology-controlled synthesis of lignin Nanocarriers for drug delivery and carbon materials. ACS Biomater Sci Eng 3:2375–2383
Yoo CG, Meng X, Pu Y, Ragauskas AJ (2020) The critical role of lignin in lignocellulosic biomass conversion and recent pretreatment strategies: a comprehensive review. Bioresour Technol 301:122784
Yue F, Lu F, Ralph S, Ralph J (2016) Identification of 4–O–5-units in softwood Lignins via definitive lignin models and NMR. Biomacromolecules 17:1909–1920
Zadeh EM, O'Keefe SF, Kim Y-T (2018) Utilization of lignin in biopolymeric packaging films. ACS Omega 3:7388–7398
Zhang X, Tu M, Paice MG (2011) Routes to potential bioproducts from Lignocellulosic biomass lignin and hemicelluloses. Bioenergy Res 4:246–257
Zhang X et al (2023) Non-cytotoxic lanthanum and nitrogen co-doped lignin-based carbon dots for selective detection of ions in biological imaging. J Environ Chem Eng 11:109881
Zheng Y, Moreno A, Zhang Y, Sipponen MH, Dai L (2024) Harnessing chemical functionality of lignin towards stimuli-responsive materials. Trends Chem 6:62–78
Zhou Y et al (2019a) Preparation of targeted lignin–based hollow nanoparticles for the delivery of doxorubicin. Nano 9:188
Zhou Y, Han Y, Li G, Chu F (2019b) Effects of lignin-based hollow nanoparticle structure on the loading and release behavior of doxorubicin. Materials (Basel) 12:1694
Zongo L, Lange H (2023) Lignin and its composites for drug delivery applications. In: Lignin-based materials. The Royal Society of Chemistry, pp 130–160. https://doi.org/10.1039/BK9781839167843-00130

Lignin-Based Hydrogels for Pharmaceutical and Biomedical Applications

13

Neelakanta Sarvashiva Kiran, Chandrashekar Yashaswini, Sudarshan Singh, and Bhupendra Gopalbhai Prajapati

Abstract

Lignin, a renewable and abundant biopolymer derived from plant cell walls, has gained attention for its remarkable mechanical strength, biocompatibility, and inherent antioxidant properties. The synthesis of lignin-based hydrogels involves the integration of lignin with other polymers or crosslinkers, resulting in versatile and tunable materials. These hydrogels exhibit excellent water retention capacity, swelling behaviour, and controlled release properties, making them promising candidates for drug delivery systems. Additionally, the inherent biodegradability of lignin-based hydrogels aligns with the increasing demand for sustainable and eco-friendly materials in the biomedical field. The antioxidant properties of lignin further contribute to their potential application in wound healing and tissue engineering. This abstract highlights the recent advancements in the development of lignin-based hydrogels, emphasizing their unique characteristics and the potential for addressing current challenges in pharmaceutical and biomedical applications, ranging from drug delivery systems to tissue engineering scaffolds. This chapter presents a comprehensive overview of the

N. S. Kiran · C. Yashaswini
Department of Biotechnology, School of Applied Sciences, REVA University, Bengaluru, Karnataka, India

S. Singh
Office of Research Administration, Chiang Mai University, Chiang Mai, Thailand

Faculty of Pharmacy, Chiang Mai University, Chiang Mai, Thailand

B. G. Prajapati (✉)
Shree S. K. Patel College of Pharmaceutical Education and Research, Ganpat University, Kherva, Gujarat, India

Centre for Research Impact & Outcome, Chitkara College of Pharmacy, Chitkara University, Rajpura, 140401, India

M. N. Collins, M. Culebras (eds.), *Sustainable Biopolymers and Composites for Biomedical Applications*, Biomaterials, Bioengineering and Sustainability 5,
https://doi.org/10.1007/978-3-031-91972-5_13

emerging field of lignin-based hydrogels and their potential applications in pharmaceutical and biomedical contexts.

Keywords

Lignin · Antioxidant · Drug delivery · Biodegradability · Wound healing · Tissue engineering

13.1 Introduction

As the fossil fuel industry's negative effects on the environment worsen, there is a rising interest in finding clean, alternative fuels that are available worldwide. Materials made of lignocellulosic biomass provide a potential remedy by lowering dependency on petrochemical resources. Researchers are paying more attention to agricultural waste because it contains a large amount of lignocellulosic biomass, which is commonly burned to generate electricity. Because it is abundant, renewable, and does not compete with food supplies, biomass is a desirable material for generating high-value goods that are also economically and environmentally sound (Barzegar et al. 2022; Domínguez-Robles et al. 2021). The main components of lignocellulosic biomass are 35–50 weight percent cellulose, 20–35 weight percent hemicellulose, and 10–25 weight percent lignin; however, the exact ratios might vary depending on the plant species, origin, and environmental factors. Various techniques have been developed to overcome the refractory character of lignocellulosic biomass, which has been related to cellulose crystal structure, lignin hydrophobic nature, and cellulose entrapment by the lignin–hemicellulose network (Terzioğlu et al. 2020). Because of its intricate propyl phenolic subunit structure, lignin is a difficult biopolymer that has drawn a lot of interest from scientists. Understanding the unique properties and physicochemical behaviour of lignin for usage in diverse formulations has been the focus of recent research. Researchers are investigating lignin's potential in creating innovative materials including hydrogels, films, nanofibers, as well as nanoparticles by utilizing its essential qualities, which include being biodegradable thermal stability, and reactivity (Domínguez-Robles et al. 2020; Ribeiro et al. 2023). Hydrogels have acquired popularity for a variety of applications, including carbon capture, agricultural water retention, biomedical usage, cleanliness, and elasticity due to their high water content, flexibility, and biocompatibility. A notable trend has been the move away from synthetic polymers and toward chemical alterations of biopolymers, which are biocompatible, biodegradable, low toxicity, and susceptible to enzymatic destruction. Among other biopolymers, lignin is a particularly good option for creating innovative hydrogels because of its low cytotoxicity, biocompatibility, antibacterial, and anti-inflammatory properties (Rico-García et al. 2020). Lignin-based hydrogels have potential uses in tissue engineering, medication delivery, wound healing, 3D bioprinting, and other biomedical fields. To improve hydrogel compositions' biological and physicochemical qualities, lignin must be included, frequently together with synthetic or biopolymers. The process of copolymerization has been utilized to guarantee superior mechanical qualities and water retention, while lignin enhances swelling as well as thermo-oxidative stability (Liu et al. 2020). There are several techniques used in the manufacture of lignin-based hydrogels, some of which include physical or chemical interactions. In certain situations, lignin functions as a crosslinked unit to create hydrogels such as lignin–cellulose, lignin–formaldehyde, or lignin–polyurethane (Nan et al. 2022). On the other hand, lignin functions as an agent of crosslinking for hydrogels that include chitosan or acrylic acid. While lignin-based hydrogels have attracted a lot of attention lately, particularly in the biomedical and pharmaceutical fields, there aren't many thorough studies on their application in 3D bioprinting, tissue engineering, wound healing, and medication administration (Karagoz et al. 2023; Hachimi Alaoui et al. 2023). By highlighting significant advancements in molecular research that have been published within the last five years, this chapter seeks to close this gap.

13.2 Lignin Biopolymer

Lignin, which comes from the Latin term "lignum," which means wood, was identified by Candolle in 1819 and makes up a sizable component of the cell wall of lignocellulosic biomass. It may be derived from a variety of materials, such as wood residuals, energy crops, and agricultural wastes (Lisý et al. 2022). Isolated lignin usually has a molecular mass of between 1000 and 20,000 g/mol. Lignin serves as a structural component that gives plant cell walls strength, stiffness, and impermeability, which facilitates the passage of water and other solutes via the vascular system. Furthermore, lignin has notable attributes such as low cytotoxicity, antibacterial and antioxidant activities, thermal resistance, anti-inflammatory effects, and biocompatibility based on the makeup of its functional groups (Sharma et al. 2020; Baloch and Labidi 2021). It is essential for protecting plants from biochemical stressors because it prevents other components from being broken down by enzymes. Lignin acts as a chemical and physical barrier to keep microbes and terrestrial animals out of plant tissues. As a result, lignin is shown to be physiologically and mechanically appropriate for the synthesis of various biomaterials, such as hydrogels. Notwithstanding its significance, the precise composition of lignin is still a mystery (Agrawal et al. 2022; Vásquez-Garay et al. 2021).

13.2.1 Methodologies for Lignin Isolation Alongside Extraction Processing

Bjokman was the first to extract lignin utilizing a dioxane–water combination in 1956. Since then, several techniques have been developed for lignin extraction from various biomass sources. Different lignin varieties have been produced using a variety of methods developed to separate lignin from additional elements in lignocellulosic biomass (Huang et al. 2020). Both the recovery yield and the physicochemical characteristics of the lignin that is recovered are strongly influenced by variables such as raw material type, ambient temperature, solvent quantity, and reaction time. Preliminary procedures such as hot-water pretreatments, acid hydrolysis, or mechanical treatments can be used to improve the process by solubilizing the fraction of hemicellulose in lignocellulosic biomass (Erdocia et al. 2021; Rodrigues et al. 2021). Lignin is produced by various extraction techniques in a variety of forms, which allows it to be classified as technical lignins that include sulfur or not. When lignin is extracted in its raw form from lignocellulosic biomass, it usually becomes fragmented into different mixes of unidentified ingredients. A range of pretreatment techniques, classified as physicochemical, enzymatic, and chemical, have been developed to investigate and expedite the separation and reclamation of lignin of lignocellulosic biomass. Processes including kraft, sulfite, alkaline in nature steam an explosion, or hydrolysis can be used to get lignin. Furthermore, "greener solvents" such as deep eutectic solvents and ionic liquids can be used to extract lignin biopolymers. Several post-treatments can be used to improve the purity of the lignins that are produced after extraction (Lobato-Peralta et al. 2021; Kienberger et al. 2021).

13.2.2 Structure and Arrangement

Coniferyl alcohol, sinapyl alcohol, and p-coumaryl alcohol are the three primary monolignols that are used to synthesize lignin, which is an aromatic biopolymer that is three-dimensional (3D), translucent, or extensively crosslinked (Fig. 13.1). Enzymatic polymerization of these monolignols results in the production of unique lignin subunits called p-hydroxyphenyl (H), as well as syringyl (S) (Zhang et al.

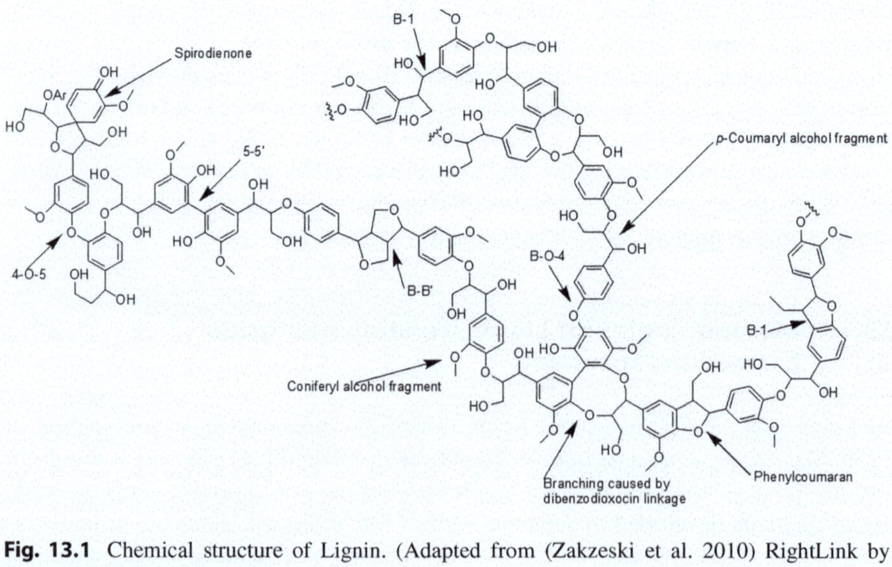

Fig. 13.1 Chemical structure of Lignin. (Adapted from (Zakzeski et al. 2010) RightLink by Copyrisht Clearance Center)

2022). The subunits function as active sites for prospective chemical changes and lignin utilization because they include a variety of chemical groups, including hydroxyl, carboxyl, and carbonyl, along with methoxy groups. The subunits differ in how many methoxy groups they contain (Liao et al. 2020; Zhang and Naebe 2021). Furthermore, through phenyl glycoside, benzene ether, and benzyl ester interactions, lignin establishes covalent bonds with hemicellulose and cellulose to create lignin–carbohydrate complexes (LCCs). Plant species, growing conditions in the environment, harvest seasons, as well as the extraction techniques used to separate lignin from lignin–carbohydrate complexes are some of the variables that affect the content and nature of lignin (Jia et al. 2023). The presence of other monolignols in tiny levels can cause extra inter-unit connections in some plant species, making it more difficult to determine the degree of polymerization. It is still difficult to understand the macromolecular framework of lignin because of its varied makeup. The majority of lignin's connections, or about 50% of all linkages, are β-O-4 ether linkages, which are an important target for several degradation pathways. Smaller percentages of other bonds in the structure include β-5 phenylcoumaran, α-O-4 ether, 4-O-5 diphenyl ethyl 5–5 biphenyl, along with β-1 diphenylmethane (Meng et al. 2021; Zheng et al. 2021).

13.2.3 Properties of Lignin for Utilisation in Medicine

Numerous studies have demonstrated the biodegradable, renewable, environmentally friendly, and safe properties of lignin as a biopolymer. Its potential uses as an antibacterial, hemostatic, antioxidant, and anti-ultraviolet agent have been noted (Shu et al. 2021; Sakagami et al. 2010). The functional groups found in lignin, such as aromatic rings, carboxyl, hydroxyl, carbonyl molecules, and methoxy groups, as well as aliphatic and phenolic groups, are responsible for these advantageous characteristics. These qualities might open the door for creative ways to formulate various materials for use in the biomedical and pharmaceutical industries (Nan et al. 2022; Spiridon 2020).

13.3 Pharmaceutical and Biomedical Application of Lignin Based Hydrogels

Lignin has become a highly promising option for the main polymer in hydrogels made for many biological applications (Table 13.1). Application areas for lignin-based hydrogels include 3D bioprinting, drug delivery systems, tissue engineering, and wound dressing (Fig. 13.2).

Table 13.1 Diverse pharmaceutical and biomedical applications of lignin-based hydrogels

Applications	Role of lignin-based hydrogels	Mechanism of action	References
Drug delivery systems	Sustained release platform	Lignin, as a hydrophilic polymer, facilitates controlled drug release through diffusion, ensuring prolonged therapeutic effects. Its structural versatility allows tailoring of release kinetics based on specific drug requirements. The inherent antioxidant properties of lignin can also contribute to the stability of certain drugs.	Das et al. (2024)
Tissue engineering	Biomimetic scaffold	Lignin-based hydrogels serve as biomimetic scaffolds, mimicking the extracellular matrix. Lignin's structural integrity, porous nature, and tunable mechanical properties support cell adhesion, proliferation, and differentiation. Additionally, lignin's phenolic groups can enhance cell-material interactions, promoting tissue regeneration.	Zheng et al. (2024)
Wound healing	Anti-inflammatory and tissue repair	Lignin's antioxidant and anti-inflammatory properties play a pivotal role in wound healing. By scavenging free radicals and modulating inflammatory responses, lignin-based hydrogels contribute to reduced oxidative stress, faster tissue repair, and accelerated wound closure. The hydrogels also provide a moist environment, conducive to optimal healing conditions.	Wu et al. (2024)
Biocompatible materials	Minimal immunogenic response	Lignin's biocompatibility arises from its natural abundance and low immunogenicity. The hydrogels exhibit compatibility with biological systems, minimizing adverse reactions. The ability to modify lignin's surface chemistry further enhances its integration with host tissues, making it a suitable material for various biomedical devices and implants.	Hu et al. (2024)
Antimicrobial applications	Pathogen inhibition	Lignin's inherent antimicrobial properties, stemming from its phenolic content, enable hydrogels to inhibit the growth of bacteria and fungi. This antimicrobial activity is valuable for preventing infections in wounds and providing a sterile environment for biomedical applications, such as catheters and implants.	Fazeli et al. (2024)

13.3.1 Tissue Engineering

In the multidisciplinary subject of tissue engineering, damaged tissues or organs from acute trauma or chronic illnesses can be preserved, replaced, enhanced, or restored using cells, growth hormones, and sophisticated scaffolds. The best scaffolds will have outstanding rheological characteristics, an interlinked porous

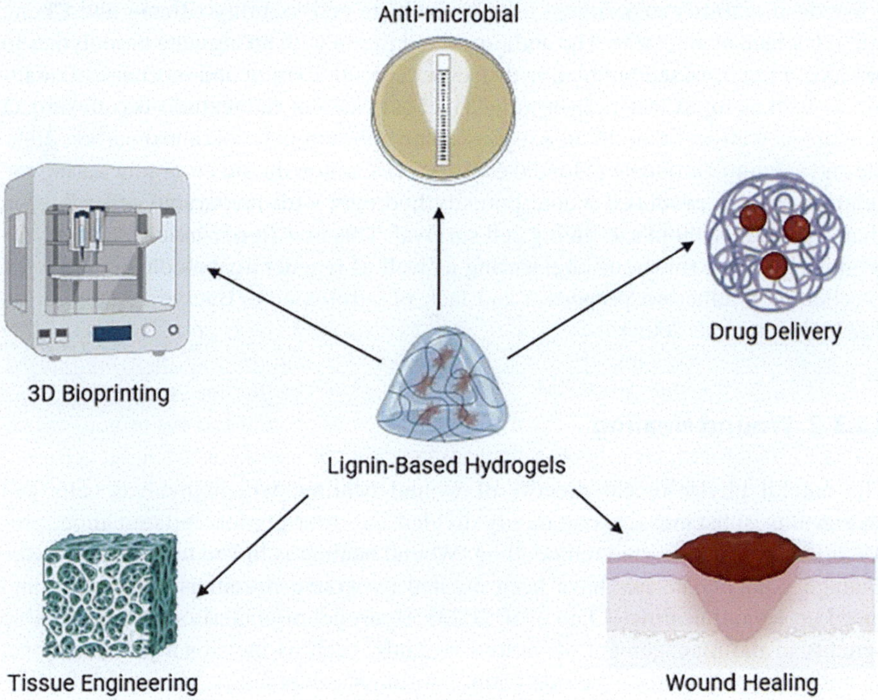

Fig. 13.2 Various applications of lignin-based hydrogels

structure, biodegradability, and possible biocompatibility (Chavooshi et al. 2023; Wang et al. 2023a). Because of their bioactivity and ability to resemble the natural extracellular matrix in three dimensions, lignin-based hydrogels are regarded as promising scaffold alternatives for tissue regeneration. Furthermore, by establishing an appropriate porosity microenvironment that promotes gas diffusion as well as metabolite exchange, these biomaterials aid in the growth and differentiation of enclosed cells. Thus, injured tissues can be restored without requiring open surgery thanks to this. For example, hydrogels made of alkali lignin and chitosan are very desired for biological applications because they have advantageous properties including biocompatibility as well as a surface with electrical conductivity for cell adhesion and development (Ribeiro et al. 2023; Lyu et al. 2023). In recent studies, a unique construction of a nontoxic hydrogel combining chitosan with alkali lignin was presented. Another lignin-based hydrogel has demonstrated remarkable mechanical and non-toxic qualities in the field of tissue engineering applications (Radotić et al. 2023). Using ultrasonic therapy for lignin nanoparticle dissolution and in situ free-radical polymerization, Chen et al. created a variety of lignin–PAAm hydrogels. Human gastroesophageal squamous carcinoma cells were then co-cultured with these hydrogels based on lignin. The cells in the hydrogels were found to have high vitality levels and to have kept their proliferative activity, according to a live/dead viability experiment used to evaluate cell viability (Zhang and Cheng 2023; Ciolacu et al. 2023). The authors mixed lignin with an alginate biopolymer to produce a lignin-based bubbled hydrogel with good textural and mechanical qualities as well as rapid water absorption. The basic idea of the method was to subject alginate as well as lignin to an aqueous-alkali solution that contained carbon dioxide and calcium carbonate (Mondal et al. 2023). Carbon dioxide foaming during the gelation process produced a dual-porosity hydrogel with favourable cell adhesion characteristics without sacrificing cell survival. This new lignin-based hydrogel is a promising option for tissue engineering as well as regenerative medicine due to its excellent cell adhesion properties and lack of cytotoxicity (Hachimi Alaoui et al. 2023; Chiani et al. 2023).

13.3.2 Wound Healing

The natural physiological process of wound healing, which involves cells and endogenous substances, is commonly divided into four phases: inflammation, proliferation, hemostasis, and remodelling. Wound healing is linked to structural tissue damage. Many materials have been created as wound dressings to improve and speed up wound healing (Chao et al. 2023). Hydrogel biomaterials provide notable benefits in the management of various wounds, such as incisional and excisional wounds, because of their porous nature, softness, adaptability, stretchability, biocompatibility, as well as elevated water content. These hydrogels can take up exudate, keep the wound wet, and transfer cells and bioactive materials. This function seeks to reduce scarring, minimize infection and desiccation, relieve pain, and stimulate immune cells to hasten recovery (Balaji et al. 2023; Balk et al. 2023). A sterile, non-toxic dressing for a wound should encourage blood flow and maintain the proper temperature. Hydrogels have developed from traditional wound dressings to efficient regenerative templates in recent years, aiding in the healing of burn injuries as well as various skin lesions and encouraging wound closure (Karagoz et al. 2023; Crivello et al. 2023). Hydrogel dressings that contain antioxidants along with antibacterial agents, including lignin biopolymers, have been shown to improve wound healing. Lignin-based hydrogels successfully eliminate unwanted substances, oppose microbial infections, and supply injury protection with an atmosphere of moisture conducive to gas exchange as well as exudate absorption (Balk et al. 2023). This is in contrast to traditional passive coverings like gauze as well as cotton, which are not able to create a damp healing environment that could result in reinjury upon removal. Crucially, it is possible to extract them without further physically harming the incision (Luo et al. 2023; Du et al. 2023; Mukheja et al. 2023).

13.3.3 Drug Delivery

Hydrogels are particularly well-researched drug delivery methods. The properties of the polymers, the composition of the formulation, and the solute all have an impact on the processes controlling drug release from hydrogels (Sanchez et al. 2023; Abdullah et al. 2023). Since lignin-based hydrogels are known for their low toxicity, chemical composition, biocompatibility, antioxidant and antibacterial activity, and stimuli-responsiveness, they have been thoroughly studied for potential use as drug delivery vehicles. By precisely and carefully administering natural substances to the damaged location, this method seeks to maximize their therapeutic efficacy while minimizing severe toxicological consequences (Zheng et al. 2023; Pathania et al. 2023; Chaudhary and Sinha 2023). The hydrogel network's density affects how quickly drugs are released. Because of their porous nature, hydrogels are especially appealing as drug delivery systems, which leads to better outcomes during therapy and a wide range of clinical uses. Hydrogels show great promise for regulated drug release via several processes contingent on the release's rate-limiting step. (i) Diffusion-controlled, depending on the drug's diffusivity through the polymeric matrix; (Nissinen and Kähäri 2014) swelling-controlled, where the amount of time needed for the solvent to diffuse through the matrix and form the gel layer is critical; and (iii) scientifically controlled, reliant on reactions taking place within the polymeric matrix (Joseph et al. 2023; Aquib 2023). Numerous hydrogels derived from polysaccharides, such as lignin, have been created for use in medication administration. Many researchers have experimented with different hydrogel formulations for drug administration by employing sodium hypophosphite and citric acid as catalysts in a reactive extrusion process with lignin, hemicellulose, and starch (Vasile and Baican 2023; Ivanova et al. 2023). Drug delivery using previously created lignin-based hydrogels showed promise. In one work, lignin was mixed with PMVE/MA as well as PEG to produce an extremely swellable hydrogel that allowed hydrophobic curcumin to be released under controlled conditions for up to four days. *S. aureus*, as well as *P. mirabilis*, showed notable decreases in adhesion when this hydrogel was used (Xu et al. 2024; Thang et al. 2023; Liu et al. 2023). Furthermore, Raschip et al. created a lignin–xanthan hydrogel with ECH as a cross-linking agent to release hydrophilic bisoprolol fumarate in a regulated manner, to treat heart failure and hypertension. Furthermore, lignin produced hydrogels with substantial swelling capabilities when mixed with cellulose along with ECH, which were then used to release polyphenols (Lu et al. 2023; Li et al. 2023a).

13.3.4 Three-Dimensional (3D) Bioprinting

3D bioprinting technology offers significant benefits over traditional tissue engineering techniques in the domains of tissue engineering as well as regenerative medicine (Wang et al. 2023b). The main difference is the use of bio-inks, which consist of layers that are deposited methodically in a pattern that resembles the architecture of natural tissues and organs. This novel method entails the in vitro as well as in vivo creation of structures packed with cells by layering bio-inks one after the other (Shah et al. 2023; Ruiz Deance et al. 2023). To create anatomically realistic biological constructions, it is a computer-assisted method that allows for exact control along with management of cellular and biological material geometries as well as their spatial distribution. This methodology's capacity to repeatedly and accurately insert tiny amounts of materials as well as cells in predetermined places in an iterative fashion is one of its primary features (Chandna et al. 2023; Jiang et al. 2023). Additionally, it makes it easier to create customized macroscopic and microscopic constructions at different scales that are matched to the anatomy of each patient. Reynolds and colleagues have presented a new microporous-structured matrix enabling embedded bioprinting, exhibiting tunable porosity, printing behaviour, and rheology. The use of these matrices offers new opportunities for the in vitro biomanufacturing of complex tissue microenvironments, with significant promise for therapeutic tissue engineering, disease modeling, and drug discovery applications (Wei et al. 2023; Lameirinhas et al. 2023). The most widely used 3D bioprinting technologies include laser-induced forward transfer, extrusion-based processes, cellular inkjet printing, and soft lithography. Because of their advantageous properties, which include functionality, physicochemical traits, and rheological qualities required to offer structural support and prevent cell injury, hydrogels have been thoroughly studied as bio-inks (Ding et al. 2023; Wan et al. 2023). Bio-inks are characterized as a combination of materials, molecules from biology, or cells appropriate for processing using automated fabrication technologies. Furthermore, because lignin biopolymer is non-cytotoxic, biocompatible, biodegradable, physically durable, and reactive, It shows promise as a hydrogel production process for three-dimensional bioprinting applications. As such, relevant literature highlights important research demonstrating the application of lignin-based hydrogels, which have improved printability and necessary functionality as biomaterial inks, in different 3D bioprinting projects (Keck et al. 2023; Bierach et al. 2023).

13.4 Future Prospects

The remarkable properties that lignin-based hydrogels display make them extremely attractive options for use in the biomedical field. Their promise in a variety of fields, including tissue engineering, medication delivery, wound healing, and 3D bioprinting, is highlighted by our thorough analysis (Feng et al. 2023; Li et al. 2023b). For example, investigated the potential uses of lignin-based hydrogels for tissue engineering as wound healing. These hydrogels are created by mixing lignin with chitosan (Afewerki and Edlund 2023; Queiroz et al. 2023). On the other hand, combined cellulose, alginate, and lignin to create hydrogels appropriate for 3D printing. Fewer researchers also created lignin-xanthan hydrogels with ECH as a coupling agent for drug delivery. Continued efforts are necessary to create new formulations or improve existing performance to further increase their usefulness in the biomedical domain. This is especially important when considering 3D bioprinting, a cutting-edge technique that has significant implications for regenerative medicine (Ariyanta et al. 2023a; Tardy et al. 2023). Numerous techniques have been developed to tackle the difficulties posed by the resistant characteristics of lignocellulosic material and enable the lignin biopolymer to be extracted more easily (Xiao et al. 2023; Ariyanta et al. 2023b; Siddiqa et al. 2023). Lignin is becoming more and more popular due to its attractive qualities, which are especially helpful when used to create high-value goods, such as hydrogels. Lignin-based hydrogels have attracted a lot of attention lately because of their unique qualities and possible uses. These hydrogels contribute to improvements in healthcare by providing a modifiable platform to overcome various obstacles in the biomedical area (Tariq et al. 2023; Wang et al. 2023c).

13.5 Conclusions

Hydrogels based on lignin have a lot of promise for use in biomedicine. By combining lignin with other polymers and biopolymers, scientists may adjust the characteristics of these hydrogels to meet certain application needs. The traits associated with mechanical durability, stable gel formation and viscoelasticity, film-forming ability, water absorption capacity, and controlled-release features are all improved by this synergistic combination. Because of these improved qualities, lignin-based hydrogels are especially appealing for use in 3D bioprinting, drug delivery, tissue engineering, and wound healing. The purpose of this work is to further improve our comprehension of lignin biopolymers as well as their potential for use as hydrogels by providing an extensive overview of the literature. It provides a comprehensive review of the many kinds of lignin-based hydrogels, including information on how they are prepared and how they are used in different biomedical fields.

Acknowledgement The authors greatly acknowledge and convey our sincere gratitude to REVA University, Chiang Mai University and Ganpat University for providing an opportunity and platform for research.

Conflict of Interest We the authors declare no potential conflict of interest.

References

Abdullah T, İlyasoğlu G, Memić A (2023) Designing lignin-based biomaterials as carriers of bioactive molecules. Pharmaceutics 15(4):1114

Afewerki S, Edlund U (2023) Combined catalysis: a powerful strategy for engineering multifunctional sustainable lignin-based materials. ACS Nano 17(8):7093–7108

Agrawal R, Kumar A, Singh S, Sharma K (2022) Recent advances and future perspectives of lignin biopolymers. J Polym Res 29(6):222

Aquib TI (2023) Lignin-based nanomaterials as drug delivery vehicles: a review. Crit Rev Ther Drug Carrier Syst 40(4):1–67

Ariyanta HA, Sari FP, Sohail A, Restu WK, Septiyanti M, Aryana N, Fatriasari W, Kumar A (2023a) Current roles of lignin for the agroindustry: applications, challenges, and opportunities. Int J Biol Macromol 240:124523

Ariyanta HA, Santoso EB, Suryanegara L, Arung ET, Kusuma IW, Taib MNAM, Hussin MH, Yanuar Y, Batubara I, Fatriasari W (2023b) Recent progress on the development of lignin as future ingredient biobased cosmetics. Sustain Chem Pharm 32:100966

Balaji S, Short WD, Padon BW, Belgodere JA, Jimenez SE, Deoli NT, Guidry AC, Green JC, Prajapati TJ, Farouk F (2023) Injectable antioxidant and oxygen-releasing lignin composites to promote wound healing. ACS Appl Mater Interfaces 15(15):18639–18652

Balk M, Sofia P, Neffe AT, Tirelli N (2023) Lignin, the lignification process, and advanced, lignin-based materials. Int J Mol Sci 24(14):11668

Baloch M, Labidi J (2021) Lignin biopolymer: the material of choice for advanced lithium-based batteries. RSC Adv 11(38):23644–23653

Barzegar S, Monfared MHA, Hubbe MA (2022) Cellulose and lignin as propitious candidates for preparation of hydrogels for pharmaceutical applications. Mater Today Commun 33:104617

Bierach C, Coelho AA, Turrin M, Asut S, Knaack U (2023) Wood-based 3D printing: potential and limitation to 3D print building elements with cellulose & lignin. Archit Struct Constr 3:157–170

Chandna S, Olivares MCA, Baranovskii E, Engelmann G, Böker A, Tzschucke CC, Haag R (2023) Lignin upconversion by functionalization and network formation. Angew Chem Int Ed 63:e202313945

Chao Y, Yu S, Zhang H, Gong D, Li J, Wang F, Chen J, Zhu J, Chen J (2023) Architecting lignin/poly (vinyl alcohol) hydrogel with carbon nanotubes for photothermal antibacterial therapy. ACS Appl Bio Mater 6(4):1525–1535

Chaudhary M, Sinha VR (2023) Lignin-based carriers for drug delivery applications: from an industrial waste to a pharmaceutical aid. Eur Polym J 195:112206

Chavooshi R, Ranjkesh MR, Hashemi B, Roshangar L (2023) Cellulose and lignin-derived scaffold and their biological application in tissue engineering, drug delivery, and wound healing: a review. Cell J (Yakhteh) 25(3):158

Chiani E, Beaucamp A, Hamzeh Y, Azadfallah M, Thanusha AV, Collins MN (2023) Synthesis and characterization of gelatin/lignin hydrogels as quick release drug carriers for ribavirin. Int J Biol Macromol 224:1196–1205

Ciolacu DE, Nicu R, Suflet DM, Rusu D, Darie-Nita RN, Simionescu N, Cazacu G, Ciolacu F (2023) Multifunctional hydrogels based on cellulose and modified lignin for advanced wounds management. Pharmaceutics 15(11):2588

Crivello G, Orlandini G, Morena AG, Torchio A, Mattu C, Boffito M, Tzanov T, Ciardelli G (2023) Lignin–Cobalt Nano-Enabled Poly (pseudo) rotaxane supramolecular hydrogel for treating chronic wounds. Pharmaceutics 15(6):1717

Das AK, Mitra K, Conte AJ, Sarker A, Chowdhury A, Ragauskas AJ (2024) Lignin-a green material for antibacterial application—a review. Int J Biol Macromol 261(Pt 2):129753

Ding R, Zúniga MG, Lee SK, Oh E, Suhr J (2023) pH and temperature responsive UV curable lignin-based hydrogels with controllable and outstanding compressive properties. Ind Crop Prod 206:117583

Domínguez-Robles J, Cárcamo-Martínez Á, Stewart SA, Donnelly RF, Larrañeta E, Borrega M (2020) Lignin for pharmaceutical and biomedical applications–could this become a reality? Sustain Chem Pharm 18:100320

Domínguez-Robles J, Cárcamo-Martínez Á, Stewart SA, Donnelly RF, Larrañeta E (2021) Fabrication of lignin-based hydrogels and their applications. In: Lignin-based materials for biomedical applications. Elsevier, pp 371–394

Du B, Li W, Chai L, Li W, Wang X, Chen X, Zhou J, Sun R-C (2023) Preparation of versatile lignin-based adsorbent for the removal of organic dyes and its application in wound healing. J Mol Liq 377:121566

Erdocia X, Hernández-Ramos F, Morales A, Izaguirre N, de Hoyos-Martínez PL, Labidi J (2021) Lignin extraction and isolation methods. In: Lignin-based materials for biomedical applications. Elsevier, pp 61–104

Fazeli M, Mukherjee S, Baniasadi H, Abidnejad R, Mujtaba M, Lipponen J, Seppälä J, Rojas OJ (2024) Lignin beyond the status quo: recent and emerging composite applications. Green Chem 26. https://doi.org/10.1039/D3GC03154C

Feng Y, Yu J, Shao C, Sun R (2023) Advances toward sustainable lignin-based gel for energy storage and smart sensing. Paper Biomater 8(2):20–36

Hachimi Alaoui C, Réthoré G, Weiss P, Fatimi A (2023) Sustainable biomass lignin-based hydrogels: a review on properties, formulation, and biomedical applications. Int J Mol Sci 24(17):13493

Hu B, Ouyang Y, Zhao T, Wang Z, Yan Q, Qian Q, Wang W, Wang S (2024) Antioxidant hydrogels: antioxidant mechanisms, design strategies, and applications in alleviating oxidative stress-related diseases. Adv Healthc Mater 13:2303817

Huang D, Li R, Xu P, Li T, Deng R, Chen S, Zhang Q (2020) The cornerstone of realizing lignin value-addition: exploiting the native structure and properties of lignin by extraction methods. Chem Eng J 402:126237

Ivanova D, Toneva M, Simeonov E, Nikolova B, Semkova S, Antov G, Yaneva Z (2023) Newly synthesized lignin microparticles as bioinspired oral drug-delivery vehicles: flavonoid-carrier potential and in vitro radical-scavenging activity. Pharmaceutics 15(4):1067

Jia G, Innocent MT, Yu Y, Hu Z, Wang X, Xiang H, Zhu M (2023) Lignin-based carbon fibers: insight into structural evolution from lignin pretreatment, fiber forming, to pre-oxidation and carbonization. Int J Biol Macromol 226:646–659

Jiang B, Jiao H, Guo X, Chen G, Guo J, Wu W, Jin Y, Cao G, Liang Z (2023) Lignin-based materials for additive manufacturing: chemistry, processing, structures, properties, and applications. Adv Sci 10(9):2206055

Joseph K, Wilson R, George G, Appukuttan S (2023) Lignin-based materials: health care and medical applications. Royal Society of Chemistry

Karagoz P, Khiawjan S, Marques MPC, Santzouk S, Bugg TDH, Lye GJ (2023) Pharmaceutical applications of lignin-derived chemicals and lignin-based materials: linking lignin source and processing with clinical indication. Biomass Conv Bioref 14:26553–26574

Keck S, Liske O, Seidler K, Steyrer B, Gorsche C, Knaus S, Baudis S (2023) Synthesis of a liquid lignin-based methacrylate resin and its application in 3D printing without any reactive diluents. Biomacromolecules 24(4):1751–1762

Kienberger M, Maitz S, Pichler T, Demmelmayer P (2021) Systematic review on isolation processes for technical lignin. PRO 9(5):804

Lameirinhas NS, Teixeira MC, Carvalho JPF, Valente BFA, Pinto RJB, Oliveira H, Luís JL, Pires L, Oliveira JM, Vilela C (2023) Nanofibrillated cellulose/gellan gum hydrogel-based bioinks for 3D bioprinting of skin cells. Int J Biol Macromol 229:849–860

Li X, Meng Y, Cheng Z, Li B (2023a) Research progress and prospect of stimuli-responsive lignin functional materials. Polymers 15(16):3372

Li K, Zhong W, Li P, Ren J, Jiang K, Wu W (2023b) Antibacterial mechanism of lignin and lignin-based antimicrobial materials in different fields. Int J Biol Macromol 252:126281

Liao JJ, Abd Latif NH, Trache D, Brosse N, Hussin MH (2020) Current advancement on the isolation, characterization and application of lignin. Int J Biol Macromol 162:985–1024

Lisý A, Ház A, Nadányi R, Jablonský M, Šurina I (2022) About hydrophobicity of lignin: a review of selected chemical methods for lignin valorisation in biopolymer production. Energies 15(17):6213

Liu R, Dai L, Xu C, Wang K, Zheng C, Si C (2020) Lignin-based micro-and nanomaterials and their composites in biomedical applications. ChemSusChem 13(17):4266–4283

Liu C, Cheng X, Zhang F, Lei F, Li P, Wang K, Jiang J (2023) Preparation and application of galactomannan-based green hydrogels initiated by lignin-Ag NPs. Mater Today Commun 34:105256

Lobato-Peralta DR, Duque-Brito E, Villafan-Vidales HI, Longoria A, Sebastian PJ, Cuentas-Gallegos AK, Arancibia-Bulnes CA, Okoye PU (2021) A review on trends in lignin extraction and valorization of lignocellulosic biomass for energy applications. J Clean Prod 293:126123

Lu F, Ni S, Meng X, Si C, Qin M, Wang Y, Fu Y, Chen X (2023) Preparation of pH-sensitive lignin nanoparticles and its application in hydrophobic drug delivery. Ind Crop Prod 202:117012

Luo J, Meng J, Zhennan C, Xueli Y, Xinran W, Ze L, Luo S, Wang L, Zhou J, Qin H (2023) Preparation and properties of lignin-based dual network hydrogel and its application in sensing. Int J Biol Macromol 249:125913

Lyu Z, Zheng Y, Zhou H, Dai L (2023) Lignin-based hydrogels for biological application. Paper Biomater 8(2):37–52

Meng Y, Contescu CI, Liu P, Wang S, Lee S-H, Guo J, Young TM (2021) Understanding the local structure of disordered carbons from cellulose and lignin. Wood Sci Technol 55(3):587–606

Mondal AK, Uddin MT, Sujan SMA, Tang Z, Alemu D, Begum HA, Li J, Huang F, Ni Y (2023) Preparation of lignin-based hydrogels, their properties and applications. Int J Biol Macromol 245:125580

Mukheja Y, Kaur J, Pathania K, Sah SP, Salunke DB, Sangamwar AT, Pawar SV (2023) Recent advances in pharmaceutical and biotechnological applications of lignin-based materials. Int J Biol Macromol 241:124601

Nan N, Hu W, Wang J (2022) Lignin-based porous biomaterials for medical and pharmaceutical applications. Biomedicines 10(4):747

Nissinen L, Kähäri V-M (2014) Matrix metalloproteinases in inflammation. Biochim Biophys Acta Gen Subj 1840(8):2571–2580. https://doi.org/10.1016/j.bbagen.2014.03.007

Pathania K, Sah SP, Salunke DB, Jain M, Yadav AK, Yadav VG, Pawar SV (2023) Green synthesis of lignin-based nanoparticles as a bio-carrier for targeted delivery in cancer therapy. Int J Biol Macromol 229:684–695

Queiroz BG, Ciol H, Inada NM, Frollini E (2023) Cross-linked bio-based hydrogels generated from solutions derived from the deconstruction of sisal fibers. J Mol Liq 369:120876

Radotić K, Spasojević D, Zmejkoski D (2023) Lignin-based materials for biomedical applications: basic requirements and properties. In: Lignin-based materials: health care and medical applications. The Royal Society of Chemistry, pp 85–105

Ribeiro AM, Santos AI, Veiga F, Figueiras A (2023) Lignin nanoparticle–based nanocomposite hydrogels for biomedical applications. In: Functional nanocomposite hydrogels. Elsevier, pp 69–90

Rico-García D, Ruiz-Rubio L, Pérez-Alvarez L, Hernández-Olmos SL, Guerrero-Ramírez GL, Vilas-Vilela JL (2020) Lignin-based hydrogels: synthesis and applications. Polymers 12(1):81

Rodrigues JS, Lima V, Araujo LCP, Botaro VR (2021) Lignin fractionation methods: can lignin fractions be separated in a true industrial process? Ind Eng Chem Res 60(30):10863–10881

Ruiz Deance AL, Siersema B, Yoe LEA-C, Wurm FR, Gojzewski H (2023) Copolymerizing lignin for tuned properties of 3D-printed PEG-based photopolymers. ACS Appl Polym Mater 5(12):10021–10031

Sakagami H, Kushida T, Oizumi T, Nakashima H, Makino T (2010) Distribution of lignin–carbohydrate complex in plant kingdom and its functionality as alternative medicine. Pharmacol Ther 128(1):91–105

Sanchez LM, Hopkins AK, Espinosa E, Larrañeta E, Malinova D, McShane AN, Domínguez-Robles J, Rodríguez A (2023) Antioxidant cellulose nanofibers/lignin-based aerogels: a potential material for biomedical applications. Chem Biol Technol Agric 10(1):72

Shah SWA, Xu Q, Ullah MW, Sethupathy S, Morales GM, Sun J, Zhu D (2023) Additive manufactured lignin-based materials: a review of current status, challenges, and future perspectives. Addit Manuf 74:103711

Sharma S, Sharma A, Mulla SI, Pant D, Sharma T, Kumar A (2020) Lignin as potent industrial biopolymer: an introduction. In: Lignin: biosynthesis and transformation for industrial applications. Springer, Cham, pp 1–15

Shu F, Jiang B, Yuan Y, Li M, Wu W, Jin Y, Xiao H (2021) Biological activities and emerging roles of lignin and lignin-based products—a review. Biomacromolecules 22(12):4905–4918

Siddiqa A, Yhobu Z, Nagaraju DH, Padaki M, Budagumpi S, Pasupuleti VR, Lim J-W (2023) Review and perspectives of sustainable lignin, cellulose, and lignocellulosic carbon special structures for energy storage. Energy Fuel 37(4):2498–2519

Spiridon I (2020) Extraction of lignin and therapeutic applications of lignin-derived compounds. A review. Environ Chem Lett 18:771–785

Tardy BL, Lizundia E, Guizani C, Hakkarainen M, Sipponen MH (2023) Prospects for the integration of lignin materials into the circular economy. Mater Today 65:122–132

Tariq Z, Iqbal DN, Rizwan M, Ahmad M, Faheem M, Ahmed M (2023) Significance of biopolymer-based hydrogels and their applications in agriculture: a review in perspective of synthesis and their degree of swelling for water holding. RSC Adv 13(35):24731–24754

Terzioğlu P, Parın FN, Sıcak Y (2020) Lignin composites for biomedical applications: status, challenges and perspectives. In: Lignin: biosynthesis and transformation for industrial applications. Springer, Cham, pp 253–273

Thang NH, Chien TB, Cuong DX (2023) Polymer-based hydrogels applied in drug delivery: an overview. Gels 9(7):523

Vasile C, Baican M (2023) Lignins as promising renewable biopolymers and bioactive compounds for high-performance materials. Polymers 15(15):3177

Vásquez-Garay F, Carrillo-Varela I, Vidal C, Reyes-Contreras P, Faccini M, Teixeira Mendonça R (2021) A review on the lignin biopolymer and its integration in the elaboration of sustainable materials. Sustain For 13(5):2697

Wan Z, Zhang H, Niu M, Guo Y, Li H (2023) Recent advances in lignin-based 3D printing materials: a mini-review. Int J Biol Macromol 253:126660

Wang X, Li X, Yadav C, Lan W, Wang L, Uraki Y, Kang J, Zhang HJ, You X (2023a) Enhancing the mechanical performance of lignin based hydrogel via lignin acetylation. Ind Crop Prod 199:116780

Wang F, Jiang M, Pan Y, Lu Y, Xu W, Zhou Y (2023b) 3D printing photo-induced lignin nanotubes/polyurethane shape memory composite. Polym Test 119:107934

Wang F, Chen C, Zhu D, Li W, Liu J, Wang J (2023c) Ultrastretchable and highly conductive hydrogels based on Fe3+-lignin nanoparticles for subzero wearable strain sensor. Int J Biol Macromol 253:126768

Wei Q, Zhou J, An Y, Li M, Zhang J, Yang S (2023) Modification, 3D printing process and application of sodium alginate based hydrogels in soft tissue engineering: a review. Int J Biol Macromol 232:123450

Wu S-H, Rethi L, Pan W-Y, Nguyen HT, Chuang E-Y (2024) Emerging horizons and prospects of polysaccharide-constructed gels in the realm of wound healing. Colloids Surf B Biointerfaces 235:113759

Xiao W, Sun R, Hu S, Meng C, Xie B, Yi M, Wu Y (2023) Recent advances and future perspective on lignocellulose-based materials as adsorbents in diverse water treatment applications. Int J Biol Macromol 253:126984

Xu X, Chao Y, Ma X, Zhang H, Chen J, Zhu J (2024) A photothermally antibacterial Au@Halloysite nanotubes/lignin composite hydrogel for promoting wound healing. Int J Biol Macromol 258:128704

Zakzeski J, Bruijnincx PCA, Jongerius AL, Weckhuysen BM (2010) The catalytic valorization of lignin for the production of renewable chemicals. Chem Rev 110(6):3552–3599. https://doi.org/10.1021/cr900354u

Zhang Y, Cheng G (2023) Lignin-containing hydrogels: transforming a low-value byproduct to absorbents, wound dressings and strain sensors. Chem Eng J 475:146460

Zhang Y, Naebe M (2021) Lignin: a review on structure, properties, and applications as a light-colored UV absorber. ACS Sustain Chem Eng 9(4):1427–1442

Zhang L, Larsson A, Moldin A, Edlund U (2022) Comparison of lignin distribution, structure, and morphology in wheat straw and wood. Ind Crop Prod 187:115432

Zheng L, Lu G, Pei W, Yan W, Li Y, Zhang L, Huang C, Jiang Q (2021) Understanding the relationship between the structural properties of lignin and their biological activities. Int J Biol Macromol 190:291–300

Zheng L, Seidi F, Wu W, Pan Y, Xiao H (2023) Dual-functional lignin-based hydrogels for sustained release of agrochemicals and heavy metal ion complexation. Int J Biol Macromol 235:123701

Zheng Y, Moreno A, Zhang Y, Sipponen MH, Dai L (2024) Harnessing chemical functionality of lignin towards stimuli-responsive materials. Trends Chem 6:62–78

Sustainable Carbon Fibres and Piezoelectric Sensors for Possible Integration in Future Biomedical Devices

14

Clotilde Techoueyres, Jean Rougé, Valeria Nico, Anne Beaucamp, and Maurice N. Collins

Abstract

Carbon fibres are strategic materials for several high values applications such as aerospace, automotive, wind turbine, sports gears, and biomedical. Nowadays, 95% of commercial carbon fibres used in these composites are made from polyacrylonitrile which notoriously impacts energy consumption, climate change, and cost. Lignin utilisation as a precursor material aims to address the challenge of reducing environmental impact while increasing sustainability and reducing the economic cost of carbon fibres allowing subsequent wider integration while maintaining mechanical performance. Despite their exceptional reinforcement properties, carbon fibre reinforced polymers exhibit poor ductility causing sudden failure without any prediction possibilities. Embedded damage detection membrane may result in improved safety and reliability while reducing costly maintenance operations. Piezoelectric materials are highly regarded for their capacity to produce electric voltage when exposed to mechanical stress, enabling failure detection in case of excessive stress to the carbon fibre structure. Nanofiber

C. Techoueyres · J. Rougé · A. Beaucamp (✉)
Stokes Labs, Bernal Institute, School of Engineering, University of Limerick, Limerick, Ireland
e-mail: anne.mcloughlin@ul.ie

V. Nico
Stokes Labs, Bernal Institute, School of Engineering, University of Limerick, Limerick, Ireland

CONNECT SFI Center, University of Limerick, Limerick, Ireland

M. N. Collins
School of Engineering, Health Research Institute and Bernal Institute, University of Limerick, Limerick, Ireland

AMBER and BiOrbic SFI Center, University of Limerick, Limerick, Ireland

M. N. Collins, M. Culebras (eds.), *Sustainable Biopolymers and Composites for Biomedical Applications*, Biomaterials, Bioengineering and Sustainability 5,
https://doi.org/10.1007/978-3-031-91972-5_14

membranes of polyvinylidene fluoride (PVDF) produced via an electrospinning process offer a solution when used as in situ sensors for integrated damage detection in carbon fibre-reinforced polymers.

Keywords

Lignin · Carbon fibres · Low cost · Carbon fibre-reinforced polymer integration · Piezoelectric nanofibres · Damaged detection

14.1 Introduction

Carbon fibres (CF) have become indispensable given their weight-to-mechanical properties ratio for structural applications and inherent suitability for functional applications. Given the rapid market expansion of carbon fibre-reinforced polymer (CFRP), forecasting 285,000 tons for 2025 (Zhang et al. 2023), CF production may conflict with initiatives aimed at mitigating global warming (Keiner et al. 2023). Currently, 95% of the worldwide CF production is produced with polyacrylonitrile (PAN) as precursor material (Beaucamp et al. 2024). PAN is a fossil-based polymer derived from the polymerisation of acrylonitrile, accounting for 53% of the total cost of CF (Beaucamp et al. 2024; Xu et al. 2020) and 37% of its environmental impact (Prenzel et al. 2024). In a global warming context, reducing the global carbon footprint has become imperative, therefore, the use of PAN precursor is being reevaluated, and sustainable alternatives are being explored. Lignin is a promising alternative for sustainable high performance and low-cost CF. Lignin is the second most abundant biopolymer on earth with approximately 50 million tons available worldwide from wood pulping processes. However, only 2% of extracted lignin is valorised into products such as dispersants, adhesives, surfactants, or antioxidants in plastics and rubbers (Jia et al. 2023). Nevertheless, lignin holds significant potential in valuable engineering applications due to its high carbon yield and aromatic structure which can be easily converted to high performance carbon materials. This in turn could pave the way for lignin CF to emerge as a cost-effective and sustainable alternative for a broader array of applications, complementing the essential role of CFRP in various high-end engineering applications (Collins et al. 2022). In addition to advancements in cost-effective CF, efforts are being made to enhance damage detection systems aimed at reducing maintenance expenses. Piezoelectric materials can be used for damage monitoring of structures allowing parts to be replaced before failure. The piezoelectric effect is the ability of a material to convert mechanical stresses into electrical energy and vice-versa. They can be categorized into three subsets: single crystals, ceramic, and polymer. PVDF is a piezoelectric polymer, whch offers significant advantages over the widely used lead zirconate titanate (PZT), which, despite its high piezoelectric coefficient, poses environmental concerns due to its lead content. PVDF, on the other hand, is presented as an alternative due to its mechanical flexibility and low cost. PVDF can be processed into nanofiber membranes through electrospinning, thereby enhancing its piezoelectric response (Gee et al. 2018). Nanofiber membranes offer the opportunity to create a piezoelectric coating on woven lignin CF, for an integrated damage sensor into CFRPs. By presenting a piezoelectric damage sensor integrated into lignin CFRP, this chapter provides various opportunities for biomedical devices such as sensors embedded within medical prostheses, implants, or mobility equipment.

14.2 Production of Carbon Fibres

14.2.1 Current Technologies for Carbon Fibres Production

Even though CF can be made from Pitch or Rayon precursor, 95% of the current production is made from PAN precursor (Beaucamp et al. 2024). PAN, originating from petroleum, is a fossil-based polymer used for its high carbon yield and its natural ability to form an organized carbon structure following thermal treatment (Khayyam et al. 2020). PAN is industrially processed through wet-spinning technique where a N,N-dimethylformamide (DMF), dimethylacetamide (DMA) or sodium thiocyanate/PAN dope solution with a concentration of 10–30 wt% (Huang 2009) is extruded in a counter-solvent coagulation bath through a spinneret to form fibre. The solvent is removed from the fibres through washing and stretching processes which also contribute to decrease their diameter, aiding in heat and mass transfer within the fibres during subsequent thermal treatment, ultimately enhancing mechanical properties (Khayyam et al. 2020). Following this, the fibres undergo thermal stabilisation in an oxygen environment and carbonisation in a nitrogen environment. This energy-intensive production process contributes to the increased cost of CF, which are initially tied to oil prices due to the use of PAN. Subsequently, the fibres undergo surface treatment and sizing (Khayyam et al. 2020) to protect the fibres, facilitate the handling and enhance the fibre/matrix interaction (Montes-Morán et al. 2002; Zhang et al. 2011).

14.2.2 Lignin as a Promising Precursor

Traditionally, lignin has been considered as a production waste from pulp and paper mill and burnt as low value fuel. However, lignin research for CF application as precursor material began in 1969 with Otani (Otani et al. 1969) and has undergone extensive research for the last 30 years due to its high carbon content surpassing 60%, cost, widespread availability, and minimal environmental footprint. Despite its great potential as a renewable and cost-effective precursor material for CF, progress has been slow until recent progress at the University of Limerick where the first scaled products have been produced (Beaucamp et al. 2024; Collins et al. 2022). Typically, lignin constitutes approximately 15–40% of plant material, playing a crucial role as a complex aromatic constituent of plant cell walls providing both strength and impermeability (Obasa et al. 2022; Tribot et al. 2019). Plant lignins can be categorised into softwood, hardwood, and grass lignins, where Softwood plants contains a higher amount of lignin in front of hardwood and grasses (Chatterjee and Saito 2015). The molecular structure of lignin is composed of three interlinked phenolic precursors with a variant distribution based on plant type and extraction technique (Beaucamp 2022). The three monolignol monomers are: *p*-hydroxyphemyl (H), guaiacyl (G), and syringyl (S), bio-synthetised from *p*-Coumaryl alcohol, Coniferyl alcohol, and Sinapyl alcohol.

14.2.2.1 Lignin Extraction

Originally, most of the extraction methods were developed for cellulose (Chatterjee and Saito 2015), leaving lignin as a low value-added co-product. As lignin applications receive an increasing interest linked to the climate change fight, recent extraction techniques tend to obtain purer lignin trying to leave the lignin structure unchanged. The isolation of lignin from cellulose and hemicellulose is driven by chemical processes resulting in four main technical lignin: kraft, sulfonated, soda, and organosolv lignin. These four technical lignins can be divided into 2 categories: sulfur-containing lignin and sulfur-free lignin (Shorey et al. 2024). Among sulfur containing lignin, kraft lignin is the most produced type of lignin with 55,000,000 tons per year (Beaucamp et al. 2022), resulting from the kraft pulping process. Lignosulfonate is also a sulfur-containing lignin produced as a by-product from sulphite pulping with a yearly production of 1,000,000 tons (Beaucamp et al. 2022; Aro and Fatehi 2017). Conversely, soda lignin, produced through the soda pulping process, and organosolv lignin, amounting respectively to 6000 and 1000 tons per year (Beaucamp et al. 2022) from pilot scale production, are sulfur-free types of lignin resulting from pulping processes that utilise solvents for lignin separation.

14.2.2.2 Lignin Fibres Production

The three main techniques considered to produce lignin precursor fibres are melt-spinning, wet spinning and electrospinning and will be presented in the next subsections. These three methods provide a wide range of possibilities leading to different diameter fibres, morphologies, and mechanical properties. Melt- and wet-spinning are used to produce micrometre fibre size for structural applications, while electrospinning method aim to produce fibres reaching the nanometre scale used in various functional applications.

Melt-Spinning

Lignin precursor fibres have predominantly been processed via melt-spinning, as it represents a more environmentally sustainable and health-conscious production method (Fang et al. 2017). Melt-spinning is a convenient, cost-effective, hazard-free, relatively straightforward and fast technique (Chaudhari 2024). Melt-spinning is a well-known technology, popularly used in the textile industry to melt thermoplastic pellets into fibres. The major lignin type exhibits thermoplastic behaviour that allows its processability through melt-spinning within a narrow range of parameters. However, due to lignin poor processability, lignin should be blended with more stable plasticising polymers to enhance its processability (Fang et al. 2017;

Rubio et al. 2022). Polymers and lignin are added in the form of pellets and powder, which are melted and extruded into fibre shape before being cooled down and collected. To be melt-spun, lignin must exhibit less than 1% impurities, no water or volatiles (Compere et al. 2004), and be within a restricted range of processability criteria (Beaucamp 2022). In addition to a low molecular weight, most lignin exhibits amorphous structure leading to potential charring at temperature higher than 200–250 °C (Jin et al. 2021). This narrow processing window presents challenges but could also pave the way for a sustainable and cheap spinning process.

Wet Spinning

Meanwhile, melt-spinning has been the most studied technique for lignin-based precursor fibres, wet-spinning holds advantages for non-fusible lignin and high *Tg* lignin grade. Wet spinning technique is characterised by the creation of a (polymer/solvent) solution extruded through a counter-solvent coagulation bath to form fibres shape. It is the main used technique for PAN based CF production because this technique leads to better quality fibres and therefore better mechanical properties. The production of lignin-based CF via wet-spinning represents a significant challenge, as this solution could potentially be directly integrated into the production lines currently used for PAN, representing a much lower risk and cost for companies. Indeed, the advancement of wet-spun lignin CF could potentially accelerate the transition towards a sustainable solution and foster greater acceptance among companies. Yet, the use of lignin as precursor material introduces novel solvent alternatives for the wet-spinning technique, not only replacing traditionally hazardous ones but also opening promising avenues for a greener production process. This includes the use of lignosulfonate, which is water-soluble and requires no stabilisation, decreasing the overall environmental impact. However, this technique remains more expensive compared to the melt-spinning, and more difficult to set as the coagulation process is not fully understood (Föllmer 2018).

Electrospinning

The electrospinning method proves to be an efficient technique for the production of carbon nanofibers (CNF) for functional applications (Kumar et al. 2019). They currently hold significant interest due to their chemical, electrical and mechanical properties for energy conversion and storage, catalysis, sensor or absorption/separation (Zhang et al. 2014). Comparably to melt- and wet-spinning, PAN is currently used as precursor material while lignin attracts extensive attention for a cheaper and sustainable solution. Lignin on its own is difficult to electrospin due to its structure and low molecular weight (Parot et al. 2022). Consequently, blending lignin with polymers such as TPU or PLA enhances its processability and facilitates the production of homogeneous fibers, or can introduce porosity, as PLA does for battery applications (Dallmeyer et al. 2010; Culebras et al. 2019). Electrospinning involves the creation of a polymer/solvent solution using a volatile solvent. An electric field is applied on a droplet of the solution extruded through a syringe generating a jet to form nanofibers. In contrast to melt- and wet-spinning techniques, using mechanical drawing, electrospinning shapes the fibre using an electric field. Furthermore, electrospinning has been the subject of numerous studies due to its capability to impart piezoelectric behaviour to certain polymer nanofibers (Ren et al. 2024). Therefore, electrospinning holds significant opportunities for sensors as it enhances the electrical response of certain piezoelectric polymers.

14.3 Piezoelectric Effect

The piezoelectric materials are widely used in dynamic sensors due to their ability to convert mechanical stress into electrical energy and vice versa. The piezoelectric effect was reported in 1880 by the Curie brothers (Curie and Curie 1880). This discovery marked the initial observation of the piezoelectric effect in quartz crystals. Piezoelectric materials can be categorized into three subsets: single crystals (quartz crystal), ceramic (zinc oxide ZnO, PZT), and polymer (PVDF, Poly L-lactic Acid PLLA, poly(vinylidene fluoride-co-trifluoroethylene) P(VDF-TrFE)) (Smith and Kar-Narayan 2021). Among piezoelectric ceramics, PZT is the most widely used due to its high piezoelectric coefficient, rigidity, and high operating temperature. However, PZT is also brittle, heavy, and toxic due to its lead content. In contrast, polymers with piezoelectric properties offer several benefits, including good mechanical properties and lightweight nature, making them suitable for structural applications while guaranteeing minimal impact on the overall weight. Conversely, their flexibility enables perfect adaptation to various shapes and forms within the system, enhancing versatility and usability. Furthermore, the biocompatibility of many piezoelectric polymers makes them suitable for safe integration for biomedical applications, expanding their potential uses in medical devices and implants (Mokhtari et al. 2021). Lastly, the production of piezoelectric polymers is considered easier compared to ceramic. There are three steps involved in producing a piezoelectric polymer: melting, mechanical stretching, and electric polarization. These stages can be easily replaced by the electrospinning process, which is a viable alternative (Kalimuldina et al. 2020).

14.3.1 State of the Art on Piezoelectricity Integration into Composite Materials

In recent years, CFRPs have been widely used to reinforce structures, subjecting them to mechanical constraints. This has provided an opportunity to integrate piezoelectric materials into composites for their unique electromechanical properties. Imparting piezoelectric behaviour to CFRPs can enable the monitoring of structural integrity throughout their lifecycle, management of vibrations, and harvesting of energy for a self-powered intelligent composite. Over the last four years, there has been significant progress in developing methods to integrate piezoelectric materials into CFRPs, as summarized in Table 14.1.

In self-sensing CFRP, while external sensors can be integrated without typically affecting the mechanical performance of the laminate, exposure to environmental

Table 14.1 Piezoelectric materials integrated into CFRP

Sensor technology	Type of sensor	Piezoelectric material	Electromechanical performances	Reference
Embedded plate sensor	Cure monitoring—damage detection	PZT	X	Liu et al. (2021)
Embedded plate sensor	Cure monitoring	PZT	X	Yu et al. (2023a)
Embedded plate sensor	Sensor and actuator, damage detection	PZT	X	Hornig et al. (2022)
Nanofibers mat integrated	Damage detection or damage localisation	P(VDF-TrFE) nanofibers	Sensitivity of 44.9 mV/kN d_{33} = 5.33 pC/N (no shield) d_{33} = 5.48 pC/N (shield)	Mongioì et al. (2024)
Nanofibers mat integrated	Damage detection—in situ pressure monitoring	P(VDF-TrFE) nanofibres	Sensitivity value of 0.14 ± 0.01 mV/N From 0.5 Hz to 20 Hz	Selleri et al. (2022)
Lead-free piezoelectric nanoparticles	Energy harvesting	Sodium potassium niobate (KNN) barium titanate (BTO)	KNN: d_{33} = 13.6 pC/N BTO: d_{33} = 12.3 pC/N	Kurita et al. (2020)
Lead-free piezoelectric nanoparticles	Damage detection and energy harvesting	KNN nanoparticles	d_{33} = 5.0 pC/N	Yu et al. (2023b)
Lead-free piezoelectric nanoparticles	Stress sensing and energy harvesting	KNN nanoparticles	d_{33} = 4.7 pC/N	Yu and Narita (2021)
Carbon fabric coating	Self-powered touch sensor	ZnO layers	Output voltage: 3.6 V Current density: 1.47 μA/cm^2 Power density of 1.8 μW/cm^2	Petrushenko et al. (2024)
Carbon fibre coating	Energy harvesting and detection variation in impact acceleration	ZnO nanorods	From 1.4 to 7.6 V under impact acceleration from 0.1 to 0.4 m s^{-2}	He et al. (2023)

conditions and electrical noise can impair their functionality and shorten their lifespan. To address these issues, several studies have explored embedding piezoelectric sensors into CFRP. The most studied approach involves embedding a PZT plate in the CFRP for cure monitoring and damage detection. However, this method is limited due to the ceramic piezoelectric material's brittleness, poor flexibility, external connection requirements, and relatively high weight. Another method, explored by Selleri et al., involves creating nanofiber mat sensors made of piezoelectric polymer and integrating them between several layers of CFRP. The nanofibers, made using the electrospinning method, enhance the flexibility and sustainability of the composites (Mongioì et al. 2024; Selleri et al. 2022). Kurita, H., et al. and Yu, Y., et al. also explored the use of lead-free piezoelectric nanoparticles integrated into the matrix to minimize the matrix/fibre interface interference (Kurita et al. 2020; Yu et al. 2023b). This approach involves incorporating piezoelectric nanoparticles directly into the matrix, thereby avoiding the need for a separate piezoelectric layer between the fibres and the matrix. As a result, the integrity of the interface is preserved, maintaining the strength and stiffness of the composite comparable to conventional CFRP. Despite the various methods available for integrating piezoelectric materials into CFRP, applying a piezoelectric coating on carbon fibres offers several advantages as experienced Bowland, C., et al., He, Q., et al., Lin, Y., et al. and Petrushenko, S.I., et al. (Petrushenko et al. 2024; He et al. 2023; Bowland et al. 2014; Lin et al. 2010). This approach protects the piezoelectric fibres from damage or fracture under mechanical loading due to the flexible nature of the polymer matrix and enhances their ability to conform to curved surfaces, thereby increasing their applicability in various fields.

While various types of piezoelectric sensors and technologies have been studied, they are designed for different applications and, therefore, are not tested under the same conditions. Additionally, the use of commercial piezoelectric materials, such as PZT plates for embedded sensors, contributes to the lack of electromagnetic performance measurements in Table 14.1, as their electromagnetic performance is already guaranteed. Moreover, there is currently no standard for piezoelectric sensors, making it very difficult to compare them. Among the technologies detailed in Table 14.1, nanofiber mats and coated fibres present a new opportunity for the use of piezoelectric polymers, offering more flexibility and sustainability compared to piezoelectric ceramics.

14.3.2 Polyvinylidene Fluoride (PVDF) as a Piezoelectric Polymer for Damage Sensor

Among piezoelectric polymers, Polyvinylidene fluoride (PVDF) has been the subject of numerous studies. PVDF is a semicrystalline biopolymer with lots of advantageous properties such as high mechanical strength, excellent flexibility, biocompatible (Laroche et al. 1995), biodegradability, and strong piezoelectricity. Due to its versatility, PVDF is used in diverse fields including energy harvesting, biomedical applications, sensors, and automotive (Yi and Liang 2008; Sukumaran et al. 2021; Husain et al. 2023). PVDF has at least five major crystalline phases, α, β, ϒ, δ and ε. The different phases of the PVDF differ by chain conformations. The α-phase is the most common and generally preferred due to its high thermodynamic stability. However, the β-phase represents the most conductive one due to its highest dipole moment, making it the phase of choice for achieving optimal piezoelectric response. Higher β-phase can be achieved using the electrospinning method (Kalimuldina et al. 2020) and remove the necessity of extra poling or mechanical stretching. Indeed, the formation of the β-phase through electrical poling is constrained by the electric field's strength, which must be uniformly distributed across

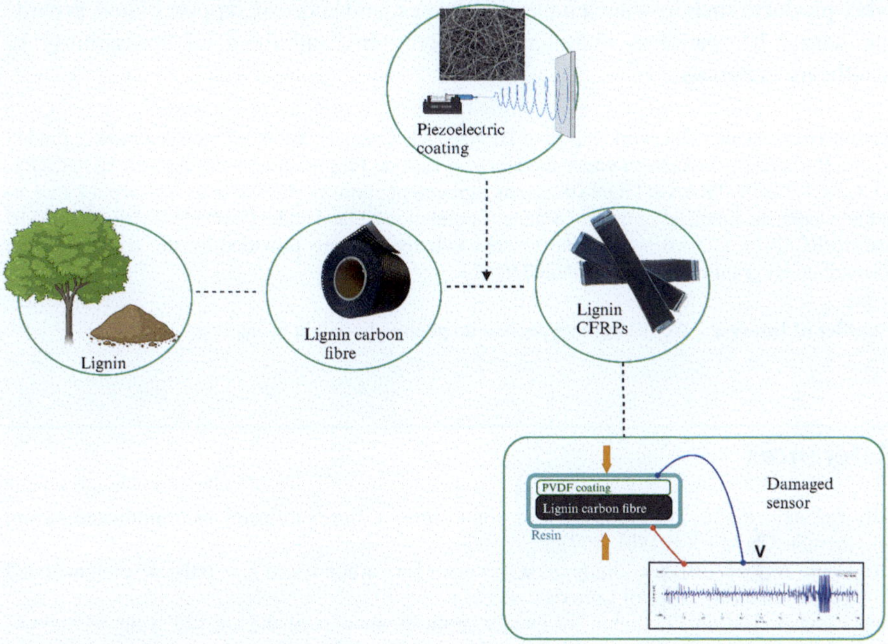

Fig. 14.1 PVDF membrane for CFRP damage sensor integration

the thickness and area of membranes. In contrast, the electrospinning charges the polymer solution during fabrication rather than post-fabrication, leading to a higher β-phase with permanent piezoelectric properties (Gee et al. 2018).

The PVDF nanofiber membrane created with electrospinning, aims to integrate a CFRP as a coating directly embedded between the weaved CF and the matrix (Fig. 14.1). represent internal electrodes. This integrated piezoelectric sensor also presents potential for biomedical applications, including failure detection in prostheses, implants, and equipment mobility.

14.4 Conclusion

Adding embedded piezoelectric coating sensors to lignin CFRPs offers the opportunity for damage sensor detection and structural health monitoring, enabling more reliable products and affordable maintenance. Electrospun PVDF nanofibres present several advantages as a piezoelectric coating material such as flexibility, lightweight nature, and environmental friendliness. This approach not only strengthens the sensing capabilities but also provides opportunities for energy harvesting, actuation, and cure monitoring, thereby expanding its utility in diverse fields. Piezoelectric sensor integration into lignin CFs reinforced polymer holds significant potential for biomedical application. As lignin CF represents a more sustainable and cheaper solution, it will leverage their properties and weight-to-strength ratio in various other products such as wheelchairs, prostheses, and surgical support plates, providing longer lifespan less maintenance operations, and financial accessibility to healthcare materials.

Acknowledgement This work is part of BIOUPTAKE project. BIOUPTAKE is a project funded by the European Commission under the Horizon Europe Programme, under the call HORIZON-CL4-2021-TWIN-TRANSITION-01, grant agreement number 101057049. VN would like to acknowledge the financial support of Science Foundation Ireland under Grants No. 21/PATHS/9510 and 13/RC/2077_P2. AB would like to acknowledge funding provided by the Irish Research Council under grant number GOIPD/2023/1012.

Conflict of Interest We the authors declare no potential conflict of interest.

References

Aro T, Fatehi P (2017) Production and application of lignosulfonates and sulfonated lignin. ChemSusChem 10(9):1861–1877

Beaucamp A (2022) Blended lignin as a precursor for carbon-based materials, development and applications. University of Limerick

Beaucamp A et al (2022) Lignin for energy applications–state of the art, life cycle, technoeconomic analysis and future trends. Green Chem 24(21):8193–8226

Beaucamp A et al (2024) Sustainable lignin-based carbon fibre reinforced polyamide composites: production, characterisation and life cycle analysis. Compos Commun 45:101782

Bowland C, Zhou Z, Sodano HA (2014) Multifunctional barium Titanate coated carbon fibers. Adv Funct Mater 24(40):6303–6308

Chatterjee S, Saito T (2015) Lignin-derived advanced carbon materials. ChemSusChem 8(23):3941–3958

Chaudhari N (2024) Carbon fiber production from lignin: a precursor of future

Collins MN, Culebras M, Ren G (2022) The use of lignin as a precursor for carbon fiber–reinforced composites. In: Micro and Nanolignin in aqueous dispersions and polymers. Elsevier, pp 237–250

Compere A et al (2004) Improving the fundamental properties of lignin-based carbon fiber for transportation applications. In Proceedings of the 36th International SAMPE Technical Conference

Culebras M et al (2019) Bio-derived carbon nanofibres from lignin as high-performance Li-ion anode materials. ChemSusChem 12(19):4516–4521

Curie J, Curie P (1880) Développement par compression de l'électricité polaire dans les cristaux hémièdres à faces inclinées. Bulletin de la Société minéralogique de France 3(4):90–93

Dallmeyer I, Ko F, Kadla JF (2010) Electrospinning of technical lignins for the production of fibrous networks. J Wood Chem Technol 30(4):315–329

Fang W et al (2017) Manufacture and application of lignin-based carbon fibers (LCFs) and lignin-based carbon nanofibers (LCNFs). Green Chem 19(8):1794–1827

Föllmer M (2018) Lignin fibres prepared by coagulation: a promising precursor for carbon fibres. Bordeaux

Gee S, Johnson B, Smith A (2018) Optimizing electrospinning parameters for piezoelectric PVDF nanofiber membranes. J Membr Sci 563:804–812

He Q et al (2023) Nano-engineered carbon fibre-based piezoelectric smart composites for energy harvesting and self-powered sensing. Adv Funct Mater 33(20):2213918

Hornig A et al (2022) Embedded sensing and actuating in CFRP composite structures—concept and technology demonstration for tailored embeddable sensor-actuator layers (TEmSAL). Smart Mater Struct 31(9):095007

Huang X (2009) Fabrication and properties of carbon fibers. Materials 2(4):2369–2403

Husain M, Singh R, Pabla B (2023) On 3D printing of PVDF composite-based sensors for biomedical applications. Natl Acad Sci Lett 47:1–6

Jia G et al (2023) Lignin-based carbon fibers: insight into structural evolution from lignin pretreatment, fiber forming, to pre-oxidation and carbonization. Int J Biol Macromol 226:646–659

Jin Y et al (2021) Lignin-based high-performance fibers by textile spinning techniques. Materials 14(12):3378

Kalimuldina G et al (2020) A review of piezoelectric PVDF film by electrospinning and its applications. Sensors 20(18):5214

Keiner D et al (2023) Techno-economic assessment of atmospheric CO2-based carbon fibre production enabling negative emissions. Mitig Adapt Strateg Glob Chang 28(8):52

Khayyam H et al (2020) PAN precursor fabrication, applications and thermal stabilization process in carbon fiber production: experimental and mathematical modelling. Prog Mater Sci 107:100575

Kumar M, Hietala M, Oksman K (2019) Lignin-based electrospun carbon nanofibers. Front Mater 6:62

Kurita H et al (2020) Fabrication and mechanical properties of carbon-fiber-reinforced polymer composites with Lead-free piezoelectric nanoparticles. Sensors Mater 32(7):2453

Laroche G et al (1995) Polyvinylidene fluoride (PVDF) as a biomaterial: from polymeric raw material to monofilament vascular suture. J Biomed Mater Res 29(12):1525–1536

Lin Y, Shaffer JW, Sodano HA (2010) Electrolytic deposition of PZT on carbon fibers for fabricating multifunctional composites. Smart Mater Struct 19(12):124004

Liu X et al (2021) Cure monitoring and damage identification of CFRP using embedded piezoelectric sensors network. Ultrasonics 115:106470

Mokhtari F et al (2021) Recent advances of polymer-based piezoelectric composites for biomedical applications. J Mech Behav Biomed Mater 122:104669

Mongioì F et al (2024) Multifunctional composite material based on piezoelectric nanofibers and Cu-CFRP electrodes for sensing applications. Compos Struct 337:118076

Montes-Morán MA, Martínez-Alonso A, Tascón JMD (2002) Effect of sizing on the surface properties of carbon fibres. J Mater Chem 12(12):3843–3850

Obasa VD et al (2022) A review on lignin-based carbon fibres for carbon footprint reduction. Atmos 13(10):1605

Otani S et al (1969) Method for producing carbonized lignin fiber. Google Patents

Parot M, Rodrigue D, Stevanovic T (2022) Electrospinning of softwood organosolv lignin without polymer addition. ACS Sustain Chem Eng 11(2):607–616

Petrushenko SI et al (2024) Carbon fabric coated with nanostructured zinc oxide layers for use in triboelectric self-powered touch sensors. J Mater Sci Mater Electron 35(6):414

Prenzel TM et al (2024) Bringing light into the dark—overview of environmental impacts of carbon fiber production and potential levers for reduction. Polymers 16(1):12

Ren K, Shen Y, Wang ZL (2024) Piezoelectric properties of electrospun polymer nanofibers and related energy harvesting applications. Macromol Mater Eng 309(3):2300307

Rubio MC et al (2022) Lignin-based carbon fibers for high-performance green composites. In: Encyclopedia of green materials. Springer, pp 1–8

Selleri G et al (2022) Self-sensing composite material based on piezoelectric nanofibers. Mater Des 219:110787

Shorey R et al (2024) Valorization of lignin for advanced material applications: a review. RSC Sustainab 2:804–831

Smith M, Kar-Narayan S (2021) Piezoelectric polymers: theory, challenges and opportunities. Int Mater Rev 67(1):65–88

Sukumaran S et al (2021) Recent advances in flexible PVDF based piezoelectric polymer devices for energy harvesting applications. J Intell Mater Syst Struct 32(7):746–780

Tribot A et al (2019) Wood-lignin: supply, extraction processes and use as bio-based material. Eur Polym J 112:228–240

Xu Y et al (2020) Current overview of carbon fiber: toward green sustainable raw materials. Bioresources 15(3):7234–7259

Yi J, Liang H (2008) A PVDF-based deformation and motion sensor: modeling and experiments. IEEE Sensors J 8(4):384–391

Yu Y, Narita F (2021) Evaluation of electromechanical properties and conversion efficiency of piezoelectric nanocomposites with carbon-fiber-reinforced polymer electrodes for stress sensing and energy harvesting. Polymers 13. https://doi.org/10.3390/polym13183184

Yu Y et al (2023a) In-situ cure monitoring of thick CFRP using multifunctional piezoelectric-fiber hybrid sensor network. Compos Sci Technol 240:110079

Yu Y et al (2023b) Carbon fiber-reinforced piezoelectric nanocomposites: design, fabrication and evaluation for damage detection and energy harvesting. Compos A: Appl Sci Manuf 172:107587

Zhang R et al (2011) Effect of the molecular weight of sizing agent on the surface of carbon fibres and interface of its composites. Appl Surf Sci 257(6):1840–1844

Zhang L et al (2014) A review: carbon nanofibers from electrospun polyacrylonitrile and their applications. J Mater Sci 49:463–480

Zhang J et al (2023) Past, present and future prospective of global carbon fibre composite developments and applications. Compos Part B 250:110463

Three-Dimensional Printing of Lignin-Based Materials

15

Sapna M. Rathod, Nisarg C. Patel, Bhupendra G. Prajapati, and Sudarshan Singh

Abstract

Additive manufacturing (AM) methods are being used in the quickly developing field of pharmaceutical additive manufacturing, commonly referred to as three-dimensional (3D) printing in the pharmaceutical business to develop consumer-centric pharmaceutical products. The potential for additive manufacturing to completely transform drug development and manufacturing by offering advantages such as personalized medicine, complex formulation systems, and production on-demand. Recently the applicability of biomaterials in 3D printing have gained significant interest among the researcher due to biodegradability and safety on use. Lignin, which is derived from lignocellulose and is the most prevalent aromatic biomass among the studied materials, is widely acknowledged as a promising biomaterial to produce pharmaceuticals using AM technology. Plant cell walls contain lignin, which has a macromolecular structure made up of

S. M. Rathod
Department of Quality Assurance and Pharmaceutical Chemistry, APMC College of Pharmaceutical Education and Research, Himatnagar, India

N. C. Patel
Department of Pharmacognosy, APMC College of Pharmaceutical Education and Research, Himatnagar, India

B. G. Prajapati
Department of Pharmaceutics, Shree S. K. Patel College of Pharmaceutical Education and Research, Ganpat University, Kherva, India

Centre for Research Impact & Outcome, Chitkara College of Pharmacy, Chitkara University, Rajpura Punjab, India

S. Singh (✉)
Faculty of Pharmacy, Chiang Mai University, Chiang Mai, Thailand

Office of Research Administrations, Chiang Mai University, Chiang Mai, Thailand

M. N. Collins, M. Culebras (eds.), *Sustainable Biopolymers and Composites for Biomedical Applications*, Biomaterials, Bioengineering and Sustainability 5, https://doi.org/10.1007/978-3-031-91972-5_15

guaiacyl, syringyl, and p-hydroxyphenyl units joined by carbon-carbon and ether bonds. These properties give lignin its unique bioactivity, amphiphilicity, and designability, which make it an intriguing candidate for use in biomedicines, ecological and engineering utility. The composition and origin of lignin, as well as its purification and the current state of 3D printed pharmaceutical products, are briefly reviewed in this chapter, which also identifies the main challenges. Additionally, summary on 3D printing technology have been presented to further understand the rapid prototyping technologies.

Keywords

Lignin · Lignocellulose · 3D printing · Additive manufacturing · Biomaterials · Bioengineering

15.1 Introduction

Any organic matter that is available again is referred to as biomass. Examples of this include aquatic plants, wood and its residues, animal wastes, agri-food and its residues, specialized energy plants and other materials. Industry-generated biomass or waste could be a great resource for creating various chemicals and composites. When compared to fossil fuels, properly managed biomass can result in a considerable decrease in net carbon emissions, making it a sustainable fuel. Reduced levels of air pollutants like Sulphur dioxide, which is a contributing factor to "acid rains," are produced by biomass fuels. An extensive range of biomass can be utilized to produce sustainable energy, including clean residues from forests and other sources of wood, organic household and agricultural wastes, industrial and public wastes, chippings from gardens and roadsides, and energy crops like poplar and willow, seed bearing oil crops, plants containing latex and common milkweed. Currently, 15% of wood is used for solid wood products, 30% is used for paper, and fuel accounts for 55% of all wood consumed worldwide. From ecological perspective, wood is a good choice than fossil fuels for energy, plastic or steel for material applications, and agricultural fibres for paper. The origin of biomass has a significant impact on its chemical makeup. Typically, 38% to 50% cellulose, 23% to 32% hemicelluloses, and 15% to 25% lignin make up biomass. The entire biorefinery is a processing plant that separates biomass (extractives) into components such as lignin, oils, and carbohydrates to create a range of compounds, like fuels and valuable chemicals or materials (Tursi 2019).

It comprises bio-composites made from forestry and agricultural biofibers (hemp, flax, and kenaf), which are employed, for instance, during fabrication of car parts and door panels, as well as for bio-rubber made from herb oils and latex, bio-foams, bioplastics obtained from herb oils and sugars. Agri-crop waste, wood and crops including, flax, kenaf and hemp are the materials utilized to make biofibers. They are renewable and biodegradable materials. Nowadays, biofibers are employed for manufacturing of superior paper and fabric materials, as well as in the construction and furniture industries for the creation of structural elements including decks, doors, and cupboards (Popa 2018).

Hemicellulose, lignin, and cellulose are the main elements of lignocellulosic materials (Deobald and Crawford 1997). The various constituents' non-covalent and covalent linkages regulate the lignocellulose structures' tertiary architecture. Microbes that are hydrolytic and fermentative are typically affixed to the surface of lignocellulosic biomass. The biodegradability of the biomass is significantly impacted by these compositional characteristics (Malherbe and Cloete 2002). The cross-linking structure between the constituents and the presence of lignin provide lignocellulosic biomass its relative resistance. These elements might then be utilized as raw materials to produce chemicals that are in high demand on the market, including organic acids and alcohols. Wood, grass, and straw are examples of lignocellulosic biomass and residues, which are plentiful non-food raw resources to produce renewable fuels and goods. The extraction of sugars from lignocellulose is a critical stage in the conversion of lignocellulosic biomass. This requirement is met by several pretreatments, including physical (size reduction), biological fragmentation, physicochemical (heating or ammonia fiber expansion) and chemical (treatment with ionic liquids or different pH media).

There are 3×10^{11} metric tons of lignin in the world and about 2×10^{11} metric tons of biosynthesis occurring each year, after cellulose, lignin is the next most common polymer (Sun 2020). Lignin is used in various synthetic and bio-derived thermoplastic polymer matrices as a copolymer, filler, or nucleating agent in the industrial setting to improve their mechanical and thermal characteristics. Three hydroxycinnamyl alcohols, often known as monolignols, are used in the biosynthesis of lignin: p-coumaryl, coniferyl, and sinapyl. Lignin makes up 15–35% of the lignocellulosic biomass generated by the timber and paper production industries (Hatakka 2001). It is composed of interconnected polyphenolic structures, which are essential to the development of cell walls and provide plants with structural support (Tsegaye et al. 2019). The majority of lignin's that are used are in the form of lignosulfonates, which are added to building materials. The remains of the lignin's are either utilized as low-grade fuel or thrown away as unused (Cao et al. 2018). Figure 15.1. Illustrate various sources for lignin and their 3D printed pharmaceutical applications.

15.2 Structure and Property of Lignin

The three primary phenylpropane units/hydroxyl cinnamyl alcohols that make up lignin's chemical structure are p hydroxyphenyl propanol (H), syringyl propanol (S), and guaiacyl propanol (G), which are connected by a variety of chemical linkages (Linger et al. 2014). Several linkages, including aryl ether, biphenyl ether, dibenzodioxocin, and phenylcoumaran, are used to join these building pieces (Lu et al. 2017). The degree to which methoxy functional groups in the aromatic rings are substituted determines the distinctions between phenylpropane units despite their comparable chemical structures. Because this polymer lacks chains with

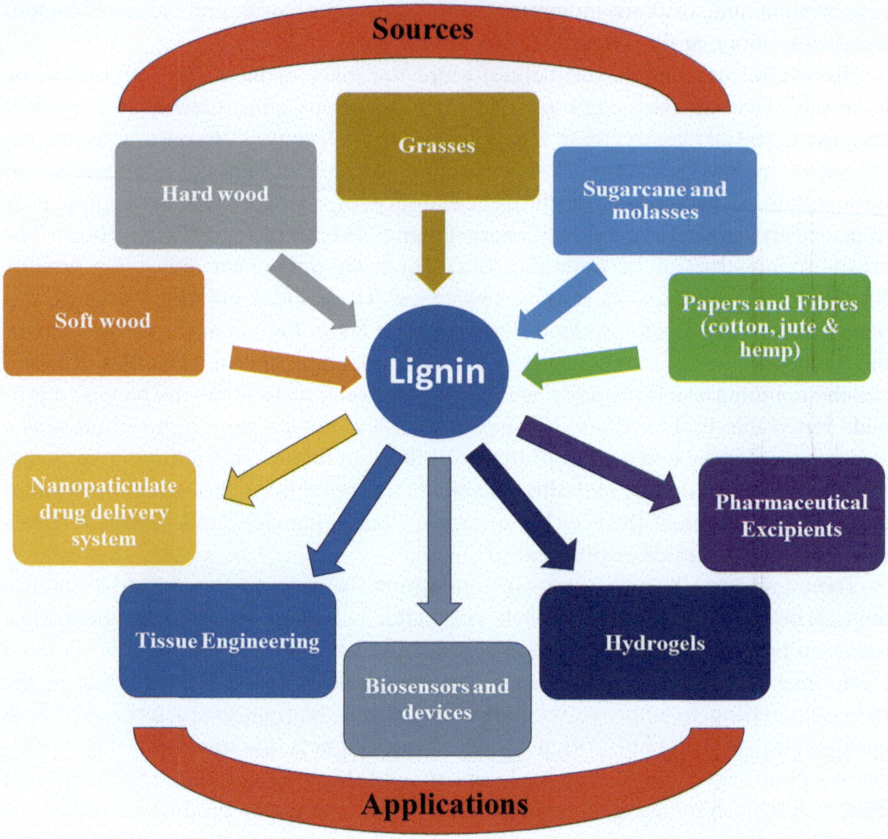

Fig. 15.1 Illustration representing various sources for lignin and their 3D printed pharmaceutical applications

repeating subunits, unlike cellulose or hemicellulose, it is very difficult to hydrolyze by enzymes. The segmentation of lignin into lignin-carbohydrate complexes and 31P NMR spectroscopic study both reveal that the structure of individual lignin molecules can vary significantly, even within the same sample (Duval and Lawoko 2014). Some molecules have a lot of branching, whereas others have a lot of linearity. As a result, the biopolymer's composition is indicated by the number of H/G/S polymeric units and the types of inter-unit linkages (Sette et al. 2011).

The side chain components of lignin also exhibit distinct conformations in stereochemistry. Through ozonation treatment, lignin's aromatic portions and double bonds can be totally broken down, converting the lignin's side chain components into simple organic acids while maintaining the side chain's native stereo structure (Xu et al. 2021). Erythron and threo are the two most prevalent lignin side chain stereochemical configurations. The erythron and threo forms of β-aryl ethers produce erythronic acid and threonic acid, correspondingly. Treatments that are physical, chemical, or biological can drastically change the structure of lignin. Organosolv lignin's, soda, and kraft which are commonly utilized commercial lignin's, are by-products of paper or biorefinery mills. Treatments of lignin that alters its linkages, polydispersity, molecular weight, and functional groups through physical, chemical, or biological means usually result in depolymerization and condensation (Abu-Omar et al. 2021).

15.3 Properties of Lignin

Studies by Faustino et al. and Azadfar et al. indicates that lignin has incredibly high levels of antioxidant properties (Azadfar et al. 2015; Faustino et al. 2010). Azadfar et al. discovered shows lignin's antioxidant qualities are on par with those of the over-the-counter antioxidants guaiacol and butylated hydroxytoluene (Azadfar et al. 2015). Several times, lignin's high concentration of phenolic groups and oxygen-containing functional groups is what gives it its antioxidant properties (Ogan et al. 2020; Kaur et al. 2017). These lignin functional groups have the ability to stop oxidative chain reactions by efficiently interacting with free radicals inside the system (Majira et al. 2019). Unchanged lignin from sugarcane bagasse was discovered by Kaur et al. to have better antioxidant activity than lignin that underwent chemical modification through acetylation and epoxidation (Kaur et al. 2017). Additionally, it was noted that lignin-based copolymers, like lignin-poly (ε-caprolactone-co-lactide) (lignin-PCLLA), maintain their antioxidant properties (Kai et al. 2017).

15.3.1 Antibacterial, Antifungal, and Antiviral

Over the years, lignin's antibacterial properties have been the subject of extensive research. Its antibacterial activity is assumed to be caused by its phenolic fragment, which has a double bond in the $C\alpha = C\beta$ position of the side chain and a methyl group in the γ position (Nada et al. 1989; Zemek et al. 1979). It was proposed that the bacterial reaction with phenolic chemicals results in bacterial lysis and cell membrane damage, which is how antibacterial activity is obtained (Sriroth and Sunthornvarabhas 2018). The lignin recovered from stover residue of maize by Dong et al. to create ethanol was found to have antibacterial activities specific to yeast and Gram-positive bacteria, but not to Gram-negative bacteria or the bacteriophage MS2 (Dong et al. 2011). Similar to this, Nada et al. have demonstrated that lignin's precipitated from pulping liquor are particularly efficient against Gram-positive bacteria like *B. subtilis* and *B. mycoides* but not against Gram-negative bacteria like *E. coli* (Nada et al. 1989). Additionally, lignin from eucalyptus, produced by the kraft approach, showed high antifungal action (fungal inhibition rates above 75%) at every level examined, while spruce extracted lignin showed antifungal effect at low concentrations only (Gordobil et al. 2018). Apple tree pruning residues were subjected to lignin extraction techniques such as autohydrolysis, organosolv, and soda. The lignin samples obtained from these processes shown antibacterial activity against Saccharomyces cerevisiae (García et al. 2017). A recent study tested lignin extracted from Caesalpinia pulcherrima leaves against a range of fungal strains, including, *Cryptococcus neoformans* (HC44), *Aspergillus furmigatus, Cryptococcus neoformans* (HC43), and *Aspergillus flavus*, as well as *Candida krusei* (ATC62), *Candida parapsilosis* (ATC22019), *Aspergillus flavus, Candida albicans* (URM49), and *Candida guilliermondii* (URM62). The antiviral activity of lignosulfonic acid or lignosulfonates, which are produced when wood is sulfite-delignified, has been studied against HIV and HSV, respectively (Gordts et al. 2015). Higher molecular weight lignosulfonates exhibited increased anti-HIV activity (Fukuchi et al. 2021). Additional research revealed that kraft lignin prevented yellowhead virus infection in black tiger shrimp and that alkaline lignin inhibited hepatitis C virus (Matsuhisa et al. 2015).

15.3.2 Ultraviolet Rays' Absorbent Properties

It is commonly known that lignin is UV-absorbent. The UV-absorbing functional groups of lignin, including ketones, phenolic and other chromophores, are thought to give it its anti-UV properties (Mehta and Kumar 2019; Park et al. 2019). Sadeghifar and Raauskas have recently conducted a thorough review of the usage of lignin as a UV barrier (Sadeghifar and Ragauskas 2020).

15.3.3 Antidiabetic

The antidiabetic potential of alkali lignin, isolated from the annually shedding *Acacia nilotica* plant, was assessed *in vitro*. The study examined the potential antidiabetic effect by blocking the uptake of glucose and inhibiting α-amylase in vivo. Degraded lignin samples were utilized to test the effect of enhanced glucose binding efficiency and inhibition of α-amylase using reduced glucose diffusion out of a dialysis tube (Barapatre et al. 2015).

15.4 Types of Lignin

The origin of lignin's can be used to categories them. Softwood lignin's are primarily made up of G, with very little S and very little H. Compared to softwood and hardwood, grass lignin's have more H units and about proportionate G and S. Hardwood lignin's are a blend of G and S, containing fewer H. Because hardwood lignin's comprises of G and S, each aromatic ring has two or three methoxy groups. There are numerous varieties of lignin that are made using various processing techniques (Azadi et al. 2013). These consist of lignosulphonates, kraft, organosolv, and soda lignin's. Of which, kraft lignin is the most prevalent, making up over 85% of the lignin generated worldwide.

Kraft (sulphate) pulping, which dissolves wood chips in white liquor (sodium sulphide and sodium hydroxide solution, pH 13–14) produces kraft lignin (Azadi et al. 2013). Solvent pulping, which has been demonstrated to be a more sustainable type of pulping than kraft and sulfite pulping, is how organosolv lignin's are created. Remaining pulp is heated to 170 °C with sodium hydroxide for about 1.5 hours to produce soda lignin's. The molecular weight of organosolv lignin and soda lignin is 4100–10,800 Da and 1300–10,400 Da respectively (Glasser et al. 1993).

15.5 Three-Dimensional Printing

The purposeful layer-by-layer deposition of ink to produce solid materials is referred to as "3D printing". Known as AM, three-dimensional printing technique superimposes printing materials in layers to create a three-dimensional item by a printer using computer control based on 3D model data (Wong and Hernandez 2012). When it comes to producing intricate 3D structures straight from design specifications, 3D printing offers more freedom and flexibility than traditional production techniques. Biological scaffolds (Liu et al. 2021), targeted drug delivery (Khosravani and Reinicke 2020), and tissue engineering (Wang and Yang 2021) can all be accomplished with the help of this technology. Materials derived from petroleum are frequently volatile, poisonous, and non-biodegradable, which looks unsuitable when considering the ecological issues. Consequently, the creation of sustainable and eco-friendly 3D printing materials is essential. Recycled or renewable resources can be used to create low-emission and ecofriendly 3D printing materials. The approach encourages the sustainable use of resources, which lessens pressure on the environment and the need for limited resources (Shuaib et al. 2021).

Because biomass-based products are renewable and biodegradable, researchers have come to appreciate them more and more in past years. The biomass that is most common on Earth is referred to as natural lignocellulose (Zoghlami and Paës 2019). Lignin is important to produce secondary cell walls in plants. It is a naturally occurring, biodegradable, biocompatible, and non-toxic polymer aromatic organic chemical (Tuck et al. 2012). The integration of lignin to AM technique gave rise to a novel area of lignin valorization known as lignin-based 3D printing (Ebers et al. 2021).

As a plentiful source of raw materials for 3D printing, lignin lessens reliance on finite fossil fuels and its adverse effects on the environment. Its strong and stiff qualities are among its excellent mechanical attributes. This makes it possible to employ it as a starting material in 3D printing process to produce printed goods that are robust and long-lasting (Mohanty et al. 2022). While creating biomass-based 3D printing materials, low-cost, biodegradable lignin and its derivatives can successfully lower manufacturing costs, improve material characteristics, and lower carbon emissions for environmental reasons (Haq et al. 2020).

15.6 Types of Three-Dimensional Printing Technologies

15.6.1 Extrusion-Based Fused Deposition Modeling

The commonly used 3D printing technology is extrusion, which is rapidly gaining favor with the world's pharmaceutical production business. The steps in the fused deposition modeling (FDM) process includes the melting of the polymer or initial material, extrusion, and gradual layer deposition. Following the material's solidification, the needed item is obtained. Raster thickness, angle, and space can be adjusted to change the object's shape and porosity (Mallikarjuna et al. 2023). Yu et al. used the 3DP to create the new fast disintegrating tablet. A cutting-edge method for creating customized dosage medication forms with regulated release patterns is fused-filament 3D printing (Yu et al. 2009). Particular release tablets are made with this technique (Goyanes et al. 2014). It was found that 3D extrusion-based printing is a potentially helpful method for creating gastric-floating devices, provided that conventional excipients and a lattice internal structure design are used (Li et al. 2018).

Employing an extrusion-based 3D printer, a single semi solid based formulation containing standard pharmaceutical excipients was employed to make acetaminophen tablets with various forms and configuration (solid ring and mesh). Khaled et al. developed 3D extrusion printing to produce paracetamol tablets with rapid release and substantial drug loading (Khaled et al. 2018).

By adopting the low-temperature FDM 3DP technology, Okwuosa and companions have developed an immediate release tablet that can be customized for each patient on demand for treatment (Okwuosa et al. 2016). A 3D printed polylactic acid (PLA) construct containing either methotrexate or gentamycin was created by Weisman and colleagues due to their antibiotic and cytotoxic properties (Weisman et al. 2015).

15.6.2 Drop on Solid Technique

The 3DP technique utilized to generate porous structure is called drop on solid (DOS). Using this technology, numerous solid formulations were created, such as implant with levofloxacin (Huang et al. 2007) or combination of isoniazid and rifampicin that showed altered or pulsatile release of the active medication. The DOS approach was used to generate acetaminophen tablets with sustained release profiles and chlorpheniramine tablets with pulsed release (Rowe et al. 2000).

15.6.3 Stereolithography Technique

It is a 3DP technique that incorporates a laser beam for transformation of product straight into a solid state without the need for liquid. The 3DP process polymerizes a liquid resin using high-energy light to create solid items. It was applied to create a formulation of drug incorporated tablets with altered release mechanisms. The releasing characteristic is contingent upon the monomer polymerization process. Stereolithography technique (SLA) 3DP 4-aminosalicylic acid (4 ASA) and paracetamol tablets were made by Wang and colleagues (Wang et al. 2016). Using SLA, Martinez and colleagues developed an ibuprofen hydrogel. The polymer is cross-linked polyethylene glycol diacrylate, or PEGDA (Martinez et al. 2017).

15.6.4 Semi-Solid Extrusion Technique

Chewable print lets are produced from the semisolid material using semi-solid extrusion printing. Using semi-solid extrusion, chewable formulations with a variety of flavors, medication combinations, and doses can be printed in any design. Khaled et al. synthesized guaifenesin polypills (bilayer tablets) by employing various polymer types (Khaled et al. 2014). The five medications included in the 3DP single pill are aspirin, ramipril, atenolol, pravastatin, and hydrochlorothiazide. The 3DP tablet features a profile of both quick and sustained release.

15.7 Three-Dimensional Printing Techniques for Lignin

In hypothesis, Polymers containing lignin should be suitable for all 3D printing processes; nevertheless, new developments indicate that lignin's complex and unique structure makes it ideal for Fused filament fabrication (FFF) and direct ink writing (DIW), stereolithography (SLA) and selective laser sintering (SLS) processes.

15.7.1 Fused Filament Fabrication

Fused filament fabrication is a widely used technique for working with polymers and composites made of polymers (Daminabo et al. 2020). Due to extensive printing rates range (50–500 mm h^{-1}), it is an easy-to-use and reasonable priced technology (Park et al. 2022). Solid polymer monofilament with a diameter of 0.5–3 mm is typically melted by a step-motor when it is pushed into a heated chamber. After that, an extrusion nozzle with a temperature-controlled setting extrudes the polymer. Because of their suitable melt rheology and low melting temperature, thermoplastic materials like ABS, nylon, and PLA as well as elastomers like polyether esters are frequently utilized as feedstocks for fluoropolymer-based foams (FFFs) (Park et al. 2022). A rotating FFF 3D printing technique was created by Raney et al. that allows short carbon fibers in an epoxy matrix to be oriented in a controlled spatial manner (Raney et al. 2018). Wu et al. developed a workable 3D structure for passive wireless sensors and integrated electronics utilizing a double-nozzle 3D printing method with a printing precision of 30 μm (Wu et al. 2015).

15.7.2 Direct Ink Writing

With the use of a layer-by-layer ink-filament deposition subsequence, DIW creates arbitrary 3D structures at a low cost and with outstanding material compatibility and spatial resolution (Saadi et al. 2022; Tagliaferri et al. 2021). There are two approaches: (1) meniscus-guided technique and (2) extrusion-based strategy. The resolution of the former can reach up to 600 nm, while the resolution of the latter can reach 1 μm (Ahn et al. 2009; Bae et al. 2020). There are two types of techniques for the extrusion-based DIW process: droplet-based and filamentary-based. Micropen direct writing and robocasting, often known as robotic deposition, are the two primary filamentary-based techniques (Anelli et al. 2022). Among the droplet-based methods are hot-melt ink (Zhang et al. 2021a) and inkjet (Guo et al. 2018; Bose et al. 2018) printing. According to Skylar-Scott et al. (Skylar-Scott et al. 2019), high resolution 3D printing using a 4-material multi-nozzle (4 × 4 nozzle) or a four-by-one two-material multi-nozzle (4 × 1) was used to design and fabricate voxelated soft matter. Peng et al. unveiled a brand-new hybrid multi-material 3D printing technology (Peng et al. 2021). Digital light processing printing and digital image writing are combined to print a variety of viscoelastic materials with intricate geometry quickly and with excellent quality. Bae et al. showed longitudinal 3D nano-printing of polymer nanowires integrated with carbon quantum dots (Bae et al. 2020). Using a multi-barrel pipet (Chen et al. 2019), a noncontact 3D nano-printing technique was devised to create clustered nanowires in parallel.

15.7.3 Stereolithography

Using a UV laser to selectively polymerize and cross-link a photo-initiator and reactive monomer, SLA also known as vat photopolymerization—creates three-dimensional materials in a liquid bath (Xu et al. 2020). In bottom-up SLA, the photosensitive material's lower surface is solidified by successively applying UV light along a predetermined path beneath the resin solution. The 3D sculpture is finished by repeating this procedure, but this time the platform ascends a certain distance to allow new, unresolved resin to restore this zone. In top-down SLA, the hardened upper surface descends to replace the fresh, uncured resin and the UV source positions over the resin bath. A wide range of nanocomposites, including biomaterials, engineering materials, electrical and magnetic materials, (Zhang et al. 2021b) and others, can be created thanks to SLA printing's excellent resolution. Lu et al. produced a robust, bright shape-memory thermoset by two-step SLA printing using chain-growth polymerization induced by UV and step-growth polymerization induced by heat (Lu et al. 2020).

15.7.4 Selective Laser Sintering

High precision and high performance are combined in SLS, a powder-based additive manufacturing technology that is commonly used for the rapid prototyping of complex 3D patterns. The heat source used in the commercially available SLS is currently mostly a CO_2 laser. As with the dual-beam approach, the Nd: YAG laser has also been utilized separately or in conjunction with the CO_2 laser (Awad et al. 2020). According to Leong et al., spherical particles between 58 and 180 μm in size are ideal for SLS printing (Leong et al. 2006). SLS printing is primarily used in the manufacturing of pharmaceuticals, including biological tissue repair and slow-release pill formulations (Awad et al. 2020). Fina et al. manufacture tablets with bilayer, gyroid lattice, and cylindrical design (Fina et al. 2017). A nano-hydroxyapatite/poly-ε-caprolactone (nano-HA/PCL) scaffold was created by Xia et al. (Xia et al. 2013) using SLS printing for bone tissue engineering purposes. The nano-HA/PCL exhibited better biocompatibility and higher new bone formation capability as compared to PCL.

15.8 Fluidity-Structure Relationship of Lignin-Based Bioink

The printability, functionality, and use of 3D scaffolds are all significantly impacted by the structure-rheology link. The main cause of a polymer's variations in printability is its rheological properties, which apply to both the solid and printing states. Additionally, the materials' characteristics and printability are altered by the polymer's addition of fillers or additives. Thus, it will be beneficial to summarise the lignin structure-rheology relationship for the purpose of material design and seamless lignin-based composite printing.

15.9 Structure-Melt Rheology Relationship in Fused Filament Fabrication

For FFF printability, it is necessary to melt the lignin to a low viscosity but adequate fluid; here, lignin's thermal durability is crucial for the filaments to print continuously. Technical lignins have low thermal stability, thus even though popular polymers like PLA (Bhagia et al. 2021) and polyether ether ketone (Sikder et al. 2022) frequently exhibit reduced viscosity with increased temperature, this method is not appropriate to them. Reduced flow or deformation is caused by lignin's huge molecular weight, which is difficult to melt at low temperatures, and its low molar mass, which breaks down to create a stiff char at high temperatures. It has been found that organosolv hardwood lignin with a high concentration of linear sinapyl alcohol units exhibits good melt stability (Sun et al. 2016). It is said that the plentiful aliphatic ether, methoxy groups and aromatic carbon groups with oxygen in hardwood lignin allow for an excellent level of molecular flexibility when rotating and bending (Holmberg et al. 2016). In a similar vein, If the purified oligomeric fraction

(≈1000 Da) is not used, kraft softwood lignin with a high concentration of condensed G units does not flow smoothly at elevated temperatures (Akato et al. 2015).

In their investigation of PEO's impact on ABS/lignin melt rheology, Akato et al. found that PEO reduces the viscosity of the blends and enhances their melt-processability (Akato et al. 2015). For FFF printing, Nguyen et al. (2018a) combined lignin with ABS and acrylonitrile butadiene rubber (NBR). Certain polymers, such PLA and nylon 12, when used by itself can help improve lignin/polymer combinations' printability for applications in 3D printing. The effects of nylon 12 on the hardwood lignin printing capability and melt rheology were thoroughly investigated by Nguyen et al. (2018b). It has been noted that the PLA matrix and the polymer nylon 12 are very compatible with organosolv hardwood lignin. For the mix to print well by FFF, lignin loading should make up 15% of the weight percentage. However, as compared to an equal softwood kraft lignin, the blend of lignin and PLA prints poorly. This is mainly because of lignin's residual soda causes PLA to degrade (Mimini et al. 2019).

15.10 Structure-Ink Rheology Relationship in Direct Ink Writing

Unlike FFF, lignin or lignin/polymer blends don't require heating up till melting point for DIW. Rather, the primary difficulty with DIW is creating a viscoelastic ink that flows within the nozzle with ease and can create a free-standing structure. Consequently, organic inks or colloidal gels with low zero shear rate compliance and good shear-thinning behaviour are especially well suited for DIW (Lewis 2006). Currently, the application of DIW on lignin is always dependent on the mixing of polymers to create colloidal formulations, like viscoelastic polymers, carbon-based polymers, cellulose nanofibers (CNFs) (Ebers and Laborie 2020; Gleuwitz et al. 2020), and cellulose nanofibers (Jiang et al. 2020; Jiang et al. 2021). The formulas and parameters of DIW for hydroxypropyl cellulose / totally bio-based OSL inks were optimised by Ebers and Laborie (2020). Zhang et al. (2020a) generated Ca^{2+}-crosslinked cellulose nanofibers -alginate- colloidal lignin particles nanocomposites via DIW using spherical colloidal lignin particles. Gleuwitz et al. also present a liquid crystalline network material created by DIW that contains lignin (Gleuwitz et al. 2020). Also, a ubiquitous, economical DIW was created for building 3D scaffolds made of lignin (Jiang et al. 2020). One crucial factor influencing the accuracy of 3D printed lignin-based materials in extrusion-based DIW is the printed structure's shrinkage as a result of post-processing or solvent evaporation, which may potentially result in the collapse of the structure. It has been shown, for instance, that lignosulfonate can reduce the printed lignin shrinkage (Shao et al. 2015). The shrinkage characteristics, process variables, and rheological behaviors of lignin-based inks must all be carefully considered for successful 3D printing.

15.11 Relationship Between Structure and Rheology in Stereolithography and Selective Laser Sintering

The authors exhibited that the 40/60 (wt. %) blended lignin/Polyamide powder may be effectively printed at 175 °C by SLS. The evaluation of the lignin/Polyamide blend's thermal characteristics also revealed that while the melting and crystallization temperatures (T_m and T_c) of the polyamide alone and lignin/Polyamide blend are relatively similar, the marginally dropped T_c was observed after mixing with lignin (Ajdary et al. 2021). The mechanical characteristics and functionality of the materials produced by SLA are significantly limited by the minimal activity and fragile nature of these free radicals, notwithstanding recent reports that lignin has a great deal of promise as a photo-initiator and that it may generate free radicals when exposed to natural light (Kim et al. 2017).

With lignin additions of ≤1 weight percent, there is only a slight improvement in tensile strength and elastic modulus; excess lignin addition (1–3 weight percent) results in a significant decline in the printed composites' performance. In order to achieve stable SLA printing and high mechanical power in the composites, lignin is chemically modified. In order to combine OSL modified with methacrylic anhydride with photopolymer resin, Sutton et al. further proved that SLA could be printed (Sutton et al. 2018). Zhang et al. synthesised alkylated de-alkaline lignin's via a straightforward single-step reaction of esterification between undecanoyl or dodecanoyl chloride and lignin (Zhang et al. 2020b). The redesigned lignin was demonstrated to be a viable medium for visible light macromolecular photoinitiation. In digital light processing 3D printing, de-alkaline lignin's -undecanoyl chloride and DAL-dodecanoyl chloride perform exceptionally well as macro photo-initiators when paired with co-initiator ethyl 4-(dimethylamino) benzoate. A viable method for obtaining value-added lignin for SLA printing and significantly enhancing the effectiveness of printed materials is lignin modification.

15.12 Pharmaceutical Three-Dimensional Printed Applications of Lignin

The characteristics of lignin are drawing attention for the advancement of oral solid dosage forms, sunscreen lotions, nanoparticles and nanotubes, hydrogels, and 3D printed materials, among other applications, even though the biological applications of lignin are still mostly unknown. Cross-linked polymer networks arranged in three dimensions are called hydrogels, and they possess the ability to take in and store enormous amounts of biological fluids or water inside of them.

Recently, bio-composite filaments for 3D printing have been effectively created by combining lignin with PLA and polyhydroxybutyrate (Tanase-Opedal et al. 2019; Lee et al. 2020). The scientific community has become interested in the application of plant-based biopolymers in 3D printing because of its attributes, which include non-cytotoxicity, biodegradability, and biocompatibility (Domínguez-Robles et al. 2019). Because of this, there has been a discernible increase in interest over the last 10 years in the creation of biomedical applications using 3D printing technology. Castor oil-coated PLA pellets can also be mixed with tetracycline, an antibiotic, and a little quantity of Kraft lignin (3 weight percent or less) to form a composite that can be used to 3D print wound dressings (Aadil et al. 2018). While continuous development in tissue engineering technology has made it possible to transplant complete organs or tissues, and it has emerged as a viable replacement for damaged tissue or portions. In order to develop regenerating tissue for use in medicine, natural biomaterials must be created (Quraishi et al. 2015). Major players in the process, biomaterials offer the appropriate foundation required for the regeneration of damaged tissue and its replacement with functional tissue (Berglund et al. 2018). Biomaterial scaffolds are employed in tissue engineering applications; they function as a template to encourage the growth and regeneration of a specific tissue and imitate the extracellular matrix (Kai et al. 2016). The utilization of lignin biopolymer in this filed to substitute, restore, and enhance the functionality of a target tissue or organ is an exciting area of research.

15.13 Advantages of Using Lignin in 3D Printing

Lignin has great potential to replace polymers based on fossil fuel like epoxy resins, polyamide, acrylonitrile butadiene styrene, and polycarbonate when printed into composites with the necessary mechanical and functional properties utilizing 3D printing processes. This is because lignin is a renewable, abundant, and non-toxic biopolymer. Personalized medicine, energy, optics, and drug delivery can all be catered for in 3D-printed lignin composites by adjusting their macro- and microstructural characteristics. Nonetheless, lignin and other polymers are thought to work with nearly every kind of 3D printing method. However, because of its intricate and distinct structure, lignin is only suitable for material extrusion (FFF and DIW), SLA, and SLS processes, according to recent study (Jiang et al. 2023). To increase its toughness, lignin is typically copolymerized with a soft segment or combined with polymer. PLA (Wasti et al. 2021), ABS (Akato et al. 2015), graphene (Mohan et al. 2021), nylon 12 (Nguyen et al. 2018b), polyhydroxy butyrate (Domínguez-Robles et al. 2019), methacrylate (Holmberg et al. 2016), and polyethylene oxide (Yu et al. 2015) are the primary components of the polymer matrix, or soft section, for FFF. For example, ABS is a polymer that is frequently blended with lignin to improve printability because of its good mechanical performance, melt characteristics, and FFF compatibility. According to a study, lignin is a suitable component for polyamide SLS that can lower costs while maintaining or improving processability and performance (Trifol et al. 2021). SLS is demonstrated as a progressive step toward lignin valorization in composites, according to Rubina Ajdary, while permitting lower costs, scalability, and facial processing (Ajdary et al. 2021). A partial substitution of lignin for polyamide demonstrates the function of the polyaromatic molecule, the potential for the addition of additional traits, and the preservation of thermomechanical properties. Lignin adds shear-thinning action and viscosity to biobased resin ink without changing the curing kinetics.

15.14 Challenges and Future Perspectives

The original and technical lignin's immiscible and brittle natures prevent their widespread use. It is believed that rather than completely exploiting lignin's unique qualities, which include redox and nutrition regulating characteristics, depolymerization or modification might increase lignin's interfacial compatibility with other polymers, which is an effective strategy to add worth to lignin. Furthermore, there are significant obstacles facing the present modification or depolymerization tactics as they attempt to concentrate on simple, low-cost, green-chemistry processes.

The out-of-order microporous structure causes complex charge transport channels, which degrades the performance of carbon-based materials derived from lignin by traditional solution processing. When integrated with 3D printing technologies, lignin is expected to function as an active functional material for added value; additive manufacturing has demonstrated that lignin-based materials can do this. Improved 3D printing methods in conjunction with targeted chemical and physical features are necessary for the development of polymers based on lignin.

The utilization of petroleum-based polymers in lignin 3D printing is excessive since it necessitates enhanced rheological properties, including viscoelasticity, modulus, and melting point. Different functional compositions are typically needed for materials used in the fields of tissue engineering and robotic applications; however, using numerous materials typically results in poor rheological behavior for a particular 3D printing technique. Owing to the intricate structure and morphology of lignin, printing lignin nanocomposites frequently results in internal defects that impair the mechanical qualities of the printed items.

Moreover, additives can modify the hydrophilic or hydrophobic surface characteristics of lignin, enhancing the adhesion and interfacial compatibility of successive printed layers. During the printing process, it may be necessary to stimulate or catalyze this in situ polymerization using external inputs like active gases or lasers. In order to reduce residual voids and inhomogeneity and to encourage the evolution of the microstructure, post printing treatment is equally desirable. Not much research has been done on how surface tension or surface energy-driven molecule segregation affects the microstructure, features, and functionality of three-dimensional structures produced through additive printing. The use of inorganic elements in lignin-based materials additive manufacturing is currently mostly understudied. The continuous development of high-quality additive manufacturing of lignin-based components requires both in situ monitoring and post-inspection. The future advancements and directions of 3D printing techniques towards the diversification of materials, structures, and procedures are highly compatible with lignin. Lignin's structural characteristics and uses still require further research.

15.15 Conclusion

Numerous investigations have shown that the printability of lignin/polymer mix inks and the performance of the resultant composites are significantly influenced by the structure-rheology correlation of lignin. The FFF, DIW, SLA, and SLS technologies can print lignin in three dimensions, but this does not imply that the material can print into three-dimensional structures with the required stability, performance, and properties. Additives are necessary for the successful construction of lignin-based three-dimensional objects, particularly macromolecules with linear structures. The lignin's molecular weight and structure are crucial for FFF printing. As was already indicated, two popular feedstocks for FFF with flexible segments and low molecular weight are oligomeric kraft softwood lignin and organosolv hardwood lignin. DIW's modifiable rheological behaviour makes it ideal for 3D printing lignin. It permits both vertical and horizontal printing of compositions. Lignin is anticipated to operate as an active purposeful material for additional value when combined with 3D printing processes; additive manufacturing has shown that this is possible for lignin-based materials. Improved 3D printing methods in conjunction with targeted chemical and physical features are necessary for the development of lignin-based polymers.

References

Aadil KR, Mussatto SI, Jha H (2018) Synthesis and characterization of silver nanoparticles loaded poly (vinyl alcohol)-lignin electrospun nanofibers and their antimicrobial activity. Int J Biol Macromol 120(Pt A):763–767. https://doi.org/10.1016/j.ijbiomac.2018.08.109

Abu-Omar MM, Barta K, Beckham GT, Luterbacher JS, Ralph J, Rinaldi R, Román-Leshkov Y, Samec JS, Sels BF, Wang F (2021) Guidelines for performing lignin-first biorefining. Energy Environ Sci 14(1):262–292. https://doi.org/10.1039/D0EE02870C

Ahn BY, Duoss EB, Motala MJ, Guo X, Park SI, Xiong Y, Yoon J, Nuzzo RG, Rogers JA, Lewis JA (2009) Omnidirectional printing of flexible, stretchable, and spanning silver microelectrodes. Science 323(5921):1590–1593. https://doi.org/10.1126/science.1168375

Ajdary R, Kretzschmar N, Baniasadi H, Trifol J, Seppälä JV, Partanen J, Rojas OJ (2021) Selective laser sintering of lignin-based composites. ACS Sustain Chem Eng 9(7):2727–2735. https://doi.org/10.1021/acssuschemeng.0c07996

Akato K, Tran CD, Chen J, Naskar AK (2015) Poly (ethylene oxide)-assisted macromolecular self-assembly of lignin in ABS matrix for sustainable composite applications. ACS Sustain Chem Eng 3(12):3070–3076. https://doi.org/10.1021/acssuschemeng.5b00509

Anelli S, Rosa M, Baiutti F, Torrell M, Esposito V, Tarancón A (2022) Hybrid-3D printing of symmetric solid oxide cells by inkjet printing and robocasting. Addit Manuf 51:102636. https://doi.org/10.1016/j.addma.2022.102636

Awad A, Fina F, Goyanes A, Gaisford S, Basit AW (2020) 3D printing: principles and pharmaceutical applications of selective laser sintering. Int J Pharm 586:119594. https://doi.org/10.1016/j.ijpharm.2020.119594

Azadfar M, Gao AH, Bule MV, Chen S (2015) Structural characterization of lignin: a potential source of antioxidants guaiacol and 4-vinylguaiacol. Int J Biol Macromol 75:58–66. https://doi.org/10.1016/j.ijbiomac.2014.12.049

Azadi P, Inderwildi OR, Farnood R, King DA (2013) Liquid fuels, hydrogen and chemicals from lignin: a critical review. Renew Sust Energ Rev 21:506–523. https://doi.org/10.1016/j.rser.2012.12.022

Bae J, Lee S, Ahn J, Kim JH, Wajahat M, Chang WS, Yoon SY, Kim JT, Seol SK, Pyo J (2020) 3D-printed quantum dot nanopixels. ACS Nano 14(9):10993–11001. https://doi.org/10.1021/acsnano.0c04075

Barapatre A, Aadil KR, Tiwary BN, Jha H (2015) In vitro antioxidant and antidiabetic activities of biomodified lignin from Acacia nilotica wood. Int J Biol Macromol 75:81–89. https://doi.org/10.1016/j.ijbiomac.2015.01.012

Berglund L, Forsberg F, Jonoobi M, Oksman K (2018) Promoted hydrogel formation of lignin-containing arabinoxylan aerogel using cellulose nanofibers as a functional biomaterial. RSC Adv 8(67):38219–38228. https://doi.org/10.1039/C8RA08166B

Bhagia S, Bornani K, Agrawal R, Satlewal A, Ďurkovič J, Lagaňa R, Bhagia M, Yoo CG, Zhao X, Kunc V, Pu Y (2021) Critical review of FDM 3D printing of PLA biocomposites filled with biomass resources, characterization, biodegradability, upcycling and opportunities for biorefineries. Appl Mater Today 24:101078. https://doi.org/10.1016/j.apmt.2021.101078

Bose S, Ke D, Sahasrabudhe H, Bandyopadhyay A (2018) Additive manufacturing of biomaterials. Prog Mater Sci 93:45–111. https://doi.org/10.1016/j.pmatsci.2017.08.003

Cao L, Yu IKM, Liu Y, Ruan X, Tsang DCW, Hunt AJ, Ok YS, Song H, Zhang S (2018) Lignin valorization for the production of renewable chemicals: state-of-the-art review and future prospects. Bioresour Technol 269:465–475. https://doi.org/10.1016/j.biortech.2018.08.065

Chen M, Yang J, Wang Z, Xu Z, Lee H, Lee H et al (2019) 3D nanoprinting of perovskites. Adv Mater 31(44):1904073. https://doi.org/10.1002/adma.201904073

Daminabo SC, Goel S, Grammatikos SA, Nezhad HY, Thakur VK (2020) Fused deposition modeling-based additive manufacturing (3D printing): techniques for polymer material systems. Mater Today Chem 16:100248. https://doi.org/10.1016/j.mtchem.2020.100248

Deobald LA, Crawford DL (1997) Lignocellulose biodegradation. In: Hurst CJ, Knudsen GR, Stetzenbach LD, Walter MV (eds) Manual of environmental microbiology, vol 1. ASM Press, Washington, DC, pp 730–737. https://doi.org/10.1023/A:1020858910646

Domínguez-Robles J, Martin NK, Fong ML, Stewart SA, Irwin NJ, Rial-Hermida MI, Donnelly RF, Larrañeta E (2019) Antioxidant PLA composites containing lignin for 3D printing applications: a potential material for healthcare applications. Pharmaceutics 11(4):165. https://doi.org/10.3390/pharmaceutics11040165

Dong X, Dong M, Lu Y, Turley A, Jin T, Wu C (2011) Antimicrobial and antioxidant activities of lignin from residue of corn Stover to ethanol production. Ind Crop Prod 34(3):1629–1634. https://doi.org/10.1016/j.indcrop.2011.06.002

Duval A, Lawoko M (2014) A review on lignin-based polymeric, micro- and nano-structured materials. React Funct Polym 85:78–96. https://doi.org/10.1016/j.reactfunctpolym.2014.09.017

Ebers LS, Laborie MP (2020) Direct ink writing of fully bio-based liquid crystalline lignin/Hydroxypropyl cellulose aqueous inks: optimization of formulations and printing parameters. ACS Appl Bio Mater 3(10):6897–6907. https://doi.org/10.1021/acsabm.0c00800

Ebers LS, Arya A, Bowland CC, Glasser WG, Chmely SC, Naskar AK, Laborie MP (2021) 3D printing of lignin: challenges, opportunities and roads onward. Biopolymers 112(6):e23431. https://doi.org/10.1002/bip.23431

Faustino H, Gil N, Baptista C, Duarte AP (2010) Antioxidant activity of lignin phenolic compounds extracted from Kraft and sulphite black liquors. Molecules 15(12):9308–9322. https://doi.org/10.3390/molecules15129308

Fina F, Goyanes A, Gaisford S, Basit AW (2017) Selective laser sintering (SLS) 3D printing of medicines. Int J Pharm 529(1–2):285–293. https://doi.org/10.1016/j.ijpharm.2017.06.082

Fukuchi K, Koshikawa T, Asai D, Inomata M, Sakagami H, Takemura H, Kanamoto T, Aimi H, Kikkawa Y (2021) Lignosulfonate rapidly inactivates human immunodeficiency and herpes simplex viruses. Medicines 8(10):56. https://doi.org/10.3390/medicines8100056

García A, Spigno G, Labidi J (2017) Antioxidant and biocide behaviour of lignin fractions from apple tree pruning residues. Ind Crop Prod 104:242–252. https://doi.org/10.1016/j.indcrop.2017.04.063

Glasser WG, Davé V, Frazier CE (1993) Molecular weight distribution of (semi-) commercial lignin derivatives. J Wood Chem Technol 13(4):545–559. https://doi.org/10.1080/02773819308020533

Gleuwitz FR, Sivasankarapillai G, Siqueira G, Friedrich C, Laborie MG (2020) Lignin in bio-based liquid crystalline network material with potential for direct ink writing. ACS Appl Bio Mater 3(9):6049–6058. https://doi.org/10.1021/acsabm.0c00661

Gordobil O, Herrera R, Yahyaoui M, İlk S, Kaya M, Labidi J (2018) Potential use of Kraft and organosolv lignins as a natural additive for healthcare products. RSC Adv 8(43):24525–24533. https://doi.org/10.1039/C8RA02255K

Gordts SC, Férir G, D'huys T, Petrova MI, Lebeer S, Snoeck R, Andrei G, Schols D (2015) The low-cost compound lignosulfonic acid (LA) exhibits broad-spectrum anti-HIV and anti-HSV activity and has potential for microbicidal applications. PLoS One 10(7):e0131219. https://doi.org/10.1371/journal.pone.0131219

Goyanes A, Buanz AB, Basit AW, Gaisford S (2014) Fused-filament 3D printing (3DP) for fabrication of tablets. Int J Pharm 476(1–2):88–92. https://doi.org/10.1016/j.ijpharm.2014.09.044

Guo Y, Peters J, Oomen T, Mishra S (2018) Control-oriented models for ink-jet 3D printing. Mechatronics 56:211–219. https://doi.org/10.1016/j.mechatronics.2018.04.002

Haq I, Mazumder P, Kalamdhad AS (2020) Recent advances in removal of lignin from paper industry wastewater and its industrial applications–a review. Bioresour Technol 312:123636. https://doi.org/10.1016/j.biortech.2020.123636

Hatakka A (2001) Biodegradation of lignin. In: Hofrichter M, Steinbüchel A (eds) Biopolymers. Biology, chemistry, biotechnology, applications. Vol 1. Lignin, humic substances and coal. Wiley-VCH, Weinheim, pp 129–180. https://doi.org/10.1002/3527600035.bpol1005

Holmberg AL, Nguyen NA, Karavolias MG, Reno KH, Wool RP, Epps TH III (2016) Softwood lignin-based methacrylate polymers with tunable thermal and viscoelastic properties. Macromolecules 49(4):1286–1295. https://doi.org/10.1021/acs.macromol.5b02316

Huang W, Zheng Q, Sun W, Xu H, Yang X (2007) Levofloxacin implants with predefined microstructure fabricated by three-dimensional printing technique. Int J Pharm 339:33–38. https://doi.org/10.1016/j.ijpharm.2007.02.021

Jiang B, Yao Y, Liang Z, Gao J, Chen G, Xia Q, Mi R, Jiao M, Wang X, Hu L (2020) Lignin-based direct ink printed structural scaffolds. Small 16(31):e1907212. https://doi.org/10.1002/smll.201907212

Jiang B, Huang H, Gong W, Gu X, Liu T, Zhang J, Qin W, Chen H, Jin Y, Liang Z, Jiang L (2021) Wood-inspired binder enabled vertical 3D printing of g-C_3N_4/CNT arrays for highly efficient Photoelectrochemical hydrogen evolution. Adv Funct Mater 31(45):2105045. https://doi.org/10.1002/adfm.202105045

Jiang B, Jiao H, Guo X, Chen G, Guo J, Wu W, Jin Y, Cao G, Liang Z (2023) Lignin-based materials for additive manufacturing: chemistry, processing, structures, properties, and applications. Adv Sci (Weinh) 10(9):e2206055. https://doi.org/10.1002/advs.202206055

Kai D, Ren W, Tian L, Chee PL, Liu Y, Ramakrishna S, Loh XJ (2016) Engineering poly (lactide)–lignin nanofibers with antioxidant activity for biomedical application. ACS Sustain Chem Eng 4(10):5268–5276. https://doi.org/10.1021/acssuschemeng.6b00478

Kai D, Zhang K, Jiang L, Wong HZ, Li Z, Zhang Z, Loh XJ (2017) Sustainable and antioxidant lignin–polyester copolymers and nanofibers for potential healthcare applications. ACS Sustain Chem Eng 5(7):6016–6025. https://doi.org/10.1021/acssuschemeng.7b00850

Kaur R, Uppal S, Sharma P (2017) Antioxidant and antibacterial activities of sugarcane bagasse lignin and chemically modified Lignins. Sugar Tech 19:678–680. https://doi.org/10.1007/s12355-017-0513-y

Khaled SA, Burley JC, Alexander MR, Roberts CJ (2014) Desktop 3D printing of controlled release pharmaceutical bilayer tablets. Int J Pharm 461(1–2):105–111. https://doi.org/10.1016/j.ijpharm.2013.11.021

Khaled SA, Alexander MR, Irvine DJ, Wildman RD, Wallace MJ, Sharpe S, Yoo J, Roberts CJ (2018) Extrusion 3D printing of paracetamol tablets from a single formulation with tunable release profiles through control of tablet geometry. AAPS Pharm SciTech 19:3403–3413. https://doi.org/10.1208/s12249-018-1107-z

Khosravani MR, Reinicke T (2020) On the environmental impacts of 3D printing technology. Appl Mater Today 20:100689. https://doi.org/10.1016/j.apmt.2020.100689

Kim KH, Dutta T, Walter ED, Isern NG, Cort JR, Simmons BA, Singh S (2017) Chemoselective methylation of phenolic hydroxyl group prevents quinone methide formation and repolymerization during lignin depolymerization. ACS Sustain Chem Eng 5(5):3913–3919. https://doi.org/10.1021/acssuschemeng.6b03102

Lee SC, Yoo E, Lee SH, Won K (2020) Preparation and application of light-colored lignin nanoparticles for broad-spectrum sunscreens. Polymers (Basel) 12(3):699. https://doi.org/10.3390/polym12030699

Leong KF, Chua CK, Gui WS, Verani (2006) Building porous biopolymeric microstructures for controlled drug delivery devices using selective laser sintering. Int J Adv Manuf Technol 31:483–489. https://doi.org/10.1007/s00170-005-0217-4

Lewis JA (2006) Direct ink writing of 3D functional materials. Adv Funct Mater 16(17):2193–2204. https://doi.org/10.1002/adfm.200600434

Li Q, Guan X, Cui M, Zhu Z, Chen K, Wen H, Jia D, Hou J, Xu W, Yang X, Pan W (2018) Preparation and investigation of novel gastro-floating tablets with 3D extrusion-based printing. Int J Pharm 535(1–2):325–332. https://doi.org/10.1016/j.ijpharm.2017.10.037

Linger JG, Vardon DR, Guarnieri MT, Karp EM, Hunsinger GB, Franden MA, Johnson CW, Chupka G, Strathmann TJ, Pienkos PT, Beckham GT (2014) Lignin valorization through integrated biological funneling and chemical catalysis. Proc Natl Acad Sci USA 111(33):12013–12018. https://doi.org/10.1073/pnas.1410657111

Liu H, Zhang H, Han W, Lin H, Li R, Zhu J, Huang W (2021) 3D printed flexible strain sensors: from printing to devices and signals. Adv Mater 33(8):2004782. https://doi.org/10.1002/adma.202004782

Lu Y, Lu Y-C, Hu H-Q, Xie F-J, Wei X-Y, Fan X (2017) Structural characterization of lignin and its degradation products with spectroscopic methods. J Spectrosc 2017:8951658–8951615. https://doi.org/10.1155/2017/8951658

Lu C, Wang C, Yu J, Wang J, Chu F (2020) Two-step 3 D-printing approach toward sustainable, repairable, fluorescent shape-memory thermosets derived from cellulose and rosin. ChemSusChem 13(5):893–902. https://doi.org/10.1002/cssc.201902191

Majira A, Godon B, Foulon L, van Der Putten JC, Cézard L, Thierry M, Pion F, Bado-Nilles A, Pandard P, Jayabalan T, Aguié-Béghin V (2019) Enhancing the antioxidant activity of technical Lignins by combining solvent fractionation and ionic-liquid treatment. ChemSusChem 12(21):4799–4809. https://doi.org/10.1002/cssc.201901916

Malherbe S, Cloete TE (2002) Lignocellulose biodegradation: fundamentals and applications. Rev Environ Sci Biotechnol 1(2):105–114. https://doi.org/10.1023/A:1020858910646

Mallikarjuna B, Bhargav P, Hiremath S, Jayachristiyan KG, Jayanth N (2023) A review on the melt extrusion-based fused deposition modeling (FDM): background, materials, process parameters and military applications. Int J Interact Des Manuf 12:1–5. https://doi.org/10.1007/s12008-023-01354-0

Martinez PR, Goyanes A, Basit AW, Gaisford S (2017) Fabrication of drug-loaded hydrogels with stereolithographic 3D printing. Int J Pharm 532(1):313–317. https://doi.org/10.1016/j.ijpharm.2017.09.003

Matsuhisa K, Yamane S, Okamoto T, Watari A, Kondoh M, Matsuura Y, Yagi K (2015) Anti-HCV effect of Lentinula edodes mycelia solid culture extracts and low-molecular-weight lignin. Biochem Biophys Res Commun 462(1):52–57. https://doi.org/10.1016/j.bbrc.2015.04.104

Mehta MJ, Kumar A (2019) Ionic liquid stabilized Gelatin–Lignin films: a potential UV-shielding material with excellent mechanical and antimicrobial properties. Chemistry 25(5):1269–1274. https://doi.org/10.1002/chem.201803763

Mimini V, Sykacek E, Syed Hashim SN, Holzweber J, Hettegger H, Fackler K, Potthast A, Mundigler N, Rosenau T (2019) Compatibility of Kraft lignin, organosolv lignin and lignosulfonate with PLA in 3D printing. J Wood Chem Technol 39(1):14–30. https://doi.org/10.1080/02773813.2018.1488875

Mohan D, Bakir AN, Sajab MS, Bakarudin SB, Mansor NN, Roslan R, Kaco H (2021) Homogeneous distribution of lignin/graphene fillers with enhanced interlayer adhesion for 3D printing filament. Polym Compos 42(5):2408–2421. https://doi.org/10.1002/pc.25987

Mohanty AK, Wu F, Mincheva R, Hakkarainen M, Raquez JM, Mielewski DF, Narayan R, Netravali AN, Misra M (2022) Sustainable polymers. Nat Rev Methods Primers 2(1):46. https://doi.org/10.1038/s43586-022-00124-8

Nada AM, El-Diwany AI, Elshafei AM (1989) Infrared and antimicrobial studies on different lignins. Acta Biotechnol 9(3):295–298. https://doi.org/10.1002/abio.370090322

Nguyen NA, Bowland CC, Naskar AK (2018a) A general method to improve 3D-printability and inter-layer adhesion in lignin-based composites. Appl Mater Today 12:138–152. https://doi.org/10.1016/j.apmt.2018.03.009

Nguyen NA, Barnes SH, Bowland CC, Meek KM, Littrell KC, Keum JK, Naskar AK (2018b) A path for lignin valorization via additive manufacturing of high-performance sustainable composites with enhanced 3D printability. Sci Adv 4(12):eaat4967. https://doi.org/10.1126/sciadv.aat4967

Ogan A, Yüce-Dursun B, Abdullah D, Beyler-Çiğil A, Kahraman MV, Çağlayan P, Birbir M, Mutlu Ö, Gülsoy N (2020) Preparation and antimicrobial properties of LL-37 peptide immobilized lignin/caprolactone polymer film. Polym Adv Technol 31(10):2222–2228. https://doi.org/10.1002/pat.4942

Okwuosa TC, Stefaniak D, Arafat B, Isreb A, Wan KW, Alhnan MA (2016) A lower temperature FDM 3D printing for the manufacture of patient-specific immediate release tablets. Pharm Res 33:2704–2712. https://doi.org/10.1007/s11095-016-1995-0

Park SY, Kim JY, Youn HJ, Choi JW (2019) Utilization of lignin fractions in UV resistant lignin-PLA biocomposites via lignin-lactide grafting. Int J Biol Macromol 138:1029–1034. https://doi.org/10.1016/j.ijbiomac.2019.07.157

Park S, Shou W, Makatura L, Matusik W, Fu KK (2022) 3D printing of polymer composites: materials, processes, and applications. Matter 5(1):43–76. https://doi.org/10.1016/j.matt.2021.10.018

Peng X, Kuang X, Roach DJ, Wang Y, Hamel CM, Lu C, Qi HJ (2021) Integrating digital light processing with direct ink writing for hybrid 3D printing of functional structures and devices. Addit Manuf 40:101911. https://doi.org/10.1016/j.addma.2021.101911

Popa VI (2018) Biomass for fuels and biomaterials. In: Biomass as renewable raw material to obtain bioproducts of high-tech value. Elsevier, pp 1–37. https://doi.org/10.1016/B978-0-444-63774-1.00001-6

Quraishi S, Martins M, Barros AA, Gurikov P, Raman SP, Smirnova I, Duarte AR, Reis RL (2015) Novel non-cytotoxic alginate–lignin hybrid aerogels as scaffolds for tissue engineering. J Supercrit Fluids 105:1–8. https://doi.org/10.1016/j.supflu.2014.12.026

Raney JR, Compton BG, Mueller J, Ober TJ, Shea K, Lewis JA (2018) Rotational 3D printing of damage-tolerant composites with programmable mechanics. Proc Natl Acad Sci 115(6):1198–1203. https://doi.org/10.1073/pnas.1715157115

Rowe CW, Katstra WE, Palazzolo RD, Giritlioglu B, Teung P, Cima MJ (2000) Multimechanism oral dosage forms fabricated by three dimensional printing. J Control Release 66(1):11–17. https://doi.org/10.1016/s0168-3659(99)00224-2

Saadi MA, Maguire A, Pottackal NT, Thakur MS, Ikram MM, Hart AJ, Ajayan PM, Rahman MM (2022) Direct ink writing: a 3D printing technology for diverse materials. Adv Mater 34(28):2108855. https://doi.org/10.1002/adma.202108855

Sadeghifar H, Ragauskas A (2020) Lignin as a UV light blocker—a review. Polymers 12(5):1134. https://doi.org/10.3390/polym12051134

Sette M, Wechselberger R, Crestini C (2011) Elucidation of lignin structure by quantitative 2D NMR. Chemistry 17(34):9529–9535. https://doi.org/10.1002/chem.201003045

Shao Y, Chaussy D, Grosseau P, Beneventi D (2015) Use of microfibrillated cellulose/lignosulfonate blends as carbon precursors: impact of hydrogel rheology on 3D printing. Ind Eng Chem Res 54(43):10575–10582. https://doi.org/10.1021/acs.iecr.5b02763

Shuaib M, Haleem A, Kumar S, Javaid M (2021) Impact of 3D printing on the environment: a literature-based study. Sustain Oper Comput 2:57–63. https://doi.org/10.1016/j.susoc.2021.04.001

Sikder P, Challa BT, Gummadi SK (2022) A comprehensive analysis on the processing-structure-property relationships of FDM-based 3-D printed polyetheretherketone (PEEK) structures. Materialia 22:101427. https://doi.org/10.1016/j.mtla.2022.101427

Skylar-Scott MA, Mueller J, Visser CW, Lewis JA (2019) Voxelated soft matter via multimaterial multinozzle 3D printing. Nature 575(7782):330–335. https://doi.org/10.1038/s41586-019-1736-8

Sriroth K, Sunthornvarabhas J (2018) Lignin from sugar process as natural antimicrobial agent. Biochem Pharmacol 7(1):239. https://doi.org/10.4172/2167-0501.1000239

Sun RC (2020) Lignin source and structural characterization. ChemSusChem 13(17):4174. https://doi.org/10.1002/cssc.202001324

Sun Q, Khunsupat R, Akato K, Tao J, Labbé N, Gallego NC, Bozell JJ, Rials TG, Tuskan GA, Tschaplinski TJ, Naskar AK (2016) A study of poplar organosolv lignin after melt rheology treatment as carbon fiber precursors. Green Chem 18(18):5015–5024. https://doi.org/10.1039/C6GC00977H

Sutton JT, Rajan K, Harper DP, Chmely SC (2018) Lignin-containing photoactive resins for 3D printing by Stereolithography. ACS Appl Mater Interfaces 10(42):36456–36463. https://doi.org/10.1021/acsami.8b13031

Tagliaferri S, Panagiotopoulos A, Mattevi CJ (2021) Direct ink writing of energy materials. Mater Adv 2(2):540–563. https://doi.org/10.1039/D0MA00753F

Tanase-Opedal M, Espinosa E, Rodríguez A, Chinga-Carrasco G (2019) Lignin: a biopolymer from forestry biomass for biocomposites and 3D printing. Materials 12(18):3006. https://doi.org/10.3390/ma12183006

Trifol J, Jayaprakash S, Baniasadi H, Ajdary R, Kretzschmar N, Rojas OJ, Partanen J, Seppälä JV (2021) 3D-printed thermoset biocomposites based on forest residues by delayed extrusion of cold masterbatch (DECMA). ACS Sustain Chem Eng 9(41):13979–13987. https://doi.org/10.1021/acssuschemeng.1c05587

Tsegaye B, Balomajumder C, Roy P (2019) Microbial delignification and hydrolysis of lignocellulosic biomass to enhance biofuel production: an overview and future prospect. Bull Natl Res Cent 43(1):1–6. https://doi.org/10.1186/s42269-019-0094-x

Tuck CO, Pérez E, Horváth IT, Sheldon RA, Poliakoff M (2012) Valorization of biomass: deriving more value from waste. Science 337(6095):695–699. https://doi.org/10.1126/science.1218930

Tursi A (2019) A review on biomass: importance, chemistry, classification, and conversion. Biofuel Res J 6(2):962–979. https://doi.org/10.18331/BRJ2019.6.2.3

Wang Z, Yang Y (2021) Application of 3D printing in implantable medical devices. Biomed Res Int 2021:1–13. https://doi.org/10.1155/2021/6653967

Wang J, Goyanes A, Gaisford S, Basit AW (2016) Stereolithographic (SLA) 3D printing of oral modified-release dosage forms. Int J Pharm 503:207–212. https://doi.org/10.1016/j.ijpharm.2016.03.016

Wasti S, Triggs E, Farag R, Auad M, Adhikari S, Bajwa D, Li M, Ragauskas AJ (2021) Influence of plasticizers on thermal and mechanical properties of biocomposite filaments made from lignin and polylactic acid for 3D printing. Compos Part B Eng 205:108483. https://doi.org/10.1016/j.compositesb.2020.108483

Weisman JA, Nicholson JC, Tappa K, Jammalamadaka U, Wilson CG, Mills DK (2015) Antibiotic and chemotherapeutic enhanced three dimensional printer filaments and constructs for biomedical applications. Int J Nanomedicine 10:357–370. https://doi.org/10.2147/IJN.S74811

Wong KV, Hernandez A (2012) A review of additive manufacturing. Int Sch Res Notices 2012:1–10. https://doi.org/10.5402/2012/208760

Wu SY, Yang C, Hsu W, Lin L (2015) 3D-printed microelectronics for integrated circuitry and passive wireless sensors. Microsyst Nanoeng 1(1):1–9. https://doi.org/10.1038/micronano.2015.13

Xia Y, Zhou P, Cheng X, Xie Y, Liang C, Li C, Xu S (2013) Selective laser sintering fabrication of nano-hydroxyapatite/poly-ε-caprolactone scaffolds for bone tissue engineering applications. Int J Nanomedicine:4197–4213. https://doi.org/10.2147/IJN.S50685

Xu X, Robles-Martinez P, Madla CM, Joubert F, Goyanes A, Basit AW, Gaisford S (2020) Stereolithography (SLA) 3D printing of an antihypertensive polyprintlet: case study of an unexpected photopolymer-drug reaction. Addit Manuf 33:101071. https://doi.org/10.1016/j.addma.2020.101071

Xu Z, Nakamura H, Akiyama T, Yokoyama T, Jin Z, Sasaki K, Matsumoto Y (2021) Syringyl ratio and its relation to the erythro ratio of β-O-4-structure in leaf cell walls. J Wood Chem Technol 41(2–3):118–127. https://doi.org/10.1080/02773813.2021.191653

Yu DG, Branford-White C, Yang YC, Zhu LM, Welbeck EW, Yang XL (2009) A novel fast disintegrating tablet fabricated by three-dimensional printing. Drug Dev Ind Pharm 35(12):1530–1536. https://doi.org/10.3109/03639040903059359

Yu Q, Bahi A, Ko F (2015) Influence of poly (ethylene oxide) (PEO) percent and lignin type on the properties of lignin/PEO blend filament. Macromol Mater Eng 300(10):1023–1032. https://doi.org/10.1002/mame.201500045

Zemek J, Košíková B, Augustin J, Joniak D (1979) Antibiotic properties of lignin components. Folia Microbiol 24:483–486. https://doi.org/10.1007/BF02927180

Zhang X, Morits M, Jonkergouw C, Ora A, Valle-Delgado JJ, Farooq M, Ajdary R, Huan S, Linder M, Rojas O, Sipponen MH, Österberg M (2020a) Three-dimensional printed cell culture model based on spherical colloidal lignin particles and cellulose Nanofibril-alginate hydrogel. Biomacromolecules 21(5):1875–1885. https://doi.org/10.1021/acs.biomac.9b01745

Zhang X, Keck S, Qi Y, Baudis S, Zhao Y (2020b) Study on modified dealkaline lignin as visible light macromolecular photoinitiator for 3D printing. ACS Sustain Chem Eng 8(29):10959–10970. https://doi.org/10.1021/acssuschemeng.0c03587

Zhang B, Nasereddin J, McDonagh T, von Zeppelin D, Gleadall A, Alqahtani F, Bibb R, Belton P, Qi S (2021a) Effects of porosity on drug release kinetics of swellable and erodible porous pharmaceutical solid dosage forms fabricated by hot melt droplet deposition 3D printing. Int J Pharm 604:120626. https://doi.org/10.1016/j.ijpharm.2021.120626

Zhang C, Li X, Jiang L, Tang D, Xu H, Zhao P, Fu J, Zhou Q, Chen Y (2021b) 3D printing of functional magnetic materials: from design to applications. Adv Funct Mater 31(34):2102777. https://doi.org/10.1002/adfm.202102777

Zoghlami A, Paës G (2019) Lignocellulosic biomass: understanding recalcitrance and predicting hydrolysis. Front Chem 7:874. https://doi.org/10.3389/fchem.2019.00874

Lignin Based Energy Materials for Biomedical Applications

16

Muhammad Muddasar, Judith Miralda Jalle,
Mario Culebras, Tadhg Kennedy, and Maurice N. Collins

Abstract

Lignin, a plentiful byproduct of paper industries and biorefineries, shows great promise for sustainable energy applications. Its low cost, carbon-rich structure, and biodegradability make it an appealing alternative to traditional materials in the development of high-performance energy storage and harvesting devices. This chapter examines its potential in next-generation supercapacitors and thermoelectric materials for the biomedical industry. Lignin-derived carbon materials offer a sustainable and high-performance alternative to traditional battery

M. Muddasar · J. M. Jalle
Stokes Laboratories, School of Engineering, Bernal Institute, University of Limerick, Limerick, Ireland

M. Culebras
Institute of Material Science (ICMUV), University of Valencia, Valencia, Spain

T. Kennedy
Department of Chemical Sciences & Bernal Institute, University of Limerick, Limerick, Ireland

Research Ireland Centre for Advanced Materials and BioEngineering Research (AMBER), Dublin, Ireland

M. N. Collins (✉)
School of Engineering, Health Research Institute and Bernal Institute, University of Limerick, Limerick, Ireland

Institute of Material Science (ICMUV), University of Valencia, Valencia, Spain

Research Ireland Centre for Advanced Materials and BioEngineering Research (AMBER), Dublin, Ireland

Research Ireland, Bioeconomy Research Centre, Dublin, Ireland
e-mail: maurice.collins@ul.ie

M. N. Collins, M. Culebras (eds.), *Sustainable Biopolymers and Composites for Biomedical Applications*, Biomaterials, Bioengineering and Sustainability 5,
https://doi.org/10.1007/978-3-031-91972-5_16

materials for supercapacitors in medical devices. These supercapacitors can be more efficient and environmentally friendly. Additionally, the chapter examines the role of lignin in thermoelectric materials, which are essential for improving energy harvesting in wearable and implantable medical devices. By fully utilizing the potential of lignin, significant advancements can be made in sustainable energy solutions for the medical field.

Keywords

Lignin · Lignin hydrogels · Lignin ionic thermoelectric materials · Lignin derived carbon · Supercapacitors

16.1 Introduction

In the healthcare industry, biomedical devices are instruments that are used to monitor biomarkers or signals. These instruments are tailored for specific systems and tissues within the body. The Apollo mission was the first time biomedical devices were used to monitor the vital signs of astronauts (Ozsahin et al. 2022). Nowadays, their use is not limited to monitoring applications as they can also be considered preventive and therapeutic instruments (Srivastava et al. 2021). Currently, biomedical devices can be found as diagnostic equipment—medical imaging devices; durable biomedical equipment—stents; therapeutic equipment—infusion pumps; life support equipment—mechanical ventilators; and medical lab equipment—PCR or antigen screening.

Several materials are used for biomedical devices, including metals, ceramics, polymers, composites, and natural polymers. The choice of material depends on various factors such as the physical principles that will be detected, design requirements, and the type of interaction that will be established with the body (Biesiekierski et al. 2020). Biocompatibility and durability are essential considerations. For devices that have direct interaction with the body but do not require significant mechanical properties, such as stents, contact lenses, and adhesives or plasters, polymers are the preferred option (Saikia and Karak 2023). Polymers can be tailored to offer good biocompatibility and specific mechanical and structural properties. In cases where mechanical properties are crucial for direct interaction with the body, composites that combine the mechanical resistance of metals and the compatibility of polymers, such as hip prostheses, can be used (Merola and Affatato 2019). For devices that will be used outside the body, material selection depends mainly on the physical principle of detection. Sensors can detect real-time physicochemical information using materials with enhanced magnetic, thermal, chemical, electrical, and mechanical properties, which can selectively target parameters thanks to their hierarchical design and nanostructures (Sulleiro et al. 2022). Surface properties and modifications are critical.

When designing and manufacturing biomedical devices, three primary challenges must be addressed: biocompatibility, degradation profile, and regulatory constraints (Huzum et al. 2021). Due to the importance of the physicochemical-related properties and the need for sterile devices, sustainability is not considered a key factor during the design and development of biomedical devices. The medical industry has strict requirements that prevent the use of devices on multiple patients. Thus, opposing the idea of a circular economy and sustainability, aggravating material scarcity, and contributing to waste generation. Sustainable materials have been designed to accommodate the needs of biomedical devices in the context of climate change.

Lignin is a promising candidate as a sustainable material because it is commonly found in the plant cell wall and accounts for 20–25% of its dry weight (Beaucamp et al. 2024; Stróżyk et al. 2024; Huerta et al. 2024). It is the second most abundant biopolymer after cellulose and the chief source of aromatic compounds. Lignin is a by-product of the pulp and paper industry, and it can be processed using various techniques to acquire materials with different and customizable properties. Despite this, lignin has not yet been utilized for valuable applications (Jia et al. 2023; Muddasar et al. 2024a, b; Beaucamp et al. 2022a). Lignin has 60% carbon content in its structure making it a sustainable carbon precursor that can be used to produce environmentally friendly energy storage and harvesting devices, once carbonized. The use of lignin to develop materials for powering biomedical devices presents an opportunity to bring sustainability and environmental awareness to this field.

This chapter begins by discussing the importance of supercapacitors in modern biomedical devices, highlighting their advantages over traditional energy harvesting methods. It examines the materials currently used in supercapacitors and explores how lignin-based materials could improve their efficiency. Following this, the chapter shifts focus to ionic thermoelectric membranes, a novel technology with potential applications in biomedical industry. It emphasizes the growing demand for sustainable materials and introduces lignin as a promising candidate. By exploring these topics, the chapter provides comprehensive insights for integrating sustainability into the development of essential biomedical technologies.

16.2 Lignin-Based Supercapacitors for Biomedical Applications

Technological advancements necessitate the development of inexpensive, green, sustainable, and high-performing energy storage devices. Supercapacitors can store a large amount of energy and release it quickly, making them ideal for various applications, including biomedical devices. They possess novel energy storage mechanisms that combine the attributes of batteries and capacitors, resulting in improved electrochemical properties such as high specific capacity, higher power density (10 kW kg^{-1}), longer life stability (>10^5 cycles), economic efficiency, environmental friendliness, safety, and faster charge–discharge rate (within seconds) (Beaucamp et al. 2022a). Supercapacitors offer two types of energy storage mechanisms: double-layer systems based on electrostatic interactions and pseudocapacitors based on electrochemical interactions (Yadlapalli et al. 2022). The most used materials for the double-layer systems are activated carbon, graphene, and carbon nanotubes. For the pseudocapacitor systems, the materials used are mainly metal oxides and conducting polymers (Chakraborty and Mary 2022).

Overall, supercapacitors are highly efficient energy storage devices that can store more energy and release it quickly, allowing potential uses in the field of biomedical devices. For instance, they can be used in pacemakers to provide a quick electric discharge when required. Another application of supercapacitors in biomedical devices is physiotherapy equipment, where they can be used for devices that selectively release low alternate currents. They can also be used for monitoring applications as they can control the quality of the energy passing through them. In the case of pacemakers, they can release an electric discharge and monitor the quality of the cardiac rhythm through assessing the electrocardiogram biosignal. Additionally, supercapacitors can be used as integrated parts of the patient's constant monitor. Supercapacitors' rapid, stable, and efficient energy charge and discharge make them ideal to power portable or implanted drug-releasing devices. In this part of the chapter, novel strategies to obtain lignin-derived carbon materials for supercapacitors are going to be exposed.

16.2.1 Sustainable Lignin-Based Tailored Porous Carbon Electrodes

Sustainable materials are key for the creation of the next generation of biomedical devices and equipment (Beaucamp et al. 2022b). Carbon-based materials obtained from lignin-derived hydrogels are being increasingly studied for supercapacitor electrodes. A study conducted at the University of Limerick in 2022 delved into this area, focusing on synthesizing highly swollen hydrogels utilizing lignin and poly(ethylene) glycol diglycidyl ether (PEGDGE) as a crosslinking agent, see Fig. 16.1a. The carbonized lignin-derived porous carbon materials were electrochemically tested for applications such as electrodes for supercapacitors. These materials can potentially be used as sustainable energy harvesting systems to power biomedical devices.

Due to its native properties, lignin is widely used for hydrogel synthesis, a technique extensively used in biomedicine. For this study, lignin was chemically crosslinked with varying PEGDGE cross-linking densities (0.4, 0.6, and 0.8 g), and a swelling degree of over 1600% was obtained. The influence of different crosslinker ratios on the structural and chemical properties of the resultant hydrogels was investigated. It was found that the cross-linker concentration modulates the lignin precursor material, modifying its structure, properties, and performance. Freeze drying, a versatile and environmentally friendly technique, was used to tailor the microstructure of the obtained hydrogels. It promoted the acquisition of hydrogels showcasing porous honeycomb-like structures, showing optimum performance levels. The obtained hydrogels were stabilized and carbonized to undergo symmetrical electrode assembly.

Sample 0.4HG exhibited results that are typical of those obtained in pseudocapacitive charge storage behavior. Pseudocapacitor behavior is crucial for

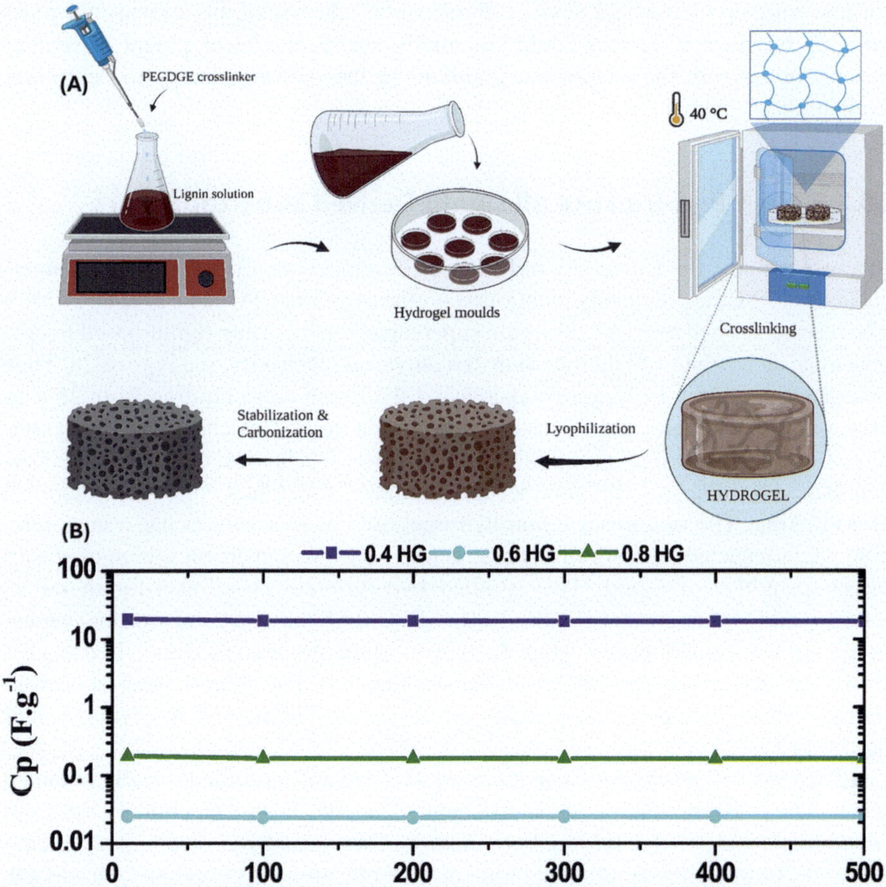

Fig. 16.1 (**a**) Schematic representation of hydrogel synthesis; (**b**) Specific capacitance for the respective hydrogels. (Adapted with permission from Beaucamp et al. (2022b))

drug-releasing devices as they function thanks to the electrochemical reactions involved in these systems. Sample 0.4HG showcases promising properties for biomedical applications and its pseudocapacitor profile can allow their use for drug-releasing devices. The specific capacitance of the hydrogels was recorded after 500 cycles, see Fig. 16.1b. Overall, the results indicate good behavior of the hydrogels in terms of specific capacitance even after 500 cycles. Long-term stability is a crucial parameter for energy storage in biomedical devices, and the hydrogels exhibited high reliability in performance over time. The average capacitance obtained for the 0.4HG, 0.6HG, and 0.8HG was 18.7, 0.02, and 0.18 $F{\cdot}g^{-1}$, respectively, measured at 1 $A{\cdot}g^{-1}$.

These results open a new avenue for lignin as a promising candidate for innovative porous carbon materials for high-performance electrode materials at low production costs and they offer a sustainable alternative to the current strategies used for powering up biomedical devices. Furthermore, the use of this strategy for powering up biomedical devices could potentially lead to the development of smaller devices optimizing the design but maintaining the performance of the currently available instruments.

16.2.2 High-Performance All Lignin-Derived Supercapacitors

In a recent study, the University of Limerick developed an all-lignin-derived supercapacitor using the previously mentioned synthesis strategy (Muddasar et al. 2024c). The research aimed to create all-lignin supercapacitors by using lignin-based hydrogels as an electrolyte and their carbon derivatives as electrodes, see Fig. 16.2a. They optimized the lignin hydrogel by increasing the lignin concentration from 25% to 40% w/v while keeping a 3:5 crosslinker to lignin ratio. This change in lignin content affected the hydrogel morphology and intrinsic mechanical and structural characteristics by altering the number of available functional sites for chemical cross-linking. The optimized lignin hydrogel used as electrolytes has a customizable interconnected network of microstructure pores, which enables them to absorb larger quantities of liquid. They studied two different crosslinker-lignin ratios, 0.65:1 (LSPC-0.65) and 1:1 (LSPC-1.00). LSPC-0.65 shows a good swelling capacity of 278% within 24 hours. After the freeze-drying process, the lignin hydrogel is converted into carbon material through carbonization. The carbon material is engineered to have nanopores arranged in a honeycomb-like pattern to optimize their performance.

LDC-0.65 had a superior capacitance of 41.7 F/g and a profile typically obtained when there is a combination of electrochemical double-layer capacitor (EDLC) and pseudocapacitance behavior, see Fig. 16.2b, c. Therefore, LDC-0.65 is a better candidate for further consideration in biomedical applications. As previously discussed, pseudocapacitance allows these materials to move from traditional energy harvesting applications towards being applied to control drug-releasing devices in novel therapeutic approaches. The tested samples show triangular GCD shapes, which indicates that there was a good transfer rate of ions, see Fig. 16.2d, e. Ease in ion transference can allow biosensors to track oxygen, glucose, and other analytes such as specific ligands for proteins inside the body. Thus, enabling selective release of drugs and promising applications in the controlled delivery and activation of those.

The study shows that lignin-derived materials are a promising approach for developing sustainable and eco-friendly supercapacitors. Thus, these materials can be safely applied in biomedical devices. LDC-0.65 exhibits superior capacitance compared to LDC-1.00 due to synergistic effects between EDLC and pseudocapacitive charge storage mechanisms. As previously discussed, pseudocapacitance allows these materials to move from traditional energy harvesting applications towards being applied to control drug-releasing devices in novel therapeutic approaches.

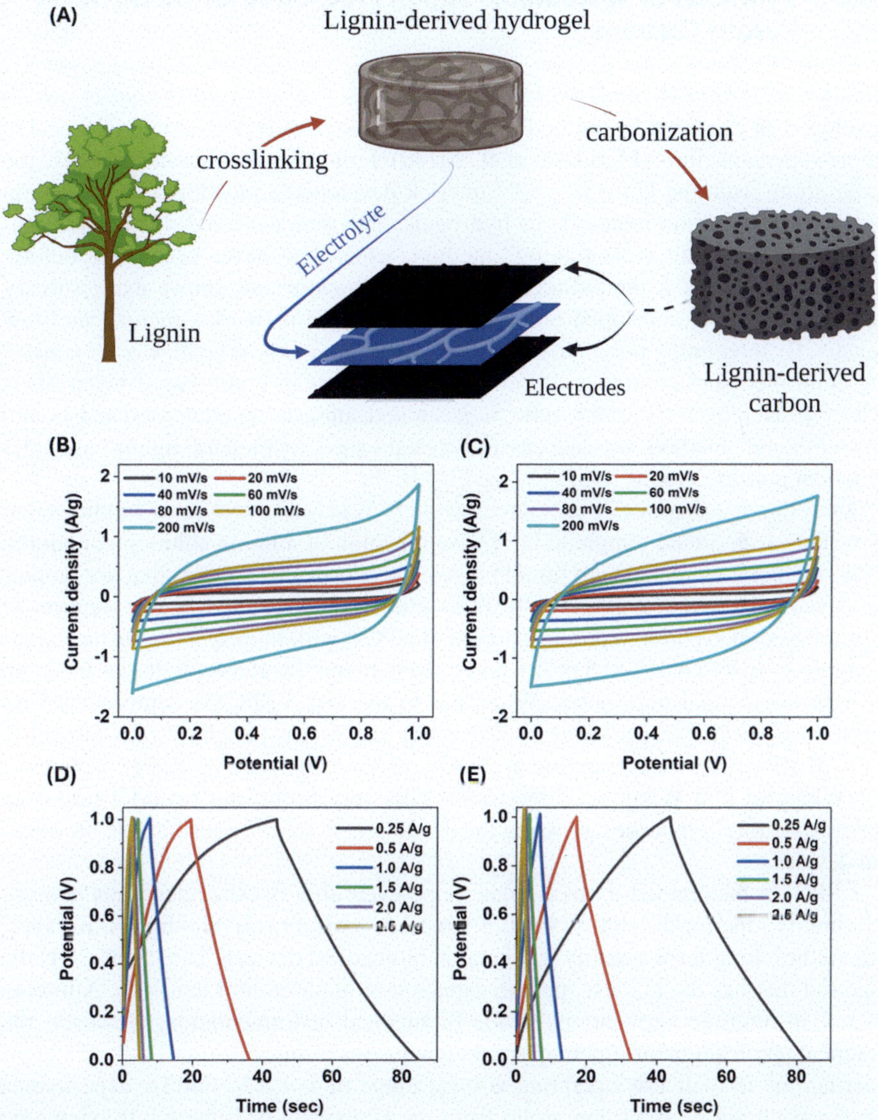

Fig. 16.2 (**a**) Schematic representation of the all-lignin supercapacitors; Electrochemical performances of the lignin-derived supercapacitors (LDSCs). (**b**, **d**) CV curves and GCD profiles of LDSC-0.65. (**c**, **e**) CV curves and GCD profiles of LDSC-1.00. (Adapted with permission from Muddasar et al. (2024c))

16.2.3 Synthesis of Sustainable Lignin Precursors for Hierarchical Porous Carbons

Another breakthrough study was conducted by the University of Limerick which developed an eco-friendly method to obtain lignin-derived carbon materials used to create supercapacitors (Muddasar et al. 2024d). Following a different approach, the same group from the University of Limerick developed a novel strategy to obtain lignin-derived carbon materials as hydrogels. This was achieved through a "template assisted in situ cross-linking" method, which had never been done before. Lignin aerogel has a three-dimensional pore structure and shows extraordinary qualities including developed porosity, multibranched network structure, and low density. By integrating polymeric templates, a unique and novel pathway for achieving controlled surface area and pore size adjustments in lignin-based materials is achieved. Herein, for the first time, a green and unique "template assisted in situ cross-linking" method was successfully established to prepare lignin-based 3D spherical porous carbons (LSPCs), see Fig. 16.3a.

Kraft lignin acts as a carbon source, while PVA acts as a self-cross-linking agent as well as a sacrificial template. Dropwise injection of a lignin solution containing PVA sacrificial templates into liquid nitrogen produces tiny spheres that are lyophilized and carbonized to produce LSPCs. The method resulted in the creation of lignin-based 3D spherical porous carbons (LSPCs) with high specific surface areas (ranging from 426.6 to 790.5 m^2/g), and tunable hierarchical morphologies made up of both micro- and mesopores. When put to the test, LSPC-28 demonstrated an impressive specific capacitance of 102.3 F/g at 0.5 A/g, excellent rate capability with 70.3% capacitance retention at 20 A/g, and a commendable energy density of 2.1 Wh/kg at 250 W/kg, see Fig. 16.3b. This very promising material improves supercapacitors' properties allowing the development of more sustainable biomedical devices.

LSPC-28 maintained its triangular shape even after 5000 cycles, thus demonstrating its superior durability, see Fig. 16.3c. As was already highlighted in previous studies, long-term stability is crucial in biomedical devices. The LSPC-28 is the material that has the highest specific capacitance at all current densities. Allowing its use in multiple applications inside biomedical instrumentation. However, the practical applications of supercapacitors in aqueous electrolytes are limited in engineering due to their low operating voltage range of 1–1.8 V. Further experiments were carried out by the same group from the University of Limerick to overcome said limitations. Yet, for some biomedical applications that deliver electric current to the body, the low operating voltage stands as a safer option.

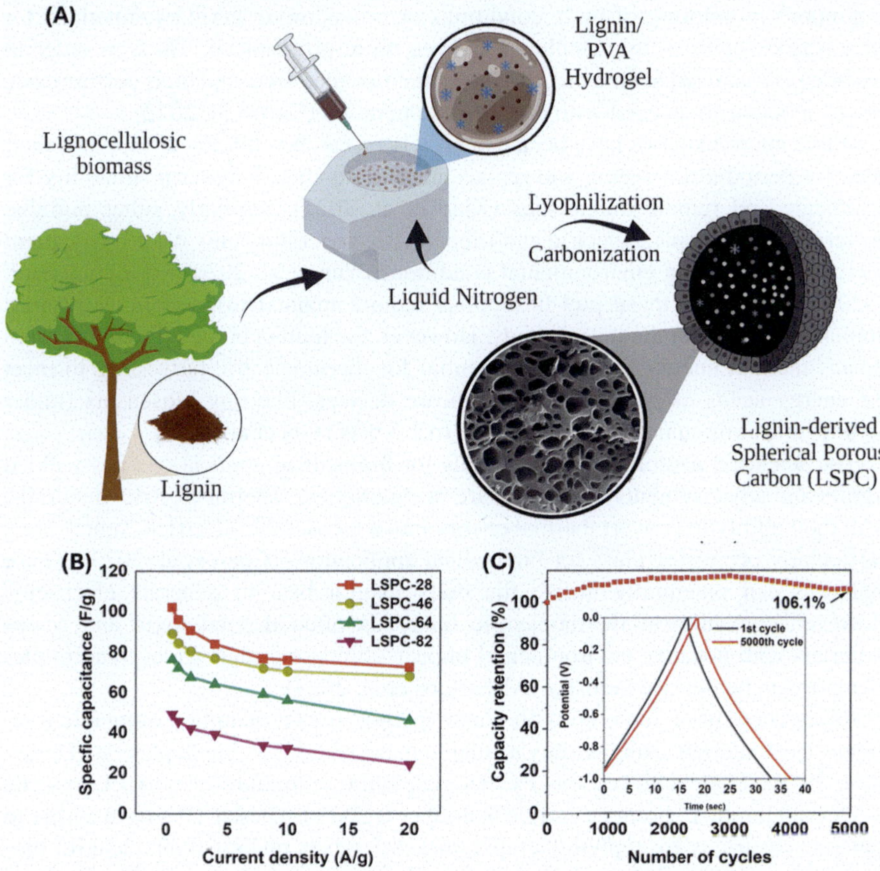

Fig. 16.3 (**a**) Schematic representation of lignin-based spherical porous carbon (LSPC) synthesis, (**b**) specific capacitance of all LSPC samples at different current densities, and (**c**) cyclic performance of LSPC-28 at 5 A/g. (Adapted with permission from Muddasar et al. (2024e))

16.3 Lignin-Based Electric Thermoelectric Materials for Biomedical Applications

Miniaturized and decentralized personalized healthcare access has gained increasing attention because it allows for the monitoring of vital signs and remote diagnostics outside of the clinical environment, which are increasingly important with the increasing demand for accessible, affordable, and quality biomedical platforms (Ray et al. 2019). In order to diagnose and treat patients more effectively, wearable and implantable platforms could continuously collect health information from their bodies (Libanori et al. 2022). Patients can benefit from personalized healthcare by removing the burden of bulky biomedical platforms and long-term hospitalizations. However, wearable and implantable healthcare devices cannot develop without reliable and portable power supplies. For implantable devices, which require continuous monitoring of body conditions or provision of auxiliary functions for long periods of time, this challenge is even more pronounced. Thus, in order to provide personalized healthcare, low-cost, maintenance-free, and high-performance power supplies are needed with continuous operation (Gao et al. 2022).

While micro batteries have been extensively researched for power supplies, their need for periodic recharging and replacement limits their long-term suitability for healthcare and remote diagnostics (Xiao et al. 2021). Similarly, other portable power sources like piezoelectric and triboelectric generators only offer intermittent energy depending on environmental conditions (Yun et al. 2020; Rodrigues et al. 2020). Importantly, these power supplies require manual inspections to support implanted devices in the human body. However, the human body continuously dissipates thermal energy, promising potential for thermoelectric harvesting to meet the energy needs of personalized healthcare devices, like tiny biosensors (under 50 μW) and communication systems (up to 1.5 mW) (Jia et al. 2021).

The scientific exploration of materials for biomedical applications has yielded significant advancements in healthcare technologies. Thermoelectric materials, with their ability to convert thermal energy into a measurable electrical signal, are a particularly promising class for biomedical applications (Chen et al. 2023). These materials can potentially utilize the body natural heat to generate electricity. However, conventional thermoelectric materials often depend toxic and scares materials with negative environmental impacts, hindering their widespread implementation in healthcare industry (Al-Fartoos et al. 2023).

Researchers have come up with a new method for fabricating sustainable thermoelectric materials using readily available materials and a simple process (Dalton et al. 2019). They achieved this by electrospinning a mixture of polyacrylonitrile (PAN) and lignin, to produce carbon nanofibers (CNFs). These CNFs have ability to generate electricity by applying temperature difference, making them ideal for biomedical sensors. Additionally, the use of lignin enhances the biocompatibility of the CNFs, making them more suitable for implantation within the body. Furthermore, the ability to precisely control the diameter and electrical properties of the CNFs through lignin content and additional treatments opens doors for designing biocompatible components with specific functionalities. Additionally, the increased flexibility due to lignin allows for CNFs that can better conform to biological tissues, reducing potential rejection by the body. This research holds promise for the development of more sustainable and efficient thermoelectric technology.

16.4 Lignin-Based Ionic Thermoelectric Materials for Biomedical Applications

The biomedical industry constantly seeks materials that exhibit excellent performance while maintaining biocompatibility and sustainability. Integrating such sustainable materials into biomedical devices can promote environmentally friendly practices without compromising performance or reliability. One particularly exciting development is the innovation of lignin-based ionic thermoelectric materials. The unique properties of lignin including biocompatibility, renewability, and affordability, make it a versatile material for various biomedical applications (Beaucamp et al. 2022a). This opens doors for the development of self-powered biomedical devices, eliminating the need for external batteries. Recent studies have demonstrated the ability of lignin-based ionic thermometric materials to generate electricity by exploiting temperature gradients. The following sections will discuss the technical details of these advancements in detail.

16.4.1 Lignin-Derived Ionic Thermoelectric Membranes

Recent research suggests wood-based ionic membranes with aligned channels hold promise for thermoelectric devices due to their high ionic Seebeck coefficient of 24 mV K^{-1} (Li et al. 2019). These typically use cellulose membranes, but these membranes are soft and break easily under pressure, limiting their use in biomedical applications. A Additionally, extracting cellulose from wood requires chemical treatments, generating lignin as a byproduct (Muddasar et al. 2022). This separation yields lignin as a by-product, an extensively available natural polymer with a three-dimensional structure. Lignin has been extensively employed in tissue engineering, drug delivery, energy storage, composites, biosensors, etc., because of its low toxicity, eco-friendliness, biocompatibility, and enzymatic degradation (Beaucamp et al. 2022b; Cao et al. 2019; Garedew et al. 2020; Meng et al. 2019; Wu et al. 2020; Azadi et al. 2013; Collins et al. 2019). Interestingly, no research has been done on creating lignin-based polymeric membranes for ionic thermoelectric applications.

Recently, a group of researchers from University of Limerick and University of Valencia have made a breakthrough in ionic thermoelectric energy harvesting (Muddasar et al. 2024f). They developed unique membranes using lignin with a special feature as they have hierarchical aligned channels. a templating strategy was employed to synthesize these membranes with channels. The strategy involved freezing and thawing a solution of lignin and polyvinyl alcohol (PVA) in a specific direction. This unidirectional freezing process formed tiny ice crystals, leaving behind nano-sized channels after thawing. The researchers then further enhanced the membrane stability through lyophilization, chemical crosslinking, and final washing and make them ready for ion infiltration for ionic thermoelectric applications.

The synthesised membranes exhibit excellent swelling capacity and also demonstrate impressive mechanical strength. With a Young's modulus ranging from 13 to 41.8 MPa and minimal deformation (12.2–18.5% under 1000 Kpa load), they offer a robust structure for potential biomedical implants. Furthermore, excellent thermal stability (up to 200 °C with minimal weight loss) suggests their suitability for sterilization procedures common in healthcare settings and are suitable for low-grade thermal energy harvesting applications.

Synthesized samples were infiltrated with aqueous KOH electrolyte at 0.5 M for ionic thermoelectric testing. One of the synthesized samples containing 69.2 wt.% of lignin results in an exceptional figure of merit (ZT_i) of ≈0.25, higher ionic conductivity (51.5 mS/cm), lower thermal conductivity (0.195 W/m·K), and remarkable ionic Seebeck coefficient of 5.71 mV/K (see Fig. 16.4). This lignin-derived membrane shows promise for revolutionizing biocompatible sensors and wearables

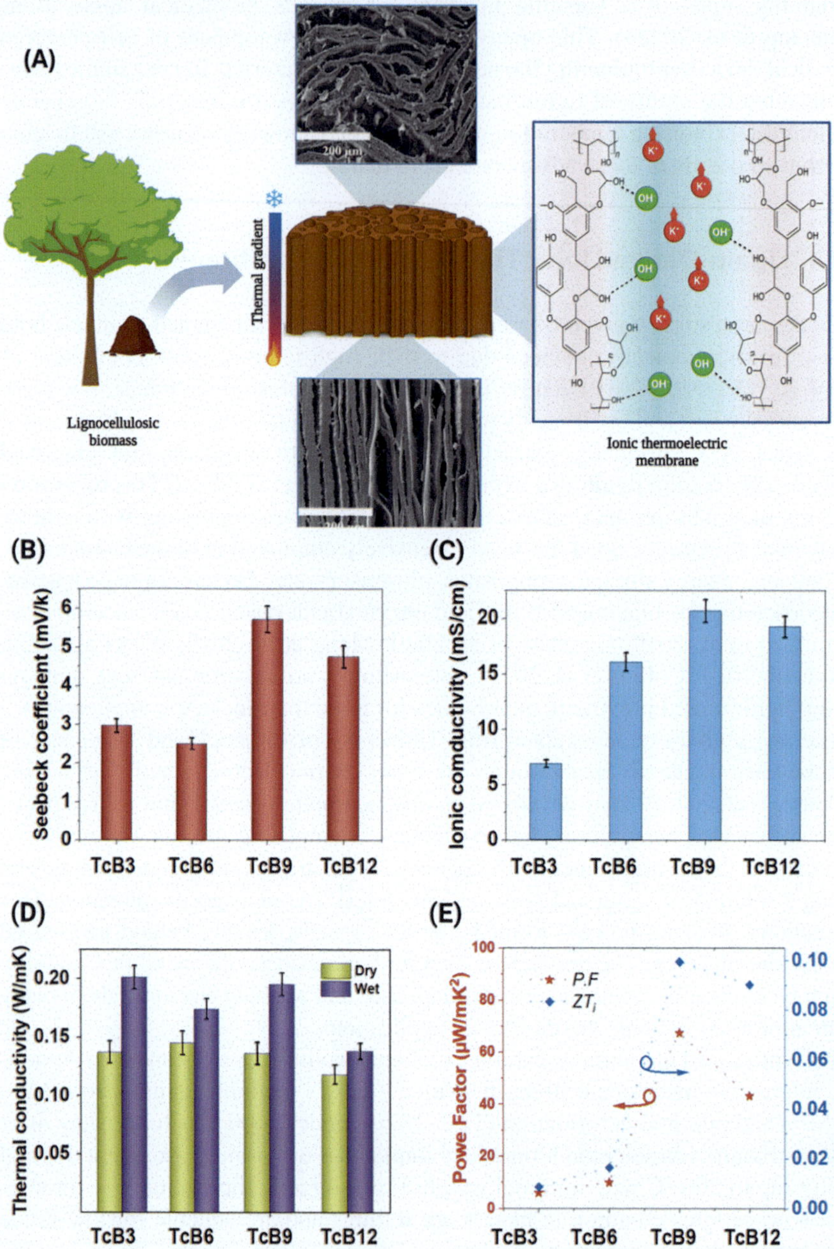

Fig. 16.4 (**a**) Lignin-derived membranes with vertically aligned channels, (**b**) Seebeck coeffeicient of all the synthesised samples, (**c**) ionic conductivity, (**d**) thermal conductivity, and (**e**) Power factor and figure of merit. (Adapted with permission from Muddasar et al. (2024f))

as they have enhanced ionic conductivity and ionic Seebeck coefficient due to the thermophoretic movement of ions in negatively charged aligned channels (Sewring et al. 2019). Furthermore, its lightweight design and ease of production make it a strong candidate for integration into comfortable and safe medical devices. With its unique properties, the lignin membrane has the potential to be a game-changer in temperature sensing and wearable technology within the biomedical industry.

16.4.2 Lignin-Derived Ionic Thermoelectric Hydrogels

A recent advancement in the field of sustainable materials has led to the development of lignin-based ionic thermoelectric hydrogels with exciting potential for use in various applications, including biomedical settings. This breakthrough follows previous research on lignin-based ionic thermoelectric materials and offers a novel approach to harnessing temperature differentials for practical purposes. In this study, researchers focused on optimizing the properties of these hydrogels by adjusting key parameters such as lignin concentration, crosslinker ratio, and electrolyte composition. Through careful experimentation, they identified an optimal formulation consisting of 9% lignin, 2.5% crosslinker, and a 6 M KOH electrolyte solution.

The resulting hydrogels demonstrated impressive characteristics, including high ionic conductivity (226.5 mS/cm), low thermal conductivity (0.29 W/mK), and a superior Seebeck coefficient (13 mV/K) as it is shown in Fig. 16.5. These properties contribute to a high-power factor (3831 $\mu W/mK^2$), indicating their effectiveness in converting temperature differentials into usable energy. These findings hold significant promise for biomedical applications. The ability of these hydrogels to effectively convert temperature differences into electricity makes them suitable for powering various biomedical sensors and wearable devices implanted or worn by patients.

Additionally, these hydrogels exhibited remarkable elasticity, ranging from 146.2% to 265.4%, thanks to the combined effects of lignin and PVA components (see Fig. 16.6). This flexibility and resilience make them well-suited for a variety of biomedical applications, including powering biomedical sensors and wearable devices where biocompatibility and adaptability are crucial. Overall, this research opens up new possibilities for sustainable energy solutions in healthcare and beyond.

16.5 Potential Applications in Biomedical Industry

Lignin-based supercapacitors and ionic thermoelectric materials are incredibly versatile in biomedicine, offering several key benefits:

- **Ultra-sensitive Temperature Sensing:** These materials can detect minute temperature fluctuations, allowing for precise monitoring of body temperature. This capability is crucial for early detection of health issues like fever or

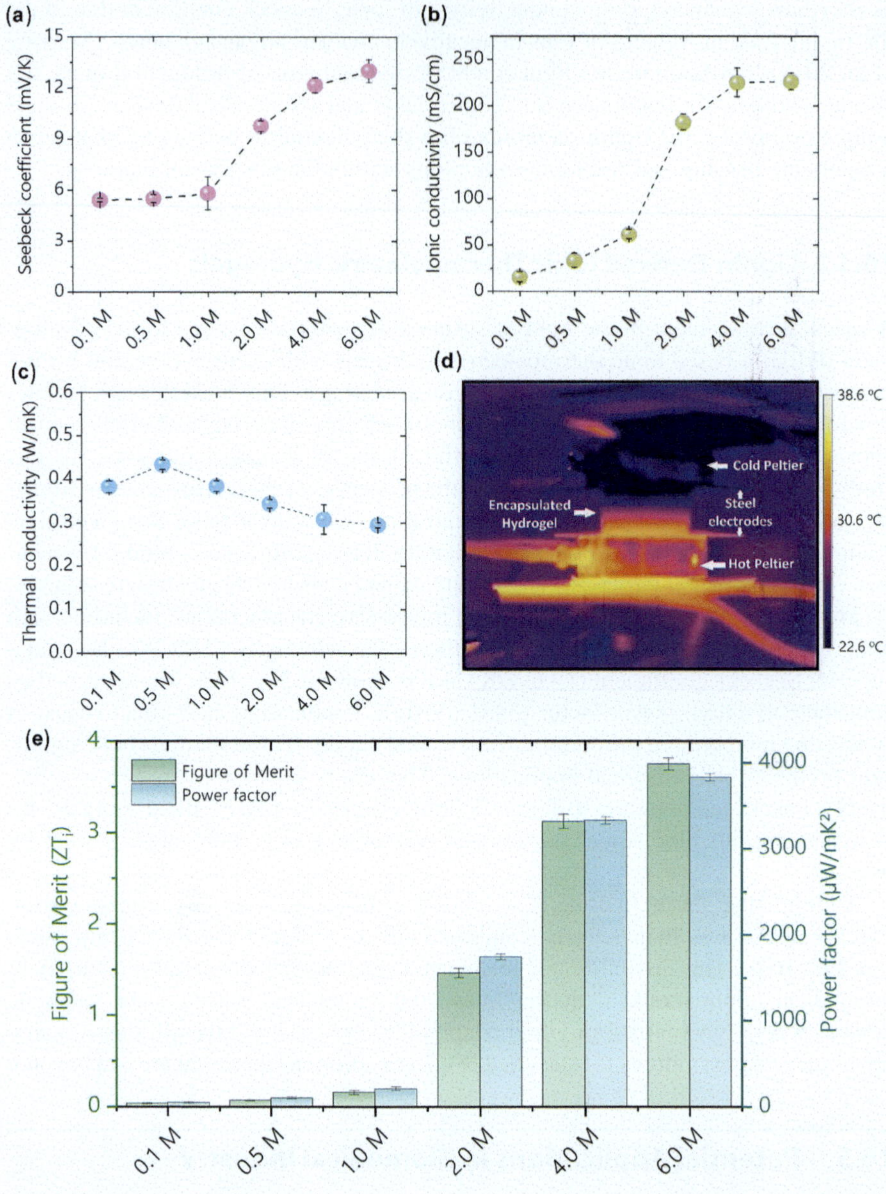

Fig. 16.5 Effect of electrolyte concentration in terms of (**a**) Seebeck coefficient, (**b**) ionic conductivity, (**c**) and thermal conductivity, (**d**) thermal camera image of hydrogel subject to axial temperature difference, (**e**) power factor and figure of merit of lignin-derived hydrogel. (Adapted with permission from Muddasar et al. (2024e))

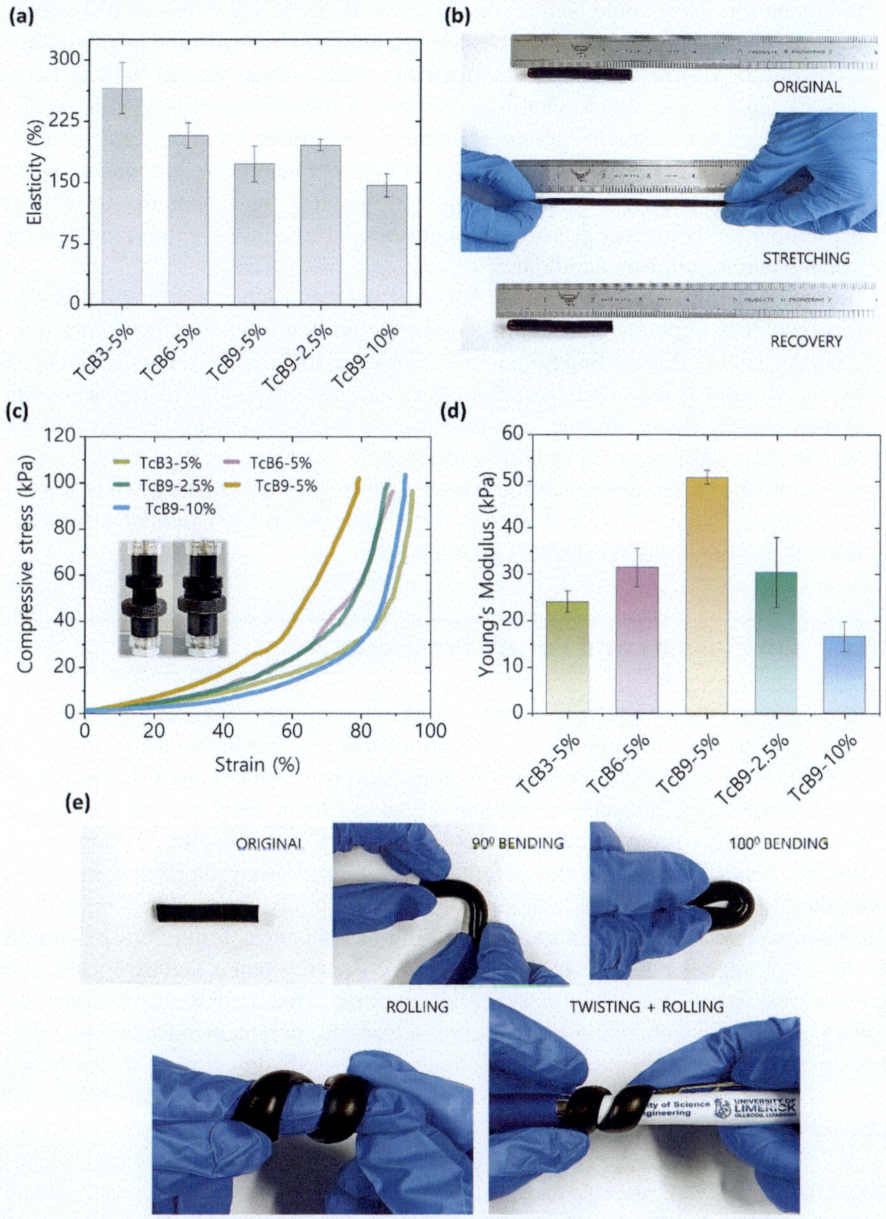

Fig. 16.6 Mechanical properties of hydrogels (**a**) elasticity, (**b**) photographs of TcB9–2.5% before, during and after stretching, (**c**) compressive stress strain curves, (**d**) Young's Modulus, and (**e**) flexibility testing of TcB9-2.5% hydrogel. (Adapted with permission from Muddasar et al. (2024e))

inflammation. They could be integrated into wearable health monitors like smartwatches or even implantable devices like pacemakers for real-time health data.

- **Continuous Wearable Health Monitoring:** These materials can harvest body heat to generate electricity, enabling continuous monitoring of vital signs without the need for frequent battery changes. This allows for uninterrupted data collection, leading to better diagnosis and improved healthcare outcomes. In the case of supercapacitors, monitoring applications rely in their ability to control the quality of the energy passing through them. Thus, making them interesting sensing and monitoring candidates.
- **Biomedical implantable devices:** Medical devices such as cardiac defibrillators, cochlear implants, cardiac pacemakers, and neurological stimulators play crucial roles in safeguarding human life. However, their effectiveness is hindered by the limited lifespan of their batteries, necessitating surgical replacements approximately every decade. Despite the relatively constant temperature of human skin, variations occur within the muscle layer due to activities, creating temperature gradients between the body's core and the skin surface. Thus, supercapacitors and ionic thermoelectric materials are promising candidates for continuous power supply for implantable devices.

16.6 Conclusions and Future Prospects

In summary, the use of lignin-based materials in supercapacitors and ionic thermoelectric membranes for biomedical applications marks a significant step forward in sustainable healthcare technology. These materials provide biocompatibility, renewability, affordability, and eco-friendliness, making them ideal for powering and improving various biomedical devices. Research in this area has demonstrated promising results, indicating the potential for lignin-derived supercapacitors and ionic thermoelectric materials to address challenges in healthcare, such as sustainable energy sources and continuous monitoring of vital signs. Future efforts should focus on optimizing synthesis methods, enhancing performance, and exploring new applications, with interdisciplinary collaborations. This collaborative approach holds potential for enhancing patient care, advancing personalized medicine, and driving sustainability in healthcare technology. Overall, integrating lignin-based materials into biomedical devices holds promise for promoting sustainability and advancing healthcare technologies.

Acknowledgement This research was conducted at the University of Limerick, Ireland, and supported by Irish Government funding via the DAFM NXTGENWOOD research program 2019PROG704. This publication has emanated from research conducted with the financial support of Science Foundation Ireland (SFI) under the SFI Research Infrastructure Programme 21/RI/9831, Grant Number 12/RC/2278_2. JMJ would like to acknowledge the support from the School of Engineering from the University of Limerick to support the research conducted. MM would also like to extend a special thanks to the Plassey Campus Centre Residential Scholarship.

Conflict of Interest We the authors declare no potential conflict of interest.

References

Al-Fartoos MMR et al (2023) Advancing thermoelectric materials: a comprehensive review exploring the significance of one-dimensional nano structuring. Nanomaterials 13(13):2011

Azadi P et al (2013) Liquid fuels, hydrogen and chemicals from lignin: a critical review. Renew Sustain Energ Rev 21:506–523

Beaucamp A et al (2022a) Lignin for energy applications – state of the art, life cycle, technoeconomic analysis and future trends. Green Chem 24(21):8193–8226

Beaucamp A et al (2022b) Sustainable lignin precursors for tailored porous carbon-based supercapacitor electrodes. Int J Biol Macromol 221:1142–1149

Beaucamp A et al (2024) Sustainable lignin-based carbon fibre reinforced polyamide composites: production, characterisation and life cycle analysis. Compos Commun 45:101782

Biesiekierski A et al (2020) 2 – Material selection for medical devices. In: Wen C (ed) Metallic biomaterials processing and medical device manufacturing. Woodhead Publishing, pp 31–94

Cao Y et al (2019) Advances in lignin valorization towards bio-based chemicals and fuels: lignin biorefinery. Bioresour Technol 291:121878

Chakraborty S, Mary NL (2022) Review—an overview on supercapacitors and its applications. J Electrochem Soc 169(2):020552

Chen L et al (2023) Super-stretching and high-performance ionic thermoelectric hydrogels based on carboxylated bacterial cellulose coordination for self-powered sensors. Carbohydr Polym 321:121310

Collins MN et al (2019) Valorization of lignin in polymer and composite systems for advanced engineering applications – a review. Int J Biol Macromol 131:828–849

Dalton N et al (2019) Thermoelectric properties of electrospun carbon nanofibres derived from lignin. Int J Biol Macromol 121:472–479

Gao W, Wang Y, Lai F (2022) Thermoelectric energy harvesting for personalized healthcare. Smart Med 1(1):e20220016

Garedew M et al (2020) Greener routes to biomass waste valorization: lignin transformation through electrocatalysis for renewable chemicals and fuels production. ChemSusChem 13(17):4214–4237

Huerta ER, Muddasar M, Collins MN (2024) Enzymatic hydrolysis lignin and Kraft lignin from birch wood: a source of functional bio-based materials. Wood Sci Technol 58:423–440

Huzum B et al (2021) Biocompatibility assessment of biomaterials used in orthopedic devices: an overview (Review). Exp Ther Med 22(5):1315

Jia Y et al (2021) Wearable thermoelectric materials and devices for self-powered electronic systems. Adv Mater 33(42):2102990

Jia G et al (2023) Lignin-based carbon fibers: insight into structural evolution from lignin pretreatment, fiber forming, to pre-oxidation and carbonization. Int J Biol Macromol 226:646–659

Li T et al (2019) Cellulose ionic conductors with high differential thermal voltage for low-grade heat harvesting. Nat Mater 18(6):608–613

Libanori A et al (2022) Smart textiles for personalized healthcare. Nat Electron 5(3):142–156

Meng Y et al (2019) Lignin-based hydrogels: a review of preparation, properties, and application. Int J Biol Macromol 135:1006–1019

Merola M, Affatato S (2019) Materials for hip prostheses: a review of wear and loading considerations. Materials (Basel) 12(3):495

Muddasar M et al (2022) Cellulose: characteristics and applications for rechargeable batteries. Int J Biol Macromol 219:788–803

Muddasar M et al (2024a) Carbon (nano)fibers and carbon materials from lignin and their applications. In: Lignin chemistry. Wiley, pp 401–431

Muddasar M, Culebras M, Collins MN (2024b) Lignin-derived materials for sustainable development of ionic thermoelectric supercapacitors. Mater Proc 17(1):25

Muddasar M et al (2024c) High performance all lignin derived supercapacitors for energy storage applications. Mater Today Sustain 26:100767

Muddasar M et al (2024d) Synthesis of sustainable lignin precursors for hierarchical porous carbons and their efficient performance in energy storage applications. ACS Sustain Chem Eng 12(6):2352–2363

Muddasar M et al (2024e) Highly-efficient sustainable ionic thermoelectric materials using lignin-derived hydrogels. Adv Compos Hybrid Mater 7(2):47

Muddasar M et al (2024f) Lignin-derived ionic conducting membranes for low-grade thermal energy harvesting. Adv Funct Mater 34(12):2306427

Ozsahin I, Ozsahin DU, Mubarak MT (2022) Chapter 1 – Introduction to biomedical instrumentation. In: Ozsahin DU, Ozsahin I (eds) Modern practical healthcare issues in biomedical instrumentation. Academic, pp 1–2

Ray TR et al (2019) Bio-integrated wearable systems: a comprehensive review. Chem Rev 119(8):5461–5533

Rodrigues C et al (2020) Emerging triboelectric nanogenerators for ocean wave energy harvesting: state of the art and future perspectives. Energy Environ Sci 13(9):2657–2683

Saikia A, Karak N (2023) Chapter 1 – Introduction to biodegradable and biocompatible polymer nanocomposites: synthesis, structure, fundamental properties, biocompatibility, and biodegradability. In: Deshmukh K, Pandey M (eds) Biodegradable and biocompatible polymer nanocomposites. Elsevier, pp 1–34

Sewring T et al (2019) Acid precipitation of kraft lignin from aqueous solutions: the influence of pH, temperature, and xylan. J Wood Chem Technol 39(1):1–13

Srivastava Y et al (2021) Chapter 18 – An overview of the various medical devices for diagnosis, monitoring, and treatment of diseases. In: Tripathi SL et al (eds) Electronic devices, circuits, and systems for biomedical applications. Academic, pp 379–403

Stróżyk MA et al (2024) Decreasing the environmental impact of carbon fibre production via microwave carbonisation enabled by self-assembled nanostructured coatings. Adv Compos Hybrid Mater 7(2):39

Sulleiro MV et al (2022) 2D materials towards sensing technology: from fundamentals to applications. Sens Bio-Sens Res 38:100540

Wu X et al (2020) Lignin-derived electrochemical energy materials and systems. Biofuels Bioprod Biorefin 14(3):650–672

Xiao X et al (2021) An ultrathin rechargeable solid-state zinc ion fiber battery for electronic textiles. Sci Adv 7(49):eabl3742

Yadlapalli RT et al (2022) Super capacitors for energy storage: progress, applications and challenges. J Energy Storage 49:104194

Yun G et al (2020) Liquid metal composites with anisotropic and unconventional piezoconductivity. Matter 3(3):824–841

Bioinspired Corona Nanomaterials for Point-of-Care Testing Sensors and Drug Delivery Systems

17

Maria Kuznowicz, Artur Jędrzak, Łukasz Klapiszewski, and Teofil Jesionowski

Abstract

Point-of-care testing (POCT) research is dedicated to the development and refinement of diagnostic technologies that enable rapid, accurate, and decentralized testing at or near the patient's location. The primary objective of POCT is to deliver precise results swiftly, thereby shortening diagnostic times and facilitating prompt decision-making by healthcare professionals. This approach eliminates the need for patient transportation to specialized facilities, a benefit that was particularly evident during the COVID-19 pandemic when access to medical units was restricted. POCT aims to enhance patient care by enabling quicker initiation of appropriate treatments, especially in critical situations, and by improving diagnostic access in remote or resource-limited settings. The focus of this chapter is on Corona-based materials a new range of materials increasingly used in the construction of biosensors and drug delivery systems. These materials use principles inspired by natural structures and processes, particularly those occurring in biological organisms, to design innovative materials with enhanced, novel properties.

Keywords

Corona nanomaterials · Biosensors · Bioinspired materials · Core-shell nanoparticles · Smart healthcare

M. Kuznowicz · A. Jędrzak · Ł. Klapiszewski · T. Jesionowski (✉)
Institute of Chemical Technology and Engineering, Faculty of Chemical Technology, Poznan University of Technology, Poznan, Poland
e-mail: teofil.jesionowski@put.poznan.pl

M. N. Collins, M. Culebras (eds.), *Sustainable Biopolymers and Composites for Biomedical Applications*, Biomaterials, Bioengineering and Sustainability 5,
https://doi.org/10.1007/978-3-031-91972-5_17

17.1 Introduction

Point-of-care testing (POCT) research focuses on creating, engineering, and refining diagnostic technologies that enable rapid, accurate, and decentralized testing at or near the patient's home. The main idea of POCT tests is to provide accurate results, shorten diagnostic time, and facilitate quick decision-making by healthcare professionals (Luppa et al. 2011). This eliminates the need to transport the patient to special facilities. Such an approach was especially visible during the COVID-19 pandemic, when movement and access to medical units were often difficult. Additionally, activities consistent with the POCT idea aim to improve patient care by enabling faster initiation and appropriate treatment, especially in critical situations, and improving access to diagnostics in remote facilities or those with limited resources (Lee et al. 2023; Etienne et al. 2021). POCT studies cover a wide range of technologies, including mobile devices, contributing to more efficient and personalized healthcare delivery (Zarei 2017; Sautter et al. 2018).

In the field of sensors and biosensors, the concept of point-of-care testing (POCT) focuses on the development and application of fast, accurate, and sensitive diagnostic devices on-site. The integration of biosensors in POCT facilitates the detection of specific biomolecules, enabling early diagnosis of diseases, rapid intervention, and monitoring of the effectiveness of treatment (Ahmed et al. 2016; Vasan et al. 2013; Srinivasan and Tung 2015). The aim of POCT in (bio)sensors is to provide real-time information about the patient's health condition using miniaturized and portable devices to analyze biological samples such as blood, saliva or urine. These types of devices enable the patient to obtain the result quickly, send it to a healthcare professional, and receive a decision on his or her treatment (Ghafar-Zadeh 2015; da Silva et al. 2017). The use of sensors, which often work in tandem with publicly available mobile devices, undoubtedly saves time compared with centralized laboratories, as is shown schematically in Fig. 17.1.

Point-of-care testing (POCT) plays a key role in drug delivery systems, providing real-time diagnostic information at the patient's bedside or in decentralized settings. In the context of drug administration, POCT allows healthcare professionals to monitor therapeutic drug levels, assess patient response to treatment, and make

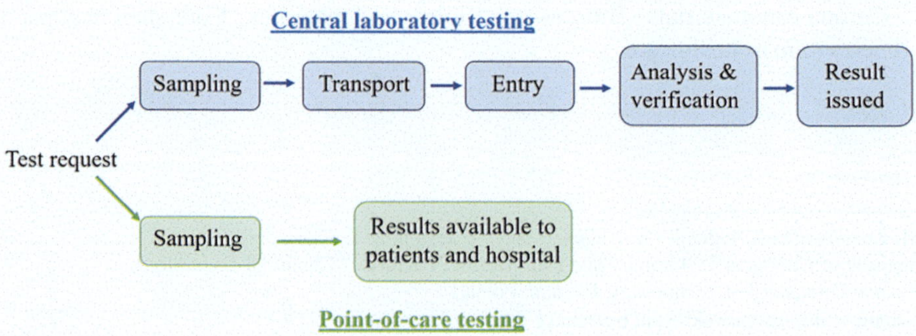

Fig. 17.1 POCT vs. central laboratory testing

timely adjustments to optimize drug delivery parameters. This approach enhances personalized medicine by tailoring treatment regimens to individual patient needs, ensuring precise dosing, and minimizing side effects (Chowdhury et al. 2021; Khadka et al. 2023).

Corona-based materials are one of the new ranges of materials increasingly used in the construction of biosensors and drug delivery systems. These materials use principles inspired by natural structures and processes, particularly those occurring in biological organisms, to design innovative materials with enhanced, novel properties (Bashiri et al. 2023; Liu et al. 2022; Meng et al. 2022).

Hybrid materials, including corona-based ones, play a key role in the development of biosensor technologies, offering unique properties that increase sensitivity, selectivity and time stability (Gómez-Romero and Sanchez 2004; Wang et al. 2013). Combining the biocompatibility of organic materials with the excellent conductivity or catalytic activity of inorganic counterparts, hybrid materials enable the creation of innovative biosensors with improved performance. Synergistic effects between the different components contribute to increasing the surface area and binding affinity of biomolecules, thus improving their properties (Kickelbick 2007; Batool et al. 2019).

17.2 Bioinspired Nanomaterials

Bioinspired materials draw inspiration from nature's design principles to develop innovative materials with novel properties and functionalities. These materials find applications in various fields, including medicine, materials science, and drug delivery (Perrett et al. 2019; Harun-Ur-Rashid et al. 2023). The study of bioinspired materials not only contributes to the development of advanced technologies, but also offers sustainable solutions by learning from the performance and resilience inherent in biological systems (Huang et al. 2015).

Bioinspired materials display unique properties, including the versatility and diversity that result from imitating complex structures found in nature. They are biocompatible, making them particularly suitable for biomedical applications (Huang et al. 2015). The possibility of self-assembly of these materials simplifies production processes, and the integration of many functionalities into one structure increases efficiency (Perrett et al. 2019; Harun-Ur-Rashid et al. 2023; Huang et al. 2015). The benefits of bioinspired nanomaterials are presented schematically in Fig. 17.2.

Increasing attention is being paid to biomaterials that are environmentally friendly and offer high specificity and sensitivity. Biomaterials are used as novel solutions in numerous biosensors, introducing new possibilities that can provide higher effectiveness, sensitivity, selectivity, and biocompatibility than their synthetic counterparts. This is of particular importance in the development of point-of-care diagnostic testing, where the superior characteristics of biomaterials promise to overcome the limitations associated with traditional materials, paving the way for more efficient and reliable biosensor technologies (Pérez et al. 2019). Additionally,

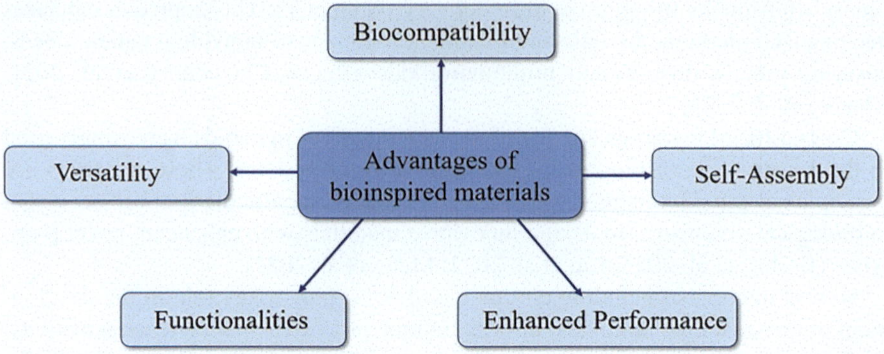

Fig. 17.2 Advantages of bioinspired nanomaterials

bioinspired nanomaterials facilitate the creation of sensor surfaces with enhanced biocompatibility, reducing the risk of unwanted interactions in biological environments. Their adaptability and ability to respond to external stimuli further enhance the real-time monitoring capabilities of biosensors (Harun-Ur-Rashid et al. 2023; Pérez et al. 2019).

Bioinspired materials have also become increasingly mainstream in the drug delivery field, offering innovative solutions to improve therapeutic outcomes. Drawing inspiration from nature's precision, these materials recreate biological structures and processes, enabling targeted and controlled drug release (Neubi et al. 2018; Alvarez-Lorenzo and Concheiro 2013). Nanoparticles, liposomes, and other bioinspired carriers mimic cellular components, facilitating interactions with biological systems. This biomimetic approach improves drug stability, solubility, and bioavailability while minimizing side effects (Tong et al. 2020). Additionally, the adaptability of bioinspired materials allows them to respond to specific stimuli, such as changes in pH or enzyme activity, resulting in precise drug release at the intended location. The biocompatibility of these materials further reduces the risk of side effects (Sabu et al. 2018).

17.2.1 Polydopamine-Based Materials

Polydopamine is a versatile biopolymer that has attracted great interest due to its unique properties. Typically, the preparation of polydopamine (PDA) occurs in alkaline conditions, at a pH of 8.5. Under these conditions, the polymerization process may take an equilibrium pathway, resulting in the formation of indole-like repeating units. These units contribute to the development of cross-linked structures in the polymer. The oxidation of dopamine is commonly triggered by an oxidizing agent, such as oxygen. This initiation process facilitates the creation of reactive quinone intermediates (Kang et al. 2017). The structure of the monomer and the final product, polydopamine, is shown schematically in Fig. 17.3.

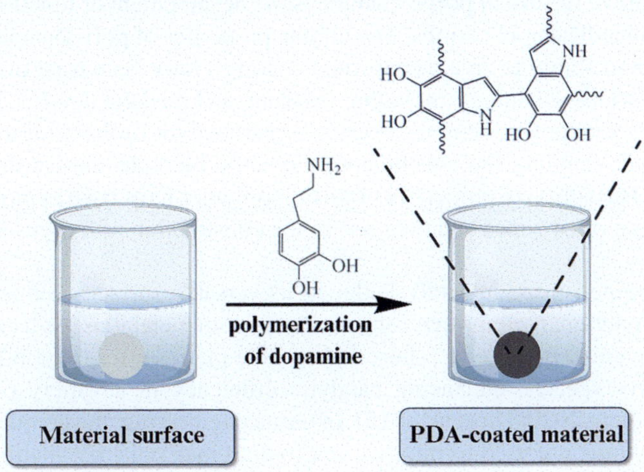

Fig. 17.3 Chemical structure of dopamine, and polydopamine

Fig. 17.4 Properties of polydopamine coatings

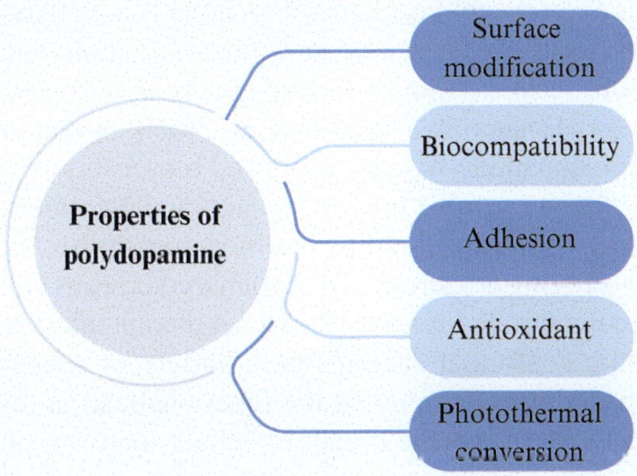

The properties of polydopamine, such as its natural hydrophilicity and adhesiveness, can be attributed to the presence of catechol and amino functional groups (Liebscher 2019). The adhesiveness of these coatings and strong binding abilities result from the presence of these groups, which facilitate strong interactions with various surfaces. Additionally, polydopamine coatings exhibit remarkable hydrophilicity, increasing their compatibility with aqueous environments (Batul et al. 2017). This feature, combined with the polymer's ability to form thin, tight-fitting layers, contributes to its effectiveness in preventing biofouling. Additionally, polydopamine coatings can serve as a versatile platform for further functionalization, enabling the introduction of tailored chemical functionalities and providing control over surface properties. Figure 17.4 illustrates the characteristics of polydopamine (Ho and Ding 2014).

An example of the use of polydopamine is the development of functional biomaterials for biomedical applications. The unique properties of polydopamine, such as its adhesion and ability to create conformal coatings, have been used to modify the surfaces of various substrates, including implants and medical devices. By coating these surfaces with polydopamine, a versatile platform for further biofunctionalization is created, enabling the attachment of specific biomolecules or drugs (Batul et al. 2017). The adhesive properties of this biopolymer have been exploited for the immobilization of enzymes and their use in the construction of biosensors (Jędrzak et al. 2018).

Polydopamine is used in catalysis due to its versatile surface chemistry and the presence of functional groups that can coordinate with metal ions. As a catalyst support, polydopamine provides a robust and tunable platform for immobilizing catalytically active species, enhancing catalytic efficiency in a variety of chemical reactions (Molnár 2020; Du et al. 2015). In tissue engineering, the unique properties of this biopolymer are used to improve scaffolding materials. By coating biomaterial scaffolds with polydopamine, researchers create a biocompatible surface that promotes cell adhesion and proliferation, thereby facilitating the development of functional tissues (Tang et al. 2021; Yan et al. 2020). The uses of polydopamine are shown schematically in Fig. 17.5.

Over recent years, polydopamine has increasingly been used in the construction of materials for sensor and biosensor applications. This biopolymer can enhance both sensitivity and selectivity, as well as augmenting the loading capacity for biological materials (Jędrzak et al. 2019). A comparison of the properties of various polydopamine-based sensors and biosensors is presented in Table 17.1.

Polydopamine has gained significant popularity in the drug delivery field, demonstrating its versatility and biocompatibility. In view of its adhesive and surface-modifying properties, polydopamine serves as an effective platform for encapsulation and controlled release of various therapeutic agents. The polymer's ability to form thin, conformal coatings on a variety of substrates enables the creation of drug-loaded nanoparticles or the functionalization of drug carriers, facilitating targeted delivery to specific tissues or cells. Moreover, polydopamine's response to external

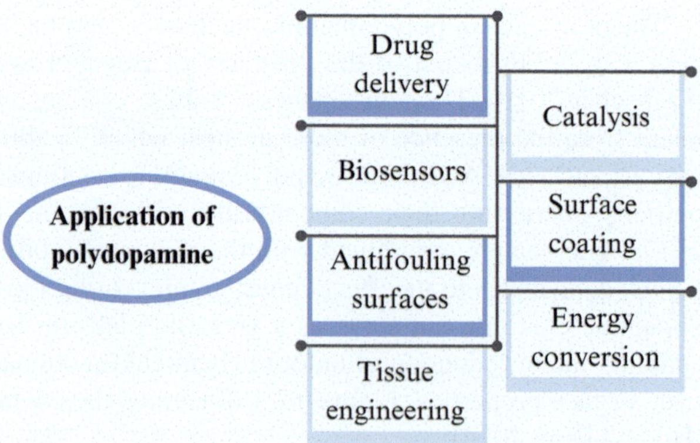

Fig. 17.5 Applications of polydopamine

Table 17.1 Comparison of polydopamine-based (bio)sensors

Electrode material	Tested analyte	Sensitivity/μA mM^{-1} cm^{-2}	LOD/ μM	Linear range/ mM	References
PDA-SPCE	Guanine	90.5	15.8	0.1–10.0	Kanyong et al. (2016)
AgNPs/PDA/ RGO	H_2O_2	140	0.68	0.005–9.97	Ma et al. (2019)
rGO/PDA/ AuNPs	Folic acid	2.75	0.025	0.0001–0.905	Mani et al. (2020)
CuNPs/ Cu(II)-PDA/Gr	Uric acid	–	6.2	0.011–0.434	Quan et al. (2021)
PDA-rGO/Au	Uric acid	–	0.7	0.002–1.0	Income et al. (2019)
Fe_3O_4/ PDA-GOx	Glucose	139.71	1.54	1.0–20.0	Kuznowicz et al. (2021a)
Fe_3O_4/PDA/ βCD-GOx	Glucose	115.74	1.55	1.0–26.0	Kuznowicz et al. (2021b)
PDA-GOD-GN	Glucose	28.4	0.10	0.001–4.7	Ruan et al. (2013)
TiO_2 NRs/PDA/ GOx	Glucose	2.80	12.96	0.2–2.4	Ma et al. (2022)

stimuli, such as changes in pH or temperature, increases its usefulness in the design of drug delivery systems (Mousavi et al. 2018; Poinard et al. 2018).

17.2.2 Poly(Caffeic Acid)-Based Materials

Poly(caffeic acid) (PCA) is a biopolymer with aromatic and catecholic characteristics, synthesized through the polymerization of its monomer, caffeic acid (3,4-hydroxycinnamic acid, CA) (Filik et al. 2013).

It has been demonstrated that the oxidation of caffeic acid (CA) on various electrode materials, such as platinum, carbon, and gold, leads to the formation of an electroactive polymer layer. This polymer has been analyzed for its electrochemical properties and potential use as a sensing material, owing to the presence of functional groups facilitating electron transfer. The oxidative coupling process initiates spontaneously in the presence of an oxidizing agent, such as hydrogen peroxide (H_2O_2) or sodium periodate ($NaIO_4$) (Makhotkina and Kilmartin 2009). The polymerization process leading to the formation of poly(caffeic acid) is shown schematically in Fig. 17.6.

Initially, the phenolic hydroxyl group of the caffeic acid monomer undergoes oxidation, forming a phenoxy radical, which subsequently reacts with another caffeic acid monomer to produce a dimer. This dimerization process continues iteratively, resulting in the formation of longer polymer chains (Fonseca et al. 2019; He et al. 2020).

Poly(caffeic acid) exhibits properties that make it an intriguing material for a variety of applications, particularly in the novel materials category. As an aromatic biopolymer, PCA has inherent antioxidant properties due to the presence of

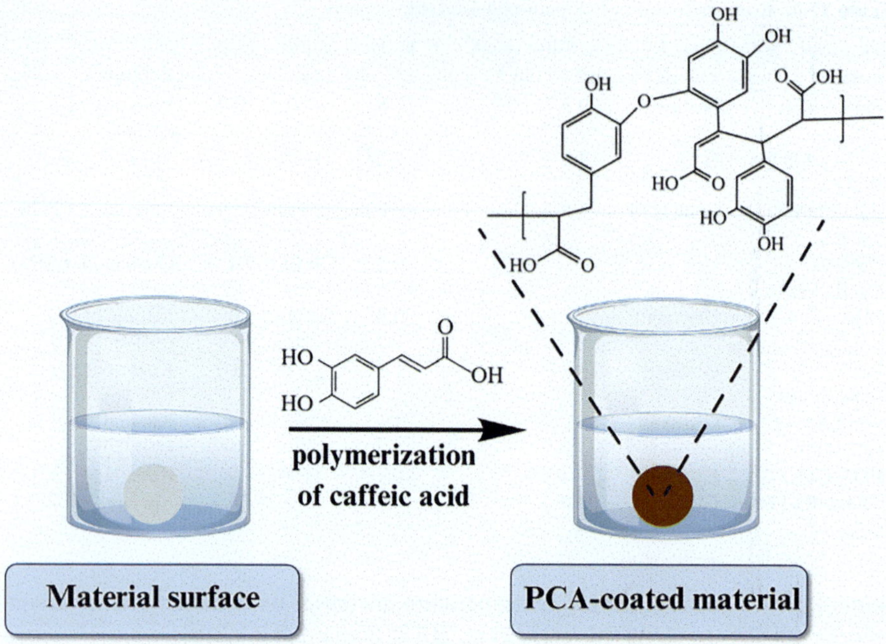

Fig. 17.6 The polymerization process leading to the formation of poly(caffeic acid)

phenolic hydroxyl groups in its structure (Zhou et al. 2019; Zare and Golabi 2000). These properties make it particularly attractive in biomedical and pharmaceutical applications, where its ability to scavenge free radicals has the potential to mitigate the damage associated with oxidative stress in biological systems. Additionally, PCA is electroactive, due to the conjugated system of π electrons in its molecular structure (Kitsati et al. 2012). This characteristic gives PCA the ability to undergo oxidation and reduction processes, making it suitable for use in electrochemical sensors such as biosensors and electrochemical devices (Bai et al. 2018). The properties of poly(caffeic acid) are presented schematically in Fig. 17.7.

Furthermore, the PCA polymerization process enables the formation of an electroactive polymer layer, especially when PCA is oxidized on different electrode materials. The resulting polymer has functional groups that enable effective electron transfer, which further increases its usefulness in electrochemical applications (Filik et al. 2013; Adhikari et al. 2023). Overall, the combination of antioxidant properties, electroactivity, and self-polymerization ability makes PCA a promising candidate for a wide range of applications, including biomedical devices, sensors, and drug delivery systems (Adhikari et al. 2023; Ishii et al. 2013).

Poly(caffeic acid) finds applications across multiple domains owing to its unique properties and functional versatility. In the biomedical field, PCA serves as a promising candidate for drug delivery systems and tissue engineering scaffolds, due to its biocompatibility and ability to interact with biological molecules (Fonseca et al.

Fig. 17.7 Properties of poly(caffeic acid)

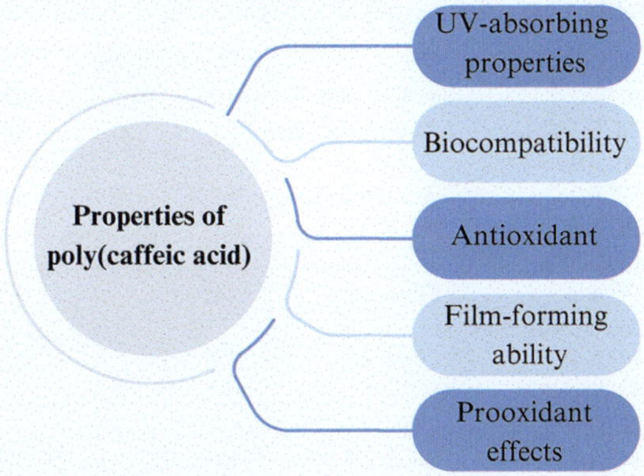

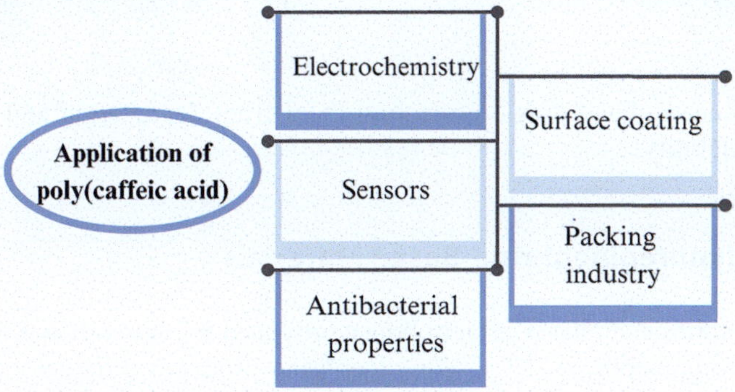

Fig. 17.8 Application of the biopolymer poly(caffeic acid)

2019; Adhikari et al. 2023; Li et al. 2008). Its antioxidant and antimicrobial properties also render it suitable for incorporation into food packaging materials to prolong shelf life and ensure food safety (Fonseca et al. 2019). Examples of applications of this biopolymer are shown schematically in Fig. 17.8.

Additionally, PCA is used in electrochemical sensors, due to its ability to increase the sensitivity and selectivity of these devices. As a bioinspired material, PCA can be functionalized on electrode surfaces to facilitate the immobilization of biomolecules including enzymes or antibodies, thereby improving the sensor's performance in detecting various analytes with high precision and efficiency (Li et al. 2008; Rębiś et al. 2021).

Table 17.2 summarizes the characteristics of enzymatic biosensors and non-enzymatic electrochemical sensors that contain poly(caffeic acid) in their structure.

To date, poly(caffeic acid) has not been widely used for drug delivery. However, these types of coatings have significant potential for applications in drug delivery systems, due to their biocompatibility, biodegradability, and ability to interact with biological molecules. PCA can be incorporated into various drug delivery vehicles such as nanoparticles, micelles, or hydrogels, offering controlled release and targeted delivery of therapeutic agents. Its antioxidant properties further increase the

Table 17.2 Comparison of poly(caffeic acid)-based sensors and biosensors

Electrode material	Tested analyte	Sensitivity/μA mM^{-1} cm^{-2}	LOD/ μM	Linear range/ mM	References
GCE/PCA/ AuNPs	Acetaminophen	–	0.014	0.05–1.0	Li et al. (2016)
GCE/PCA-CoP	Acetaminophen	–	0.01	0.00005–0.05	Li et al. (2021)
PCA@ MWCNT	NADH	85.7	0.12	0.0005–3.0	Rębiś et al. (2021)
PCA@ MWCNT-CuO	Glucose	2412.0	0.43	0.002–9.0	Kuznowicz et al. (2022)
PCA@ MWCNT-$Ni(OH)_2$	Glucose	232.70	0.29	0.05–10.0	Kuznowicz et al. (2023)
PCA@ Fe_3O_4-GOx	Glucose	1198.0	5.23	0.05–25.0	Kuznowicz et al. (2023)
pCAF-GCE	L-DOPA	–	0.14	0.001–0.050	Rohanifar et al. (2016)

stability of encapsulated drugs, protecting them from degradation and improving their bioavailability.

17.2.3 Polynorepinephrine-Based Materials

Polynorepinephrine (PNE) is a biopolymer produced by autoxidation of the catecholamine norepinephrine (NE). Norepinephrine produces ultra-smooth coatings with thinner and more uniform coverage than polydopamine. This is due to the presence of the beta-hydroxyl group, which is responsible for the extensive oxidative degradation of the catecholamine side chain during oxidation (Baldoneschi et al. 2020). Similarly to dopamine and L-DOPA, norepinephrine possesses the ability to undergo self-polymerization under oxidative and alkaline conditions, resulting in the formation of nanometric films that adhere well to various surfaces, including synthetic polymers, silicates, and metals (Jeon and Kang 2013; Jędrzak et al. 2022). The polymerization process of polynorepinephrine is presented schematically in Fig. 17.9.

Polynorepinephrine presents adhesive properties, creating strong and versatile coatings on a variety of substrates as a result of an effective oxidative polymerization process. Additionally, this polymer is biocompatible, making it suitable for biomedical applications, including drug delivery systems, tissue engineering scaffolds, and surface coatings for medical implants (Park et al. 2014). It commonly undergoes further functionalization, enabling the attachment of biomolecules, polymers or nanoparticles for tailored applications. Polynorepinephrine exhibits good mechanical properties and chemical reactivity, and its film-forming ability enables protection against corrosion, contamination and biological deposits, making it promising for use in a variety of industrial and biomedical applications (Kang et al. 2009; Hong et al. 2013). Moreover, PNE exhibits inherent hydrophilicity, eliminating the need for organic solvents or anhydrous conditions during cross-linking and

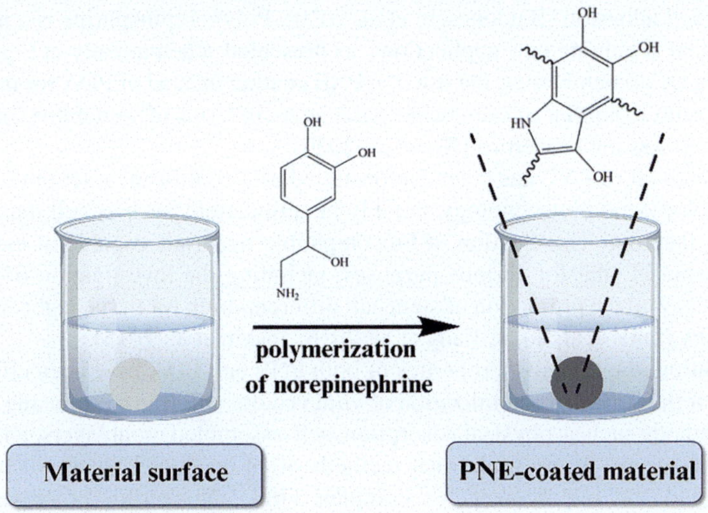

Fig. 17.9 Polymerization of polynorepinephrine

Fig. 17.10 Properties of a polynorepinephrine biopolymer coating

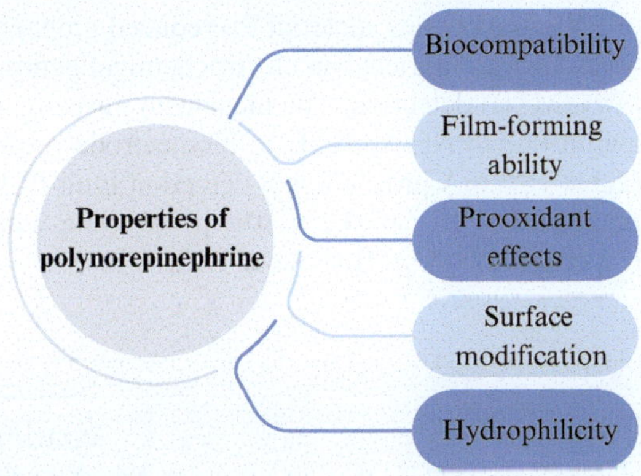

deposition processes, thus rendering it compatible with aqueous environments. Another studied feature of PNE is its electron transfer capability, facilitated by the catechol/quinone redox equilibrium involving two electrons and two protons. During the polymerization process, the catechol groups of NE undergo oxidation, while the resultant quinone moieties (Baldoneschi et al. 2020).

The properties of polynorepinephrine coatings are shown schematically in Fig. 17.10.

Polynorepinephrine is a biopolymer from the catecholamine group. It is an excellent material for creating functional coatings, especially on inorganic compounds, offering good biocompatibility and hydrophilicity, and excellent adhesion. A PNE coating has been found to produce a smoother and thinner surface than PDA, which formed irregular aggregates on the fiber surface, potentially having a detrimental effect on cell adhesion (Baldoneschi et al. 2020). Polynorepinephrine is a new biopolymer that is gaining new applications, as presented schematically in Fig. 17.11.

In the case of membranes, the use of a PNE coating instead of PDA for modification can result in similar or even better parameters in terms of wettability, morphology, and antifouling properties (Xia et al. 2020).

The potential of PNE has been demonstrated as a significant asset in the realms of cell biology and biotechnology, notably in applications such as cell therapy and tissue engineering. The creation of biocompatible materials capable of enhancing cell adhesion is vital for various purposes, including the investigation of cellular mechanisms and the promotion of stem cell differentiation for tissue regeneration or cell therapy (Park et al. 2014; Jiang et al. 2016; Taskin et al. 2015).

In addition, the adhesive properties of both PNE and PDA have been effectively utilized for the surface immobilization of viral vectors, offering a promising alternative to methods such as physical adsorption, self-assembled monolayers, and chemical modifications. These traditional methods often encounter issues such as low stability and the requirement for complex virus engineering processes (Kim et al. 2014).

Polynorepinephrine can be a binding agent used to coat various surfaces, for example in the construction of modern biosensors. Bisht et al. explored the potential of PNE as a coating material for reduced graphene oxide (RGO) and gold nanoparticles (Au) to fabricate an electrochemical genosensor for *Mycobacterium tuberculosis* (MTB) detection. The biosensing investigations conducted using the ssDNA/avidin/RGO/PNE/Au/GCE bioelectrode demonstrated high sensitivity (2.3×10^{-3} mA μM^{-1}), a low detection limit (0.1×10^{-7} μM) and a wide detection range (0.1×10^{-2} to 0.1×10^{-7} μM), along with excellent selectivity and a short response time (5 s) (Bisht et al. 2023).

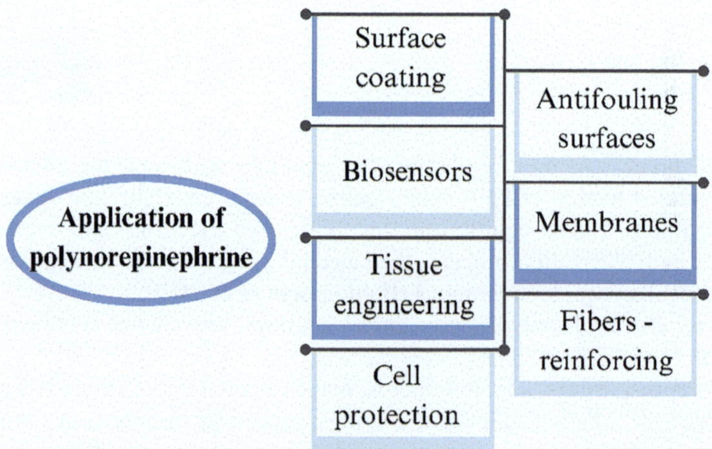

Fig. 17.11 Application of polynorepinephrine

In another study, Jędrzak et al. introduce a novel nanoplatform constructed from polynorepinephrine (PNE) grafted onto magnetite nanoparticles (Fe_3O_4), incorporating glucose oxidase (GOx) sourced from *Aspergillus niger* to create Fe_3O_4@ PNE-GOx. This innovative system is integrated with a smartphone analyzer, presenting a potential point-of-care testing (POCT) biosensor for glucose measurement. Functionalizing the magnetite surface with the biomimetic polymer polynorepinephrine significantly enhances the efficiency of enzyme immobilization, achieving an impressive 38.40 mg g^{-1}, compared with 17.30 mg g^{-1} on bare magnetite. The Fe_3O_4@PNE-GOx nanoplatform is then applied onto a screen-printed electrode (SPE) forming a cohesive setup for glucose measurement. This biosensor exhibits a wide range of linearity (0.2–24 mM), a low detection limit (6.1 μM), and excellent sensitivity (97.34 μA mM^{-1} cm^{-2}) (Jędrzak et al. 2022).

In further work by Jędrzak et al., the proposed magnetite@polinorepinephrine system was enriched with the addition of β-cyclodextrins as nanocontainers. The proposed hybrid nanomaterial was used for the immobilization of glucose oxidase and then for the construction of a biosensor based on a screen-printed SPE electrode. The SPE/Fe_3O_4@PNE@βCD-GOx biosensor displayed impressive capabilities, allowing measurements across a broad concentration range (0.1–30.0 mM), and exhibiting enhanced sensitivity(204.82 μA mM^{-1} cm^{-2}), a low limit of detection (3.2 μM), and a rapid response time (2.6 s) (Jędrzak et al. 2024).

17.3 Application of Bioinspired Core-Shell Materials in Drug Delivery Systems

Core-shell materials have emerged as promising platforms for drug delivery systems, offering unique advantages in encapsulation, protection, and controlled release of therapeutic agents (Ghosh Chaudhuri and Paria 2012).

These materials typically consist of a core in which the delivered drug is encapsulated, surrounded by a coating that acts as a protective barrier. The core can be composed of various materials such as polymers, lipids, or inorganic nanoparticles, providing stability and controlling the release kinetics of the loaded drug molecules (Gawande et al. 2015; Zhong and Maye 2001). The coating protects the encapsulated drug from premature degradation or removal, allowing sustained and targeted delivery to the desired site of action. Additionally, the coating can be designed to respond to specific stimuli, such as pH, temperature, or enzymes, enabling the triggered release of the drug payload in response to physiological signals (Mandal et al. 2013).

Core-shell materials present a multitude of benefits compared with conventional dosage forms, such as protection of the drug from biodegradation, precise direction of the drug to its site of action, and mitigation of the side effects associated with chemotherapy (Wong and Melendez 2006). These advantages are presented schematically in Fig. 17.12.

Additionally, these materials offer several significant benefits when used in drug delivery systems. They protect drugs against biodegradation or oxidation, thus

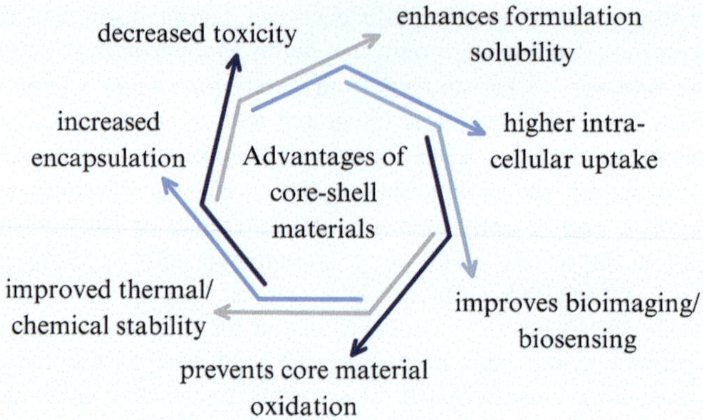

Fig. 17.12 Advantages of core-shell materials for medical applications

increasing their stability and extending their shelf life. They enable precise targeting of drugs to specific sites of action in the body, increasing therapeutic effectiveness while minimizing systemic side effects (Gawande et al. 2015). Core-shell structures enable the controlled release of drugs over time, leading to improved patient compliance and reduced dosing frequency. Additionally, they offer the versatility to incorporate different drugs and therapeutic agents into the same carrier system, facilitating combination therapy and synergistic effects (Zhong and Maye 2001; Chatterjee et al. 2014).

17.4 Summary

The corona-based hybrid nanomaterials reviewed here—for example, those based on catechol compounds—offer unique properties that are causing them to gain more and more importance in materials chemistry and in the immobilization of biomolecules. As a result, the number of works reporting their use in (bio)sensors and drug delivery systems is increasing year by year.

The use of corona-based biopolymers in hybrid materials represents a promising avenue for the development of various applications in many branches of science, medicine and industry. These types of biopolymers offer unique properties, including increased surface energy, improved wettability, and compatibility with other materials. Therefore, their integration with hybrid materials may lead to the development of biocompatible coatings, and scaffolds for tissue engineering or drug delivery systems. The described mechanical properties of these compounds may be beneficial in applications in packaging, textiles and building materials, where strength and elasticity are necessary. Biopolymers derived from renewable resources offer environmental benefits over traditional petroleum-based polymers. The use of corona-treated biopolymers in hybrid materials aligns with sustainability goals by reducing dependence on fossil fuels and minimizing environmental impact. In summary, further research into corona-based hybrid materials may lead to a wide range of applications in many sectors. Taking advantage of their unique properties and versatility, innovative solutions can be developed, in particular for use in (bio)sensors and drug delivery.

Acknowledgments *The work was financed and prepared by the Poznan University of Technology research grant no. 0912/SBAD/2506.*

References

Adhikari S, Sunder GSS, Poudel A, Asfaha TY, Lawrence JG, Kandage MM, Marszewski M, Kirchhoff JR (2023) Application of poly(caffeic acid) for the extraction of critical rare earth elements. ACS Appl Mater Interfaces 15:24892–24900

Ahmed MU, Hossain MM, Safavieh M, Wong YL, Rahman IA, Zourob M, Tamiya E (2016) Toward the development of smart and low cost point-of-care biosensors based on screen printed electrodes. Crit Rev Biotechnol 36:495–505

Alvarez-Lorenzo C, Concheiro A (2013) Bioinspired drug delivery systems. Curr Opin Biotechnol 24:1167–1173

Bai R, Yu Y, Wang Q, Fan X, Wang P, Yuan J, Shen J (2018) Laccase-catalyzed poly(ethylene glycol)-templated 'zip' polymerization of caffeic acid for functionalization of wool fabrics. J Clean Prod 191:48–56

Baldoneschi V, Palladino P, Scarano S, Minunni M (2020) Polynorepinephrine: state-of-the-art and perspective applications in biosensing and molecular recognition. Anal Bioanal Chem 412:5945–5954

Bashiri G, Padilla MS, Swingle KL, Shepherd SJ, Mitchell MJ, Wang K (2023) Nanoparticle protein corona: from structure and function to therapeutic targeting. Lab Chip 23:1432–1466

Batool R, Rhouati A, Nawaz MH, Hayat A, Marty JL (2019) A review of the construction of nano-hybrids for electrochemical biosensing of glucose. Biosensors 9:46

Batul R, Tamanna T, Khaliq A, Yu A (2017) Recent progress in the biomedical applications of polydopamine nanostructures. Biomater Sci 5:1204–1229

Bisht N, Patel M, Dwivedi N, Kumar P, Mondal DP, Srivastava AK, Dhand C (2023) Bio-inspired polynorepinephrine based nanocoatings for reduced graphene oxide/gold nanoparticles composite for high-performance biosensing of Mycobacterium tuberculosis. Environ Res 227:115684

Chatterjee K, Sarkar S, Rao KJ, Paria S (2014) Core/shell nanoparticles in biomedical applications. Adv Colloid Interf Sci 209:8–39

Chowdhury NK, Choudhury R, Sonawane GA, Mavinamar S, Lyu X, Pandey RP, Chang C-M (2021) Nanoparticles as an effective drug delivery system in COVID-19. Biomed Pharmacother 143:112162

da Silva ETSG, Souto DEP, Barragan JTC, Giarola J de F, de Moraes ACM, Kubota LT (2017) Electrochemical biosensors in point-of-care devices: recent advances and future trends. ChemElectroChem 4:778–794

Du Y, Yang H-C, Xu X-L, Wu J, Xu Z-K (2015) Polydopamine as a catalyst for thiol coupling. ChemCatChem 7:3822–3825

Etienne EE, Nunna BB, Talukder N, Wang Y, Lee ES (2021) COVID-19 biomarkers and advanced sensing technologies for point-of-care (POC) diagnosis. Bioengineering 8:98

Filik H, Çetintaş G, Avan AA, Aydar S, Koç SN, Boz I (2013) Square-wave stripping voltammetric determination of caffeic acid on electrochemically reduced graphene oxide-Nafion composite film. Talanta 116:245–250

Fonseca AC, Lima MS, Sousa AF, Silvestre AJ, Coelho JFJ, Serra AC (2019) Cinnamic acid derivatives as promising building blocks for advanced polymers: synthesis, properties and applications. Polym Chem 10:1696–1723

Gawande MB, Goswami A, Asefa T, Guo H, Biradar AV, Peng D-L, Zboril R, Varma RS (2015) Core–shell nanoparticles: synthesis and applications in catalysis and electrocatalysis. Chem Soc Rev 44:7540–7590
Ghafar-Zadeh E (2015) Wireless integrated biosensors for point-of-care diagnostic applications. Sensors 15:3236–3261
Ghosh Chaudhuri R, Paria S (2012) Core/shell nanoparticles: classes, properties, synthesis mechanisms, characterization, and applications. Chem Rev 112:2373–2433
Gómez-Romero P, Sanchez C (2004) Hybrid materials, functional applications. An introduction. Funct Hybrid Mater:1–14
Harun-Ur-Rashid M, Jahan I, Foyez T, Imran AB (2023) Bio-inspired nanomaterials for micro/nanodevices: a new era in biomedical applications. Micromachines 14:1786
He Y, Chen Q, Zhang Y, Zhao Y, Chen L (2020) H_2O_2-triggered rapid deposition of poly(caffeic acid) coatings: a mechanism-based entry to versatile and high-efficient molecular separation. ACS Appl Mater Interfaces 12:52104–52115
Ho C-C, Ding S-J (2014) Structure, properties and applications of mussel-inspired polydopamine. J Biomed Nanotechnol 10:3063–3084
Hong S, Kim J, Na YS, Park J, Kim S, Singha K, Im G, Han D, Kim WJ, Lee H (2013) Poly(norepinephrine): ultrasmooth material-independent surface chemistry and nanodepot for nitric oxide. Angew Chem Int Ed 35:9187–9191
Huang J, Lin L, Sun D, Chen H, Yang D, Li Q (2015) Bio-inspired synthesis of metal nanomaterials and applications. Chem Soc Rev 44:6330–6374
Income K, Ratnarathorn N, Khamchaiyo N, Srisuvo C, Ruckthong L, Dungchai W (2019) Disposable nonenzymatic uric acid and creatinine sensors using pad coupled with screen-printed reduced graphene oxide-gold nanocomposites. Int J Anal Chem 2019:1–11
Ishii D, Maeda H, Hayashi H, Mitani T, Shinohara N, Yoshioka K, Watanabe T (2013) Effect of polycondensation conditions on structure and thermal properties of poly(caffeic acid). ACS Symp Ser 1144:237–249
Jędrzak A, Rębiś T, Klapiszewski Ł, Zdarta J, Milczarek G, Jesionowski T (2018) Carbon paste electrode based on functional GOx/silica-lignin system to prepare an amperometric glucose biosensor. Sens Actuators B Chem 256:176–185
Jędrzak A, Rębiś T, Kuznowicz M, Jesionowski T (2019) Bio-inspired magnetite/lignin/polydopamine-glucose oxidase biosensing nanoplatform. From synthesis, via sensing assays to comparison with others glucose testing techniques. Int J Biol Macromol 127:677–682
Jędrzak A, Kuznowicz M, Rębiś T, Jesionowski T (2022) Portable glucose biosensor based on polynorepinephrine@magnetite nanomaterial integrated with a smartphone analyzer for point-of-care application. Bioelectrochemistry 145:108071
Jędrzak A, Kuznowicz M, Jesionowski T (2024) Mobile-assisted diagnostic biosensor for point-of-care glucose detection in real human samples with rapid response and long-live stability. J Appl Electrochem 54:163–174
Jeon YJ, Kang SM (2013) Chemically stable poly(norepinephrine) coatings on solid substrates by post-oxidation. Polym Degrad Stab 98:1271–1273
Jiang X, Li Y, Liu Y, Chen C, Chen M (2016) Selective enhancement of human stem cell proliferation by mussel inspired surface coating. RSC Adv 6:60206–60214
Kang SM, Rho J, Choi IS, Messersmith PB, Lee H (2009) Norepinephrine: material-independent, multifunctional surface modification reagent. J Am Chem Soc 131:13224–13225
Kang X, Cai W, Zhang S, Cui S (2017) Revealing the formation mechanism of insoluble polydopamine by using a simplified model system. Polym Chem 8:860–864
Kanyong P, Rawlinson S, Davis J (2016) Fabrication and electrochemical characterization of polydopamine redox polymer modified screen-printed carbon electrode for the detection of guanine. Sens Actuators B Chem 233:528–534
Khadka B, Lee B, Kim K-T (2023) Drug delivery systems for personal healthcare by smart wearable patch system. Biomolecules 13:929
Kickelbick G (2007) Introduction to hybrid materials. Hybrid Mater 1:2

Kim E, Lee S, Hong S, Jin G, Kim M, Park KI, Lee H, Jang J-H (2014) Sticky "delivering-from" strategies using viral vectors for efficient human neural stem cell infection by bioinspired catecholamines. ACS Appl Mater Interfaces 6:8288–8294

Kitsati N, Fokas D, Ouzouni M-D, Mantzaris MD, Barbouti A, Galaris D (2012) Lipophilic caffeic acid derivatives protect cells against H_2O_2-induced DNA damage by chelating intracellular labile iron. J Agric Food Chem 60:7873–7879

Kuznowicz M, Jędrzak A, Leda A, Rębiś T, Jesionowski T (2021a) Measurements of working parameters of external mediators for biodetectors based on the polydopamine@magnetite nanoparticles. Measurement 184:1–10

Kuznowicz M, Jędrzak A, Rębiś T, Jesionowski T (2021b) Biomimetic magnetite/polydopamine/β-cyclodextrins nanocomposite for long-term glucose measurements. Biochem Eng J:108127

Kuznowicz M, Rębiś T, Jędrzak A, Nowaczyk G, Szybowicz M, Jesionowski T (2022) Glucose determination using amperometric non-enzymatic sensor based on electroactive poly(caffeic acid)@MWCNT decorated with CuO nanoparticles. Microchim Acta 189:159

Kuznowicz M, Rębiś T, Jędrzak A, Nowaczyk G, Jesionowski T (2023) Facile fabrication of a selective poly(caffeic acid)@MWCNT-Ni$(OH)_2$ hybrid nanomaterial and its application as a non-enzymatic glucose sensor. Chemosensors 11:452

Lee S, Bi L, Chen H, Lin D, Mei R, Wu Y, Chen L, Joo S-W, Choo J (2023) Recent advances in point-of-care testing of COVID-19. Chem Soc Rev 52:8500–8530

Li NB, Ren W, Luo HQ (2008) Simultaneous voltammetric measurement of ascorbic acid and dopamine on poly(caffeic acid)-modified glassy carbon electrode. J Solid State Electrochem 12:693–699

Li T, Xu J, Zhao L, Shen S, Yuan M, Liu W, Tu Q, Yu R, Wang J (2016) Au nanoparticles/poly(caffeic acid) composite modified glassy carbon electrode for voltammetric determination of acetaminophen. Talanta 159:356–364

Li R, Zhai T, Zhao L, Zhang N, He M, Tan L (2021) Preparation of poly(caffeic acid)-CoP nanoparticle film on electrode surface and sensitive voltammetric detection of acetaminophen. Colloids Surf A 627:127173

Liebscher J (2019) Chemistry of polydopamine—scope, variation, and limitation. Eur J Org Chem 2019:4976–4994

Liu Z, Liu Q, Zhang H, Zhang X, Wu J, Sun Z, Zhu M, Hu X, Qi T, Kang H (2022) Genetically engineered protein corona-based cascade nanozymes for enhanced tumor therapy. Adv Funct Mater 32:2208513

Luppa PB, Müller C, Schlichtiger A, Schlebusch H (2011) Point-of-care testing (POCT): current techniques and future perspectives. TrAC Trends Anal Chem 30:887–898

Ma ZM, Wang BT, Cui KY, Wan Y, Li SJ (2019) The preparation of Ag nanoparticles/graphene nanocomposites with polydopamine as coupling agent for enhanced detection of H_2O_2. Int J Electrochem Sci 14:6840–6854

Ma J, Zhang M, Su W, Wu B, Yang Z, Wang X, Qiao B, Pei H, Tu J, Chen D, Wu Q (2022) Photoelectrochemical enzyme biosensor based on TiO_2 nanorod/TiO_2 quantum dot/polydopamine/glucose oxidase composites with strong visible-light response. Langmuir 38:751–761

Makhotkina O, Kilmartin PA (2009) Uncovering the influence of antioxidants on polyphenol oxidation in wines using an electrochemical method: cyclic voltammetry. J Electroanal Chem 633:165–174

Mandal B, Bhattacharjee H, Mittal N, Sah H, Balabathula P, Thoma LA, Wood GC (2013) Core–shell-type lipid–polymer hybrid nanoparticles as a drug delivery platform. Nanomedicine 9:474–491

Mani V, Balamurugan TST, Huang S-T (2020) Rapid one-pot synthesis of polydopamine encapsulated carbon anchored with au nanoparticles: versatile electrocatalysts for chloramphenicol and folic acid sensors. Int J Mol Sci 21:2853

Meng Y, Chen J, Liu Y, Zhu Y, Wong Y-K, Lyu H, Shi Q, Xia F, Gu L, Zhang X (2022) A highly efficient protein corona-based proteomic analysis strategy for the discovery of pharmacodynamic biomarkers. J Pharm Anal 12:879–888

Molnár Á (2020) Polydopamine – its prolific use as catalyst and support material. ChemCatChem 12:2649–2689

Mousavi S, Zarei M, Hashemi S (2018) Polydopamine for biomedical application and drug delivery system. Med Chem 8:218–229

Neubi GMN, Opoku-Damoah Y, Gu X, Han Y, Zhou J, Ding Y (2018) Bio-inspired drug delivery systems: an emerging platform for targeted cancer therapy. Biomater Sci 6:958–973

Park M, Shin M, Kim E, Lee S, Park KI, Lee H, Jang J-H (2014) The promotion of human neural stem cells adhesion using bioinspired poly (norepinephrine) nanoscale coating. J Nanomater 2014:2

Pérez JAC, Sosa-Hernández JE, Hussain SM, Bilal M, Parra-Saldivar R, Iqbal HMN (2019) Bioinspired biomaterials and enzyme-based biosensors for point-of-care applications with reference to cancer and bio-imaging. Biocatal Agric Biotechnol 17:168–176

Perrett S, Buell AK, Knowles TPJ (2019) Biological and bio-inspired nanomaterials. Springer

Poinard B, Neo SZY, Yeo ELL, Heng HPS, Neoh KG, Kah JCY (2018) Polydopamine nanoparticles enhance drug release for combined photodynamic and photothermal therapy. ACS Appl Mater Interfaces 10:21125–21136

Quan DP, Thao BTP, Van Trang N, Le Huy N, Dung NQ, Ahmed MU, Lam TD (2021) The role of copper nanoparticles decorating polydopamine/graphene film as catalyst in the enhancement of uric acid sensing. J Electroanal Chem 893:115322

Rębiś T, Kuznowicz M, Jędrzak A, Milczarek G, Jesionowski T (2021) Design and fabrication of low potential NADH-sensor based on poly(caffeic acid)@multi-walled carbon nanotubes. Electrochim Acta 386:138384

Rohanifar A, Devasurendra AM, Young JA, Kirchhoff JR (2016) Determination of l-DOPA at an optimized poly(caffeic acid) modified glassy carbon electrode. Anal Methods 8:7891–7897

Ruan C, Shi W, Jiang H, Sun Y, Liu X, Zhang X, Sun Z, Dai L, Ge D (2013) One-pot preparation of glucose biosensor based on polydopamine–graphene composite film modified enzyme electrode. Sens Actuators B Chem 177:826–832

Sabu C, Rejo C, Kotta S, Pramod K (2018) Bioinspired and biomimetic systems for advanced drug and gene delivery. J Control Release 287:142–155

Sautter RL, Earnest DM, Halstead DC (2018) What's old is new again: laboratory oversight of point of care testing—guidelines, challenges, and practical strategies. Clin Microbiol Newsl 40:191–198

Srinivasan B, Tung S (2015) Development and applications of portable biosensors. J Lab Autom 20:365–389

Tang Y, Tan Y, Lin K, Zhu M (2021) Research progress on polydopamine nanoparticles for tissue engineering. Front Chem 9:727123

Taskin MB, Xu R, Zhao H, Wang X, Dong M, Besenbacher F, Chen M (2015) Poly(norepinephrine) as a functional bio-interface for neuronal differentiation on electrospun fibers. Phys Chem Chem 17:9446–9453

Tong Q, Qiu N, Ji J, Ye L, Zhai G (2020) Research progress in bioinspired drug delivery systems. Expert Opin Drug Deliv 17:1269–1288

Vasan ASS, Mahadeo DM, Doraiswami R, Huang Y, Pecht M (2013) Point-of-care biosensor system. Front Biosci–Schol 5:39–71

Wang S, Kang Y, Wang L, Zhang H, Wang Y, Wang Y (2013) Organic/inorganic hybrid sensors: a review. Sens Actuators B Chem 182:467–481

Wong WSF, Melendez AJ (2006) Frontiers in research reviews: cutting-edge molecular approaches to therapeutics. Clin Exp Pharmacol Physiol 33:480–481

Xia L, Vemuri B, Gadhamshetty V, Kilduff J (2020) Poly(ether sulfone) membrane surface modification using norepinephrine to mitigate fouling. J Membr Sci 598:117657

Yan J, Wu R, Liao S, Jiang M, Qian Y (2020) Applications of polydopamine-modified scaffolds in the peripheral nerve tissue engineering. Front Bioeng Biotechnol 8:590998

Zare HR, Golabi SM (2000) Caffeic acid modified glassy carbon electrode for electrocatalytic oxidation of reduced nicotinamide adenine dinucleotide (NADH). J Solid State Electrochem 4:87–94
Zarei M (2017) Advances in point-of-care technologies for molecular diagnostics. Biosens Bioelectron 98:494–506
Zhong CJ, Maye MM (2001) Core–shell assembled nanoparticles as catalysts. Adv Mater 13:1507–1511
Zhou Q, Yan B, Xing T, Chen G (2019) Fabrication of superhydrophobic caffeic acid/Fe@cotton fabric and its oil-water separation performance. Carbohydr Polym 203:1–9

Sustainable Marine-Based Biopolymers and Biocomposites for Advanced Biomedical Applications

18

Thi Nga Tran, Binh T. Mai, and John Santigie Conteh

Abstract

Marine algae are sustainable and natural abundant resource that are rich in structural cell wall and storage polysaccharides. Marine polysaccharides are macromolecules with high diversity in monosaccharide composition, glycosidic linkages, structural configuration, molecular weight, and wide ranges of functional groups. Marine-originated polysaccharides have extensively employed in the development of advanced medical devices thanks to their biodegradability, biocompatibility, high mechanical strength, antitumor, anticoagulant, antiviral, antioxidant, and antimicrobial properties. These advantages combined with natural biodiversity of the marine polysaccharides are intriguing for the development of new generation of advanced biomaterials and medical devices. Furthermore, the use of natural biopolymers offers more sustainable, greener pathway for polymeric production and less dependent on the non-renewable fossil petroleum resource. Intriguingly, the properties of marine-based polysaccharide can be leveraged by the hybridization with different synthetic and natural materials, leading to the discovery of biocomposites with unprecedented performances. With a strong focus on sustainability, this chapter will discuss the therapeutic potential and biomedical applications of biocomposites derived from major natural marine polysaccharides from various brown and red algae focusing on alginate, agarose and sulfated galactan-carrageenan.

T. N. Tran (✉)
School of Biological and Chemical Sciences, University of Galway, Galway, Ireland
e-mail: Thinga.Tran@universityofgalway.ie

B. T. Mai · J. S. Conteh
School of Biological and Chemical Sciences, University of Galway, Galway, Ireland

CÚRAM, SFI Research Centre for Medical Devices, University of Galway, Galway, Ireland
e-mail: Binh.Mai@universityofgalway.ie; john.conteh@universityofgalway.ie

M. N. Collins, M. Culebras (eds.), *Sustainable Biopolymers and Composites for Biomedical Applications*, Biomaterials, Bioengineering and Sustainability 5,
https://doi.org/10.1007/978-3-031-91972-5_18

Keywords

Polysaccharide · Algae · Alginate · Agarose · Carrageenan · Biomedical device · Bioapplication

18.1 Introduction

With the coverage of about 70% surface of the earth, marine realm is the largest ecosystem containing over 80% of plant and animal species on earth (Zhang et al. 2023; Park et al. 2022). Polysaccharides are the most abundant biomass in our planet, both on land and under marine environment (Tran et al. 2016). The terrestrial and marine polysaccharides are different in term of chemical structures of the polymeric backbone and the functional groups. Marine environment contains a higher concentration of sulfate compared to freshwater and soil, resulted on distinct sulfation functional groups on the structure of the marine polysaccharides. The ability of ionization of marine polysaccharides, mostly sulfation, offers marine plants strong resistant to desiccation, osmotic stress, heavy metal toxicity, extreme temperature and pH environment (Bloch et al. 2010; Ciarlantini et al. 2024). Marine algae, also known as seaweed, are generally divided into three major groups including brown algae (Phaeophyceae), red algae (Rhodophyceae) and green algae (Chlorophyceae). Depending on the species and geographical conditions, the chemical compositions of algae are varied with polysaccharides (15–76%), proteins (5–47%), minerals (7–36%), and lipids (1–5%) (Yang et al. 2023; Ijaz et al. 2022). The two types of algal polysaccharides are cell wall and storage polysaccharides. A wide ranges algal polysaccharides can be found depending on the algae species, as shown in Fig. 18.1, namely alginate from brown algae, agarose and carrageenan from red algae. The chemical structure and composition of polysaccharides vary substantially based on the type of algae. The most investigated sulfated marine polysaccharides are extracted from the cell walls of macroalgae due to the industrial interest in their hydrocolloid features (Bajpai and Kaarthikeyan 2024). Alginate, the most common used marine polysaccharides, is generally produce from brown algae. Sulfated galactans, including mainly carrageenan, are found in red algae.

In human body, skin is the largest and most essential organ holding important function to protect internal tissues from mechanical damage, microbial infection, and ultraviolet radiation. Different damages (mechanical, heat, chemical, etc.) on the skin create wound (Ghorbani et al. 2023; Kamoun et al. 2017). Generally, the wound healing process involves of various stages including hemostasis, anti-inflammation, cell proliferation, angiogenesis, and tissue regeneration. The serious wound that cannot heal in good time manner will lead to infection and eventually chronic wounds (Lokhande et al. 2018). Wound treatment is one of the major challenges for health care systems around the world. Due to the disruption of the dermal layer, the healing of chronic wound is very limited and required additional medical treatments. Wound dressings play a crucial role in the treatment of large and deep chronic wounds. The wound dressing materials are ideally biocompatible and

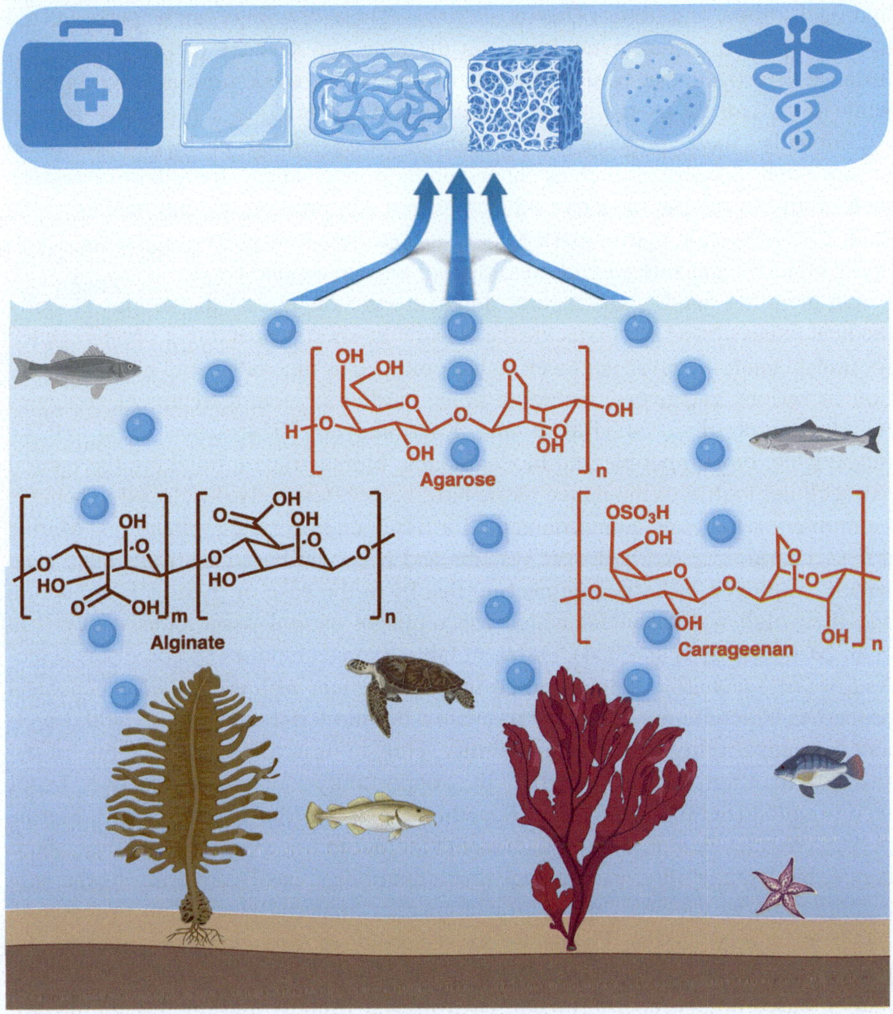

Fig. 18.1 The structures of polysaccharide biopolymers from brown and red algae and their applications in different biomedical devices

biodegradable, offer good moisture environment, remove exudate, protect the wound from pathogens, exhibit good breathability and moisture permeability, promote cell proliferation and accelerate wound healing (Samadi et al. 2020; Wang et al. 2023). Interestingly, for wound dressing application, marine-derived polysaccharides provide several benefits such as promoting wound healing by providing a moist environment that facilitates cell migration and proliferation. They can also act as a barrier against external contaminants and provide a protective layer to prevent further damage to the wound. Plethora studies have shown that marine-derived polysaccharides can be used to develop different types of wound dressings such as hydrogels, films, and fibres (Zhao et al. 2023). These dressings can be personalized to meet specific requirements based on the type and severity of the wound. For instance, hydrogels can be used for deep wounds to provide a moist environment, while films can be used for superficial wounds to provide a protective barrier. Additionally, these polysaccharides can be compounded in biocomposites to improve their properties, such as enhancing their mechanical strength or increasing their ability to release bioactive molecules that can promote wound healing (Mao et al. 2023). Overall, marine-derived polysaccharides show great promise for developing effective and safe wound dressings for various wound types.

On the other hand, a shortage of donated organs is one of the serious globally medical issues nowadays. To tackle the worldwide shortages of donor organs needed for transplantation, tissue engineering has emerged as innovative and effective solution in various endeavors, including bone, cardiac or neural treatment strategies (Ciarlantini et al. 2024; Bajpai and Kaarthikeyan 2024; Chen et al. 2024). Sustainable, biocompatible and biodegradable biomaterials mimicking the natural extracellular matrix of the native tissue have been extensively developed to achieve biomimicry regenerative environments for tissue engineering applications. Marine polysaccharide-derived hydrogel systems and hydrogel-based scaffolds have been widely employed in tissue engineering thanks to the ease of hydrogel production and their high water content which can replicate natural tissue consistency (Liu et al. 2020; Qamar et al. 2024). Different fabrication techniques and precisely selection of polysaccharide types resulted in the materials with controlled mechanical properties which mimic the native tissue in a biomimicry manner along with excellent biocompatibility and biodegradability. This, in turn, accelerates the rate of tissue regeneration, while offering the opportunity for cells/bioactive factor incorporation (Serafin et al. 2023; Tripathi et al. 2009; Martin et al. 2013). Marine polysaccharides feature numerous benefits including low cost, renewability, abundance, biodegradability, exceptional biocompatibility, easily adhering to the skin making them as valuable sources for biomedical material production (Yang et al. 2023; Jafari et al. 2024). Thanks to the versatility in their chemical structure and processing, different synthetic and natural components can be incorporated into marine-based polysaccharides using environment-friendly and low hazardous procedure, leading to development of advanced biomaterials platform for biomedical application such as drug delivery, wound healing, and tissue engineering. In the context of sustainability, marine-derived materials and composites are highly sought after as they hold great promise to implement the concept of circular economy in biomedical sectors. This chapter will discuss marine polysaccharides-derived composites regarding their preparation and biomedical applications. The spotlight will be focused on the biocomposites derived from the most common marine polysaccharides, including alginate, agarose, and carrageenan that can be prepared using simple water-based process.

18.2 Alginates

In the species Laminaria, Ascophyllum, and Fucus of brown algae family, the structural polysaccharide in cell walls and the intercellular matrix are mainly made of common natural alginate. Alginate is commercially available in a wide range of molecular weight making it suitable for different material development for specific applications (Ghorbani et al. 2023; Mao et al. 2023). Alginates are generally the water-soluble salts of alginic acid. The chemical structure of alginate composes of linear copolymers of β-d-mannuronic acid and α-l-guluronic acid linked by 1–4 glycosidic bonds (Fig. 18.1) (Serafin et al. 2023). Alginate hold great potential in various biomedical applications, especially wound dressing, thanks to the high absorption capacity, biocompatibility, biodegradability, ease to fabricate, and economic efficiency.

One of appealing feature of alginate is the capability to form hydrogels in aqueous solutions upon the addition of bivalent metal salts. Such cations can create the coordination bond between carboxylate functional groups in alginate chains, resulting in the crosslinking. Interestingly, it has been demonstrated the formation of alginate hydrogel can be induced by abundant and endogenous bivalent cations such as Ca^{2+} and Mg^{2+}, making it an intriguing candidate for applications in tissue engineering and wound dressings. Depending on the chemical compositions (the ratio between β-d-mannuronic acid and α-l-guluronic acid monomers) of alginate macromolecule, the mechanical stiffness of the obtained hydrogel is varied (Yang et al. 2023; Bajpai and Kaarthikeyan 2024). In particular, the hydrogels containing more β-d-mannuronic acid moiety are softer, whereas the harder hydrogels are achieved with higher content of α-l-guluronic acid monomer. In addition, the combination of alginates with other natural biopolymers (such as chitosan, hyaluronic acid, collagen, fibrin, gelatin, and cellulose) can also offer an interesting approach in the preparation of biocomposites with wide range of bioactivities for diverse bioapplications (Saraiva et al. 2023). Notably, alginate-derived biocomposites are sterilizable using conventional sterilizing techniques which is a critical characteristic for the their clinical translations. In the context of wound dressing, alginate-based composites are patient friendly since they do not cause any pain to patients when being applied and removed from wounds without causing significant tissue damage. Such composites have great ability to promote epithelial cell proliferation and tissue development, absorb exudate, protect wounds from maceration, provide high gas exchange, and keep moist wound environment (Mao et al. 2023). They also offers the possibility to incorporate active agents such as antioxidants and antimicrobial compounds, obtaining the multifunctional wound dressings materials and devices. This, in turn, provides an aid in medicine administration *via* the skin, reducing bacterial infections and faster healing of inspected wounds (Yang et al. 2023; Wang et al. 2023; Mao et al. 2023).

18.2.1 Alginates-Based Biocomposites for Wound Healing Applications

One of the first example of the all-marine-originating biocomposites were developed by Yang et al. (2023). In this study, novel wound dressings biocomposites made of alginate and chitosan with optimized compositional and structural design that could adapt to different wound area were developed. The marine polymeric microcapsules with alginate core and chitosan shell were formed through polyelectrolyte complexation and glutaraldehyde cross-linking using microfluidic electrospray method. The obtained microcapsule showed great biocompatibility and antibacterial capacity. In addition, vascular endothelial growth factor was loaded into the microcapsules and able to release in a prolong period. These advanced microcapsules offered several benefits when applied to wound sites such as inhibiting bacterial growth and promoting angiogenesis during wound closure demonstrating the values of the microcapsules as drug delivery vehicles in wound dressing in clinical practice (Yang et al. 2023).

Alginates were compounded in a biocomposites with amino acid and inorganic ion to achieve the hydrogel for wound dressing (Mao et al. 2023). The dried films composed of sodium alginate and arginine were obtained by simple and scalable solvent casting method and then crosslinked with zinc ion to form sodium alginate-arginine-zinc ion hydrogel. The zinc ion chelated hydrogel showed high swelling capacity, great antioxidant activity, strong antibacterial inhibition against *E. coli* and *S. aureus*, and ability to promote the proliferation of fibroblasts. Interestingly, they also down-regulated the expression of inflammatory factors (TNF-α and IL-6) and promoted the growth factor levels (VEGF and TGF-β1). Thanks to such characteristics, these hydrogels can reduce wound inflammation and accelerate re-epithelialization, angiogenesis and wound healing. In the *in vivo* test on rat skin, the alginate-based hydrogels featured better wound healing efficacy in comparison with other conventional dressings. The wound was completely closed after 14 days since applying the hydrogel. Hence, with a simple but effective fabrication technique, such alginate-derived hydrogel represents a promising and sustainable wound dressing materials in a large scale (Mao et al. 2023).

To obtain the hydrogel with improved biocompatibility and bioactivity, the biocomposites of alginate and other bio-derived materials were also investigated. Wang et al. developed a dual-component hydrogel system composed of sodium alginate and platelet-rich plasma through a simple one-step thrombin activation process for wound healing treatment. In this approach Fe^{3+} ions were used as crosslinker to crosslink sodium alginate in the presence of coagulated platelet-rich plasma activated by thrombin. The hydrogels demonstrated excellent biocompatibility, particularly in term of hemocompatibility, cytocompatibility, and histopathology. These traits are desirable for the acceleration of the wound healing process. Indeed, such alginate-derived hydrogel showed the ability to assist cell proliferation and vascular regeneration. In fact, *in vivo* wound healing test revealed that the hydrogel exhibited effectively wound closure on the full-thickness defected skin of rats, demonstrating the potential of the developed alginate-based hydrogels for clinical wound healing treatment (Wang et al. 2023).

Nanocomposites comprising of hydroxyapatite and zinc oxide nanoparticles and alginate as the matrix were also extensively investigated for wound dressing application. In an conventional fabrication technique, such NPs are dispersed in alginate solution, followed by cross-linking using chitosan and/or different metal ions including Ca^{2+}, Zn^{2+}, and Cu^{2+} (Yang et al. 2023). The presence of metal ion led to slightly acidic environment which is beneficial for wound healing process. The alginate-derived nanocomposites showed effective antimicrobial effect against *E. coli* and *S. aureus* as well as promoted the proliferation of the fibroblasts, increased the amount of collagen fibers, along with new arterial and venous capillaries. These novel marine-derived featured great adsorption of exudate, maintaining necessary wound humidity, biocompatibility, increased antimicrobial activity, ensuring integrity and painless dressing removal making them suitable materials for a wide range of wound care applications (Yang et al. 2023).

It was also demonstrated that the introduction of alginate into innovative electroactive hydrogel could offer significant restoring wound currents, promoting cell proliferation, thus accelerating the wound healing process (Zhao et al. 2023). Zhao et al. had developed novel hydrogel system composed of electroactive oxidized sodium alginate, carboxymethyl chitosan and silver nanoparticles without the need of conductive fillers or synthesized conductive polymers. The electroactive hydrogels exhibited injectability, self-healing properties, along with excellent biocompatibility and high antibacterial activities against both *S. aureus* and *E. coli*. Showing tunable gelation time and high swelling ratio, such hydrogels can readily fit to the irregular-shaped wound without compromising a full absorption of the exudates. In addition, the developed hydrogels significantly enhanced the proliferation of L929 cells *in vitro* under electrical stimulation. Intriguingly, such hydrogels can facilitate collagen deposition and angiogenesis with less inflammatory infiltration *in vivo*. In addition to the capability of inducing anti-inflammation, promoting the fibroblasts proliferation, and angiogenesis, the alginate-based hydrogel significantly accelerated the wound healing process in the full-thickness and defected skin model. This new polyelectrolyte polysaccharides-based electroactive hydrogels provided promising advanced and improved therapeutic approach for chronic wounds treatment (Zhao et al. 2023).

18.2.2 Alginates-Based Biocomposites for Tissue Engineering Applications

In addition to wound dressing applications, alginate has also been extensively employed in the development of novel materials for tissue engineering applications (Serafin et al. 2023). Serafin et al. had comprehensively investigated different hydrogel formulations made of popular biopolymers including alginate, hyaluronic acid and gelatin for various targeted tissue engineering strategies. Pure alginate hydrogels showed a quick degradation and high swelling property, but lack of cell binding sites. These features are suitable for medical devices coating as such gels can limit the initial cellular infiltration while being implanted *in situ*. The incorporation of gelatin to the alginate matrix did not significantly alter mechanical, morphological, or swelling behaviors of the obtained hydrogels although the existence of gelatine as extracellular matrix mimic might promote the cell adhesion. On the other hand, the hydrogel composed of alginate and hyaluronic acid featured intricate and controlled pore size, similar swelling profiles to the pure alginate hydrogel. The variation of physico-chemical properties of these alginate, gelatin and hyaluronic acid hydrogels offer the possibility to identify the most suitable natural polysaccharides hydrogel system for different targeted tissue engineering applications (Serafin et al. 2023).

In order to improve the mechanical and biological properties of alginate-derived hydrogels, Ghorbani et al. reported the dual crosslinking of alginate, oxidized alginate and silk fibroin *in situ* through simultaneous ionic gelation using $CaCO_3$-(Glucono-Delta-Lactone) ($CaCO_3$-GDL) and Schiff-base reaction (Ghorbani et al. 2023). Fibroin protein for possessing cell-binding sites was grafted to oxidized alginate through the Schiff-base reaction. The mechanical properties of the hydrogel can be modulated by using in situ encapsulated CaCO3-GDL as reservoir to slowly release Ca^{2+} ions, leading to the controlled gelation time by ionic crosslinking. Thanks to the covalent imine bond formation and the incorporation of silk fibroin and oxidized alginate, the mechanical strength of alginate-based hydrogels considerably improved with the compressive modulus increased from 28 to 67 kPa in comparison with the physically crosslinked alginate hydrogel. A high biocompatibility of the developed materials enables the encapsulation of bone marrow mesenchymal stem cells into hydrogel scaffolds for bone tissue regeneration. Interestingly, encapsulated cells showed more differentiation into bone tissue in case of composite hydrogel scaffold in compared to the case of physically crosslinked alginate hydrogel, demonstrating high potential of the developed composite scaffold for bone tissue engineering applications (Ghorbani et al. 2023).

In another approach, the bioactive and biomimetic scaffolds composed of alginate-chitosan polyelectrolyte complexes were fabricated by freeze-drying techniques following by crosslinking with $CaCl_2$. The structural and mechanical properties of the scaffolds can be tuned by varying molar ratios of alginate and chitosan components. After the crosslinking step, the scaffolds showed a less porous structure and higher elastic modulus. To obtain the scaffolds with bioactive and biomimetic features, the alginate-based scaffold was further functionalized with 3,4-dihydroxyhydrocinnamic acid and then with $PySO_3$ or Heparin to introduce groups/molecules mimicking the extracellular matrix, thus promoting the cell attachment. The functionalize scaffolds showed high cell viability when tested on fibroblasts, represented by the capability of cells to grow in cluster in high population. These functionalized scaffolds presented significant high antioxidant capacity, higher porosity with more interconnected pore and more regularity of the pore size and as well as improved hydrophilicity, resulting in an excellent penetration and proliferation of fibroblasts into the scaffold. This innovative alginate-derived scaffolds have high potential to be used as novel biocomposites for tissue engineering, especially for the regeneration of skeleton muscle disease (Ciarlantini et al. 2024).

18.3 Sustainable Biocomposites Based on Agarose

Agarose, also known as agar, is the major polysaccharide of the cell wall of some red algae species (Fig. 18.1), including mainly *Gelidium* and *Gracilaria*. The extraction of agarose from such seaweeds species involves multi alkaline and acid pretreatment and hot extraction processes along with bleaching step. Agarose can be extracted using ionic liquid and/or deep eutectic solvent which might offer a more efficient and greener approach. The constituted unit of agarose is a disaccharide of β-D-galactose and 3,6-anhydro-α-L-galactopyranose. Due to a medium molar mass of 100,000 g/mol and a good balance between hydrogen bonding donor and acceptor in its structure, agarose can undergo the gelation based on temperature by creating intermolecular hydrogen bonding. Interestingly, the unique chemical structure also offers agarose hydrogel with a self-healing feature by simply tuning the temperature. In comparison to other polysaccharides, agarose is very appealing as the gelation can occur without the need of any toxic and hazardous crosslinkers. The formation of gel usually occurs when a hot solution of agarose in water is cooled to below 35–45 °C. The obtained gels remain stable at temperatures up to 85 °C. Notably, the gel formation can be achieved at a concentration as low as 0.1% weight, offering versatility for the formulation with other components in biocomposites development. The global production of agarose is estimated to be 10,000 tons per annum. Although the primary application of agarose is still centered in food industry as thickening agents, its unique physiochemical properties and biocompatibility are promising for various applications, including but not limited to environmental engineering, tissue engineering, bioimaging, drug delivery systems, cancer therapy, and biosensors. Along with its abundant and renewable nature, agarose represents an appealing building block for the development of sustainable composites for advanced applications in biomedical research.

18.3.1 Agarose-(In)organic Particle Biocomposites for Biomedical Applications

Several pioneer studies have demonstrated the potential of agarose as innovative materials for different biomedical applications. Various fabrication approaches based on physical treatment such as wet spinning, freeze-drying, electrospinning, gas foaming and emulsion templating have been used to prepared fiber, hydrogels, scaffold and micro capsules of agarose. The properties of obtained materials can be finely tuned to meet the demand for different applications including tunable morphology and biocompatibility. Agarose-based hydrogels exhibit excellent biocompatibility along with controlled microstructures have been found for various applications including islet implantation, drug delivery device and scaffolds for tissue regeneration. One of the first examples of agarose-based hydrogel was reported by Iwata et al. It was demonstrated that a formulation of agarose microbeads and pancreas islets could be injected *in vivo*, resulting in the alloislets in diabetic mice with improved stability. Notably, the encapsulation of the islets in agarose gels diminishes the need of using immunosuppressants. Other studies also showed hydrogel made of agarose can be used as scaffold to promote the growth of human chondrocytes, offering the allogenic cartilage implants for osteoarthritis treatment. Later, Tuszynski and coworkers showed that the freeze-dried agarose scaffold with multi lumen and linear morphology provided a proper axonal regeneration, leading to the improvement of spinal cord injury treatment. Nevertheless, materials made of entire agarose suffer a very slow biodegradability, low cell attachment, and modest mechanical properties which remain bottlenecks in the context of translational research. To overcome such intrinsic drawbacks, the incorporation of other components into agarose matrix to leverage the performance of resulting composites has been a highly sought after approach. Indeed, the development of agarose-based composites for biomedical application has been a very active research field with tremendous potential in the last decade. Given its versatile processing, different components can be incorporated into agarose matrix, mainly including metal-based nanoparticles, clay/ceramic particles, carbon-based materials and other polymers.

Metal-based NPs can be introduced into agarose matrix by simply mixing the two components at different mass ratio. The other approach is *in situ* synthesis in which the metal ions are impregnated in agarose hydrogel matrix, followed by their reduction/oxidation using additional chemical reagents. Using these approaches, a wide range of different metal-based NPs have been successfully incorporated in agarose-based composites. They include pure metal (Pd, Cu, Pt, Ag, and Au), metal oxide (NiO, ZnO, TiO_2, Fe_3O_4, and Co_3O_4), and chalcogenide (ZnS). The incorporation of metal-based NPs not only improves the mechanical properties of agarose gel but also results in biocomposites with interesting characteristics that are desirable for biomedical applications. Indeed, due to their antimicrobial activities, NPs made of Ag, ZnO and TiO_2 have been widely incorporated in agarose gels for wound healing applications. Chen and coworker employed a green approach by using agarose as reducing agent and capping agent to prepare Ag NPs nanocomposites. The versatility of such composites offers the capability to load odorranain A, an antimicrobial peptide, which led to a superior wound healing performance *in vivo* (Chen et al. 2021).

In comparison to noble metal-based, the use of abundant and natural clay/ceramic to prepare advanced composite of agarose is a very appealing avenue in the context of sustainability. It has been widely demonstrated that such biomineral nano/microparticles can harness the mechanical properties of agarose due to a good interaction between agarose polymer chains and their hydrophilic surfaces. In addition, the microstructure of resulting composites such as porosity and pore connectivity can be modulated by finely tuning the fabrication process. Although different types of clay/ceramic nano/micro-particles can be introduced in agarose matrix, montmorillonite (MMT) and hydroxyapatite (HAP) have been of great interest due to their abundance and excellent biocompatibility. Due to its layered microstructures, the introduction of MMT into agarose gels has been found to improve the loading capacity of curcumin thanks to the intercalation within the layered structures (Samadi et al. 2020; Jayrajsinh et al. 2017; ul Haque and Nasar 2018). Samadi and coworkers showed that incorporating MMT in chitosan-agarose hydrogels improved the loading capacity from 49% to 62% (Samadi et al. 2020). Interestingly, a sustained release of curcumin from such composites over the course of 96 h can be achieved while pH can be used as a means to trigger a faster release. Such composite shows great promise in the treatment of breast cancer in an *in vitro* model (Samadi et al. 2020). MMT containing agarose-based composites have also been found for potential in wound dressing applications (Zhang et al. 2023; Polat et al. 2020). Indeed, Polat and coworkers proposed the applications of agarose/κ-carrageenan/MMT as robust and versatile biomaterials to load and deliver both analgesic lidocaine hydrochloride and antibiotic chloramphenicol to the wound simultaneously (Polat et al. 2020). Along with excellent antibacterial properties and mechanical flexibility, the obtained composite represents an interesting candidate for advanced wound dressing. In another approach, Zhang and coworker impregnated agarose/MMT sponge gels with silver ion to afford the antimicrobial properties (Zhang et al. 2023). The developed gel sponge featured a good mechanical strength and good water retention as MMT can serve as the cross-linker between agarose chains. Thanks to such properties, the resulting sponge gels offered a good wound healing performance and a promising capability to prevent blood bleeding even in an *in vivo* model (Zhang et al. 2023). In addition to MMT, HAP is also of great interest to develop sustainable composite based on agarose. As an abundant biomineral found in human and animal bones, HAP has been highly sought after for bone regeneration applications (Shashvatt et al. 2017; Szcześ et al. 2017; Sánchez-Salcedo et al. 2008). Indeed, Akashi's group prepared the agarose/HAP gels by soaking process in which HAP crystals were formed in situ within agarose matrix (Tabata et al. 2003, 2005). The obtained composites featured a good biocompatibility, adhesiveness, leading to the osteoconductive and hemostatic capabilities. Fascinatingly, the developed composite could serve as bone-grafting materials, inducing bone regeneration in an *in vivo* primate model. This study suggested that gels made of agarose and HAP might offer a novel approach to regenerate lost periodontal tissue. The potential of HAP-agarose composite as drug delivery system has also been studied (Samadi et al. 2021). Samadi and coworkers incorporated HAP nanoparticles into agarose/polyvinylpyrrolidone hydrogels to boost the loading of quercetin, a potent anticancer agent, up to 61% (Samadi et al. 2021). Thanks to a unique interactions between HAP, quercetin and polymer chains, the release of quercetin is rather low at physiological conditions while an accelerated release can be achieved at mild-acidic pH. This, in turn, might potentiate the potential of quercetin in the treatment of solid tumor. Composites made of agarose and mesoporous HAP were also appealing for the delivery of antibiotics such as amoxicillin and gentamicin (Kolanthai et al. 2015, 2016, 2017). A prolonged and controlled release of such antibiotics can be achieved by fine tuning the morphology and doping density of HAP (Kolanthai et al. 2015, 2016, 2017).

Carbon-based materials such as carbon nanotubes (CNT) and graphene/graphene oxide (GO) are promising for biomedical applications thanks to their unique structures (Islam et al. 2022; Ku et al. 2013; Shin et al. 2016). The abundance of sp^2 carbon in such materials is appealing for the loading of different bioactive compounds thanks to the π-π stacking interaction, being of interest in the context of drug delivery (Yazdi et al. 2020). The incorporation of such materials into agarose gels offers a high biocompatibility of the resulting composites with a higher level of control over the release of therapeutics. Indeed, such composites have emerged as an interesting class of materials for controlled drug delivery systems applications (Dong et al. 2021; Najafi et al. 2024; Rajabzadeh-Khosroshahi et al. 2022). Recently, composite made of graphene oxide, chitosan, and agarose has been developed recently to deliver 5-fluororacil (Rajaei et al. 2023). The obtained composites featured a pH-triggered release trait that could be promising for breast cancer treatment (Rajaei et al. 2023). Ones of the most intriguing properties of CNT/graphene and GO are their intrinsic conductivity and excellent mechanical properties (Islam et al. 2022; Ku et al. 2013; Shin et al. 2016). They are highly sought after materials to reinforce the mechanical properties of the scaffolds made of biopolymers such as polysaccharides, gelatin, hyaluronic acid and collagens. In addition, their conductivity was found to be essential for neural and cardiac tissue engineering, and injured spinal cord repair (Islam et al. 2022; Ku et al. 2013; Shin et al. 2016; Jalilinejad et al. 2023). In a pioneer study, it was shown that composite fiber made of agarose and CNT were biocompatible and non-toxic (Lewitus et al. 2011). Fascinatingly, such fibrous composites were shown to facilitate attachment and response of neural cells both *in vitro* and *in vivo*, representing an advanced materials platform for neural engineering and interfacing (Lewitus et al. 2011). Later, it was shown that scaffolds made of conductive multiwall CNT-agarose having multi-microchannel can trigger the growth of neuron following electrical stimulation (Park et al. 2022; Liu et al. 2020). It is of note that most carbon-materials-based agarose composites have been developed towards energy storage, food packaging and waste water treatment. In the context of cardiac tissue engineering and injured spinal cord repair, the potentials of such materials remained an untaped research avenues, yet to be further explored (Park et al. 2022; Chen et al. 2024).

18.3.2 Alginates-Based Polymeric Biocomposites for Biomedical Applications

Due to its versatility and robustness in processing, agarose can be compounded with different polymers including the synthetic and natural ones. The hybrid materials made of agarose and other synthetic polymers such as poly(caprolactone) (PCL), poly(ethylene glycol) (PEG), poly(methyl methacrylate) (PMMA), poly(*N*-dimethyl aminoethyl methacrylate) (PDMAEMA), polyvinyl alcohol (PVA), poly(aniline) (PAN), and polydopamine (PDOPA) have been reported, showing intriguing physiochemical properties including pH-responsiveness, tunable mechanical properties, amphiphilicity, and conductivity. These properties are desirable for various applications, ranging from drug delivery to tissue engineering and biosensors. However, due to a drastic difference in chemical structure which leads to a low compatibility between such polymers with agarose, the hybridization protocol often involves multiple chemical modification steps with the need of many toxic and hazardous reagents. This, in turn, makes such materials less appealing in the context of sustainability.

On the other hand, the similarity in water solubility and the abundance of hydroxy groups of biopolymers, for instance other polysaccharides, enables a straightforward hybridization between agarose and such polymers. The involved processes are usually water-based without the need of multiple chemical modifications, offering a highly sustainable fabricating approach. The incorporation of other polysaccharide results in the alteration between agarose and other loaded molecules along with the improvement in mechanical properties of the obtained composites. These features are of interest for controlled drug delivery applications. It has been shown that agarose can be used to improve the mechanical properties of calcium alginate hydrogels beads (Yin et al. 2018). The swelling of gel beads can be controlled by tuning the amount of doped agarose, leading to a sustained release of indomethacin within 720 min. Interestingly, the gel beads exhibited a pH-dependent swelling characteristic, making them interesting candidate for gastric-intestine tract delivery (Yin et al. 2018). Later, Zhang and coworkers developed mixed hydrogels made of agarose and κ-carrageenan (Zhao et al. 2020). The incorporation of κ-carrageenan was found the alter the mechanism of agarose gels formation while a remarkable increase in the loading of metformin hydrochloride could be achieved (Zhao et al. 2020). In the context of cancer therapy, composites based on agarose/chitosan doped with graphitic carbon nitride and γ-alumina have been also developed and used as delivery systems for curcumin and 5-fluororacil, respectively (Rajabzadeh-Khosroshahi et al. 2022; Bayat et al. 2023). In addition to polysaccharides, proteins including mainly gelatin and fibrin have also been studied. The introduction of such proteins usually provide the composite materials with enhanced mechanical properties along with a good cell attachment (Tripathi et al. 2009; Gupta et al. 2014; Bhat and Kumar 2012). The first example was reported by Bloch and coworkers in which agarose cryogel scaffolds grafted with gelatin were prepared by a two-step subsequent freezing/thawing procedure (Bloch et al. 2010). Thanks to wide porous structures, the implanted cryogel scaffolds promote the formation of new blood vessels in diabetic mice model, demonstrating their potential in vascularization (Bloch et al. 2010). Kumar's group used cryogelation technology to prepare different types of binary and trinary biopolymers scaffolds made of agarose-gelatin and agarose-gelatin-chitosan with controlled porosity (Tripathi et al. 2009; Gupta et al. 2014; Bhat and Kumar 2012). The agarose-gelatin offered good attachment of fibroblast cells along with excellent biocompatibility (Tripathi et al. 2009). Whilst, agarose-gelatin-chitosan cryogel scaffolds can support the regeneration of the skin and cardiac tissue by an enhancement of biocompatibility and cell attachment (Bhat and Kumar 2012). Fascinatingly, the same cryogel scaffolds can be used to repair of subchondral cartilage defects even in rodent models (Gupta et al. 2014). Once being implanted in the cartilage of New Zealand white rabbit, cryogel scaffolds does not provoke any undesirable immune response and severe inflammation, leading to a good cartilage regeneration performance (Gupta et al. 2014). In addition to gelatin, fibrin has also been subjected to the development of agarose-protein composites (de la Cruz Cardona et al. 2011; Ionescu et al. 2011). One of the first examples of agarose-fibrin composites was reported by Perez and coworkers (de la Cruz Cardona et al. 2011). The authors showed that the hydrogels made of such composites exhibited an excellent optical transparency in visible range. Along with a good biocompatibility tested on keratocytes, such hydrogel represents an interesting candidate for cornea stroma substitutes (de la Cruz Cardona et al. 2011; Ionescu et al. 2011, 2017; Alaminos et al. 2006). The same hydrogel platform was also tested on rabbit cornea model, showing the capability of promoting the formation of stratified layer of epithelial cells along with stromal keratocytes proliferation (Alaminos et al. 2006). The same group also demonstrated that agarose-fibrin hydrogels can be used as scaffolds for generating the artificial oral mucosa (Martin et al. 2013; Rodríguez et al. 2012).

18.4 Carrageenan Biopolymer

Carrageenans (CGs) are an interesting family of biopolymers with linear sulphated polysaccharides that are extracted from the Florideophyceae class of red algae (Pacheco-Quito et al. 2020). Their chemical structure comprise basic disaccharide unit consisting of alternating 3-linked β-D-galactopyranose and 4-linked α-D-galactopyranose residue units. With notable differences in their anhydro moiety and the number or position of the sulphate group (s) in their monosaccharides, three groups of commercially relevant CGs have been identified namely, kappa- (κ-), iota- (ι-), and lambda- (λ-) carrageenan, which have one, two, and three sulphate groups in their basic disaccharide units, respectively. CGs are biocompatible and are generally recognized as safe (GRAS) by the FDA (Liu et al. 2023).

In addition, they do also possess unique physicochemical gel forming attribute that positions them for applicability mostly in the food and cosmetic industries, where they have been widely used as gelling and thickening agents. Apart from their thermally reversible gelation property, CGs are also known to be water soluble, viscoelastic and have high zeta potential. They also exhibit strong bioactivity with proven immunomodulatory, anticoagulation, and antiviral potentials. Moreover, the ability to chemically modify their structures *via* sulfation, methylation, glycosylation, or by substituting their functional groups with other polymeric materials enhances their utility in forming functional biocomposites (Jiang et al. 2021). All these characteristic properties render carrageenan biopolymers to be suitable candidate for a number of biomedical applications such as targeted drug delivery, wound healing dressings, bone/cartilage regeneration in tissue engineering, 3D bioprinting, biosensing device fabrication, to name just a few (Pacheco-Quito et al. 2020). The solubility of CGs is made possible by the presence of hydroxyl and sulphate functionalities in their native structure, and their dissolution rate is dependent on not only the type of carrageenan but also on parameters such as the medium's pH, temperature, and type cation present in solution. On the other hand, the presence and amount of the 3,6-anhydrogalactose ring in their structures dictates the extent of their hydrophobicity (Alba and Kontogiorgos 2018). With a trend of 3,6-anhydrogalactose content being kappa > iota > lambda-carrageenan, it therefore stands to reason why κ-carrageenan dissolves more slowly than their λ- and ι-carrageenan counterparts (Qamar et al. 2024). These characteristics have a strong impact on the processing step in the preparation of carrageenan-based biocomposites. The ability of CGs to form gel upon interaction with metal ions like calcium and potassium is one of the most important features, accounting for their pharmaceutical and commercial significance. This gelling attribute arise due to the interaction between the negatively charged sulphate groups of CGs and the metallic cationic species upon cooling the solution, as these ions act as crosslinking agents, helping to stabilize the gel's helical network structure. The nature of the gel formed, be they clear or turbid, rigid or elastic, tough or soft, and heat stable or thermally reversible, is dependent not only on the cationic and CG type, but also on presence of co-solutes and amount of sulphate groups present in their structure (Pacheco-Quito et al. 2020; Necas and Bartosikova 2013). In this later case, the lower the amount of sulphate groups, the better their chance of gelation. Thus, κ-carrageenan with one sulphate group forms harder and brittle gels, I-carrageenan (two sulphate groups) produces weak and soft gels, whereas λ-carrageenan barely produces viscous non gel liquids in the presence of mono or bi cationic species. However, recent studies show they (λ-CGs) can form gels in the presence of trivalent ions like ferric ions (Fe^{3+}) and aluminum ions (Al^{3+}) (Pacheco-Quito et al. 2020; Liu et al. 2023). Viscoelasticity is a notable feature of CGs. Such properties originate from the varying motion of their polymeric chains as they interact and glide past each other. When the chains strongly interact, they become viscous, which represent a state of resistance to flow. On the other hand, when CGs are subjected to an applied stress or shear force they become less viscous (thixotropic). This attribute makes CG biopolymer and their derived composites useful candidates for 3D bioprinting applications. The viscoelastic property of CG biopolymers is influenced by the ion concentration and carrageenan type, and can thus be enhanced by adding other polymeric or nanomaterials to alter their ionic interactions, gelation and structural properties (Liu et al. 2023).

Another feature of CG is that they are negatively charged biopolymers due to the presence of their ionizable sulfate groups in their native structures. This attribute accord CGs the ability to interact with several other positively charged molecules by means of electrostatic interaction, offering different therapeutic perspectives (Li et al. 2014).

18.4.1 Carrageenan in Drug Delivery (DD) Application

Carrageenan being a biocompatible biopolymer with interesting gelling, hydrolysable glycosidic bonds, negatively charged sulphate groups for electrostatic interaction, and the presence of hydroxyl groups as site for chemical modifications with other polymeric materials, are regarded as prospective biomaterials for drug delivery systems. For this application, CG's rapid swelling, tunable stimuli responsiveness of their gel and notable biodegradation, which result to their rapid removal from living systems after administration further outlines their usefulness. To enhance their DD performance, various combinations of CGs with other types (e.g., *ι*-, *λ*-, *κ*-) or with different bio/synthetic polymers including mostly Chitosan, Sodium alginate, psyllium, pectin, polyacrylamide, poly vinyl alcohol, hyaluronic acid etc. by means of either electrostatic interaction, cross linking chemistries or related chemical modifications have been employed.

For instance, Sobia Noreen and team reported the preparation of Chitosan/κ--Carrageenan/sodium tripolyphosphate CS/CG/STPP polymeric nanoparticle (NPs) composites to which Naproxen, a drug known to cure pain, inflammation, and arthritis related stiffness but with formidable gastrointestinal tract side effects, were loaded using polyelectrolyte complexation technique (Noreen et al. 2021). Here, they explored the positive charged amino groups of CS and the negative charges on the sulphate and phosphate groups of CG and STPP (added as crosslinker), respectively. These NPs were further encapsulated into a Carbopol 940 (Ca-940) gel system, before evaluating their therapeutic drug delivery capability. By *in vitro* study of drug permeation done using full-thickness rat skin, about 88.6% of drug permeated from the Naproxen loaded Carrageenan-based nanocomposites, while *in vivo* study done on Wistar rats revealed them to be more effective in treating arthritis-related stiffness with no observed skin irritation. In a similar direction, Kulkarni et al. (2012) using polyacrylamide grafted on k-CG and sodium alginate developed an intestine targeting pH-sensitive carrageenan-based hydrogel beads. The obtained hydrogel beads were further loaded with ketoprofen, a drug used as painkiller and to treat osteoarthritis. By means of *in vitro* pulsating swelling study, 10% of the drug was reportedly released in acidic medium (pH 1.2), contrasting to 90% released in alkaline pH 7.4, suggesting a very promising intestinal delivery platform. On the other hand, follow up stomach histopathology studies done *in vivo* on albino rats with Ketoprofen loaded CG-based platform confirmed significant reduction in previously observed gastrointestinal side effects of the free drug including ulceration, hemorrhage, and erosion of the gastric mucosa. In another study aimed at control delivery of meropenem, an antibacterial drug used to treat a wide range of bacterial infections, Uzma Ijaz et al. developed a thermoreversible injectable hydrogel platform based on *k*-carrageenan/hyaluronic acid biopolymers (Ijaz et al. 2022). This gel system was prepared using the solvent casting method. By means of an *in vitro* study done on the developed meropenem loaded hydrogel, controlled release of about 96.1% and 94.7% of meropenem in phosphate buffer saline (PBS pH 7.4) and simulated wound fluid at pH 6.8 within 24 h were respectively confirmed. The study also shows the platform's strong bacterial inhibition effects on P. aeruginosa, S. aureus, and E. coli. Following *in vivo* study on Sprague Dawley rats, the meropenem loaded carrageenan-based thermogels demonstrated an accelerated wound closure (90%) in comparison to the 60% observed in the negative control group (treated with saline) over 14 days, highlighting the CG-based thermogel's synergistic wound-healing potential.

18.4.2 Carrageenan in Wound Healing Applications

One of the notable applications of CGs-based biocomposites is wound healing application. To support wound healing, the excellent biocompatibility, good water holding capacity, and potent bioactivity of carrageenan-based hydrogels are the main driving force to their adoption as wound dressings alternatives to the traditional bandages and wools. They have been shown to enhance cell migration or re-epithelialization (Kamoun et al. 2017; Qamar et al. 2024).

For such wound healing application, Lokhande and colleagues reported the development of κCG-based hydrogel to which they loaded nanosilicate (Lokhande et al. 2018). The introduction of the nanosilicate was found to improve the hydrogel stability *in vitro*. Such biocomposite also boosted the wound healing process, through improved cellular interaction with the composites surface, suppressed release of entrapped vascular endothelial growth factor (VEGF), and aid tissue regeneration. Hydrogels for wound healing applications were also produced using cyclic β-(1→3) (1→6) glucan/carrageenan (CBG/Car) composites (Nair et al. 2016). The film derived from the gel was loaded with a hydrophobic drug, ciprofloxacin. The addition of CBG, a molecule with inherent immunomodulatory activities improves the resulting gel's porosity, drug-loading tendency and as well enhance cell proliferation. By means of *in vitro* cellular and *in vivo* excision wounds study performed in rats, the hydrogel films show much accelerated wound closure compared to the control experiment. As an approach to address diabetic wounds, Sohail et al. reports the development of carrageenan-based biopolymer hydrogel composites for use as wound dressing (Khaliq et al. 2022). The composite consists of chitosan HCl, κ-carrageenan and polyvinyl alcohol PVA, and cefotaxime sodium, a potent anti-bacterial drug known for its effectiveness to both Gram-positive and negative bacteria. To form this hydrogel platform, the solvent casting approach was adopted. The obtained gel was shown to have Oxygen permeability values greater than 8.2 mg/ml. Further *in vitro* studies revealed that loaded cefotaxime drug can be sustainably released from the hydrogel system, suppressing bacterial proliferation. Fascinatingly, *in vivo* experiments conducted on diabetic burn rat model indicated that cefotaxime loaded hydrogel membrane could support wound healing by promoting re-epithelization and tissue formation, when compared to other control groups.

In another approach, carrageenan and polyethylene oxide composite films were prepared by J.S. Boateng et al. exploring the solvent casting film technique (Boateng et al. 2013). Glycerol was used as plasticizer to improve the flexibility of obtained composites films. Streptomycin and diclofenac were separately loaded with the aim to treat chronic wound infections and regulate the inflammatory phase of the wound healing process, respectively. By means of a series of *in vitro* experiments, the mucoadhesion, drug dissolution and antibacterial properties of these drug loaded films were evaluated. Indeed, the films absorbed significant amount of the simulated wound fluid and adhered well to protect the wound surface. Upon controlled release of both drugs within 72 h, a strong bacteria inhibition growth was observed on

S. aureus, *P. aeruginosa* and *E. coli*, being superior to the individual drugs inhibition levels.

18.4.3 Carrageenan in Tissue Engineering Applications

In addition to drug delivery and wound healing application, their bio-availabilities makes carrageenan-derived biocomposites promising candidate for tissue engineering. Indeed, the composites made of nanoparticles and/or other polymeric materials have found great applicability in tissue engineering, targeting the regeneration of in hard/soft tissue. In recent years, CG-based hydrogels have been proposed as bio-ink in 3D printing of organs thanks to their ability to incorporate and support the growth of cells (Qamar et al. 2024; Khan et al. 2020; Murphy and Atala 2014).

In the context of hard tissues regeneration such as bones and teeth, CG-based hydrogels, in particular iota-CG origin, have gained tremendous interest thanks to their high viscosity, interconnected porosity that enhance tissue cells vascularization along with their ability to produce bone like apatite comprising calcium-phosphate and type I collagen (Zhang et al. 2018; Daniel-da-Silva et al. 2007).

With the aim to regenerate bone tissue, Bajpai D. et al. in 2024 developed carrageenan-alginate calcium chloride interconnected scaffolds to combat particularly Periodontitis, a condition that result in the deterioration of both soft and hard tissues of the periodontium (Bajpai and Kaarthikeyan 2024). In comparison to the conventional PerioCol®, the developed material, displayed superior properties in terms of its rate of degradation, losing only 8% of its initial weight in 28 days as oppose to the 12% in the control scaffold (PerioCol®) *in vitro*. In parameters such as percentage bone volume, tensile strain and object surface density, the carrageenan-based scaffolds also outperform the conventional material, thus making them suitable bone regeneration candidates. In another effort, Shakir et al. (2023) developed a ternary carrageenan based nanocomposites comprising nanohydroxyapatite/κ--carrageenan/silica doped polyvinyl alcohol for bone regeneration application. In addition to a rough surface, this composite also displayed impeccable thermal stability, optimum swelling capability, anti-bacterial activity and above all deposited significant layer of apatite, rendering it as prospective nanocomposite implant candidate for orthopedic applications. In an attempt to address intervertebral disc degeneration, a condition that starts in the nucleus pulposus that is a cartilage tissue, Jayakumar et al. developed κ-carrageenan hydrogel (Dinesan et al. 2024). This gel was cross-linked with potassium chloride and loaded with kartogenin, a chondrogenic factor. The viscoelastic properties of the resulting gel, as well as its ability to sustainably release kartogenin, proves pivotal for nucleus pulposus regeneration.

In recent years, 3D printing of human organs to address an elevating demand and supply mismatch has been a very active and fast-growing field. Hydrogels of carrageenan or carrageenan composites are currently under consideration as appealing biomaterials to produce the bio-ink needed to print vital organs in a well-controlled fashion. In this context, the biocompatibility of CG-gels together with their tunable viscosity, ionic, mechanical and functional chemical properties are highly desirable

(Murphy and Atala 2014; Zhang et al. 2019). As an example, Li et al. in 2018 demonstrated the use of *k*CG-gelatin hydrogels made of gelatin and k-carrageenan for bioink applications employing simple and sustainable layer-by-layer approach. The mechanism of hydrogel formation is due to the electrostatic interaction between the positively charges amine groups of gelatin and the negatively charged sulphate groups in k-carrageenan (Li et al. 2018). In comparison to either bilayer of singular k-CG or gelatin, the resulting printed gel construct made of composites had greater interfacial force with good biocompatibility and structural integrity at physiological temperature (37 °C). Recently, Jafari et al. (2024) developed polyvinyl alcohol, gelatin and carrageenan PVA/Gelatin/Carrageenan based bioink for the 3D printing of heart valves, to tackle valvular heart diseases. The printed valves were profoundly studied for their biocompatibility, immune responsiveness, mechanical strengths and hydrodynamic features in physiological conditions in *in vitro* and *in vivo* models. Remarkably, such 3D valve constructs were shown to have similar properties compared to the natural ones. Notably, the *in vivo* studies done *via* subcutaneous implantation of the valves found them to be not prone to induce chronic inflammation with minimal hemolysis and thrombogenic tendencies. Owing to its tremendous potential, many more carrageenan-based hydrogel composites tailored for 3D printing have been and will be explored to produce better tissue and organs, fulfilling the demand of human transplantation.

18.4.4 Carrageenan in Biosensors

CG biopolymers, given their biocompatibility, bioreactivity and ease of chemical modification are currently being used in the development of biodevices (biosensors). A typical example of such application was reported by Peerasak et al. (2021) were they fabricated a biosensor device by drop casting polyaniline (PANI) and carbon dots (CDs) derived from i-carrageenan on a glassy carbon electrode (GCE). This reusable electrochemical CDs-PANI/GCE device could quantitatively detect 17βestradiol, a hormone known to affect female physiology and pathology. In comparison to the conventional high-performance liquid chromatography (HPLC) instrument used for such quantification, this device is easily deployable for real time monitoring of 17βestradiol within 2 min and relatively cost effective. Such devices are promising for decentralized health care systems thanks to the ease of distribution and operation. Similarly, Narayan and team developed *a Glucose biosensor device using* carbon dots synthesized from κ-carrageenan and later functionalized with phenyl boronic acid (PBA) (Das et al. 2019). This PBA molecule binds covalently to the cis-diol moiety of glucose to cause the quenching of the carbon dot's fluorescence intensity as the glucose concentration increase. The detection limit of this glucose sensor was 1.7μM. Interestingly, this device can simultaneously deliver a loaded anti-diabetic drug, Metformin, in response to a high glucose level.

Despite the interesting attributes and potential applications of Carrageenan based biopolymer materials, the presence of sulphate groups in their native structure do pose adverse blood coagulation and uncontrolled immune response. This consideration must be taken when developing blood-contacting products, as in the case for CG-based drug delivery platforms (Zia et al. 2017). They can as well be lethal to human colonic epithelial cells at concentrations in the range of 1–10 mg/L, as evidenced by the necrotic cell death observed when these cells were incubated with CG for up to 8 days (Bhattacharyya et al. 2008). With these been said, thorough epidemiological studies and clinical assessments are needed to evaluate the safety of carrageenan-based materials for any intended biomedical use. Table 18.1 summarizes the *in vivo* research employing Carrageenan biopolymers.

18.5 Conclusion and Future Prospective

The development of innovative and sustainable marine polysaccharides-derived biocomposites have successfully provided a wide range of advanced materials for various biomedical applications. Although a variety of applications in biomaterials and medical devices can be achieved, the major focuses of scientific community in the last decade are centralized at drug delivery systems, wound healing, and tissue engineering. Indeed, the effectiveness and benefits of common marine-originated polysaccharides, including alginate, agarose and carrageenan, in wound healing and tissue engineering have been proven in numerous recent research and clinic practice. They demonstrated the ability to accelerate healing and rebuild skin through improved cell proliferation and migration as well as to provide the moist environment for effective wound healing. In addition, the biodegradable, biocompatible, antibacterial and anti-inflammatory properties of these developed marine polysaccharide wound dressing offer the prevention of infections and the reduction of inflammation at wound site. Furthermore, the hydrogels and scaffolds based on marine polysaccharides also featured excellent cell growth and tissue regeneration as well as increased biomechanical signals, cellular activity, biological and biochemical signals. The marine-derived polysaccharides also improved the mechanical performances including tensile strength and elasticity of the obtained biocomposites. Hence, marine polysaccharides offer great natural and sustainable materials in wound healing and tissue engineering applications. The advancement in materials science have been also pivotal in the quest of marine-polysaccharide composites development, including the production by extraction processes, structural and physical properties characterizations, and composite fabrication techniques using sustainable approaches. The versatility in chemical structure of such marine polysaccharides can offer a wide range of sustainable approaches to incorporate different synthetic and other natural components, resulting in tailor-made biocomposites with desirable and controlled properties.

Nevertheless, due to their natural origin, the structure and biological activities of marine polysaccharides are significantly impacted by the extraction processes (such as acid, basic and hydrothermal extractions). In addition to that, the chemical, biological and mechanical performances of marine polysaccharides might vary depending on the harvest season, period, and location. This has become a more pressing issue due the impact of climate change in the last decade. Thus, the industrial

Table 18.1 The *in vivo* research employing Carrageenan biopolymers

Polymers	Biocomposites composition	Material form	Bioactivities	Application	References
k-Carrageenan	Chitosan/κ-Carrageenan/sodium tripolyphosphate	Nanoparticles	–	Drug delivery	Noreen et al. (2021)
k-Carrageenan	Polyacyamide/k-CG/alginate	pH hydrogels	–	Drug delivery	Kulkarni et al. (2012)
k-Carrageenan	Hyaluronic acid/k-CG	Thermoresponsive hydrogel	Antibacterial	Wound healing/drug delivery	Ijaz et al. (2022)
k-Carrageenan	k-CG	Hydrogel	–	Wound healing/drug delivery	Lokhande et al. (2018)
k-Carrageenan	Cyclic β-glucan/k-CG	Film	–	Wound healing/drug delivery	Nair et al. (2016)
k-Carrageenan	Chitosan/k-CG/polyvinyl alcohol	Hydrogel	Antibacterial	Wound healing/drug delivery	Khaliq et al. (2022)
k-Carrageenan	Polyethylene oxide/	Film	Antibacterial	Wound healing/drug delivery	Boateng et al. (2013)
k-Carrageenan	Alginate/k-CG	Scaffolds	–	Tissue engineering	Bajpai and Kaarthikeyan (2024)
k-Carrageenan	Nanohydroxyapatite/κ-carrageenan/silica doped polyvinyl alcohol	Nanocomposite	–	Tissue engineering	Fatima et al. (2023)
k-Carrageenan	k-CG	Hydrogel	–	Tissue engineering	Dinesan et al. (2024)
k-Carrageenan	k-CG/Gelatin	Hydrogel	–	3D bioprinting	Li et al. (2018)
k-CG	Polyvinyl alcohol/Gelatin/k-CG	Hydrogel	–	3D bioprinting	Jafari et al. (2024)
i-CG	Polyaniline/carbon dots from i-carrageenan	Film device	–	Biosensor	Supchocksoonthorn et al. (2021)
k-CG	Phenyl boronic acid/carbon dots from k-carrageenan	Film device	–	Biosensor/drug delivery	Das et al. (2019)

large-scale extraction and purification of marine polysaccharides may provide polydisperse macromolecule ranges. This, in turn, can lead to the variation of biomedical treatment outcomes. In the context of sustainability, the extraction of polysaccharide from marine biomass might be problematic due to the involvement of different hazardous chemicals and require a large consumption of energy. As such, the emergence of new extraction technique using deep eutectic solvent and/or ionic liquids that are natural and abundant could offer more sustainable approaches. Furthermore, a low compatibility between marine polysaccharides and other components in biocomposites can be also a pitfall, leading to an inconsistent performance from batch to batch. This, in turn, will impair their translation perspective. Therefore, the development of novel fabrication approach to overcome this challenge might leverage the performances of such biocomposites drastically.

From biomedical application standpoint, most of the marine polysaccharides-based materials for biomedical application are still in the preclinical stage, showing promising proof of concept data however lacking the clinical evidence. Although the *in vivo* experiments have demonstrated the potential of these materials on small animals, the compositions of skin and tissues of the small animal are different from human's ones. Therefore, the future research will focus on the development of appreciable biotesting method as well as on the evaluation of the clinical efficacy in human. To realize the potential of such marine biocomposites, rigorous studies involving profound investigation in terms of long-term toxicity and immune response are crucial. This challenge will require collective efforts with transdisciplinary expertise including chemistry, material science and engineering, clinical practitioner, and even regulatory authority. In addition to that, widening the applications of such biocomposites to emerging biomedical research frontiers such as biosensors, blood toxin removal, and nano/microbots might be also foreseen. In near future, marine biocomposites will be essential materials in medical devices with multifunctionality that can tackle some of the most challenging issues in human health such as cancers and lab-grown organs. Eventually, life on Earth originated from the ocean and looking back into marine resource might offer unprecedented solutions to solve the emerging and pressing issue in human healthcare and sustainable development.

References

Alaminos M et al (2006) Construction of a complete rabbit cornea substitute using a fibrin-agarose scaffold. Invest Ophthalmol Vis Sci 47(8):3311–3317

Alba K, Kontogiorgos V (2018) Seaweed polysaccharides (agar, alginate carrageenan). Elsevier

Bajpai D, Kaarthikeyan G (2024) Development and evaluation of alginate-and carrageenan-incorporated scaffold for bone regeneration: an in vitro study. Cureus 16(5):e61139

Bayat F et al (2023) Improving release profile and anticancer activity of 5-fluorouracil for breast cancer therapy using a double drug delivery system: chitosan/agarose/γ-alumina nanocomposite@ double emulsion. J Clust Sci 34(5):2565–2577

Bhat S, Kumar A (2012) Cell proliferation on three-dimensional chitosan–agarose–gelatin cryogel scaffolds for tissue engineering applications. J Biosci Bioeng 114(6):663–670

Bhattacharyya S et al (2008) Carrageenan induces cell cycle arrest in human intestinal epithelial cells in vitro3. J Nutr 138(3):469–475
Bloch K et al (2010) Vascularization of wide pore agarose–gelatin cryogel scaffolds implanted subcutaneously in diabetic and non-diabetic mice. Acta Biomater 6(3):1200–1205
Boateng JS, Pawar HV, Tetteh J (2013) Polyox and carrageenan based composite film dressing containing anti-microbial and anti-inflammatory drugs for effective wound healing. Int J Pharm 441(1–2):181–191
Chen X et al (2021) Agarose oligosaccharide-silver nanoparticle-antimicrobial peptide-composite for wound dressing. Carbohydr Polym 269:118258
Chen K et al (2024) Biomaterial-based regenerative therapeutic strategies for spinal cord injury. NPG Asia Mater 16(1):5
Ciarlantini C et al (2024) Design of bioactive and biomimetic scaffolds based on chitosan-alginate polyelectrolyte complexes for tissue engineering. Carbohydr Polym 327:121684
Daniel-da-Silva AL et al (2007) Synthesis and characterization of porous κ-carrageenan/calcium phosphate nanocomposite scaffolds. J Mater Sci 42:8581–8591
Das P et al (2019) Biocompatible carbon dots derived from κ-carrageenan and phenyl boronic acid for dual modality sensing platform of sugar and its anti-diabetic drug release behavior. Int J Biol Macromol 132:316–329
de la Cruz Cardona J et al (2011) Transparency in a fibrin and fibrin–agarose corneal stroma substitute generated by tissue engineering. Cornea 30(12):1428–1435
Dinesan A et al (2024) Biomimetic kartogenin containing κ-carrageenan hydrogel for nucleus pulposus regeneration. Int J Biol Macromol 276:133868
Dong Y et al (2021) Smart MXene/agarose hydrogel with photothermal property for controlled drug release. Int J Biol Macromol 190:693–699
Fatima T et al (2023) Combinatorial approach to fabricate silica doped polyvinyl alcohol/hydroxyapatite/carrageenan nanocomposite for bone regeneration applications. Polym Adv Technol 34(7):2272–2285
Ghorbani M et al (2023) Dual-crosslinked in-situ forming alginate/silk fibroin hydrogel with potential for bone tissue engineering. Biomater Adv 153:213565
Gupta A et al (2014) Evaluation of three-dimensional chitosan-agarose-gelatin cryogel scaffold for the repair of subchondral cartilage defects: an in vivo study in a rabbit model. Tissue Eng A 20(23–24):3101–3111
Ijaz U et al (2022) Biofunctional hyaluronic acid/κ-carrageenan injectable hydrogels for improved drug delivery and wound healing. Polymers 14(3):376
Ionescu A-M et al (2011) Investigating a novel nanostructured fibrin–agarose biomaterial for human cornea tissue engineering: rheological properties. J Mech Behav Biomed Mater 4(8):1963–1973
Ionescu AM et al (2017) Optical properties of an anterior lamellar human cornea model based on fibrin-agarose. In: Third international conference on applications of optics and photonics. SPIE
Islam M et al (2022) Carbon-based materials for articular tissue engineering: from innovative scaffolding materials toward engineered living carbon. Adv Healthc Mater 11(1):2101834
Jafari A et al (2024) Formulation and evaluation of PVA/gelatin/carrageenan inks for 3D printing and development of tissue-engineered heart valves. Adv Funct Mater 34(7):2305188
Jalilinejad N et al (2023) Electrically conductive carbon-based (bio)-nanomaterials for cardiac tissue engineering. Bioeng Transl Med 8(1):e10347
Jayrajsinh S et al (2017) Montmorillonite nanoclay as a multifaceted drug-delivery carrier: a review. J Drug Delivery Sci Technol 39:200–209
Jiang J-L et al (2021) Insight on structure-property relationships of carrageenan from marine red algal: a review. Carbohydr Polym 257:117642
Kamoun EA, Kenawy E-RS, Chen X (2017) A review on polymeric hydrogel membranes for wound dressing applications: PVA-based hydrogel dressings. J Adv Res 8(3):217–233
Khaliq T et al (2022) Self-crosslinked chitosan/κ-carrageenan-based biomimetic membranes to combat diabetic burn wound infections. Int J Biol Macromol 197:157–168

Khan MUA et al (2020) Development and in vitro evaluation of κ-carrageenan based polymeric hybrid nanocomposite scaffolds for bone tissue engineering. RSC Adv 10(66):40529–40542
Kolanthai E et al (2015) Effect of solvent; enhancing the wettability and engineering the porous structure of a calcium phosphate/agarose composite for drug delivery. RSC Adv 5(24):18301–18311
Kolanthai E et al (2016) Synthesis of nanosized hydroxyapatite/agarose powders for bone filler and drug delivery application. Mater Today Commun 8:31–40
Kolanthai E et al (2017) Agarose encapsulated mesoporous carbonated hydroxyapatite nanocomposites powder for drug delivery. J Photochem Photobiol B Biol 166:220–231
Ku SH, Lee M, Park CB (2013) Carbon-based nanomaterials for tissue engineering. Adv Healthc Mater 2(2):244–260
Kulkarni RV et al (2012) pH-responsive interpenetrating network hydrogel beads of poly (acrylamide)-g-carrageenan and sodium alginate for intestinal targeted drug delivery: synthesis, in vitro and in vivo evaluation. J Colloid Interface Sci 367(1):509–517
Lewitus DY et al (2011) Biohybrid carbon nanotube/agarose fibers for neural tissue engineering. Adv Funct Mater 21(14):2624–2632
Li C et al (2014) Enhancement in bioavailability of ketorolac tromethamine via intranasal in situ hydrogel based on poloxamer 407 and carrageenan. Int J Pharm 474(1–2):123–133
Li H, Tan YJ, Li L (2018) A strategy for strong interface bonding by 3D bioprinting of oppositely charged κ-carrageenan and gelatin hydrogels. Carbohydr Polym 198:261–269
Liu Z et al (2020) Preparation of multiwall carbon nanotubes embedded electroconductive multi-microchannel scaffolds for neuron growth under electrical stimulation. Biomed Res Int 2020(1):4794982
Liu F, Duan G, Yang H (2023) Recent advances in exploiting carrageenans as a versatile functional material for promising biomedical applications. Int J Biol Macromol 235:123787
Lokhande G et al (2018) Nanoengineered injectable hydrogels for wound healing application. Acta Biomater 70:35–47
Mao G et al (2023) Preparation and evaluation of a novel alginate-arginine-zinc ion hydrogel film for skin wound healing. Carbohydr Polym 311:120757
Martin SS et al (2013) The effects of fibrin and fibrin-agarose on the extracellular matrix profile of bioengineered oral mucosa. J Tissue Eng Regen Med 7(1):10–19
Murphy SV, Atala A (2014) 3D bioprinting of tissues and organs. Nat Biotechnol 32(8):773–785
Nair AV, Raman M, Doble M (2016) Cyclic β-(1 → 3)(1 → 6) glucan/carrageenan hydrogels for wound healing applications. RSC Adv 6(100):98545–98553
Najafi M et al (2024) Physicochemical and in vitro characterization of Agarose based nanocarriers incorporated with Graphene Quantum Dots/α-Fe2O3 for targeted drug delivery of Quercetin to liver cancer treatment. Mater Chem Phys 320:129333
Necas J, Bartosikova L (2013) Carrageenan: a review. Vet Med 58(4):187–205
Noreen S et al (2021) Optimization of novel naproxen-loaded chitosan/carrageenan nanocarrier-based gel for topical delivery: ex vivo, histopathological, and in vivo evaluation. Pharmaceuticals 14(6):557
Pacheco-Quito E-M, Ruiz-Caro R, Veiga M-D (2020) Carrageenan: drug delivery systems and other biomedical applications. Mar Drugs 18(11):583
Park J et al (2022) Conductive hydrogel constructs with three-dimensionally connected graphene networks for biomedical applications. Chem Eng J 446:137344
Polat TG, Duman O, Tunc S (2020) Agar/κ-carrageenan/montmorillonite nanocomposite hydrogels for wound dressing applications. Int J Biol Macromol 164:4591–4602
Qamar SA et al (2024) Carrageenan-based hybrids with biopolymers and nano-structured materials for biomimetic applications. Starch-Stärke 76(1–2):2200018
Rajabzadeh-Khosroshahi M et al (2022) Chitosan/agarose/graphitic carbon nitride nanocomposite as an efficient pH-sensitive drug delivery system for anticancer curcumin releasing. J Drug Delivery Sci Technol 74:103443
Rajaei M et al (2023) Chitosan/agarose/graphene oxide nanohydrogel as drug delivery system of 5-fluorouracil in breast cancer therapy. J Drug Delivery Sci Technol 82:104307

Rodríguez I et al (2012) Rheological characterization of human fibrin and fibrin–agarose oral mucosa substitutes generated by tissue engineering. J Tissue Eng Regen Med 6(8):636–644
Samadi A et al (2020) Curcumin-loaded chitosan-agarose-montmorillonite hydrogel nanocomposite for the treatment of breast cancer. In: 2020 27th National and 5th international Iranian conference on biomedical engineering (ICBME). IEEE
Samadi A et al (2021) Ameliorating quercetin constraints in cancer therapy with pH-responsive agarose-polyvinylpyrrolidone-hydroxyapatite nanocomposite encapsulated in double nanoemulsion. Int J Biol Macromol 182:11–25
Sánchez-Salcedo S, Nieto A, Vallet-Regí M (2008) Hydroxyapatite/β-tricalcium phosphate/agarose macroporous scaffolds for bone tissue engineering. Chem Eng J 137(1):62–71
Saraiva MM et al (2023) Alginate/polyvinyl alcohol films for wound healing: advantages and challenges. J Biomed Mater Res B Appl Biomater 111(1):220–233
Serafin A, Culebras M, Collins MN (2023) Synthesis and evaluation of alginate, gelatin, and hyaluronic acid hybrid hydrogels for tissue engineering applications. Int J Biol Macromol 233:123438
Shashvatt U, Aris H, Blaney L (2017) Evaluation of animal manure composition for protection of sensitive water supplies through nutrient recovery processes. In: Chemistry and water. Elsevier, pp 469–509
Shin SR et al (2016) Graphene-based materials for tissue engineering. Adv Drug Deliv Rev 105:255–274
Supchocksoonthorn P et al (2021) Facile fabrication of 17β-estradiol electrochemical sensor using polyaniline/carbon dot-coated glassy carbon electrode with synergistically enhanced electrochemical stability. Talanta 235:122782
Szcześ A, Hołysz L, Chibowski E (2017) Synthesis of hydroxyapatite for biomedical applications. Adv Colloid Interf Sci 249:321–330
Tabata M et al (2003) Osteoconductive and hemostatic properties of apatite formed on/in agarose gel as a bone-grafting material. J Biomed Mater Res B Appl Biomater 67(2):680–688
Tabata M et al (2005) Apatite formed on/in agarose gel as a bone-grafting material in the treatment of periodontal infrabony defect. J Biomed Mater Res B Appl Biomater 75(2):378–386
Tran TN et al (2016) Transparent and flexible amorphous cellulose-acrylic hybrids. Chem Eng J 287:196–204
Tripathi A, Kathuria N, Kumar A (2009) Elastic and macroporous agarose–gelatin cryogels with isotropic and anisotropic porosity for tissue engineering. J Biomed Mater Res A 90(3):680–694
ul Haque S, Nasar A (2018) Montmorillonite clay nanocomposites for drug delivery. In: Applications of nanocomposite materials in drug delivery. Elsevier, pp 633–648
Wang T et al (2023) Sodium alginate hydrogel containing platelet-rich plasma for wound healing. Colloids Surf B: Biointerfaces 222:113096
Yang C et al (2023) Marine polymers-alginate/chitosan composited microcapsules for wound healing. Chem Eng J 456:140886
Yazdi MK et al (2020) Agarose-based biomaterials for advanced drug delivery. J Control Release 326:523–543
Yin Z-C, Wang Y-L, Wang K (2018) A pH-responsive composite hydrogel beads based on agar and alginate for oral drug delivery. J Drug Delivery Sci Technol 43:12–18
Zhang K et al (2018) Advanced smart biomaterials and constructs for hard tissue engineering and regeneration. Bone Res 6(1):31
Zhang Y et al (2019) Biomaterials based on marine resources for 3D bioprinting applications. Mar Drugs 17(10):555
Zhang J et al (2023) Montmorillonite/agarose three-dimensional network gel sponge for wound healing with hemostatic and durable antibacterial properties. ACS Appl Nano Mater 6(18):17263–17275
Zhao J et al (2020) Studies on the physicochemical properties, gelling behavior and drug release performance of agar/κ-carrageenan mixed hydrogels. Int J Biol Macromol 154:878–887
Zhao L et al (2023) Electroactive injectable hydrogel based on oxidized sodium alginate and carboxymethyl chitosan for wound healing. Int J Biol Macromol 230:123231
Zia KM et al (2017) A review on synthesis, properties and applications of natural polymer based carrageenan blends and composites. Int J Biol Macromol 96:282–301

The manufacturer's authorised representative in the EU is Springer Nature Customer Service Centre GmbH, Europaplatz 3, 69115 Heidelberg, Germany. If you have any concerns regarding our products, please contact ProductSafety@springernature.com

Printed and bound by CPI Group (UK) Ltd, Croydon, CR0 4YY
05/10/2026
02228133-0005